NEUROMUSCULAR FUNCTION AND DISORDERS

To patients with neuromuscular
disorders

Neuromuscular Function and Disorders

Alan J. McComas, BSc, MB, BS, FRCP(C)
Professor and Director of Neurology in the Department of Medicine at
McMaster University
Member, Medical Research Council's Developmental Neurobiology Research Group,
McMaster Medical Centre, Hamilton, Ontario

BUTTERWORTHS
LONDON - BOSTON
Sydney - Wellington - Durban - Toronto

THE BUTTERWORTH GROUP

ENGLAND

Butterworth & Co (Publishers) Ltd
London: 88 Kingsway, WC2B 6AB

AUSTRALIA

Butterworths Pty Ltd
Sydney: 586 Pacific Highway, Chateswood, NSW 2067
Also at Melbourne, Brisbane, Adelaide
and Perth

SOUTH AFRICA

Butterworth & Co (South Africa) (Pty) Ltd
Durban: 152–154 Gale Street

NEW ZEALAND

Butterworths of New Zealand Ltd
Wellington: 26–28 Waring Taylor Street, 1

CANADA

Butterworth & Co (Canada) Ltd
Toronto: 2265 Midland Avenue,
    Scarborough, Ontario, M1P 4S1

USA

Butterworths (Publishers) Inc
Boston: 19 Cummings Park, Woburn,
    Mass. 01801

First published 1977

© Butterworth & Co (Publishers) Ltd, 1977

ISBN 0 407 00058 5

Library of Congress Cataloging in Publication Data
McComas, A. J.
  Neuromuscular function and disorders.

  Bibliography: p.
  Includes index.
  1. Neuromuscular diseases. 2. Myoneural
junction. I. Title. [DNLM: 1. Neuromuscular
diseases. 2. Neuromuscular junction—
Physiology. WE500 M129n]

  RC925.5.M26   616.7'4   76-10185
  ISBN 0-407-00058-5

Printed and Bound in England by Chapel River Press, Andover, Hants.

INTRODUCTION

A new book on neuromuscular disorders appears desirable for a number of reasons. Most important of these is the need for a radically different approach and, in particular, one which describes the various disease processes in terms of disordered neuromuscular function. Descriptions have also been given of neurophysiological techniques which, following their successful application to man, have made this conceptual advance possible. For the results in patients to be understood fully it is obviously important that adequate accounts of the normal anatomy and physiology of peripheral nerve and muscle should be given and this material comprises the first half of the book. Included within this section are descriptions of the ionic mechanisms responsible for the resting and action potentials of nerve and muscle, the sequential stages in neuromuscular transmission, excitation–contraction coupling, the sliding filament mechanism of myofibrillar shortening, and the morphological and functional properties of motor units. In addition there are critical reviews on the neurophysiology of exercise and muscle fatigue and on the nature of the trophic influences exerted by the motoneurone and muscle fibre upon each other. Accounts have also been given of the changes in the neuromuscular apparatus during development and as part of the normal ageing process.

The second half of the book deals entirely with various diseases of peripheral nerve and muscle. Although each of these has been analysed in terms of disordered neuromuscular function, adequate clinical descriptions have also been submitted; in several instances it has seemed fitting to quote from the classical early papers. Also included are succinct summaries of diagnostic procedures and therapeutic management. In the full accounts of disordered morphology and function which follow, attempts have been made to answer certain key questions. Most important of these is the pathogenesis of the various disease states. Thus the book contains detailed consideration of such topics as the nature of the membrane defects in myotonia and familial periodic paralysis, the disorder of neuromuscular transmission responsible for myasthenia gravis and the various pseudo-myasthenic syndromes, and the disorders of Schwann cell function which cause demyelination. A consistent theme in the second half of the book has been the recent recognition of neural abnormalities in diseases hitherto considered as primary disorders of the muscle fibre. Much of the evidence has come from the estimations of numbers and sizes of functioning motor units in human muscles using techniques developed in the laboratory of the author. An objective evaluation of the reliability of the method has been given in one of the appendices.

The clinical section of the book contains a number of hypotheses. These have been submitted in the recognition that many, perhaps most, will eventually be shown to be false or at least not wholly accurate Their value lies in providing tentative explanations in situations where less plausible or conflicting hypotheses exist. It is hoped that the newer ideas will prove of value in stimulating new lines of experimental research. One theoretical concept which has already attracted considerable interest is the 'sick motoneurone hypothesis' of various muscle diseases. In view of the active controversy presently surrounding the hypothesis, the original account has been included in Chapter 13. Inasmuch as the hypothesis relates to muscular dystrophy in animals, it now appears that certain qualifications must be made. Thus, although there appears to be a neural inductive influence on the genesis of dystrophy, there is no evidence of the defective trophic influence previously postulated to be present in the adult animal. Whether the findings of the animal studies are applicable to the human varieties of dystrophy is less certain, since in addition to species differences there is the much longer embryonic development of the neuromuscular apparatus to take into account. Other hypotheses in the book concern the role of ageing in motoneurone disease, the presence of multiple axonal lesions in entrapment neuropathies, the transneuronal degeneration of motoneurones following lesions at higher levels, and the development of 'silent' synapses during the course of motoneurone dysfunction.

The book includes a large number of illustrations, some of which are original while others have been taken from certain key papers. In order not to disrupt the coherence of the text, matters of unusual interest have been deferred to the appendix; these include such items as the discovery of myotonic goats and Captain Cook's adventure with tetrodotoxin.

It is hoped that the book will have a wide appeal. It should be of value to medical students, especially since the integration of anatomy and physiology with disease processes is a strong feature of the new curricula. Neurologists who are either in training or already established should also benefit from the availability of a comprehensive modern account of neuromuscular function in health and disease. The reviews of the motor unit studies undertaken in the author's laboratory include much unpublished material which will be of interest to research workers in neuromuscular diseases. Finally, it is hoped that the broad scope of the book will attract students and research scientists in physiology, zoology, pharmacology, kinesiology and physical education.

There are many acknowledgements to make. I have been unusually fortunate in having a number of extremely able and enthusiastic colleagues during these crucial years of muscle study; in chronological order they are Sahib Mossawy, Peter Payan, Konstanty Mrożek, Peter Fawcett, Malcolm Campbell, Roberto Sica, Adrian Upton, Frank Petito, Peter Law, Mario Caccia, Kazutaka Toyonaga, Carlos de Faria, Jean Delbeke and Jerzy Kopec. Adrian Upton accompanied the author to McMaster University and helped to establish a neurology section within the Department of Medicine. The double crush syndrome (Chapter 23), although described jointly, was really his inspiration. Roberto Sica must also be singled out for special gratitude in view of his sacrifice in leaving home and family in Buenos Aires for six months in order to help the McMaster group during their early days. Many valuable discussions have been held with Ethel Cosmos, Michel Rathbone and Alan Peterson at McMaster University and the author is grateful to Vanda Lennon of the Salk Institute and to Edson Albuquerque of the University of Maryland for their generosity in making available their most recent experimental results. The author is also indebted to his clinical colleagues, first at Newcastle upon Tyne and then in Hamilton, for having referred so many interesting cases. All these persons helped to create this book through the ideas and the results which they gave so freely over the years. The author also wishes to acknowledge the helpful and stimulating influence which Professor Sir John Gray, Professor John Walton and Professor Jack Diamond exerted upon him at different times during his formative years. He is also indebted to Ms Irene Csatari and Mrs Norma Zimmerman for typing the manuscript in its draft and completed forms. Klaus Fabich deserves much credit for his fine artistic craftsmanship shown in the illustrations and the author is obliged to Judy Leon for technical assistance. The Editorial Staff of Butterworths must be complimented on their patience and editorial help. As with any book, however, the real heroes and heroines are the members of one's family. The author apologizes for neglecting them and promises to make amends in the future.

SYMBOLS, UNITS OF MEASUREMENT AND ABBREVIATIONS

Length
m = metre
cm = centimetre (10^{-2}m)
mm = millimetre (10^{-3}m)
μm = micrometre (10^{-6}m)
Å = Ångstrom (10^{-10}m)

Mass
g = gram
kg = kilogram

Time
s = second
ms = millisecond (10^{-3}s)
μs = microsecond (10^{-6}s)

Velocity
m/s = metres per second

Frequency
Hz = hertz (cycles per second)

Electrical
A = ampere
C = capacitance
E = e.m.f. (electromotive force)
I = current
Ω = ohm
R = resistance
V = volt
mV = millivolt (10^{-3}V)
μV = microvolt (10^{-6}V)

Chemical
mEq = milliequivalent
mM = millimolar

[ ] = concentation of
ACh = acetylcholine
AChE = acetylcholinesterase
AChR = acetylcholine receptor
ADP = adenosine diphosphate
AMP = adenosine monophosphate
ATP = adenosine triphosphate
BTX = bungarotoxin
Ca = calcium
ChE = cholinesterase
Cl = chlorine
CPK = creatine phosphokinase
CSF = cerebrospinal fluid
DFP = diisopropyl fluorophosphate
DNA = deoxyribonucleic acid
EDB = extensor digitorum brevis
EEG = electroencephalogram
EMG = electromyogram
EPP = end-plate potential
FHL = flexor hallucis longus
FSH = facioscapulohumeral (dystrophy)
Hg = mercury
HRP = horseradish peroxidase
K = potassium
LG = limbgirdle (dystrophy)
M(wave) = maximum evoked muscle response
m.e.p.p. = miniature end-plate potential
Na = sodium
PAS = periodic acid Schiff (stain)
RNA = ribonucleic acid
SMA = spinal muscular atrophy
SOL = soleus
STX = saxitonin

Statistical treatment
Unless otherwise stated, means have been expressed with standard deviations. Significances of differences between means have been estimated by the Student 't' test.

CONTENTS

PART 1: MUSCLE FIBRES AND MOTONEURONES

1 The Muscle Fibre   3
2 The Motoneurone and its Axon   8
3 Resting and Action Potentials   16
4 The Neuromuscular Junction   27
5 Muscle Contraction   35
6 Motor Units   47
7 Exercise and Fatigue   63
8 Trophic Interactions of Nerve and Muscle: Denervation and Reinnervation   72
9 Use and Disuse   80
10 Trophic Influence of Muscle on Nerve   89
11 Muscle Growth   92
12 Ageing   101

PART 2: DISORDERS OF MUSCLE AND NERVE

13 Neuropathic and Myopathic Disorders: Sick Motoneurone Hypothesis   111

Disorders of Muscle Fibre Membranes
14 Myotonia   123
15 Familial Periodic Paralysis   133

Disorders of Muscle Fibre Contents
16 The Muscular Dystrophies   143
17 Polymyositis, Malignant Hyperthermia and other Myopathies   179

Disorders of Neuromuscular Junctions
18 Myasthenia Gravis   193
19 Pseudomyasthenic Syndromes and other Synaptic Defects   209

Disorders of Nerve Fibres
20 Wallerian Degeneration and Fibre Regeneration   221
21 Demyelination and Remyelination   233
22 Nerve Compression   243
23 The Double Crush Syndrome   253

Disorders of Motoneurones
24 Motoneurone Degeneration   263
25 Toxic and Metabolic Neuropathies   274
26 Reversible Motoneurone Dysfunction in Thyrotoxicosis   285

27 Trans-synaptic Motoneurone Degeneration   289

28 Conclusions   295

Appendices   303
References   319
Index   351

PART 1

MUSCLE FIBRES AND MOTONEURONES

Chapter 1

THE MUSCLE FIBRE

The 'voluntary' muscles are composed of muscle fibres, of which two types are found. By far the commonest are those fibres which make up nearly all the bulk of the muscle and are described as *extrafusal*. This term distinguishes them from the much smaller muscle fibres which are found inside the muscle spindles; because of their location these last fibres are referred to as *intrafusal*. The special structure and function of the intrafusal fibres are of considerable interest and have been reviewed elsewhere (Matthews, 1972). This book will deal only with the extrafusal muscle fibres, however, for it is these fibres about which most is known in disease and it is their ineffectiveness which is ultimately responsible for the cardinal symptom of weakness.

NUMBERS AND SIZES OF MUSCLE FIBRES

Because of the time-consuming nature of the task involved, there are very few values for the numbers of extrafusal fibres in human voluntary muscles. On the basis of fibre counts in samples taken from cadaveric tissue, Feinstein *et al.* (1955) made the estimates set out in Table 1.1.

The long gestation period in man allows sufficient time for the precursors of the muscle fibres to have finished dividing and to have formed the adult complement of fibres before birth (MacCallum, 1898). In species with a shorter gestation period the number of fibres continues to increase in the neonatal period. At birth the human fibres are slender, measuring about 10–20 μm in diameter. Throughout childhood, and particularly during the growth spurt in puberty, the sizes increase and eventually attain adult dimensions, with most diameters in the 40–80 μm range (see Figure 1 of Brooke and Engel, 1969). So far as length is concerned, it is assumed that individual fibres run from one end of the muscle to the other; in the human sartorius muscle such fibres may not be functionally continuous; certainly the thigh muscles possess more than one innervation zone and it is possible that long fibres may be composed of two or more shorter fibres arranged end-to-end.

STRUCTURE OF THE MUSCLE FIBRE

Sarcolemma (plasmalemma)

All living cells are bounded by a membrane; that of the muscle fibre is termed the *sarcolemma* and is some 75 Å thick. The sarcolemma resembles the membrane of the nerve fibre in possessing the special property of excitability, enabling electrical impulses to be transmitted down the length of the cell (see page 20). In the region of the innervation zone (motor end-plate) the sarcolemma is highly convoluted, due to the presence of junctional folds (page 27). Elsewhere along the surface of the fibre the membrane displays much shallower folds; these result from slackness of the membrane when the fibre is in its resting or contracted states and they disappear if the fibre is passively stretched. There are also numerous very small in-pocketings of membrane, the *caveolae*,

TABLE 1.1
Number of Muscle Fibres in Various Human Muscles (results given to nearest 50)

Muscle	No. of muscle fibres	Author
First lumbrical	10 250*	Feinstein *et al.* (1955)
External rectus	27 000	Feinstein *et al.* (1955)
Platysma	27 000	Feinstein *et al.* (1955)
First dorsal interosseous	40 500	Feinstein *et al.* (1955)
Sartorius	128 150*	MacCallum (1898)
Brachioradialis	129 200*	Feinstein *et al.* (1955)
Tibialis anterior	271 350	Feinstein *et al.* (1955)
Medial gastrocnemius	1 033 000	Feinstein *et al.* (1955)

* Average values

which are connected to the surface membrane by narrow necks; their function is uncertain though they can also act as reserve sources of membrane during stretching of the fibre (Dulhunty and Franzini-Armstrong, 1975). Biochemical and ultrastructural investigations indicate that the sarcolemma is largely composed of lipid molecules arranged perpendicularly to the surface of the fibre and forming two layers (*Figure 1.1, upper*; see also Capaldi, 1974). The hydrophilic 'heads' of the lipid molecules form the internal and external surfaces of the membrane while the hydrophobic 'tails' make up the interior of the membrane. The membrane also contains proteins, of which two types are generally recognized; these are referred to as extrinsic and intrinsic. Extrinsic proteins are only attached at the internal or external surfaces of the membrane and can be dislodged relatively easily by chemical means. In contrast, intrinsic proteins penetrate the full thickness of the membrane and are difficult to remove. Among the special proteins known to be localized in the sarcolemma are (*a*) *transport systems* for sugars, lipids and amino acids; (*b*) *kinases* for phos-

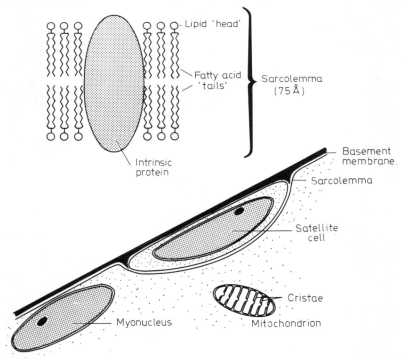

Figure 1.1 (Upper) Structure of the sarcolemma, showing the double layer of lipid molecules and an 'intrinsic' protein (see text). (Lower) Membranes, nuclei and organelles seen at the surface of a muscle fibre; the mitochondrion would measure about 1.5 μm in its long diameter

phorylating various membrane proteins; (c) *adenylate cyclase*, responsible for synthesizing cyclic AMP; (d) *ATPase* enzymes for pumping cations across the membrane (one type for sodium and potassium and another for calcium and magnesium); and (e) *carrier molecules* (*ionophores*), each of which can select one species of ion (sodium, potassium or chloride) and transfer it across the membrane (see page 24). In the end-plate region the sarcolemma also contains two special proteins which combine with acetylcholine; these are the *acetylcholine receptor* and the hydrolytic enzyme, *acetylcholinesterase*. Since much of the membrane lipid has a melting point below body-temperature the sarcolemma would be expected to have fluid properties. By labelling a spot of membrane with a fluorescent dye and then observing its enlargement under the microscope Fambrough *et al.* (1974) were able to show that this was indeed the case.

Basement membrane

Just outside the sarcolemma and clearly visible in electronmicrographs is the *basement membrane* (*Figure 1.1, lower*). This membrane is about 500 Å thick and is composed of proteins and polysaccharides. It is probable that the basement membrane provides a special ionic milieu for the muscle fibre by restricting the further diffusion of electrolytes once these have crossed the sarcolemma. In addition the basement membrane helps to maintain the shape of the muscle fibre by providing external support. If the muscle fibre is damaged the membrane may be spared and can then guide the regenerating myoblasts in the formation of a new fibre.

Nuclei

Each muscle fibre contains numerous nuclei (*myonuclei*) which, in health, are dispersed along the inner surface of the sarcolemma, particularly in the region of the motor end-plate. The nucleus is bounded by two membranes, the outer one of which may join the sarcoplasmic reticulum (*Figure 1.1, lower*).

Indistinguishable from the myonuclei with the light microscope are the nuclei of the *satellite cells*. These cells probably account for less than 1 per cent of the muscle fibre nuclei in the adult. They can only be differentiated from the myonuclei by the electronmicroscope, which reveals the presence of twin membranes separating the cytoplasm of the satellite cell from that of the muscle fibre.

The satellite cells are of particular importance for the regeneration of muscle following disease or injury (page 100).

Myofibrils

The most obvious structures within the muscle fibre are the myofibrils, which are the units responsible for contraction and relaxation of the fibre (*Figure 1.2*). Each myofibril is about 1 μm in diameter and, even with the light microscope, can be seen to have a banded, or striated, appearance. The 'dark' and 'light' striations are termed the A- and *I-bands* respectively; in the relaxed muscle fibre the centre of the A-band has a light region, the *H-zone*, which is itself bisected by a 'dark' *M-line*. In the centre of the I-band is a dark *Z-line* (*Z-disc*). The striations are caused by the fact that the part of the myofibril in the A-band has a refractive index which is substantially higher than that of the fluid medium, or *sarcoplasm*, in which the myofibrils are embedded. The pattern of one dark band followed by one light band is repeated every 2.2 μm (measured with the muscle in the relaxed state), the segment between two successive Z-lines being termed a *sarcomere*. All the myofibrils within a healthy muscle fibre are in register, such that the light and dark bands of one myofibril are adjacent to the corresponding bands of neighbouring myofibrils, giving the whole muscle fibre a striped appearance. A satisfactory explanation for these muscle striations is now possible in terms of the disposition of the contractile macromolecules along the axis of the myofibril (page 35).

Tubular systems

Early in the present century Veratti (1902) was able to stain a fine interlacing network within the muscle fibre (*Figure 1.2*). It was only many years later, with the aid of the electronmicroscope, that the details of this structure could be resolved into a tubular system comprising two parts (see, for example, Franzini-Armstrong and Porter, 1964).

The sarcoplasmic (endoplasmic) reticulum. An elaborate system of channels runs in the long axis of the muscle fibre and largely surrounds individual myofibrils. Through side branches the longitudinal channels enveloping one myofibril are connected to each other and to those around other myofibrils. When the muscle fibre contracts the longitudinal channels become shorter and wider.

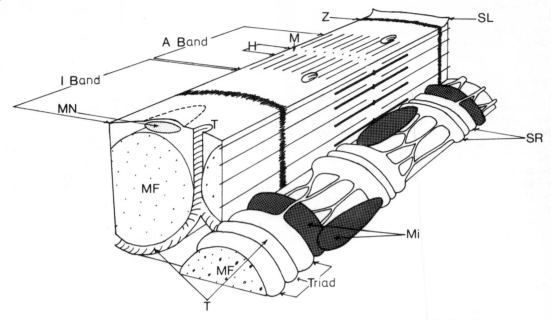

Figure 1.2. Part of the periphery of a muscle fibre. Of the several hundred myofibrils in the fibre the section shows only three (MF); their structure has been simplified and the foreground myofibril reflected slighty upwards. H, H-zone; M, M-line; Mi, mitochondrion; MN, myonucleus; SL, sarcolemma; SR, sarcoplasmic reticulum; T, transverse tubular system; Z, Z-line (see text)

The transverse tubular (T) system. This lies perpendicular to the long axis of the muscle fibre in the form of narrow zones of channels which encircle the myofibrils at regular intervals. In mammalian muscle fibres, including those of man, there are two zones of transverse tubules in each sarcomere; they lie at the junctions of the A- and I-bands. Interestingly, in cardiac muscle fibres and in the fibres of frogs, there is only one T-zone for each sarcomere and this is situated at the Z-line. As the T-tubules encircle the myofibrils they interrupt the longitudinal channels of the sarcoplasmic reticulum. At these points of contact the sarcoplasmic reticulum is somewhat dilated to form *lateral sacs* (or *terminal cisterns*); neighbouring sacs are connected together. *Figure 1.2* shows that each of the relatively narrow T-tubules is embraced on either side by a lateral sac; the three elements are referred to as a *triad*. Electron-microscopy reveals that the membranes of the T-tubules and sarcoplasmic reticulum, although closely apposed at the triads, remain intact. According to Peachey (1965) approximately 80 per cent of the transverse tubular system in a frog muscle fibre is surrounded by the sarcoplasmic reticulum. At the surface of the muscle fibre the T-tubules form small openings at the junctions of the A- and

I-bands and their membranes become confluent with the sarcolemma. By examining muscle fibres bathed in solutions containing electron-dense material or fluorescent dyes, it has been shown that the T-tubules contain extracellular fluid. The principal function of the tubules is to conduct impulses from the surface to the interior of the muscle fibre. Each inwardly conducted impulse causes calcium ions to travel from the lateral sacs along the sarcoplasmic reticulum to the region of the myofibrils where the contraction will take place; afterwards the calcium ions are returned to the lateral sacs (page 40).

Sarcoplasmic components

Mitochondria

The mitochondria (sarcosomes) are ovoid structures, measuring some 1–2 μm in their longest diameters. They have a double membrane, of which the inner one is repeatedly folded to form *cristae*; these folds bulge into the central compartment of the mitochondria (*Figure 1.1, lower*). The mitochondria house the enzyme systems required for the Krebs tricarboxylic acid cycle which breaks down pyruvate to carbon dioxide and water. A large part of the energy released by the successive reactions is captured by a chain of cytochromes which enable ATP to be formed. There is now good evidence that the cytochrome chain is located on the membrane of the cristae. Mitochondria are found especially between the myofibrils in the region of the Z-line and also in relation to the nuclei and the motor end-plate. Although the mitochondria appear oval in longitudinal sections of muscle fibres, some are not ovoid but are much more complex; extremely bizarre shapes may occur in disease.

Ribosomes

These are small spheres some 150 Å in diameter which may occur singly or else in groups (poly-ribosomes). They are especially numerous in immature muscle fibres and in regenerating ones, being concerned with the synthesis of proteins; they are composed of RNA (ribonucleic acid).

Glycogen granules

Glycogen granules, some 250–400 Å in diameter, are scattered throughout the sarcoplasm and are the major sources of energy for the muscle fibre.

Lipid droplets

These are often to be found close to mitochondria and contain fatty acids or triglycerides; they form important supplementary sources of energy.

Chapter 2

THE MOTONEURONE AND ITS AXON

When a muscle is required to contract it is sent the necessary instructions in the form of nerve impulses (action potentials) by large cells lying in the ventral grey matter of the spinal cord (or in a corresponding region of the brainstem). These cells are the *motoneurones,* each of which consists of a cell body (soma, perikaryon) and special processes termed the dendrites and the axon (*Figure 2.1*). The *soma* contains the nucleus of the cell together with various structures which will be considered later. The function of the *dendrites* is to receive signals from other neurones while the major role of the *axon* is to transmit a resulting message to the muscle fibres. The lengths of the axons vary considerably. In the case of a man 180 cm tall, an axon running from the lumbosacral region of the spinal cord to one of the plantar muscles would be about 125 cm long. In contrast, the fibres passing in the cranial nerves to the external ocular muscles, or to the muscles of the face or tongue, would only measure about one-tenth of this length. As the axon nears the muscle it begins to divide with each branch dividing further, so that eventually a single parent axon is able to make contact with many muscle fibres. The contact region between an axonal twig and a muscle fibre is termed a *synapse,* or *neuromuscular junction.* The synapse possess special structural and functional features which enable the impulse in the nerve fibre to be translated into an impulse in the muscle fibre through the action of a chemical link, the transmitter *acetylcholine.* In the normal adult mammal each muscle fibre has only one neuromuscular junction area and is innervated by only one motoneurone. Sherrington (1929) pointed out that a single motor nerve fibre and the colony of muscle fibres which it supplied could be considered as a functional entity, since each time the nerve fibre discharged an impulse the muscle fibres of the colony would be excited together; Sherrington described this entity as a *motor unit* (see Chapter 6).

Many methods have been used to study the structure of the motoneurone. For example, Haggar and Barr (1950) examined serial sections of cat spinal cord and were able to make three-dimensional models of the soma and dendrites. Another technique, also using a light microscope, was devised by Chu (1954). Pieces of ventral horn were dissected from recent autopsy specimens of human spinal cord and were made into a crude suspension with physiological saline. Within this suspension a proportion of the motoneurones were completely dissociated from other tissue and yet retained considerable lengths of axon and dendrites suitable for examination. More recently a technique for injecting the dye *procion yellow* through a micropipette into the soma of a neurone has been applied to motoneurones; the dye diffuses into the dendrites and proximal axon, enabling the full extent of the cell to be visualized (Kellerth, 1973). For information concerning the fine structure of the motoneurone it has been necessary to turn to the electronmiscroscope and several comprehensive reports are now available (see, for example, Bodian, 1964). The various parts of the motoneurone will now be considered in more detail.

THE MOTONEURONE AND ITS AXON
Soma

Within the ventral grey matter of the spinal cord, the cell bodies of the motoneurones are arranged in columns parallel to the long axis of the cord. The cells supplying the extrafusal muscle fibres are termed *alpha*-motoneurones in order to distinguish them from the *gamma*-motoneurones (fusimotoneurones) innervating the small fibres within the muscle spindles. The cell bodies of the alpha-

motoneurones are much larger than those of the gamma type and may have diameters of 100 μm; an average value would be about 70 μm.

The most prominent feature of the soma is the relatively large *nucleus* which is bounded by a wavy double membrane and contains nucleoplasm and a nucleolus. Within the nucleoplasm are the chromosomes, themselves made up of many genes, each of which consists of DNA. It is the genes which are ultimately responsible for directing the metabolic

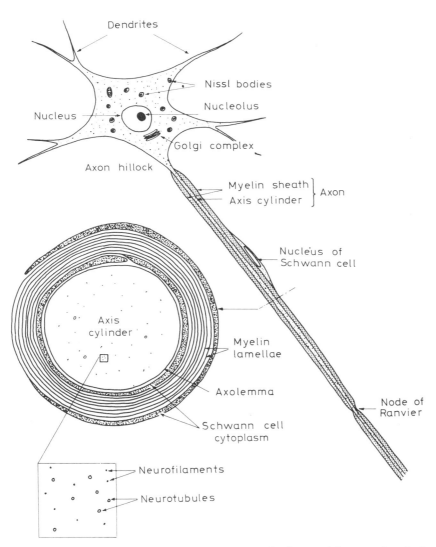

Figure 2.1. (Upper) A motoneurone and the proximal part of its axon (see text). (Middle) A transverse section through the axon to show the arrangement of the myelin lamellae in relation to the axis cylinder and the cytoplasm of the Schwann cell. (Lower) Part of the axis cylinder, enlarged to show the neurotubules and neurofilaments

activities of the neurone. They do so by sending instructions, in the form of messenger RNA, out into the cytoplasm of the cell, possibly through the pores in the nuclear membrane which can be seen with the electronmicroscope. Since human motoneurones do not multiply after birth the chromosomes cannot be distinguished in the nucleoplasm of the motoneurone; all that can be seen in the latter are irregularly distributed particles, 10–20 μm in diameter. Within the nucleus the *nucleolus* appears as a large structure, measuring about 4 μm across and consisting mostly of ribosomal RNA. This RNA is made on the DNA templates of the genes and is eventually passed out from the nucleolus into the cytoplasm to take part in the synthesis of proteins.

Cytoplasm

The cytoplasm of the motoneurone soma contains several different types of organelle, the most prominent of which is the *Nissl body*. These bodies range from 0.5 to 3 μm in diameter and electronmicrographs show them to be composed of tightly packed arrays of endoplasmic reticulum. The membranes of the reticulum are studded with ribosomes, giving them a rough appearance. Acting on instructions received through messenger RNA, the ribosomes engage in the synthesis of proteins. Their behaviour during the reactions of the cell following injury to the axon is of great interest (page 89).

In addition to the Nissl bodies, the cytoplasm of the motoneurone contains many mitochondria (page 6). There are also *neurotubules* and *neurofilaments*, most of which enter the dendrites and the axon. The *Golgi apparatus* is the name given to a system of flattened tubular channels to be found near the nucleus; one of its functions is thought to be the 'packaging' of proteins prior to their delivery into the axon (page 12). Finally, with advancing age, the motoneurone cytoplasm contains increasingly large masses of pigment, the *'lipofuscin' granules*; the significance of this material is unknown.

Dendrites

The motoneurone possess several dendrites which radiate from the cell body in dorsal, superior and inferior directions; the dendrites become progressively narrower and also divide into several branches. As already stated, the function of the dendrites is to receive information from other nerve cells. They do so by establishing synaptic connections with the terminal twigs of the axons from these cells. The fine structure of these synapses is similar to that of the neuromuscular junction (Chapter 4); the terminations of the axon twigs are expanded to form 'boutons' inside which many synaptic vesicles can be distinguished. The packing density of the boutons on the dendritic membrane increases as the dendrites narrow; more proximally there are gaps into which processes from the glial cells project. Some synapses are also found on the membrane of the soma.

Glial cells

The glial cells of the central nervous system do not conduct impulses and therefore have no direct role in signalling. Their importance lies in their various supportive functions; they provide a structural matrix for the neurones and also control the passage of substances from the capillaries into the neuronal milieu. In addition it appears that the metabolism of the glial cells is at least partly linked to that of the neurones. In the case of the motoneurone, several oligodendroglial cells can be seen clustered around its periphery and occupying any spaces available between the synaptic knobs (boutons) of the incoming fibres.

Axon

The axon arises from a conical protrusion of the motoneurone soma known as the *axon hillock* and extends to the muscle as a long *axis cylinder.* The cylinder is bounded by a membrane, the *axolemma,* which has structural and functional features similar to those of the muscle fibre sarcolemma (page 3). Within the cytoplasm of the axis cylinder is an array of small *neurotubules* and *neurofilaments* which run in the long axis of the fibre between the soma and the many neuromuscular junctions. The neurotubules are about 200 Å wide while the neurofilaments are rather smaller, being approximately 70 Å thick. An interlacing system of rather wider tubules forms the *endoplasmic reticulum.* All the motor axons have lipid coverings surrounding the axis cylinders; these are the *myelin sheaths* and they are derived from a type of satellite cell known as the *Schwann cell.* The motor axons in man are not quite as thick as those in the cat and monkey; if the myelin sheaths are included in the measurements, their diameters range from approximately 2 to 14 μm. In the ventral roots, which contain motor fibres only, the axon diameters fall into a bimodal distribution with a separation at about 7 μm. The population of fibres with large (7–14 μm) diameters corresponds to the *alpha*-motor axons supplying the extrafusal muscle fibres; the smaller axons are the *gamma* or 'fusimotor' axons innervating the intrafusal muscle fibres inside the muscle spindles.

The myelin sheath has been studied with the electronmicroscope and has been shown to consist of spiral wrappings of tightly-packed membranes laid down by the Schwann cell (Geren, 1954). The myelin sheath is not a continuous structure but is interrupted at regular intervals by the *nodes of Ranvier*. The distance between two successive nodes is an *internode* and corresponds to the

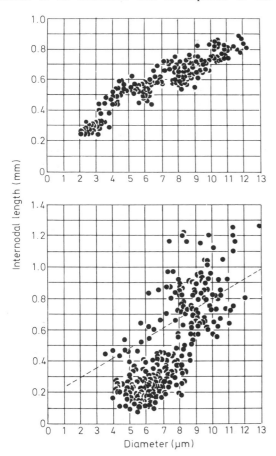

Figure 2.2. Measurements of internodal length (distance separating two successive nodes of Ranvier) made on teased fibres of anterior tibial nerves from an 18-year-old girl (upper) and an 80-year-old man (lower). Notice the linear relationship between fibre diameter and internodal length in the younger subject and the deviation from this relationship (— — — —) in the older one. (From Vizoso (1950) by courtesy of the author, and the Editor and publishers of Journal of Anatomy)

territory of a single Schwann cell. At birth the internodes measure about 230 μm in human motor nerves; as the limbs grow so the lengths of the internodes increase, since the number of Schwann cells remains the same. Vizoso (1950) found that the longest internodes in the ulnar and anterior tibial nerves of an 18-year-old subject were 1100 and 980 μm respectively, indicating that there had been a fourfold increase in their lengths. If, during the course of a disease process, the myelin sheath is destroyed and then remade, or if the axon is damaged and then regenerates, many of the newly formed internodes are much shorter than in the normal adult (*Figure 2.2*). The explanation for this discrepancy is that during the recovery process the Schwann cells divide and thereby increase their number; each new cell occupies a smaller length of axon.

The electronmicroscope has also been invaluable in revealing the ultrastructure of the nodes of the Ranvier. *Figure 2.3* summarizes, in diagram form, the findings of Williams and Landon (1967). On the left-hand side of the figure the axon has been bisected by a vertical incision and a segment removed; to the right of the node some of the basement membrane has been peeled away. It can be seen that the myelin sheath on the other side of the node (*paranodal* region) is furrowed and that the superficial grooves are filled with columns of Schwann cell cytoplasm rich in mitochondria. As these columns approach the node they first become confluent and then send finger-like processes toward the nodal portion of the axolemma. The processes are embedded in an amorphous extracellular material known simply as 'gap substance'. Studies by Landon and Langley (1971), among others, have demonstrated that the gap substance is composed of mucopolysaccharides, and that the anionic groups of these molecules exert a powerful electrostatic attraction for cations. Landon and Langley further suggest that the gap substance may serve to maintain a high concentration of sodium ions available for flow across the axolemma during the action potential. Similarly the gap substance might limit the diffusion of potassium from the vicinity of the node following an impulse and hold it in readiness for active transportation back into the fibre subsequently (page 21). It is also tempting to assign a functional role to the Schwann cell processes which project to the nodal axolemma. It is possible that these convey ATP to the nerve membrane from the mitochondria in the columns of Schwann cell cytoplasm; the ATP might then be used to supply the energy required for sodium ion pumping (see Landon and Langley, 1971). Another interesting feature of the myelin sheath are the *Schmidt–*

Lanterman incisures (clefts). At each of these regions a narrow cytoplasmic process is sent from the Schwann cell to the axis cylinder. The projection does not actually penetrate the myelin wrappings but instead winds its way around the axon, following the plane of separation between the myelin lamellae. Using time-lapse cinematography Gitlin and Singer (1974) have observed that the Schmidt–Lanterman clefts are not static

thick coat of connective tissue which invests the whole nerve trunk; this is the *epineurium*.

AXOPLASMIC FLOW

The function of the axon is to act as a communication pathway between the spinal cord and muscle. Rapid signalling to the periphery is required if the

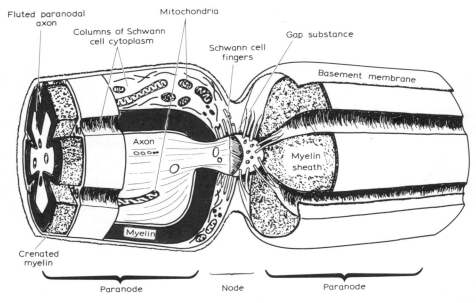

Figure 2.3. Structure of a node of Ranvier and the adjacent regions of nerve fibre (paranodes). See text for description. (From Williams and Landon (1967), courtesy of the authors, and the Editor and publishers of Gray's Anatomy*)*

structures but can be open or closed at different times. It is possible that the open phase enables materials to be passed between the axis cylinder, on the one hand, and the Schwann cell and the endoneurial space of the nerve fibre, on the other. Even the remainder of the myelin sheath is not stationary but can be seen to develop small indentations which then regress; possibly this type of movement is related to some component of axoplasmic flow (see below and Weiss, 1969).

In considering the structure of a peripheral nerve, mention must also be made of the connective tissue. Each of the nerve fibres is enclosed in a sheath of connective tissue, or *endoneurium*. Within the nerve trunk the fibres are collected into a number of bundles or *fasciculi*, each being bounded by a condensation of connective tissue termed the *perineurium*. Lastly, there is a relatively

muscle is to contract and is achieved by the nerve impulses; the ionic mechanisms underlying this event are considered in detail on page 21. Equally important, however, is a slow signalling system which enables messages, coded in the form of chemicals, to be sent in both directions between the cell body of the motoneurone and the muscle fibres which it innervates. These messages are of paramount importance for the maintenance of the normal structure and cellular metabolism of both the muscle fibre and the motoneurone; the integrity of the Schwann cells and of the axon itself are also dependent on this chemical signalling system. These controlling effects are described as 'trophic' and they are analysed in Chapters 8, 9 and 10. Of immediate concern is the nature of the axoplasmic transport which makes this chemical signalling system possible. It will be shown that in the centrifugal direction (from motoneurone to muscle) there are both fast and slow transport systems while in the reverse (centripetal) direction the axoplasmic flow has an intermediate velocity.

Centrifugal transport

'Slow' axoplasmic flow

The earliest intimation that there was normally a flow of cytoplasm from the cell body of the motoneurone outwards along the axon came from a series of experiments by Weiss and his colleagues in the 1940s (Weiss, 1944; Weiss and Davis, 1943; Weiss and Hiscoe, 1948); the results of these and later experiments have recently been summarized by Weiss (1969). The technique employed by these workers was to apply a gentle constriction to the sciatic nerve of an animal by investing the nerve with a sleeve of artery. As the arterial cuff gradually contracted, due to its own elasticity, the nerve fibres underwent compression to varying extents and the chronic effects of this were studied after several months. It was found that the segment of nerve abutting the proximal end of the constriction was swollen, partly because of oedematous fluid between the nerve fibres but mainly on account of distortions and distensions of the axons themselves. With the light microscope the axis cylinders appeared to be either beaded or else ballooned, telescoped or 'corkscrewed'. Within and beyond the constriction the axis cylinders were narrowed. To Weiss and his colleagues the appearances of the axons suggested that there had been a 'damming up' of axoplasm at the site of constriction; this conclusion implied that, under normal circumstances, axoplasm must be manufactured in the cell body and somehow propelled down the axon. Supporting evidence for Weiss's interpretation came from a subsidiary experiment in which the constriction was removed (Weiss and Cavanaugh, 1959). The dammed-up material was then released and could be observed to travel down the axon as a wave with a velocity between one and several millimetres per day. Even during the period of the constriction, however, there had been a small flow of axoplasm distally from the core of the swollen proximal region of nerve. To Weiss these results indicated that the axons were perpetually growing from the cell bodies of the motoneurones and that the contents of the new axoplasm were then consumed distally as part of a continual replenishment process. The relatively large amount of material requiring synthesis would account for the high turnover of RNA in the cell bodies of the motoneurones (and other neurones).

Although some of the conclusions reached by Weiss and his colleagues have been challenged recently by Spencer (1972), on the basis of electronmicrographs of ligated nerve, the existence of 'slow' axoplasmic flow is not seriously doubted. The study by Weiss and Cavanaugh (1959) has already been cited and further supporting evidence has come from the results of isotope experiments. For example, Droz and Leblond (1963) showed unequivocally that protein labelled with [^{3}H]-leucine moved distally in rabbit sciatic nerve with a velocity of about 1 mm per day.

'Fast' axoplasmic flow

After the clear demonstration of axoplasmic flow with the 'damming' experiments described above, attempts were made to explore the phenomenon more fully by labelling the axoplasm with radioactive isotopes and then studying their passage down the axon. The first experiments involved radioactive phosphorus while later ones employed labelled carbon in glucose and amino acids; these methods have been superseded following the availability of tritiated amino acids. At present a commonly used strategy is to injected [^{3}H]-leucine into the ventral grey matter of the lumbar region of the spinal cord; the amino acid is then taken up by the cell bodies of neighbouring motoneurones and rapidly incorporated into newly synthesized proteins. At a given time after injection the sciatic nerve is excised and cut into segments of uniform length. The amount of radioactivity in each segment is then measured with a scintillation counter and expressed as a function of distance from the spinal cord. An example from the work of Ochs and Ranish (1969) is given in *Figure 2.4,* the lower curve of which shows the distribution of radioactivity in the sciatic nerve of the cat 6 hr after injection of [^{3}H]-leucine into the L7 segment of the cord. Included for comparison, and displayed in the upper curve, are the results for sensory nerve fibres following an injection given at approximately the same time into the L7 dorsal root ganglion on the opposite side. The peak of radioactivity in the sensory fibre curve corresponds to isotope remaining in the ganglion; similarly the high value at the left of the motor fibre curve denotes the activity left in, and around, the cell bodies of the motoneurones. The arrows at the bottoms of the two curves indicate the advancing fronts of the labelled axoplasm; the spatial disparity corresponds to the extra length of the motor pathway due to the inclusion of the L7 ventral root. Studies such as these have demonstrated that, in addition to the slow movement of axoplasm already described, there is a very much faster flow with a maximum velocity, in mammals, of about 410 mm/day. Another technique is to produce a temporary arrest of axoplasmic flow by cooling a short length of nerve; the transported material then accumulates in, and proximal to, the cooled region. Upon rewarming the nerve, the movement

can increase the rate fivefold (Boegman, Wood and Pinaud, 1975). Such a finding raises the obvious possibility that the flow can be modulated under physiological circumstances, but this remains to be proven (see, however, page 86). Finally, it should be noted that the neurone soma sends cytoplasm not only into the axon but also out into the various dendrites and their branches.

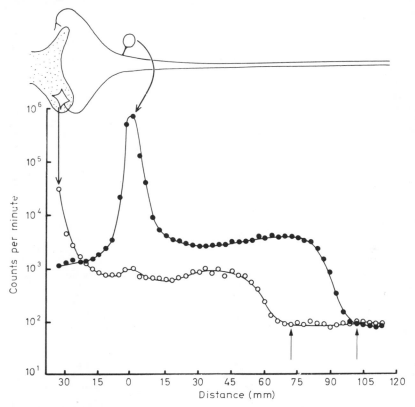

Figure 2.4. Centrifugal transport of radioactive leucine in sensory nerve fibres (●) and motor fibres (O) of cat sciatic nerve, measured 6 hr after injection of labelled material into dorsal root ganglion and ventral horn. See text for description of technique and results. (Modified from Ochs and Ranish (1969) courtesy of the authors, and the Editor and publishers of Journal of Neurobiology)

of the material is resumed and its velocity can be determined. This 'stop-flow' method has been used by Brimijoin (1975) to study the passage of the enzyme dopamine-β-hydroxylase in rabbit sciatic nerve; a flow rate of 300 ± 17 mm/day was found. The presence of a 'fast' axoplasmic flow is a property of all the motor and sensory axons which have been tested to date. Although the velocity of the 'fast' axoplasmic flow is independent of fibre diameter it now appears that it can be influenced quite markedly by certain drugs; for example pargyline, a monoamine oxidase inhibitor,

Mechanism of fast axoplasmic flow

By injecting inhibitors of protein synthesis such as puromycin or cycloheximide it has been shown that the motoneurone soma is able to complete its synthesis of protein within 10–20 minutes of the arrival of the labelled precursor, [³H]-leucine. Not all the amino acid is converted into protein since polypeptides are also labelled and there is a large fraction which is taken up by small axoplasmic particles.

Other studies have shown that lipids and polysaccharides are also rapidly conveyed down the axon. Included among the transported proteins are the enzymes acetylcholinesterase and choline acetyltransferase (page 31); in addition Miledi and Slater (1970) have shown that a fast-travelling factor(s) is necessary for the maintenance of the axon terminal at the neuromuscular junction. Other substances, as yet unidentified, supervise the metabolic machinery of the axon, Schwann cells and muscle fibres in keeping with the 'trophic' role of the motoneurone (see page 72). Of the particulate matter transported down the axon, the most prominent fraction is the mitochondria and these can be observed in motion with the phase-contrast and interference microscopes. The suggestion has been made that the mitochondria are transported to the axon terminal for the synthesis of acetylcholine, and that their ageing components are continually resynthesized from proteins conveyed by fast axoplasmic transport.

A further proposal is that the Golgi apparatus of the cell body acts as a 'gate' by controlling the delivery of the material into the axon (Ochs, 1972). So far as the transport mechanism itself is concerned, a number of observations are relevant. First, axoplasmic flow is able to proceed in both directions at a normal rate even when the axon has been removed from the body; this finding indicates that the transport system obtains its energy from local sources in the axon (or the Schwann cell). Secondly, on the basis of experiments utilizing metabolic blocking agents such as DNP (dinitrophenol) it is likely that ATP (backed up by creatine phosphate) provides this energy.

There is general acceptance of the idea that the neurotubules and neurofilaments within the axon are somehow involved with fast axoplasmic transport but there is no agreement as to mechanism by which this is effected. One proposal, that by Ochs (1972, 1974), is that the materials are conveyed on 'transport filaments', rather like wagons on a railway track. In this case the 'track' would be a neurotubule or neurofilament from which projecting cross bridges, energized by ATP, would move the 'wagon' onwards. The concept is thus very similar to the sliding filament mechanism of muscle contraction (page 35) and it is relevant to the hypothesis that actomyosin has been shown to be component of brain tissue (Berl and Puszkin, 1970). It is also probable that the system of fine interlacing longitudinal channels within the axis cylinder, the endoplasmic reticulum, is important in transporting material along the axon (Droz et al., 1975).

So far no consideration has been given to the axoplasmic flow which occurs in a centripetal direction, that is, from the muscle fibre to the motoneurone. Evidence for such a movement has come from several sources. For example, Lubinska and Niemierko (1970) have found that acetylcholinesterase is transported proximally as well as distally; the rate of the centripetal flow is about one half of the centrifugal one. Other workers have observed particles, probably mitochondria, being carried in axons away from the periphery. Proof that some of the material reaches the cell bodies of the motoneurones has been obtained by Glatt and Honegger (1973) who injected albumin coupled with the fluorescent dye, Evans blue, into triceps muscles of the rat forelimb and were able to detect dye in the ventral horns some 12 hr later. In the study by Kristensson and Olsson (1971) horseradish peroxidase was used as a marker instead. This substance had the advantage that it could produce an electron-dense reaction product and, with the electronmicroscope, its intracellular location was seen to be in small cytoplasmic granules around the nucleus. Just as the centrifugal axoplasmic flow largely mediates the trophic control of axon, Schwann cell and muscle fibre by the motoneurone, so the centripetal flow exerts a trophic influence on the motoneurone soma by the periphery. Interruption of this trophic influence, as in cutting the axon, sets in train the phenomenon of chromatolysis in the motoneurone (see page 89).

Chapter 3

RESTING AND ACTION POTENTIALS

It has been known for more than a century that a difference in electrical potential normally exists between the inside of a cell and its fluid environment. During the past three decades it has been possible to determine this potential difference directly by inserting a microelectrode through the cell membrane into the interior of the fibre and connecting the other terminal of the voltage measuring device to a reference electrode in the fluid bathing the cell (see Appendix 3.1 for methods). In the case of inactive mammalian muscle the inside of the cell has been found to be some 85 mV negative with respect to the outside; this potential difference is termed the *resting membrane potential* (*Figure 3.1, left*).

IONIC BASIS OF THE RESTING MEMBRANE POTENTIAL

An understanding of the resting membrane potential requires knowledge of the ions present on the two sides of the membrane. Inside the muscle fibre the most common cation is potassium; the anions are supplied by phosphate, sulphate and bicarbonate together with amino acids, polypeptides and proteins. Outside the cell the interstitial fluid has a composition similar to plasma; sodium and choloride are the dominant cation and anion respectively and smaller amounts of potassium, calcium, magnesium, bicarbonate and phosphate are also present.

The concentrations of the various ions in mammalian skeletal muscle and in its extracellular fluid are given in Table 3.1. The intracellular values should be recognized as very approximate ones for there is difficulty in determining the proportion of muscle fluid which is intracellular rather than extracellular. Further, even if the intracellular value was accurately established it would only reflect a gross average for the various organelles, myofibrils, tubular systems and cytoplasm of the fibre.

There are two reasons why the compositions of the intracellular and extracellular fluids are so different. First, a large proportion of the organic anions in the interior of the fibre are part of the cell structure and are therefore unable to migrate. Second, the resting membrane is only semipermeable; it allows potassium and chloride ions to diffuse through but it impedes the passage of sodium. The internal anions exert an electrostatic attraction for cations which can only be satisfied by a high internal concentration of potassium, since sodium ions are unable to cross the resting membrane. The external sodium ions will, however, be effective in balancing the anions of the extracellular fluid, the most prevalent of which is chloride. This unequal distribution of potassium and chloride ions is termed a *Donnan equilibrium,* such that

$$\frac{[K]_o}{[K]_i} = \frac{[Cl]_i}{[Cl]_o} \qquad (1)$$

where the brackets signify the concentration of the ion inside (i) or outside (o) the cell.

The potential difference across the membrane arises because the potassium ions, although attracted into the cell by the electrical force generated by the internal anions, are required to move 'uphill' against their concentration gradient. Hence the internal potassium concentration does not quite balance the anions present within the cell; the slight excess of the latter is responsible for the internal negativity of the resting membrane potential. The size of this electrical potential is related to the concentration of potassium on the two sides of the membrane by the *Nernst equation*, in which

$$E_K = \frac{RT}{F} \log_e \frac{[K]_0}{[K]_i} \tag{2}$$

where E_K is termed the potassium equilibrium potential, R is the universal gas constant, T is the absolute temperature and F is the Faraday constant. For a mammalian muscle at 37 °C the equation can be simplified by inserting values for the various constants and transforming the logarithms so that,

$$E_K = 60 \log_{10} \frac{[K]_0}{[K]_i} \tag{3}$$

Assuming values of 5 and 150 mM respectively for external and internal concentrations of potassium, E_K would be -89 mV, which is approximately the value observed for the resting membrane potential. A more rigorous test of the postulated ionic basis of the resting membrane potential would be to observe the effect of altering $[K]_0$, the concentration of potassium in the fluid surrounding the muscle fibre. Provided pre-

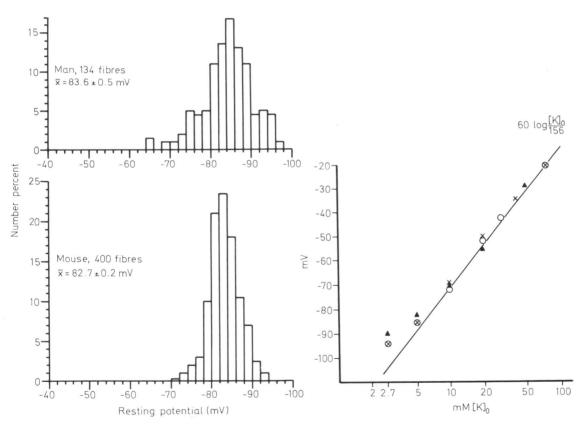

Figure 3.1. (Left) Resting membrane potentials recorded in situ from the brachial biceps and quadriceps muscles of three healthy human subjects (upper) and from the gracilis muscles of normal mice (lower). The greater scatter of the human results probably resulted from unavoidable damage to some of the fibres during removal of the superficial connective tissue. Data of McComas et al. (1968b). (Right) Membrane potential in three different specimens of human intercostal muscle, studied in vitro. The effect of varying the external concentration of potassium is shown. The straight line is a plot of the potassium equilibrium potential for $[K]_i = 156$ mM at 37 °C. Each point represents the mean value from five fibres. The small deviation between the observed and predicted values, when the $[K]_0$ is less than 10 mM is due to sodium permeability of the membrane; the latter is effectively abolished by adding protein to the bathing solution; see text. (From Ludin (1970) courtesy of the author, and the Editor and publishers of European Neurology)

cautions are taken to include protein in the bathing fluid, the membrane potentials of frog and mammalian muscle fibres correspond precisely to the potassium equilibrium potentials calculated from the Nernst equation (Kernan, 1963). Thus, an increase in the external potassium concentration causes the resting potential to fall (*depolarization*) while a reduction in concentration induces a rise in potential (*hyperpolarization*; *Figure 3.1, right*). In

TABLE 3.1

Ionic Compositions of Mammalian Skeletal Muscle Fibres and of the Interstitial Fluid Surrounding Them

	Interstitial fluid *mEq/1*	*Intracellular fluid* *mEq/kg water*
Sodium	145	10
Potassium	4	160
Calcium	5	2
Magnesium	2	26
Total cations	156	198
Chloride	114	3
Bicarbonate	31	10
Phosphate	2	100
Sulphate	1	20
Organic acids	7	—
Proteins	1	65
Total anions	156	198

From Maxwell and Kleeman (1962)

the same way, equilibrium potentials can be calculated for both chloride and sodium ions. It is found that the equilibrium potential for chloride has the same value and polarity as the potassium potential. Further, since the membrane is freely permeable to chloride, one would expect the resting potential to be affected by changes in external concentration of the ion. Hodgkin and Horowicz (1959) were able to show that this was so but that the effect was shortlived because diffusion of chloride, potassium and water subsequently took place until the previous concentration gradient for chloride was restored. In effect the chloride ion had been redistributed so as to form a new Donnan equilibrium with potassium. In the case of sodium the calculated equilibrium potential has a polarity opposite to the resting membrane potential. This discrepancy indicates that sodium ions cannot be contributing toward the resting potential and is in keeping with the impermeability of the membrane to sodium described previously. It follows that an alteration of the external sodium concentration should be without effect on the membrane potential and experimentally this can be shown to be so.

The theoretical basis for these observations can

also be stated using the 'constant field' equation of Goldman (1943),

$$E_m = \frac{RT}{F} \log_e \frac{P_K[K]_o + P_{Na}[Na]_o + P_{Cl}[Cl]_i}{P_K[K]_i + P_{Na}[Na]_i + P_{Cl}[Cl]_o} \quad (4)$$

where P denotes the permeability of the membrane for an ion species and E_m is the resting potential. Since at rest P_{Na} is very low, and the effects of changes in chloride concentration are transient, the behaviour of the resting membrane will be that of a potassium electrode, and the equation will simplify to eqs. (2) and (3). Suppose, however, that the permeability of the membrane to sodium were to increase as a result of electrical or chemical stimulation. Under these circumstances the potential would depolarize to reach a value between E_{Na} on the one hand and E_K and E_{Cl} on the other. If the membrane permeability to sodium increased still further, so that the potassium and chloride permeabilities were comparatively small, the membrane potential would approximate to E_{Na}, the sodium equilibrium potential. In fact, this is precisely what happens at the summit of the action potential, which will be considered later.

Another way of analysing the behaviour of the membrane is to depict it as an electrical analogue (*Figure 3.2*). The various equilibrium potentials can be represented as batteries, with the polarity of the sodium battery opposite to those of the potassium and chloride cells. The permeability of the membrane for an ion may be symbolized as an

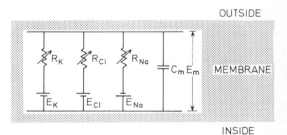

Figure 3.2. Electrical analogue of membrane. E_m, membrane potential; C_m, membrane capacity. E_K, E_{Cl} and E_{Na} are ionic equilibrium potentials and R_K, R_{Cl}, R_{Na} the corresponding membrane resistances

electrical resistance since the latter is a measure of the ease, or difficulty, with which that ion will traverse the membrane. A highly permeable membrane would therefore be shown as having a low electrical resistance. The arrow over each resistance in *Figure 3.2* emphasizes that the resistances are not fixed but may vary, depending on whether the membrane is at rest or participating in impulse activity. From the figure it is obvious that if any one resistance becomes very small (permeability very high) in comparison with the others, the potential appearing across the membrane will be that of the corresponding ionic equilibrium potential.

The net resistance of the membrane to the various ions may be determined experimentally by measuring the change in potential produced by passing current through the membrane from an intracellular stimulating electrode. According to Ohm's law, the fibre *resistance* will be equal to the induced *potential* divided by stimulating *current*. In *Figure 3.4* the smallest of the three currents, 2.5×10^{-8} A, produced a depolarization of 12 mV (trace *a*), which would give a value for the resistance of 0.48 MΩ. The resistance measured in this way is the 'input' resistance of the fibre; it depends on the resistance of the fibre interior as well as on that of the membrane. The contribution of the various species of ion toward the membrane resistance may be determined by replacing each, in turn, with an impermeant substance. For example, by replacing chloride in the external bathing solution with methylsulphate, Hutter and Noble (1960) were able to show that the resting membranes of frog muscle fibres were twice as permeable to chloride as to potassium.

Finally, it should be noted that the electrical analogue shown in *Figure 3.2* includes the symbol for capacitance (C_m). This is required because the lipid membrane of the fibre acts as a dielectric between two conducting media, namely the interstitial fluid and the sarcoplasm. Each time a depolarizing current is made to flow across the membrane the capacitor has to be discharged; hence the change in membrane potential is never instantaneous but takes place exponentially, as in *Figure 3.4* for the smallest current (response *a*). Similarly there is an exponential decline in potential as the stimulus is terminated, caused by the recharging of the membrane capacity. The time constant of the membrane, τ_m, is a measure of the capacity of the membrane, being equal to the product of the capacity and the membrane resistance. It can be determined experimentally by measuring the time taken for the membrane potential to reach 84 per cent of its final value following the onset of the rectangular pulse of current. The capacity of the mammalian muscle fibre membrane is 4–5 μF/cm^2 of surface membrane (Lipicky, Bryant and Salmon, 1971) and is much larger than that estimated for nerve fibre membrane (about 1 μF/cm^2). This increased capacity of the muscle fibre is due to the substantial invaginations of membrane which form the transverse tubular (T) system. Convincing proof of the supposition came from the experiments of Gage and Eisenberg

(1969a) in which glycerol was used to disrupt the connections of the T-tubules to the sarcolemma; the membrane capacity was decreased by a factor of almost 3.

So far the membrane of the resting muscle fibre has been discussed as if it was a homogeneous structure with the permeability of one region similar to that of another. It turns out that this is not so. One of the first indications of such a variation came from the experiments of Hodgkin and Horowicz (1959), already mentioned, in which the ionic composition of the solution bathing single frog muscle fibres was changed abruptly. These authors discovered that whereas alterations in chloride concentration produced an immediate alteration in membrane potential, the effects of potassium were slower, particularly when the external concentration was being reduced. Hodgkin and Horowicz suggested that the reason for the slowness of the potassium effect was that the membrane permeability for this ion was restricted to the transverse tubules and that diffusion into, and out of, these channels would be retarded because of their narrowness.

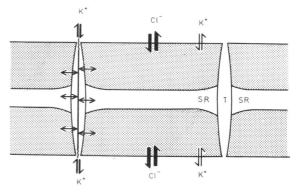

Figure 3.3. Passive fluxes of potassium and chloride through the membranes of the muscle fibre at rest. The thickness of an arrow indicates the relative size of the flux. S.R., sarcoplasmic reticulum; T, transverse tubular system; sarcoplasm shown by stippling

Eisenberg and Gage (1959) put this hypothesis to direct test by measuring the potassium and chloride permeabilities of muscle fibres after the necks of the transverse tubules had been disconnected from the sarcolemma by treatment with glycerol. They found that the chloride permeability was restricted to the sarcolemma but that the potassium permeability was shared by the sarcolemma and T-system, the permeability of the latter being twice as high as that of the former (*Figure 3.3*). The slow diffusion of potassium out of the T-system is responsible for two other effects. The first of these is the high resistance displayed by the muscle fibre to the movement of potassium ions *outwards* through the membrane, as when an intracellular stimulating electrode is used to pass current. By discriminating between inward and outward potassium currents the membrane is said to act as a *rectifier*. The second

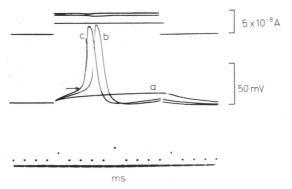

Figure 3.4. *Responses evoked in a normal human muscle fibre in situ, using intracellular stimulation through a Wheatstone bridge circuit. At top are shown three rectangular current pulses of different intensities; the middle section displays the corresponding changes in membrane potential. Response a, produced by the smallest current, is subthreshold but in b and c the depolarizations are large enough to reach the firing level (arrow) for an action potential. (Modified from McComas et al. (1968) by courtesy of the Editor and publishers of* Journal of Neurology, Neurosurgery and Psychiatry*)*

effect of the T-system is that, during impulse activity, there is an efflux of potassium from the muscle fibre into the T-system (page 6). Since this potassium is slow to diffuse away, the concentration gradient for potassium will be reduced across the tubular membrane and so the potassium equilibrium potential, E_K, will be correspondingly smaller (page 17). This, in turn, will cause the membrane potential to fall provided the potassium permeability of the fibre is significantly larger than that of chloride; normally the reverse is true (page 19). The condition of a high potassium permeability occurs during and immediately after the spike component of the action potential. Because of the accumulation of potassium in the tubules, the membrane potential will remain partially depolarized for a few milliseconds, producing a *negative after-potential*. This potential is more obvious in frog muscle fibres than in mammalian ones (see, however, *Figure 3.5*) and it is enhanced by cooling or by repetitive impulse activity (since there is a greater accumulation of potassium). Sometimes the negative after-potential

becomes so large that it triggers off a spontaneous impulse.

These observations are also relevant to a consideration of the disease phenomenon of *peripheral myotonia* (page 125) in which the fibres are hyper-excitable, discharging long trains of impulses spontaneously and after transient mechanical or electrical stimulation of the fibre membrane. It has been shown that in the myotonic fibre the chloride permeability is greatly reduced (page 128); hence potassium in the T-system is likely to be effective in reducing the resting potential and thereby bringing the membrane to the threshold for firing spontaneous impulses. A similar situation would be predicted to occur if all the chloride were removed from a solution bathing a normal muscle fibre; such fibres do indeed become hyperexcitable and exhibit myotonic-like behaviour.

THE ACTION POTENTIAL

The ability of their membranes to develop transient changes in potential, which can be transmitted from one point to another, confers upon nerve and muscle fibres the special property of excitability. The propagated change of membrane potential is the *action potential,* or *impulse;* in order to record its full amplitude it is necessary to measure, during excitation, the potential developed between an electrode in the cytoplasm of the fibre and an external electrode. In *Figure 3.4* the same electrode was used simultaneously to stimulate and record from a human muscle fibre and a Wheatstone bridge circuit was employed to nullify the stimulus artefact. It can be seen that the smallest rect-

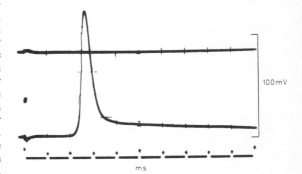

Figure 3.5. *Response of a mouse tibialis anterior muscle fibre in situ to stimulation of the sciatic nerve. The action potential reached the recording point 2 ms after the stimulus had been delivered (artefact at left of trace) and had an overshoot of 39 mV; the resting potential was −80 mV. Note the negative after-potential following the spike*

angular pulse of current produced only a small maintained depolarization of the membrane (*a*). In contrast each of the two larger pulses evoked reversals of membrane potential (*b*, *c*), such that the inside of the fibre became 13 mV positive with respect to the outside for about 1 ms. One of the advantages of the intracellular stimulation technique is that it enables measurement to be made of the critical amount of membrane depolarization required to trigger off the action potential mechanism. From *Figure 3.4* it can be seen that the 12 mV depolarization induced by the weakest stimulus was insufficient whereas depolarizations of 14 mV produced by the two larger stimuli were adequate. In one case the onset of the action potential from the evoked depolarization has been indicated by an arrow. *Figure 3.5* shows, for comparison, the action potential set up in a muscle fibre following electrical stimulation of its motor axon; the transient reversal of membrane potential and the negative after-potential following the spike are both clearly shown.

Like the resting membrane potential the action potential has an ionic basis, depending on the permeability of the membrane to the ions on its inner and outer surfaces, as well as upon the concentrations of those ions. Many years ago it was realized that sodium ions had an important role since nerves and muscles bathed in sodium-free solutions lost their excitability. The key to our present understanding of the ionic mechanisms involved in the action potential was the *voltage clamp experiment* of Hodgkin and Huxley (1952a). These authors chose to study the giant axon of the squid for its large diameter, about 0.5 mm, permitted them to insert both a stimulating and a recording electrode into the axoplasm; the stimulating and recording circuits were completed by two external electrodes in the artificial seawater bathing the fibre (*Figure 3.6, upper*). Their technique was to rapidly change the potential across the membrane to any desired level by passing current between the stimulating electrodes. By using a feedback circuit from the recording electrodes they were able to keep the membrane potential steady at its new level. The amount of current necessary to clamp the membrane in this way was equal to, and opposite in sign to, the ionic current which would have normally been flowing through the membrane if the depolarization had been a naturally-occurring one. Hodgkin and Huxley then determined the contribution of sodium ions to the total current by substituting choline, an impermeant cation, in the bathing solution. They were able to show that as the membrane potential was reduced there was an initial flow of sodium ions into the cell and

that this was followed by a flow of potassium ions in the opposite direction (outwards).

It is obvious that the membrane permeability must have changed during the action potential since under resting conditions the membrane is impermeable to sodium. During the action potential the sodium permeability not only increases but the increase becomes self-regenerative. The explanation for this phenomenon is that, as the membrane becomes permeable to sodium, these ions will diffuse into the fibre down their concentration gradient and also under the attraction of the internal negativity of the cell. However, the entry of sodium ions will depolarize the membrane further for, being positively charged, the ions make the inside of the cell less negative. In turn, the further depolarization causes the membrane to become even more permeable to sodium and the cycle is repeated (*Figure 3.7*). From a consideration of the electrical analogue of the membrane (*Figure 3.2*) and of the Goldman field equation (page 18) it is apparent that a membrane which is much more permeable to sodium than to potassium or chloride should have a potential across it equal to the sodium equilibrium potential, E_{Na}. The fact that the recorded potential is rather less than E_{Na} is due to two additional properties of the membrane; first, the sodium permeability mechanism is soon switched off and second, the membrane increases its permeability to potassium as that to sodium declines. The time courses of these changes are shown in *Figure 3.6, lower*. It is the increase in potassium permeability which is responsible for the delayed outward current recorded in the voltage clamp experiment. In the normal 'unclamped' fibre the increased potassium permeability serves to restore the membrane potential to its resting level. Thus, at the end of an action potential the fibre will have gained a little sodium and lost some potassium. The quantities are so small, however, that a motor nerve axon or muscle fibre can conduct several thousand action potentials without difficulty. In a very small muscle fibre or axon the situation is rather different, for appreciable changes in internal sodium concentration would occur after fewer impulses.

During periods of rest the changes in ionic composition of the fibre are corrected by means of a membrane 'pump' which actively extrudes sodium (Thomas, 1972). By expelling positive charges the pump increases the negativity of the interior of the fibre and is therefore 'electrogenic'. However, the extrusion of sodium appears to be loosely coupled with an inward movement of potassium such that two ions of potassium enter for every three ions of sodium expelled. Since both sodium and

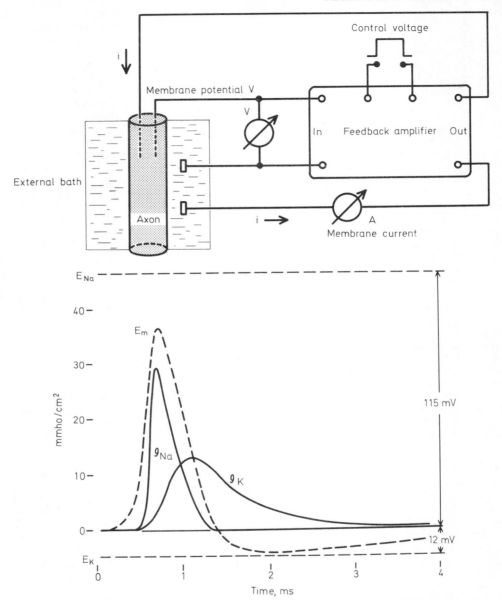

Figure 3.6. (Upper) Experimental arrangement used in the voltage clamp studies of Hodgkin and Huxley (1952a, b) on the squid giant axon. The potential between an intracellular and an extra-cellular electrode is measured (V) and compared with a controlling voltage; any difference is automatically eliminated by the passage of a current (i) through another pair of electrodes situated on either side of the membrane. (Modified from Katz (1966), courtesy of the author and McGraw-Hill Ltd). (Lower) Time courses of the ionic permeability changes during an action potential, as determined by the voltage-clamp experiment. The permeabilities of the membrane to sodium and potassium are indicated by the corresponding conductances (g); E_m, is the action potential recorded when the clamp was no longer applied. (Since the recordings were made from an axon, in which the T-system is not present, there is no negative after-potential; the hyperpolarization recorded instead is a consequence of the fact that the potassium equilibrium potential, E_K, may be larger than the resting membrane potential if the fibre is not in an optimal condition). (Modified from Hodgkin and Huxley (1952b), courtesy of the authors, and the Editor and publishers of Journal of Physiology)

potassium are being transported 'uphill', against their respective concentration gradients, energy must be expended by the pump and this is supplied by ATP. Inhibitors of cell metabolism interfere with the pump by depriving it of ATP while cardiac glycosides, such as ouabain, inhibit the pump

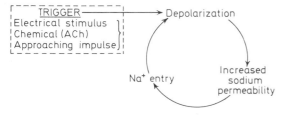

Figure 3.7. The regenerative nature of the increase in sodium permeability of the membrane

directly. The fact that ouabain also causes the membrane to depolarize by about 20mV suggests that the pump generates part of the resting potential (Locke and Solomon, 1967). It is now possible to make preparations of cell membrane which exhibit the properties of a pump, that is, they contain an ATPase enzyme which is Na:K dependent (Skou, 1957).

The ionic hypothesis of the resting and action potentials has now been verified in a strikingly elegant series of experiments by Baker, Hodgkin and Shaw (1962a, b). These authors were able to extrude the axoplasm from a squid giant axon and to fill the 'bag' of membrane left behind with solutions of any desired composition. By altering the constituents of the extracellular fluid as well, they could alter the resting potential at will. For example, if the external concentration of potassium was higher than the internal one, the resting membrane potential reversed its sign and became positive inside the fibre, in agreement with predictions from the Nernst equation (page 17).

MECHANISM OF THE INCREASED SODIUM PERMEABILITY

One of the outstanding problems to be solved is the molecular nature of the change in sodium permeability which takes places in the membrane during the genesis of the action potential. It now appears that the sodium system has two parts. First, there is a component which senses the difference in potential across the membrane; this molecular complex then regulates the accessibility of sodium ions to the second component, which is the sodium

channel itself. The sodium channel can be inactivated by *tetrodotoxin* (TTX), a powerful toxin produced by the Japanese puffer fish (Appendix 3.2), and also by *saxitonin* (STX), a similar poison derived from the dinoflagellate *Gonyalaux catenella* (Kao, 1966). The latter organism lives in the sea and when rapidly multiplying forms a 'red tide'; if infected shellfish are eaten by man paralysis supervenes. By using very dilute solutions of TTX or STX, and also by labelling these compounds, it has been possible to estimate the density of the sodium channels in excitable membranes. It appears that the channels are remarkably sparse; for example, in lobster axons there are probably fewer than 13 sodium channels per square micrometre of membrane (Moore, Narahashi and Shaw, 1967) while for rat diaphragm the corresponding figure is about 21 channels (Colquhoun, Rang and Ritchie, 1974). Such low densities imply that during the impulse sodium ions must flow through each channel at a very high rate, probably in the region of 100 million ions per second (Keynes, Ritchie and Rojas, 1971). This flow is too high to be accounted for simply by the opening up of pores in the membrane and it is necessary to postulate instead that the entry of sodium ions is facilitated by the action of special *carrier molecules* (ionophores). The part of the molecule facing outwards (away from the fibre) is presumed to have a high affinity for the sodium ion which, having been seized, is then transported rapidly to the inner surface of the membrane before being released. The nature of the conformational change in the carrier molecule which is associated with the transport of sodium ions is unknown. Clearly, from the quantitative data already presented, the cycle must be completed very rapidly and then repeated several thousand times during a single impulse. Another type of carrier, working in the reverse direction, would be responsible for the movement of potassium out of the cell during the later stages of the action potential. Although the evidence for the existence of sodium and potassium carrier molecules is increasing, most authorities exercise caution and still prefer to describe the permeability pathways as 'sites', 'gates' or 'channels', and to speak of them as opening and closing.

Other substances will also interfere with the sodium permeability mechanism. *Local anaesthetics* are the best known example for the abolition of the nerve impulse is, of course, responsible for the loss of sensation which is used clinically. Competitive binding experiments on nerve have shown that local anaesthetics do not act at the same point in the sodium channel as TTX and STX. The latter compounds, being water soluble, probably bind at the external opening of the channel whereas local anaesthetics, being lipid soluble, act within the membrane. *Batrachatoxin,* a highly lethal paralytic poison produced by a Brazilian species of frog, also has an action inside the membrane. The alkaloid *veratrine* differs from the other substances considered so far in having an excitatory action. By acting on the inside of the membrane the veratrine alkaloids (including germine acetate; see page 198) induce a slow secondary rise in sodium permeability following the impulse; this may be so marked as to cause repetitive firing of the membrane.

The sodium permeability system has an added significance in that it underlies the phenomena of the *refractory period* and *accommodation.* The refractory period of a nerve or muscle fibre is the length of time following an impulse during which there is a depression of membrane excitability. At first the fibre is *absolutely* refractory and cannot respond with an impulse to a testing stimulus, no matter how large the latter is. This phase is succeeded by the *relatively* refractory period in which the fibre is able to fire an action potential provided the stimulus intensity has been increased beyond its initial threshold value. In man the absolutely refractory periods of muscle fibres vary from 2.2 to 4.6 ms (Farmer, Bucthal and Rosenfalck, 1960) while that for the largest motor axons is about 0.5 ms. The explanation of the absolutely refractory period is that all the sodium channels are still firmly closed while the potassium ones remain open. In the relatively refractory period some, but not all, of the sodium sites have recovered and are available for participation in a further action potential.

A member is said to display *accommodation* if it fails to fire an action potential in response to a slowly-rising current pulse even though a rapidly-increasing pulse is effective. In terms of the sodium permeability hypothesis one can envisage that, during the slowly-rising pulse, some channels are starting to close while others have yet to be opened; in addition the potassium channels will already be opening. During the rapidly-rising pulse more sodium channels will be opened initially and, through the regenerative action of the resulting depolarization, will be more effective in causing others to open.

PROPAGATION OF THE ACTION POTENTIAL

So far only the events which take place locally in the nerve or muscle fibre membrane have been considered. The functional significance of the action potential mechanism is that, once an impulse has been initiated, excitatory changes automatically take place in neighbouring regions of the membrane and so cause the impulse to travel the length of the fibre. This spread of excitation depends on the difference in potential which exists between the region of membrane at which the action potential is momentarily located and more distant regions which are still in the resting state. At the crest of the action potential the interior of the fibre is some 30 mV positive with respect to the exterior while farther along the fibre will exhibit the normal resting membrane potential such that the inside of the fibre is some 85 mV negative to the outside. Because of this difference in potential current will flow between the two regions of membrane; the resting membrane is said to act as a 'source' of current for a 'sink' at the site of the action potential. This current comes from the discharge of the membrane capacity in the resting membrane. It is usual to state the direction of a current by indicating the movement of the positive charges; in this situation cations will flow inwards through the membrane at the sink. As the resting ('source') membrane discharges the potential will fall to the critical depolarization necessary for local impulse generation; in this way the excitatory disturbance is transmitted along the fibre.

In *Figure 3.8* the situation has been displayed as an electronic circuit. The resting membrane potential at the source is shown as a battery of -85 mV which is in series with a membrane resistance, R_m, and in parallel with a membrane capacity, C_m. Similarly the action potential is depicted as a battery of $+30$ mV in series with another resistance, $R_{m'}$, and a second capacity, C. Finally, R_i and R_e represent the resistances of the interior of the fibre and of the extracellular fluid respectively. For a muscle fibre R_e is small because of the large volume of fluid surrounding the fibre; $R_{m'}$ is also small because of the huge increase in sodium permeability during the action potential. Therefore, the potential E_m will drop to a value intermediate between -85 mV and $+30$ mV, approximately given by $R_m (30-85)/(R_m + R_i)$ mV. The speed with which this depolarization takes place will depend on the product of the membrane capacity, C_m, and the series resistances $R_i + R_{m'} + R_e$; of these only R_i is significant. *Figure 3.8* serves to draw attention to the fact that the velocity with which the impulse propagates will depend on the dimensions of the fibre, being lower for a small muscle fibre than for a larger one. The reason for this is that the smaller fibre will have a narrower core of sarcoplasm and hence a higher electrical resistance, R. In turn this means that the internal current, i, flowing between source and sink will be relatively small and that it will take rather longer for the membrane capacity of the source to

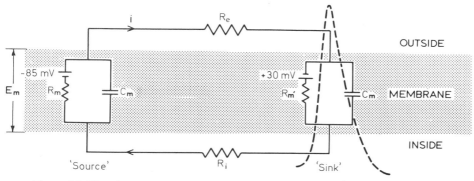

Figure 3.8. Electrical analogue of the membrane during passage of an action potential

discharge to the threshold potential required for an impulse. In the case of muscle fibres the conduction velocities have been measured either by stimulating and recording at different points along the same fibre (Buchthal, Guld and Rosenfalck, 1955) or alternatively by timing the passage of a 'volitional' action potential across successive small electrode surfaces arranged in line (Stålberg, 1966). Both methods indicate that there is a range of velocities, the respective mean values for the brachial biceps muscle being 4.02 ± 0.13 m/s (Buchthal, Guld and Rosenfalck, 1955) and 3.37 S.D. ± 0.67 m/s (Stålberg, 1966); the latter author obtained rather lower values for the smaller fibres of the frontalis muscle. In a condition such as Duchenne muscle dystrophy, in which abnormally large and small muscle fibres are present, one would expect the range of conduction velocities to be increased. Surprisingly, no abnormality was found by Buchthal, Rosenfalck and Erminio (1960) although work from the same laboratory has indicated that the atrophied fibres of denervated muscle may have 50–75 per cent reductions in velocity (Buchthal and Rosenfalck, 1958).

In nerve fibres a modification of structure enables the action potential to be conducted much more efficiently than in muscle fibres. This modification is the incorporation of a special lipid insulating layer around the nerve fibre membrane; this extra coat is the *myelin sheath* and is formed by the Schwann cells (page 10). At regular intervals the myelin sheath is interrupted by the *nodes of Ranvier* at which the nerve membrane, *the axolemma*, is exposed to the extracellular fluid and *gap substance*. The effect of the myelin sheath is to prevent current from leaking across the axolemma, that is, R_e in *Figure 3.8* becomes very large in relation to the other resistances in the circuit. Thus, as the action potential advances, only the axolemma

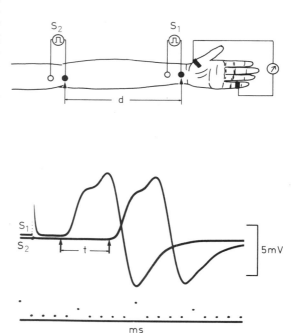

Figure 3.9. Determination of the maximum impulse conduction velocities in motor axons of the median nerve. The nerve is maximally stimulated at two sites by the electrode pairs S_1 (wrist) and S_2 (elbow). The corresponding muscle responses are recorded by a stigmatic electrode over the thenar muscles and an indifferent electrode on the little finger. A ground electrode is placed on the dorsum of the hand. The distance, d, separating the cathodal electrodes (●) at the wrist and elbow respectively is divided by the difference, t, between the latencies of the two evoked muscle potentials (lower figure); the result is the impulse velocity of the fastest-conducting motor axons (v). In this example d = 25 cm and t = 4.2 ms, giving a conduction velocity of approximately 60 m/s

at the next nodes of Ranvier will be able to depolarize to the levels necessary for impulse initiation. In this way the action potential jumps from node to node, skipping the intervening myelinated segments of axon. This form of propagation is termed *saltatory conduction* and it enables the impulse to travel much faster than in unmyelinated structures. Saltatory conduction has the additional advantage of restricting the ionic exchange during the impulse to the nodes of Ranvier; as a result the fibre expends less energy in pumping out sodium in exchange for potassium. Not all mammalian nerve fibres are myelinated; in fact both cutaneous and muscle nerves contain more unmyelinated fibres than myelinated ones. The unmyelinated fibres (C-fibres) are thin, most being less than 1 μm in diameter, and they are arranged in small colonies within the cytoplasm of individual Schwann cells. However, so far as muscle is concerned, all the nerve axons supplying the extrafusal muscle fibres have myelin sheaths. In man the largest of these axons have diameters

of about 14 μm, including the thicknesses of the myelin sheaths; rather thicker axons are found in some of the other mammals. The impulse velocity in the motor axons can readily be determined by successively stimulating a nerve at two points and measuring the time elapsing before the muscle fibres are excited on each occasion. The difference between these times is then divided into the extra distance that the impulses had to travel when the stimulating electrodes were placed at the site on the nerve farthest from the muscle (*Figure 3.9*). The impulse conduction velocities are rather higher in the upper limb than in the lower limb, being about 50–65 m/s for the median and ulnar nerves in the forearm and 40–55 m/s for the tibial and peroneal nerves below the knee. These values are the velocities in the fastest conducting axons only, since the time measurements are made from the earliest responses in the muscle. To measure the impulse velocities in the slowest conducting fibres requires special techniques, two of which are described in Appendix 3.3.

Chapter 4

THE NEUROMUSCULAR JUNCTION

MORPHOLOGY (*Figures. 4.1 and 4.2*)

As the motor axon approaches the muscle fibre it loses its myelin sheath and divides into several small twigs. These twigs lie in shallow grooves on the surface of the muscle fibre and run short distances before terminating. The region of the muscle fibre under these twigs is termed the *motor end-plate*; it includes the sarcolemma and also a mound of sarcoplasm, the *sole-plate*. Within the sole-plate are collected a number of muscle fibre nuclei as well as many mitochondria, ribosomes and pinocytic vesicles. Lying over the whole end-plate are membrane-covered cytoplasmic processes derived from the Schwann cells. With the electron-miscroscope it can be seen that the membrane of the axon terminal is separated from the sarcolemma by a distinct gap measuring about 500 Å; this is the *primary synaptic cleft*. The primary cleft is interrupted by repeated invaginations of the sarcolemma into the sole-plate; each fold forms one *secondary synaptic cleft*. The secondary clefts are approximately 0.5–1 μm deep and are rather wider (700–900 Å) at their terminations than at their necks (500 Å). The electronmicroscope also shows that the *basement membrane* on the outside of the sarcolemma (page 5) runs through both primary and secondary clefts to emerge on the far side of the junction.

Like the muscle fibre, the axon is also highly specialized at the neuromuscular junction. The axon terminations contain large numbers of small spheres with membranous linings; they measure some 300 Å across and are typically clustered opposite the secondary synaptic clefts. These spheres are the *synaptic vesicles* and contain the transmitter substance, *acetylcholine*. It has been suggested that the vesicles are formed by the pinching-off of neurotubules or endoplasmic reticulum within the axon terminal (Blumcke and Niedorf, 1965); alternative possibilities are that they arise from mitochondria or from invaginations of the axolemma. The axoplasm also contains two other types of vesicle, though in much smaller numbers. The *dense-cored vesicles* (700–1100 Å) resemble those known to contain monoamine transmitters in the central nervous system and it is conceivable that their contents are similar at the neuromuscular junction; an alternative suggestion is that they contain some of the neurotrophic messenger molecules (see page 80). The *coated vesicles* apparently form by in-pouching of the axolemma and presumably enable the axon terminal to take up impermeant molecules from the synaptic cleft. Also within the axon terminal are large numbers of mitochondria which probably provide most of the energy, in the form of ATP, required for the synthesis of acetylcholine. Finally the axon terminal contains large numbers of neurotubules and neurofilaments which enter from the axon fibre.

NEUROMUSCULAR TRANSMISSION

The structure of the neuromuscular junction has now been described as have the ionic mechanisms underlying the resting and action potentials. Using this framework, and with the addition of

27

experimental observations on the junction itself, it is now possible to give an account of the synaptic events which enable excitation to spread from the motor axon to the muscle fibre. The account is a

able to record a propagated potential with an extra-cellular microelectrode positioned close to the axon terminal. As expected on theoretical grounds (page 24) the conduction velocity of the impulse was much

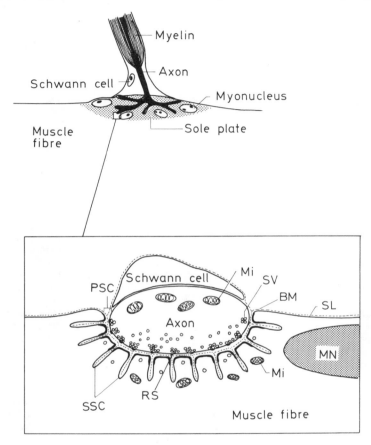

Figure 4.1 (Upper) Gross structure of neuromuscular junction (see text). (Lower) Part of the neuromuscular junction shown at much higher magnification; dimensions of structures as given in the text. BM, basement membrane; Mi, mitochondrion; MN, myonuclei: PSC, primary synaptic cleft; SSC, secondary synaptic cleft; SV, synaptic vesicles. Note the thickening of the muscle fibre membrane in the primary synaptic cleft, which corresponds to the distribution of the acetylcholine receptors; small ridges can be seen on the opposing axon membrane and are the acetylcholine release sites (RS) (see text)

satisfying one, not only because many details of the transmission process are understood, but also because many structural features of the synapse can now be correlated with function.

The first step in synaptic transmission (Figure 4.3) is, of course, the propagation of the action potential into the distal regions of the motor axon. It now appears that the impulse travels all the way to the synapse itself since Katz and Miledi (1965) were

lower in the fine terminal branches of the axon than in the main trunk. In the frog the velocity distally was 0·3 m/s, and may be compared with the usual value of about 20 m/s for motor axons within a peripheral nerve of the same species.

When the impulse invades the axon terminal, it depolarizes the axon membrane in the usual way (page 21). During this depolarization sodium crosses the membrane into the axoplasm but of greater

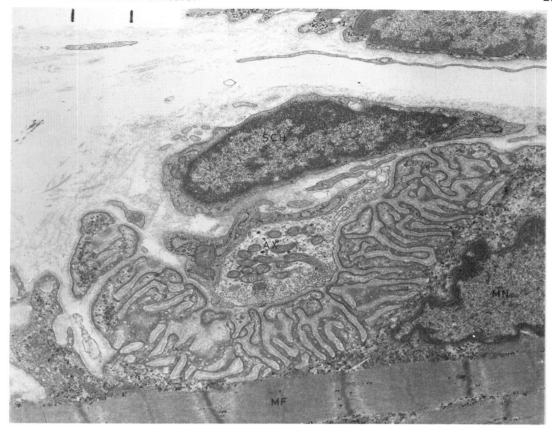

Figure 4.2. Electron micrograph of neuromuscular junction. The dispositions of the Schwann cell (SCH), axon terminal (AX) and myonucleus (MN) are similar to those in Figure 4.1 (lower). With the aid of Figure 4.1 the basement membrane, mitochondria, synaptic vesicles, primary and secondary synaptic clefts can easily be recognized. A shortened myofibril (MF) is also seen (×17,500). (Courtesy of Dr A. G. Engel)

importance is the *entry of calcium ions* from the extracellular fluid. It has been shown that neuromuscular transmission will cease if calcium ions are omitted from the bathing fluid or alternatively if the concentration of magnesium is raised. At the neuromuscular junction the magnesium ions appear to compete for the same receptors as calcium and, in this way, can block the normal effects of calcium. The action of calcium inside the axon terminal is not known for certain but the presence of these ions is clearly necessary for the release of the transmitter substance, *acetylcholine*. Since most of the transmitter is contained within the synaptic vesicles, one hypothesis of calcium action is that the ions activate sites on the inside of the axolemma which allow fusion to take place between this membrane and those of the vesicles. The vesicles are then opened and discharge their acetylcholine into the synaptic cleft (*Figure 4.4*). Most of the *synaptic delay* between the excitation in the nerve and its subsequent appearance in the muscle fibre is due to the calcium-mediated release of transmitter; for the frog neuromuscular junction this delay is of the order of 0·5 ms but at mammalian junction the value is rather smaller (about 0·2 ms). Experiments with double or multiple stimuli have shown that, for the first 100 ms or so following an impulse, the axon terminal is in a hyperexcitable state. Thus, although 100–200 vesicles will have been emptied of acetylcholine, the transmitter remaining is more available for release by a second impulse. This facilitation is attributed to increased 'mobilization' of transmitter; whether the remaining vesicles stay momentarily closer to the axolemma or whether some other effect of the admitted calcium ions persists for a while is not clear.

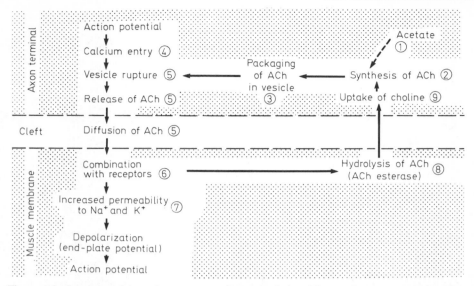

Figure 4.3. Summary of steps in neuromuscular transmission. The numbers correspond to those in Figure 4.4 which displays the same events pictorially

Once the acetylcholine is discharged into the cleft it diffuses very quickly to combine with receptors in the muscle fibre membrane. That the receptors are on the outer surface of the membrane is known from experiments in which acetylcholine was released iontophoretically from a micropipette. When the tip of the pipette was inside the fibre no response to ejected acetylcholine could be detected whereas external application of the substance produced a rapid fall in muscle fibre membrane potential.

The fall in muscle fibre membrane potential following an impulse in the motor axon is termed an *end-plate potential* (EPP). The EPP results from an increase in the permeability of the membrane to both sodium and potassium which is brought about by the combination of acetylcholine with its receptor (Takeuchi and Takeuchi, 1960). If the full EPP could be examined, it would be seen to have an amplitude of 70–80 mV, a value which lies between the equilibrium potentials for sodium and potassium and is slightly smaller than the resting potential. Under normal circumstances, however, the developing EPP is overtaken by an action potential which arises as soon as the critical membrane potential has been exceeded (Fatt and Katz, 1951). The impulse is set up in the membrane in, and immediately adjacent to, the synapse and then propagates in both directions along the fibre.

The sequence of events in the transmission pro-

cess is concluded by the hydrolysis of acetylcholine by the enzyme *cholinesterase* into choline and acetate. Now that the overall features of neuromuscular transmission have been described, certain steps may be considered in more detail.

Impulse invasion of the axon terminal

On the basis of *in vitro* studies of the rat phrenic nerve-diaphragm preparation Krnjevic and Miledi (1958) concluded that the preterminal axon was especially susceptible to the effects of anoxia. By electrical stimulation of single motor axons they had been able to show that, on occasion, end-plate potentials were completely absent in some muscle fibres while still present in other fibres of the same motor unit (see also page 68). It now appears that a failure of impulse invasion also underlies the paralysis exhibited by mice of the *motor end-plate disease (Med)* strain (Duchen and Stefani, 1971) and a similar deficit could conceivably occur in any human diseases in which the terminal axons were unusually tortuous or thin. Such deformities can arise in a neuropathy as a result of collateral re-innervation, segmental demyelination or axon regeneration; unusual terminal axons have also been noted in myasthenia gravis and in muscular dystrophy (Cöers and Woolf, 1959).

Synthesis of acetylcholine in the axon terminal

The synthesis of acetylcholine is undertaken by the enzyme *choline acetyltransferase* which, as its name implies, transfers an acetyl group (from acetyl-Coenzyme A) to choline. This enzyme is found in the axon terminal and at least some will have been carried there from the motoneurone soma (Jablecki and Brimijoin, 1974). The axon terminal obtains its supply of choline by uptake from the extracellular fluid; part is derived from the plasma and part from the hydrolysis of acetylcholine by the enzyme cholinesterase on the muscle fibre membrane. The choline uptake can be inhibited by the substance *hemicholinium* (HC–3) and use has been made of this in the experimental analysis of acetylcholine synthesis.

The most widely held view is that the synthesis of acetylcholine occurs in the axoplasm and that the transmitter is then taken up and concentrated by the synaptic vesicles. The rate of synthesis is apparently geared to the amount of impulse activity in the terminal but a small amount of synthesis continues even in the resting state.

A more complete understanding of the distri-bution of acetylcholine in the nerve terminal has come from experiments using repetitive nerve stimulation; these have indicated that the acetylcholine can be visualized as existing in three compartments. The first of these comprises the acetylcholine which is readily available for release; electronmicrographs suggest that this corresponds to the synaptic vesicles found bordering the synaptic region of the axolemma. The second compartment is the large remaining population of vesicles found more centrally within the terminal; these form the 'main store' of acetylcholine. Finally there is an appreciable amount of acetylcholine within the cytoplasm of the terminal; isotope studies have shown that this exchanges freely with the acetylcholine in the vesicles. As already stated, acetylcholine can be synthesized quickly and in surprisingly large amounts by the terminal during continuous impulse activity; it appears that the newly-formed transmitter is largely directed into the 'readily available' compartment.

The synaptic vesicles

As described earlier, the synaptic vesicles are spherical structures, some 300 Å in diameter, which are always to be seen in electronmicrographs of the axon terminal (*Figures 4.1 and 4.2*). The possibility that the vesicles contain acetylcholine was first considered when electrophysiological experiments indicated that the transmitter was released from the axon terminal in small packets, or 'quanta'. Even at rest there is a continuous and random release of acetylcholine, each quantum producing a small depolarization of the muscle fibre membrane (*Figure 4.5*); the latter were referred to as *miniature end-plate potentials* (m.e.p.p.s.) by Fatt and Katz (1952), who described them first. By using raised concentrations of magnesium in the bathing fluid, so as to reduce the release of acetylcholine from the axon terminal, it can be shown that the end-plate potential following a nerve impulse is normally the summation of many m.e.p.p.s. It has also been shown that the spontaneous release of acetylcholine probably reflects the resting level of calcium ions within the nerve terminal and that this is regulated by calcium uptake and release from the mitochondria (Alnaes and Rahamimoff, 1975).

The validity of the vesicle hypothesis is supported by combined biochemical and electron-microscopical studies on tissue homogenates. Both in brain and in the electric organ of the electric eel it has been possible to prepare cell fractions which are rich in vesicles and contain large amounts of acetylcholine (Whittaker, Michaelson and

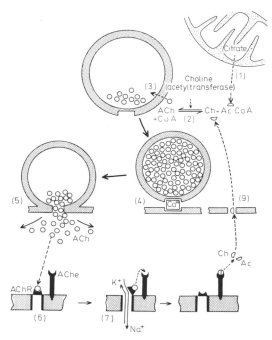

Figure 4.4. Summary of steps in neuromuscular transmission: the axon terminal is shown at top and the muscle fibre membrane below. See text and Figure 4.3 for explanation of steps. ACh, acetylcholine; AChE, acetylcholinesterase; AChR, acetylcholine receptor; CoA, coenzyme A; Ch, choline.

Kirkland, 1964). Unfortunately a similar experiment cannot be performed on motor nerve terminals because of the difficulty in obtaining satisfactory preparations of vesicles without contamination from subcellular components of muscle.

A second important test of the vesicle hypothesis is to demonstrate a reduction in their number following massive release of acetylcholine by the nerve terminal. In the experiments of Jones and Kwanbunbumpen (1970) the rat phrenic nerve was stimulated repetitively and resynthesis of

be necessary to account for a m.e.p.p. of 0.3 mV in a frog muscle fibre. However, the number of molecules in a vesicle must be rather larger than this for additional molecules will be lost by diffusion out of the synaptic cleft and by hydrolysis with cholinesterase. Potter (1970), using radioactively-labelled ACh, calculated that a single impulse in a phrenic motor nerve fibre released about 4×10^6 molecules of transmitter from the axon terminal; he considered that a typical vesicle might contain 4000–9000 molecules of ACh.

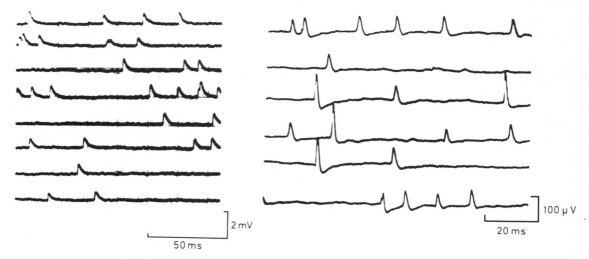

Figure 4.5. Miniature end-plate potentials (m.e.p.p.s.) recorded in situ with an intracellular microelectrode from a mouse gracilis muscle fibre (left) and with a coaxial needle electrode from the vastus medialis muscle of a normal subject (right). Since in the latter instance the recording electrode is effectively extracellular, the potentials appear much smaller (note amplification).

acetylcholine was prevented by hemicholinium (see above). The authors found that a significant depletion of vesicles had occurred in the zone of axoplasm bordering the synaptic cleft and the residual vesicles were reduced in size. A further observation, of uncertain significance, was that the mitochondria were redistributed around the periphery of the axon terminal, many appearing degenerative. Another, and rather interesting, technique for depleting the nerve terminals of acetylcholine is to expose them to the venom of the black widow spider. Once again it has been possible to demonstrate a reduction in the numbers of vesicles within the nerve terminal (Clark, *et al.,* 1970).

The number of acetylcholine (ACh) molecules inside a single vesicle has been determined in various ways. For example, Katz and Miledi (1972) analysed membrane potential 'noise' during the delivery of ACh from a micropipette; they estimated that a single molecule of ACh produced a depolarization of about 0.3 μV and that at least 1000 would

Possibly the most accurate estimate of quantal size has been made by Kuffler and Yoshikami (1975) who devised a highly sensitive bioassay system to determine the amount of ACh delivered from a micropipette on to the exposed subsynaptic membrane in the frog and snake; these authors concluded that a quantum of transmitter contained fewer than 10 000 molecules of ACh. A comparison of the sizes of m.e.p.p.s with those of endplate potentials in curarized nerve-muscle preparations would indicate that at least 100 quanta are emptied from a terminal by each nerve impulse. A better estimate, obtained by a different technique which avoided the use of curare, is that 200–300 quanta are released per impulse (Hubbard and Wilson, 1973).

The functional advantage of containing the transmitter in a vesicle, rather than in the axoplasm, is probably twofold. First, the acetylcholine is protected from the small amount of cholinesterase which is normally to be found within the nerve terminal. Secondly, the influx of calcium during the impulse is only able to activate a certain number of sites on the inner surface of the axolemma and it is therefore advantageous to deliver an optimal quantity of acetylcholine to each site. Electronmicroscopic studies on freeze-fractured membranes have enabled 'vesicle release sites' to be identified; these sites border distinctive ridges on the membrane of the motor axon terminal (Heuser, Reese and Landis, 1974).

One interesting question concerns the fate of the vesicles after they have discharged their acetylcholine into the synaptic cleft. If the membranes of the vesicles fuse with the axolemma, as electronmicrographs suggest, the area of the axolemma would be increased to such an extent that some later mechanism would have to be available for removing the excess membrane. By using extracellular markers Heuser and Reese (1973) have shown that 'recycling' takes place, the presynaptic membrane being reformed into vesicles towards the periphery of the synapse.

The acetylcholine receptor

The chemical identity of the acetylcholine receptor is currently under investigation. The most promising approach has been to label radioactively certain compounds which are thought to react specifically with the receptor and to apply these to the membrane; the membrane components bearing the label can then be isolated and purified. Such substances include *alpha-bungarotoxin,* derived from a snake venom, and *histrionicotoxin,* produced by a poisonous species of frog, as well as *curare.* From the electric organ of the electric eel, *Electrophorus electricus,* a protein has been isolated with a molecular weight of approximately 250,000.

According to Albuquerque *et al.* (1973a) the combination of acetylcholine with its receptor activates an associated 'ion conductance modulator' (possibly a carrier molecule) which then brings about the observed permeability change in the membrane. In recent studies α-bungarotoxin, labelled with either [^{3}H] or horseradish peroxidase, has been used to map out the distribution of the acetylcholine receptors at the neuromuscular junction. Contrary to earlier expectations the receptors are largely restricted to the muscle fibre membrane facing the motor nerve terminal, that is, within the primary synaptic cleft. The infoldings of sarcolemma which form the secondary clefts contain few receptors except in their uppermost regions (Barnard *et al.,* 1975; Lentz, Rosenthal and Mazurkiwicz, 1975). In the receptor-rich areas the postsynaptic membrane is thickened and

electronmicrographs have shown that it contains particles some 110–140 Å in diameter, possibly the receptor-complexes themselves (Heuser, Reese and Landis, 1974). Porter and Barnard (1975) have estimated that in these regions of membrane there are 20 000–25 000 receptors per μm^2 of membrane. Barnard and colleagues (1975) further conclude that there is a considerable surplus of receptors since approximately ten are available for each molecule of acetylcholine released following a single nerve impulse. Katz and Miledi (1972) calculate that each of the activated receptor channels allows 5×10^4 univalent ions to be transferred across the membrane; most of these will be sodium ions entering the fibre down the electrical and concentration gradients (page 21). In addition to the large population of receptors at the neuromuscular junction the muscle fibre contains smaller receptor colonies at its ends, where these join the tendons of origin and insertion. In the slow twitch fibres of mammals there is also a sparse scattering of receptors along the membrane intervening between the neuromuscular junction and the ends of the fibre. Using cultured chick myotubes it has been shown that there is a continual turnover of receptors in the muscle fibre membrane. The receptors are first prepared on internal membranes and are then transported to the sarcolemma where they remain for an average period of 22 hr (Devreotes, 1975). They are then removed and carried back into the interior of the fibre within secondary lysosomes (degradation vacuoles).

A recent finding of great interest, but of uncertain functional significance, is that acetylcholine receptors are also present on the presynaptic membrane of the axon (Lentz *et al.,* 1975), though they were not observed by Barnard and his associates (1975), using a rather different marking technique.

Acetylcholinesterase

The muscle fibre contains three types of esterase, namely one which is specific for acetylcholine, one which will hydrolyse other choline esters as well, and a non-specific esterase. All three types are found at the neuromuscular junction on the synaptic surface of the muscle fibre; in addition both acetylcholinesterase (AChE) and cholinesterase (ChE) can be demonstrated in the synaptic region of the axolemma (Davis and Koelle, 1967). There is good evidence that the acetylcholinesterase in the axon terminal has been transported there from the motoneurone soma by axoplasmic flow. Although the muscle fibre is also able to synthesize enzyme, it is apparent from denervation experiments that much of this synthesis is under the 'trophic' control of the motoneurone. Using labelled substrate, Barnard and colleagues (1975) have found that there are about 3000 AChE and 6000 ChE molecules per μm^2 in the postsynaptic membranes at mouse end-plates. Unlike the acetylcholine receptors, the cholinesterase molecules are distributed evenly throughout the primary and secondary synaptic clefts. The cholinesterase molecules also differ in that they can be easily removed from the synaptic clefts following digestion with proteolytic enzymes. It is therefore probable that the AChE molecules lie within the cleft substance and that their protein 'tails' have only a weak attachment to the sarcolemma.

OTHER DRUG ACTIONS

The actions of a number of drugs at the neuromuscular junction have already been considered: these drugs include (i) the transmitter substance, acetylcholine (ii) hemicholinium, which blocks the synthesis of transmitter, and (iii) α-bungarotoxin, which blocks the combination of acetylcholine with its receptors. It is now appropriate briefly to consider certain other drugs.

Tubocurarine is an alkaloid which can be prepared from crude extracts of the plant toxin, curare. By competing for the same post-synaptic receptors as acetylcholine, tubocurarine diminishes the action of the transmitter. Since the drug does not produce depolarization of the muscle fibre membrane itself, it is classified as a non-depolarizing blocking agent. Experimentally, microelectrode recordings from single muscle fibres reveal progressive reductions in the sizes of the end-plate potentials as the latter continue to fall below the level required for impulse initiation. In man the action of tubocurarine usually lasts about 30 minutes; *gallamine* is another drug with a similar type of action.

Decamethonium and *suxamethonium* are quaternary ammonium compounds which also block neuromuscular transmission by combining with acetylcholine receptors; unlike the drugs considered above they mimic acetylcholine by producing a depolarization. As the depolarizing action commences the muscle fibres begin to twitch spontaneously, indicating that their membrane potentials have fallen to the critical level for action potential initiation. As depolarization proceeds, the muscle fibres become refractory to motor nerve excitation and paralysis ensues. In comparison with the natural transmitter, acetylcholine, the action of these drugs is prolonged and this enables them to be used as muscle relaxants during surgery; suxamethonium can be administered by intravenous drip in the form of its chloride *(succinylcholine)*.

Anticholinesterase drugs potentiate neuromuscular transmission by preventing the hydrolysis of acetylcholine by the cholinesterases attached to the postsynaptic muscle fibre membrane. Consequently, acetylcholine released from a nerve terminal exerts a larger and more prolonged depolarization of the muscle fibre. Examples of anticholinesterases are *neostigmine, pyridostigmine bromide* (Mestinon, Roche Ltd.) and *edrophonium chloride* (Tensilon, Roche Ltd.). While the first two drugs have a clinical use in the treatment of patients with myasthenia gravis (page 193), the last drug, because of the rapid onset and short duration of its action, is valuable in the diagnosis of this disorder (page 195).

Chapter 5

MUSCLE CONTRACTION

In order to understand the molecular basis of muscle contraction it is necessary to review briefly the microanatomy of the muscle fibre (see *Figure 1.2*). It will be recalled that the muscle fibre itself, and all the myofibrils within it, have a striated appearance due to the alternation of dark (A) bands with light (I) bands. In the centre of the A-band is a pale region, the H-zone, with a dark (M) line in its middle. The I-band is divided into two by a dark (Z) line; the segment of muscle fibre between two successive Z-lines is referred to as one *sarcomere*.

In early studies with the electronmicroscope it was shown that each myofibril was composed of many *myofilaments* and that the latter were of two types, thick and thin. In cross-sections of muscle fibres each thick filament was seen to be surrounded by a hexagonal array of thin filaments (*Figure 5.1, f*); in longitudinal sections the thick filaments of a myofibril were found in register with each other (*Figure 4.2, MF* and *Figure 5.1, d*). For a long time it had been known that the contractile proteins of muscle were *myosin* and *actin* and next it was shown that these proteins corresponded to the thick and thin filaments respectively. This step was achieved by dissolving the myosin in potassium chloride solution and demonstrating that the thick filaments were no longer visible on electronmicroscopy.

At the same time that H. E. Huxley was undertaking these important studies, A. F. Huxley was using the interference microscope to examine the muscle striations of living frog muscle fibres during contraction and relaxation. He observed that during contraction the I-(light) band became shorter while the A-(dark) band remained the same length;

within the A-band, however, the pale H-zone narrowed and might disappear completely. Quite independently the Huxleys proposed that their respective findings could be explained by a sliding movement of the actin and myosin filaments past each other (Huxley and Niedergerke, 1954; Huxley and Hanson, 1954; see also Huxley, 1959a and 1974). This *sliding filament hypothesis* is now accepted as being correct and is displayed diagrammatically in *Figure 5.1 (d, e)*.

From inspection of this figure (and also *Figure 1.2*) it can be seen that the I-band is the region of fibre where only actin filaments are present; the A-band corresponds to the position of the myosin filaments. In the relaxed state, although there is some overlap between the actin and myosin filaments, opposing actin filaments are separated from each other along the myosin filament; the gap between the actin filaments is responsible for a pale region (H-zone) at the centre of the A-band.

When the muscle contracts the opposing actin filaments are propelled toward each other and slide along the intervening myosin filament. As they near each other they cause the H-zone to become narrower; similarly as more of each actin filament is drawn into the space between the myosin filaments, the I-band becomes shorter. Since the myosin filaments do not alter their shape, the length of the A-band stays unchanged.

The function of the Z-line, or Z-disc, is to tether the actin filaments together while the M-line in the centre of the A-band corresponds to bridges linking the myosin filaments; both types of structure maintain the orderly geometrical relationship of the filaments to one another.

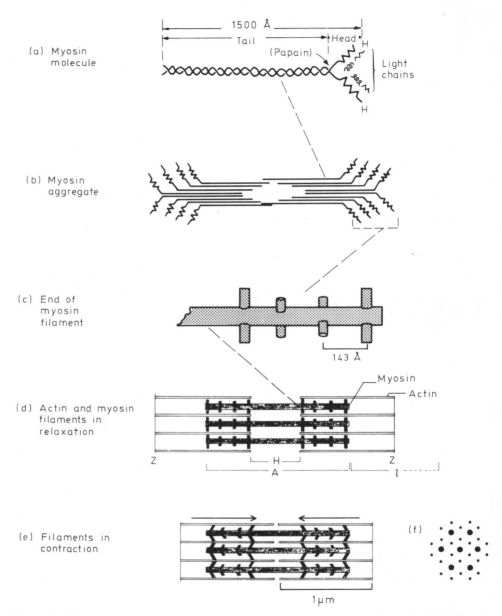

Figure 5.1. The basis of muscle contraction, shown in terms of the myosin molecule (a) and the combination of many myosin molecules to form an aggregate (b) or a filament (c). The sliding movement of the actin filaments over the myosin filaments is shown in (e). The appearance of the overlapping filaments in transverse section is portrayed in (f); note the hexagonal array of the actin filaments around each myosin filament. Compare with Figure 1.2, which shows a larger part of the muscle fibre

Recent advances in biochemistry and electron-microscopy have added to the original sliding filament hypothesis by indicating the probable molecular configurations of the actin and myosin molecules. The *myosin molecules* appear as structures some 1500 Å long, each consisting of a globular head and a relatively long tail. The head and tail can be snapped apart by digestion with the proteolytic enzyme, papain. The tail is an alpha-helix while the head is composed of two heavy chains and four light chains (*Figure 5.1, a*).

by 180 degrees; the next pair is always 143 Å away with its axis rotated through 60 degrees (*Figure 5.1, c*). The attachment of the cross-bridge to the actin filament is probably followed by a conformational change in the myosin head which causes the cross-bridge to flex and so move the actin filament onwards. At some stage ATP is split into ADP and phosphate by the cross-bridge, releasing the energy needed for the movement to take place. The cross-bridge now becomes disengaged but it quickly reattaches itself to the actin filament at

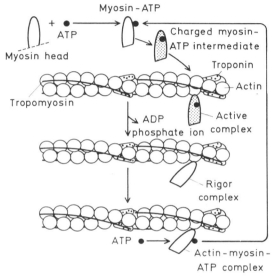

Figure 5.2. The molecular events which take place at the cross-bridge during a single contraction; see text (Modified from Murray, and Weber (1974), courtesy of the authors, and the Editor and publishers of Scientific American)

It is evident that many myosin molecules must aggregate to form a single myosin filament since the length of the latter (about 1.5 μm) is considerably greater than the molecular dimension (0.15 μm) and the filament is also much thicker than the molecule. The likeliest estimate is that several hundred molecules are combined to form a single filament. The probable form of this aggregation has been determined by observations on myosin precipitated from solution. The molecules cluster together to form rods; the rods consist of two groups of myosin molecules facing away from each other and joined at their tails; within each group the tails overlap (*Figure 5.1, b*).

The role of the myosin head is to slide the actin filament past during muscle contraction. It does so by temporarily attaching itself to the actin filament; the attachment is seen as a *cross-bridge* projecting from the myosin filament. The cross-bridges are arranged on the myosin filament as pairs separated

another point; the cycle of events is repeated many times in a single contraction. Since the myosin heads are grouped at opposite ends of the filament with their tails in the centre, the two ends will propel their respective actin filaments towards each other, in keeping with the sliding filament hypothesis.

A considerable amount is also known about the *actin filaments* and this new knowledge has led to a better understanding of the operation of the cross-bridges. The actin filaments are about 1 μm in length and contain between 300 and 400 actin molecules. These small molecules are spherical in shape and are arranged in series so as to form a double strand twisted about its own axis (*Figure 5.2*). The actin filament also contains two other proteins; these have important regulatory roles and are termed *tropomyosin* and *troponin*. The tropomyosin molecules are long thin filaments which lie on the surfaces of the actin strands; each tropomyosin molecule spans about seven actin

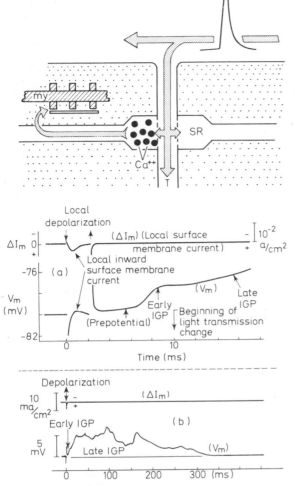

Figure 5.3. (Upper) Summary of the two key events in excitation–contraction coupling: first, the spread of the action potential down the T-system (T), and second, the movement of calcium ions from the sarcoplasmic reticulum (SR) to the cross-bridges on the myosin filament (my). (Lower) Intracellular generated potentials (IGP), recorded with an intracellular microelectrode from a frog muscle fibre and using local stimulation through a voltage-clamp circuit. The lower record has been made at a slower sweep speed than the upper one; in each case the IGP is displayed on the lower of the two traces. (From Strickholm (1974), courtesy of the author, and Editor and publishers of Journal of Neurobiology)

molecules. Attached to each tropomyosin molecule near one end is a short, globular molecule of troponin (*Figure 5.2*). Tropomyosin and troponin have an inhibiting action for, unless acted upon, they prevent a contraction from taking place; possibly the tropomyosin molecule physically impedes the attachment of cross-bridges to the actin molecules.

This inhibiting action is overcome by the presence of *calcium ions* which, in the intact fibre, are brought by the sarcoplasmic reticulum.

The calcium ions combine with one of the three subunits of troponin and thereby cause the attached tropomyosin molecule to move to a 'neutral' position (see Cohen, 1975). This displacement of the tropomyosin molecule now permits the cross-bridges, that is, the heads of the myosin molecules, to attach themselves to the actin molecules. Each cross-bridge carries a molecule of ATP, since the myosin head has a great affinity for the ATP molecules freely available in the sarcoplasm. The combination of myosin–ATP and actin forms an '*active complex*'; the ATP is now rapidly hydrolysed to ADP and phosphate with the release of energy. This energy is used to produce a conformational change in the head of the myosin molecule which is seen externally as a flexion of the corresponding cross-bridge. The actin filament is correspondingly carried onwards for about 100 Å. Provided ATP is freely available in the sarcoplasm— as it normally is—the myosin head will take up a further molecule and, at the same time, disengage from the actin filament. After the myosin head (cross-bridge)–ATP returns to its initial position it can attach itself to a new site on the actin filament and repeat the movement cycle described above, provided calcium ions are still available to overcome the troponin–tropomyosin inhibition. It is probable that each cross-bridge undergoes many such cycles in the course of a single twitch.

EXCITATION–CONTRACTION COUPLING

Having described the way in which the myofibril shortens, it remains to consider the mechanism by which the signal to contract is communicated to the myofibrils from the action potential travelling along the surface of the fibre. The process by which this is done is termed *excitation–contraction coupling*; it occupies less than 1 ms and consists of two steps: (*a*) depolarization of the transverse tubules; and (*b*) migration of calcium ions from the sarcoplasmic recticulum to the myofilaments (*Figure 5.3, upper*).

Depolarization of the transverse tubules (T-system)

The detailed structure of the T-system has been determined with the electronmicroscope. The tubules are situated at regular intervals along the muscle fibre and run inwards toward its centre, meeting with each other to form a continuous structure (see Peachey, 1965 and *Figure 1.2*). In the frog the tubules are situated in the vicinity of the Z-disc and this occurs once in each sarcomere. In mammals, however, the tubules are to be found at the junctions of the A- and I-bands, giving two tubular arrays per sarcomere. Electronmicrographs have revealed that the tubules open on to the surface of the muscle fibre so that the tubular membrane becomes continuous with the sarcolemma. The existence of such openings has been confirmed by the ability of relatively large molecules to pass into the T-system from solutions bathing the muscle fibre. The substances chosen for this type of experiment have included ferritin (Huxley, 1964), and fluorescent dyes (Endo, 1966), as well as albumin, thorium dioxide and horseradish peroxidase.

The key role of the T-system in excitation–contraction coupling was shown by two contrasting experimental approaches. First, Huxley and Taylor (1958) applied weak stimulating currents at different points along the surface of frog muscle fibres. They found that local contractions of myofibrils only occurred when the electrode tip was over the I-band, in the centre of which the T-tubules are situated (see above). In the second type of experiment Gage and Eisenberg (1969b) demonstrated that action potentials were unable to elicit twitches in muscle fibres treated with glycerol. In these experiments glycerol was added to the physiological bathing fluid and penetrated the muscle fibres. When the fibres were returned to a glycerol-free solution the T-tubules swelled and broke off from the sarcolemma (Appendix 5.1).

The speed with which the signal to contract travels into the fibre has been measured by Gonzales-Serratos (1971). The technique used was to embed single frog semitendinosus fibres in gelatin-Ringer and to compress them longitudinally; the myofibrils then became wavy. The fibre was stimulated electrically and the contractions of the myofibrils were photographed with a high-speed ciné camera; in shortening, they became straight instead of wavy. It was found that the evoked action potential caused the superficial myofibrils to contract first and the central ones last. At 20 °C the velocity of inward spread of activation was 7 cm/s.

By themselves, the measurements of this velocity and of its change with temperature do not enable the nature of the inward spread to be determined. In theory two such mechanisms are possible. One is a passive 'electrotonic' spread of depolarization along the T-system while the other possibility is that the tubules propagate action potentials into the centre of the fibre. One approach to this problem has been to abolish any propagated action potentials with tetrodotoxin and to depolarize the sarcolemma

using an intracellular stimulating electrode. In this way only the effects of electrotonic spread are observed. Adrian, Costantin and Peachey (1969) found that when brief stimuli were used the superficial myofibrils would only contract when the fibre membrane had been depolarized to zero mV; larger surface depolarizations were necessary to make the central myofibrils shorten. In an ingenious extension of their work the same authors imposed an 'artificial' action potential on the membrane by using a voltage clamp circuit driven by an action potential in another fibre. It appeared that the reversal of membrane polarity during the spike was just sufficient to activate the central myofibrils by electrotonic spread along the T-system. If, however, the same type of experiment is carried out on toad muscle at 20 °C, it is found that the surface action potential only produces about 30 per cent of the normal twitch tension, the remaining 70 per cent presumably requiring a propagated impulse in the T-tubules (Bastian and Nakajima, 1974).

Other indirect evidence for a T-impulse has come from the work of Costantin (1970) who investigated the responses of single frog muscle fibres to focal stimulation through a microelectrode. By reducing the concentration of sodium in the solution bathing the fibre the initiation of an action potential in the sarcolemma was prevented. Costantin found that the central and superficial myofibrils had very similar thresholds for contraction, suggesting that an action mechanism was present and still effective in the T-system even though it was absent at the fibre surface. This conclusion was strengthened by the results of experiments involving tetrodotoxin in which the superficial myofibrils now had lower thresholds than the central ones and were the first to shorten. Under these last conditions only passive electrotonic depolarization of the fibre interior could have taken place. Perhaps the best evidence for a propagated potential in the T-system has come from the recent study by Strickholm (1974). By using a special voltage-clamping technique (page 21) he found it possible to record small 'internal' potentials from frog muscle fibres following surface excitation. Similar results were obtained by Natori (1975) in 'desheathed' fibres and the authors gave reasons for supposing that they were the electrical responses of the tubular systems within the fibre (*Figure 5.3, lower*).

The conclusions from these various studies are that the myofibrils are normally activated by inwardly-propagating action potentials within the T-system and, rather more tentatively, that the sarcoplasmic reticulum may have an active mechanism for depolarization too (see also Costantin and Podolsky, 1967).

The role of calcium

It has been known that calcium ions play an important role in muscle contraction ever since Ringer (1883) showed that the frog heart would stop beating if this element was omitted from the bathing solution. Mines (1913) was able to demonstrate that the quiescent heart still generated action potentials, indicating that calcium ions must

('grana') seen with the electronmicroscope. When the depolarization invades the T-system a large fraction of the current will flow across the membranes of the lateral sacs since 80 per cent of the T-system lies within the triads (Peachey, 1965). Some of the inward current will be carried by calcium ions and it now appears that this entry causes further calcium to be released from the lateral sacs of the sarcoplasmic reticulum; the concentration of calcium

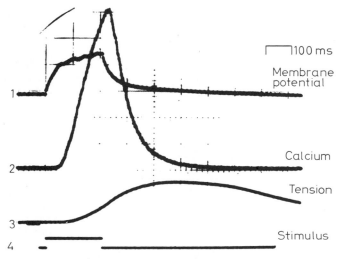

Figure 5.4. Simultaneous recordings from a single barnacle muscle fibre of (1) the change in membrane potential, (2) the appearance of intracellular calcium ions, and (3) the generation of tension, during electrical stimulation (4). (Modified from Ashley and Ridgway (1970), courtesy of the authors, and the Editor of Journal of Physiology)

have been required for some step beyond the excitation of the fibres. Similarly, in the case of skeletal muscle, Frank (1958) showed that frog muscle fibres would not develop contractures when placed in potassium-rich solutions unless calcium was also present. Further evidence for the important role of calcium was that injections of this ion into a muscle fibre through a micropipette evoked local contractions; sodium, potassium and magnesium ions were ineffective (Heilbrunn and Wiercinski, 1947). Another experiment has been to 'desheath' a muscle fibre by removing the sarcolemma and then to induce a contraction by applying calcium ions directly to myofibrils with a micropipette (the Natori preparation; see Podolsky, 1964).

The importance of calcium ions, as revealed by these experiments, is that they provide the second step in the excitation—contraction coupling process. During inactivity the calcium is retained in a bound form within the lateral (terminal) sacs of the sarcoplasmic reticulum, probably in the granular material

ions increases rapidly through this regenerative mechanism (Ford and Podolsky, 1972).

The mobilized calcium ions leave the sarcoplasmic reticulum and move into the myofibrils where they combine with troponin on the actin filaments (*Figure 5.3, upper*). The inhibitory action of tropomyosin is removed and the sliding movement between the actin and myosin filaments occurs (see page 38). After the contraction has taken place the calcium is removed from the myofibrils and returned to the lateral sacs of the sarcoplasmic reticulum.

The time during which the calcium is available in its ionic form within the fibre has been measured by Ashley and Ridgway (1968, 1970). These authors injected large single muscle fibres of barnacles with *aqueorin*, a protein which luminesces in the presence of calcium ions. Following direct stimulation the light emitted by the fibre was detected by a photomultiplier tube and the electrical output from the latter was amplified and displayed on an oscilloscope; the membrane depolarization and the force generated by the fibre were also recorded (*Figure 5.4*). The authors were able to show that the calcium ions were released between the onset of the membrane response and the start of the muscle contraction, as would be expected for a coupling mechanism. The concentration of calcium ions increased rapidly during the membrane response and began to fall on completion of the latter. The change in muscle tension ran a much slower course,

binding protein). The efficiency of the sarcoplasmic reticulum is impressive; it can reduce the concentration of free calcium ions from 5×10^{-6}M to less than 10^{-7}M with extreme rapidity. Electronmicroscopic studies have known that the ATPase is a globular particle with a diameter of about 100 Å. One of the interesting aspects of this work is that the purified ATPase, when combined with phospholipid and proteolipid, spontaneously forms hollow

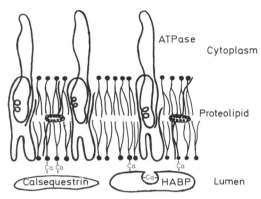

Figure 5.5. Interrelationship between ATPase, proteolipid, calsequestrin and HABP in sarcoplasmic reticulum; see text (MacLennan, personal communication)

with relaxation beginning at a time when the calcium ion concentration had already returned to the resting value (*Figure 5.4*). This last observation is of considerable interest for it might indicate that relaxation does not result simply from the removal of calcium but may also involve an intermediary step. Very similar results to these have since been obtained by Rüdel and Taylor (1973) from single amphibian muscle fibres which had been injected with aqueorin. Rather more is known concerning the recapture of calcium by the sarcoplasmic reticulum than about its release (MacLennan and Holland, 1975). The membrane of the reticulum has been found to contain an ATPase which requires both calcium and magnesium ions. The initial step in the calcium-transport process is a calcium-dependent phosphorylation of membrane protein by ATP; this is followed by a magnesium-dependent dephosphorylation. As a result of these two steps calcium ions are transported from the outside of the sarcoplasmic reticulum into its interior, with a movement of magnesium ions taking place in the reverse direction. The maintenance of a downhill calcium concentration gradient across the membrane is achieved by removal of the free ions once they have reached the inside of the membrane. This sequestration is achieved by two proteins with great calcium-binding activity, *calsequestrin* and *HABP* (high affinity

vesicular membranes of regular structure. MacLennan has suggested that, within the sarcoplasmic reticulum, the ATPase, proteolipid, HABP and calsequestrin are arranged as in *Figure 5.5*.

Active state

In considering the contraction of muscle it is useful to recognize the concept of an 'active state'. In effect this is the phase following excitation of the fibre in which the actin and myosin filaments interact with each other. As a result of this interaction the muscle fibre will either shorten or develop tension, or do both, as already considered (page 35). In the case of tension measurements the maximum value actually recorded following a single stimulus is diminished because of the presence of the *series elastic component* (page 46) and the time course of the recorded twitch is prolonged for the same reason. The active state is therefore considerably shorter than the contraction time actually measured.

In terms of excitation–contraction coupling the duration of the active state probably corresponds fairly closely to the time during which calcium ions are present in the vicinity of the myofibrils. To determine the full isometric tension that a muscle fibre can produce it is necessary to prolong the active state and so overcome the effect of the series elastic component. One way of achieving this is to give a series of rapidly-repeated stimuli (a *tetanus*) to the muscle fibre so that the effects of successive active states can add together (see *Figure 5.10*). Even after the tetanus has been stopped the twitch responses to single shocks, given during the next few seconds, remain enlarged. This behaviour has been termed *post-tetanic potentiation* and is again probably due to a temporary alteration in the intensity or duration of the active state. Another interesting phenomenon with a similar underlying basis is the *positive staircase,* which was originally observed in the frog gastrocnemius muscle but has now been demonstrated in the human adductor pollicis muscle by Slomić, Rosenfalck and Buchthal (1968). It consists of a progressive enlargement of isometric twitches when stimuli are given at a low repetition rate, such as 2 Hz.

The active state may also be extended by cooling the muscle fibre or by applying a variety of chemical agents (see Sandow, 1965 for review). *Lyotropic anions* such as bromide, nitrate and methylsulphate seem to act by reducing the mechanical threshold of the fibre. Thus the active state is prolonged because the contractile machinery is switched on at a lower membrane depolarization during the action potential. *Divalent metal ions* such as zinc and uranyl can augment the twitch tension by a factor of 2–3 times; they do so by increasing the duration of the action potential and hence of the active state. *Caffeine* in low concentrations (above 5 mM for frog muscle) will produce a maintained shortening of the muscle (the caffeine contracture). This alkaloid produces its effect by releasing calcium from the sarcoplasmic reticulum and then preventing its subsequent recapture by the calcium pump.

In contrast, the intensity of the active state process can be *diminished* by reducing the availability of calcium ions to the myofibrils. One method is to bind the calcium as an organic salt by injecting potassium citrate or potassium oxalate into the fibre. Another technique is to immerse the fibre in *hypertonic saline;* although the fibre shrinks the T-tubules and the lateral sacs become dilated. This behaviour would be expected of the T-system since this is really an extracellular space which will draw water from the fibre by osmosis (page 39); the sarcoplasmic reticulum appears to behave as an intermediate compartment between the intra- and extra-cellular fluids. Evidently the end-result of the distension of the triads is to reduce the release of calcium from the lateral sacs (Ashley and Ridgway, 1970). The effect of *adrenaline* is to shorten the active state and thereby to speed up the isometric twitch; in

theory, the tension developed should be rather smaller but Marsden and Meadows (1970) observed little change in the human soleus muscle. These authors interpret their findings in terms of an action of adrenaline upon β-receptors within the muscle fibres themselves.

Dantrolene sodium. This drug has been shown to reduce the isometric twitch without affecting the surface action potential and has recently been found of value in the treatment of spasticity. The mechanism by which dantrolene is apparently able to interfere with excitation–contraction coupling has not yet been determined though Ellis and Carpenter (1972) have suggested that it reduces the calcium released into the sarcoplasm.

CONTRACTURE

A contracture differs from a contraction in that the shortening of the myofibrils is prolonged in the absence of action potential activity in the sarcolemma. One method of producing a contracture is to immerse the fibre in a solution rich in potassium ions. By reducing the potassium equilibrium potential (page 17) these ions maintain the membrane in a depolarized state and thereby cause a lasting release of calcium ions from the sarcoplasmic reticulum. Another technique is to add caffeine to the bathing solution; the nature of this drug action has been described in the previous section. Contractures may also occur as part of a disease process; in *McArdle's syndrome* (myophosphorylase deficiency, page 187) the muscle fibres stay shortened and swell after physical exertion, at a time when impulse activity in the membrane has ceased. In this condition a failure of the calcium pump has been postulated, even though there is a plentiful supply of ATP available (Gruener *et al.,* 1968). An even more dramatic example of a clinical contracture is *malignant hyperthermia* (page 184). In this hereditary disorder the muscles of the affected patient may go into a contracture under the influence of certain anaesthetics or depolarizing drugs. So severe is the contracture that unless the anaesthetic is stopped immediately and vigorous cooling of the patient instituted, death will inevitably supervene. Once again, it would appear that the calcium pump is ineffective.

It should be noted that the term 'contracture' has been used here in a physiological sense. Unfortunately the term is also applied by clinicians to permanent shortening of muscle produced by excessive growth of fibrous tissue within the muscle belly and possibly by resorption of sarcomeres as well (Tabary *et al.,* 1972). One of the best examples of this type of contracture is the severe shortening of the calf muscles which affects boys with advanced Duchenne muscular dystrophy (page 145). In such cases it is best to refer to the phenomenon as a 'pathological' contracture to avoid confusion with the 'physiological' type considered.

Rigor

In rigor there is also a maintained shortening which is independent of action potential activity. In this condition, unlike a contracture, the fibre is depleted of ATP. Because of this deficiency, the cross-bridges on the myosin molecules cannot be detached from the actin filaments (*Figure 5.2*) and the myofibrils are consequently unable to relax. A rigor state eventually supervenes after death once the ATP in the fibre has been consumed by the various autolytic reactions which take place during the early degenerative processes.

ISOMETRIC AND ISOTONIC CONTRACTIONS

In experimental situations it is usual to study the contractile behaviour of muscle fibres under either isometric or isotonic conditions, since the analysis of the results is made considerably easier. In an *isotonic* contraction the muscle is able to shorten and to lift whatever load has been attached to its tendon. Under these circumstances external work is performed, being equal to the product of the load and the distance through which it has been moved (i.e. work = load × distance). In an *isometric* contraction the muscle is prevented from shortening by fixing both its ends. Instead of performing external work the muscle develops tension at its points of attachment; the energy expended in the contraction is released as heat. In everyday life there are many examples of contractions which are purely isotonic or isometric. Isotonic contractions include cycling, combing the hair, placing objects on shelves, and loading a grocery cart. An isometric contraction would be an unsuccessful attempt to lift a heavy object, providing a counter force to prevent an object from toppling over, or simply maintaining one's posture against gravity. Other activities are more complicated. For example, in walking the forward swing of the leg is checked by the action of the gluteal muscles which thus develop tension while being *lengthened*. Again, consider a situation in which progressively larger loads required to be lifted. It is a well-known experience that the lift becomes increasingly slow as the load is made larger. In the laboratory

this phenomenon may be investigated by stimulating the muscle repetitively (tetanically) and measuring the velocity of muscle shortening for different loads (*Figure 5.6*). It can be seen that, not only is the velocity of shortening reduced when a relatively large load is applied, but there is a latent period before the object is moved at all. During this latent period the muscle is contracting isometrically until sufficient tension has been produced to equal the load. *Figure 5.6* also shows that, not only is the rate of shortening reduced for heavy loads, but the amount of shortening is also decreased.

A point to be emphasized is that, irrespective of the circumstances of the contraction—isotonic,

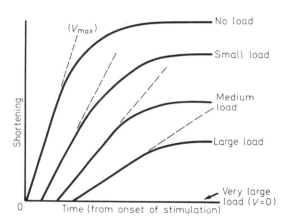

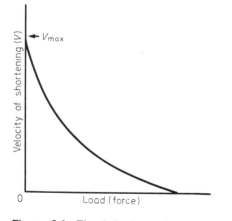

Figure 5.6. The behaviour of a muscle when it is stimulated tetanically and required to lift increasingly large loads: (upper) relationship between load and amount of shortening; (lower) relationship between load and the maximum velocity of shortening (— — — — in upper part of figure); this is commonly referred to as the 'force–velocity' curve. Note that if the load is very large it will not be lifted and the velocity will be zero

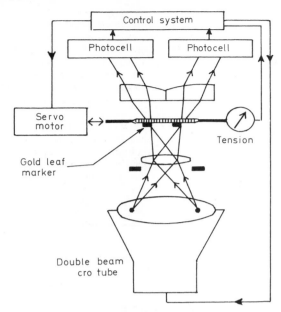

Figure 5.7. Experimental arrangement used to measure the tension developed by a single muscle fibre at controlled sarcomere lengths. See text for description. (Modified from Gordon, Huxley and Julian (1966) courtesy of the authors, and the Editor and publishers of Journal of Physiology)

isometric or lengthening—the action of the myofilaments remains the same. That is, the cross-bridges on the myosin filaments engage sites on the actin filaments and attempt to slide the latter along (page 37). In an isotonic contraction the sliding movement is large and the myosin filaments become completely overlapped by actin. In an isometric contraction the amount of overlap will obviously depend on the length at which the muscle is fixed prior to stimulation. In order to investigate this point precisely Gordon, Huxley and Julian (1966) examined small regions of single muscle fibres in the frog. They fixed two small pieces of gold leaf to the fibre and used these to interrupt two beams of light passing from oscilloscope tube 'spots' to two photocells (*Figure 5.7*). The output from the photocells was fed into a control circuit which operated a servo-motor attached to one end of the muscle fibre. The other end of the fibre was attached to a strain gauge. By using negative feedback the system enabled the length of the fibre between the gold leaf markers to be kept at a pre-set value while the tension developed during tetanic stimulation was measured. In some of their experiments Gordon and colleagues stretched the muscle fibre so far that there was no overlap between the myosin and actin filaments. Since the myosin cross-bridges were unable to reach the actin filaments no tension

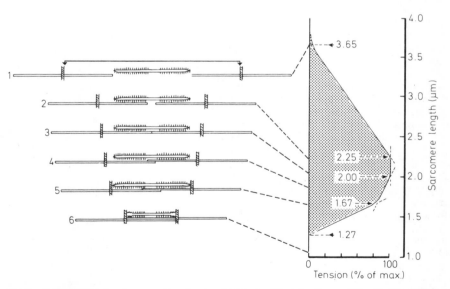

Figure 5.8. Length-tension results of experiment depicted in figure 5.7. At the left is shown a single sarcomere, the arrows in 1 indicating the two Z-lines. The amount of overlap of the actin and myosin filaments at different sarcomere lengths is shown in 2–6, and the corresponding tensions developed are displayed at the right. Critical sarcomere lengths are indicated by arrows. (Modified from Gordon et al. (1966) courtesy of the authors, and the Editor and the publishers of Journal of Physiology)

could be developed (*Figure 5.8; 1*). This is exactly the situation which is thought to obtain in the cardiac failure associated with ventricular distension. Whether excessive lengthening can ever take place in normal skeletal muscles is doubtful for the permissible ranges of joint movement are possibly too small. In diseased muscles the possibility of hyperextension seems more likely since the partial replacement of muscle fibres by relatively inelastic fibrous tissue could well allow surviving segments of fibres to be stretched excessively. Gordon, Huxley and Julian (1966) also investigated isometric contractions elicited at muscle lengths which permitted

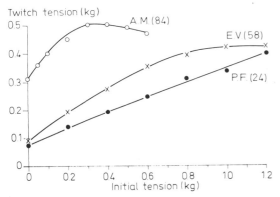

Figure 5.9. *The effect of stretch on the isometric twitch tensions developed by the extensor hallucis brevis muscles of three adult males, P.F., E.V. and A.M., aged 24, 58, 84 years respectively. Note that, for experimental convenience, the stretch has been indicated by the tension applied to the muscle rather than the muscle length (which would have been better). (From Sica and McComas (1971a) courtesy of the Editor and publishers of* Journal of Neurology, Neurosurgery and Psychiatry)

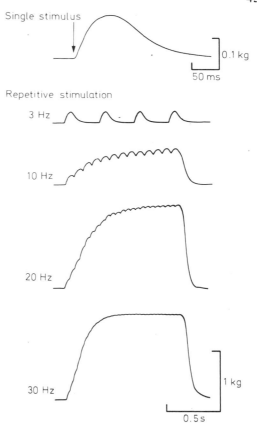

Figure 5.10. *Tension developed in the human abductor pollicis brevis muscle following maximal stimulation of the median nerve once and at 3, 10, 20 and 30 Hz*

some overlap of actin and myosin filaments. They observed that, over a certain range, the tension developed was proportional to the degree of overlap and hence to the number of active cross-bridges on the myosin filaments (*Figure 5.8; 2*). If further shortening was allowed, such that opposing actin filaments now overlapped each other as well as the underlying myosin filament, the isometric tension declined (*Figure 5.8; 4*). It is possible that the overlapping actin filaments interfered with the cross-bridge mechanism at these short sarcomere lengths.

When the isometric contraction of a whole muscle fibre is considered the situation becomes more complicated for the two ends of the fibre will tend to shorten at the expense of the middle region. In view of this complexity, studies of whole muscles have rather less significance than those of single fibres. Nevertheless, because it was carried out on man, mention should be made

of a study on the triceps muscles of patients whose arms had been amputated at a level above the elbow (University of California, 1947). A strain gauge was attached to the triceps tendon and the patient was asked to make maximal contractions when the muscle had been fixed at different lengths. It was possible to demonstrate a length–tension curve with a distinct optimal value and a shape generally similar to that shown for the isolated muscle fibre in *Figure 5.8*. That is, the isometric tension increased as the muscle was stretched and then, beyond an optimal length, the tension declined. In another study Sica and McComas (1971a) studied isometric twitches in extensor hallucis brevis muscles of healthy subjects of various ages. In a young adult (P.F. in *Figure 5.9*) they found the greatest stretch which could be applied to the muscle, by plantar-flexing the great toe, was still insufficient for the muscle to develop its maximum isometric twitch tension. In older adults an optimum length of muscle could be demonstrated (E.V. in *Figure 5.9*), and this appeared to decrease with advancing age. One consequence of this was that an 'elderly' muscle developed a much larger tension in the neutral position of the joint, that is, without any stretch being applied (A.M. in *Figure 5.9*). The likeliest interpretation of these results is that parts of the muscle-tendon complex become increasingly inelastic during ageing so that more and more of the stretch is undertaken by still normal regions of the muscle fibres.

The concept of 'elasticity' in muscle is a very important one for not only does it affect the length-tension relationship of the whole muscle, as discussed above, but it also influences the form of the mechanical response recorded from the muscle. If it were not for the *series elastic component* the tension recorded during a single isometric twitch would rise very rapidly to the maximum value commensurate with the permitted degree of overlap between the actin and myosin filaments. Instead much of the mechanical energy liberated by the sliding action of the filaments is expended in stretching the elastic component within the muscle and tendon rather than in developing tension at the attachments of the tendon. If, in place of a single shock, the muscle is stimulated repetitively (*tetanically*), sufficient time becomes available for the elastic component to be fully stretched and for the full tension developed by sliding filaments to be recorded (*Figure 5.10*). In mammals such as the rat and cat, the ratio between the tensions developed in a single twitch and in a tetanus (*the twitch: tetanus ratio*) is about 0.2 (Buller and Lewis, 1965; Close, 1972), but rather lower values, around 0.1, have been obtained for the human adductor pollicis (Slomić, Rosenfalck and Buchthal, 1968; data of Desmedt *et al.*, 1968; see also *Figure 5.10*). Where is this elasticity situated? Clearly, not only in the tendon for it can still be demonstrated experimentally if the tendon is excised and the strain gauge attached directly to the muscle. It now seems probable that the major part of the elasticity resides within the myosin cross-bridges (Huxley and Simmons, 1971). Thus the same elements which perform mechanical work through their attachments to the actin filaments may also confer upon the muscle its elastic features.

Chapter 6

MOTOR UNITS

So far the muscle and nerve fibres have been treated largely as single cells. It is time to consider the anatomical and physiological relationships between these two types of cell and then to study the way in which the body makes use of the neuromuscular system. To begin with, it is necessary to introduce the concept of the *motor unit*; this term describes a single motoneurone and the many muscle fibres to which its axon runs. As Sherrington (1929) appreciated, all the varied reflex and voluntary contractions of a muscle are achieved by different combinations of active motor units. Expressed differently, all movements are planned by the central nervous system in terms of motor units rather than individual muscle fibres. Some of the more important aspects of motor unit function can now be discussed.

NUMBERS OF MOTOR UNITS

One of the problems which has repeatedly interested anatomists concerns the numbers of motor units in individual muscles. In animals the simplest approach has been to cut dorsal roots distal to their ganglia and to allow time for degeneration of the severed sensory nerve fibres. If the nerve to a muscle is then examined the surviving nerve fibres will be those which left the cord in the ventral roots and are motor in function. Until the important study of Leksell (1945) it was not realized that the smallest motor axons in the ventral roots, the 'gamma' axons, were those passing from fusimotor neurones to the small muscle fibres inside spindles. In the earliest studies the numbers of motor units

estimated were therefore too high, in most cases by 20–40 per cent (see, for example, Eccles and Sherrington, 1930). Even in these early studies, however, it was clear that there were considerable differences in the numbers and sizes of motor units between muscles within the same animal.

For obvious reasons it has not been possible to determine numbers of motor units in human muscles with the same precision as that of the animal studies. Some indication of the probable human values may be obtained from experimental investigations on large primates (for example, Wray 1969; Table 6.1). The best that can be done in man is to count the number of large myelinated fibres in a muscle nerve and to assume that a certain proportion of these are 'alpha'-motor and that the remainder are sensory fibres from spindles and tendon organs. The uncertainty introduced by this assumption is evident from the painstaking work of Boyd and Davey (1968) who showed that the proportion of large fibres that are motor varied between 40 and 70 per cent in different muscle nerves in the cat hind limb. In the study of Feinstein *et al.* (1955) it was assumed that 60 per cent of the large diameter fibres were alpha-motor. This value was chosen on the basis of observations on the muscle nerves of a patient dead from severe poliomyelitis; no motor axons were thought likely to have been left. Leaving aside the questionable validity of this assumption there is no doubt that Feinstein and colleagues (1955) have provided the best anatomical data for the numbers and sizes of human motor units. Table 6.1 includes most of the results obtained by these authors; it emphasizes the considerable differences between limb muscles such that the

TABLE 6.1

Number of Sizes of Motor Units in Various Muscles of Man and Baboon

Species	Muscle	No. of motor units	Muscle fibres/unit	Author
Man	Ext. rectus	2 970	9	Feinstein et al. (1955)
Man	Platysma	1 096	25	Feinstein et al. (1955)
Man	1st lumbrical	96*	108	Feinstein et al. (1955)
Man	1st dorsal interosseous	119	340	Feinstein et al. (1955)
Man	Brachioradialis	333*	>410	Feinstein et al. (1955)
Man	Tibialis anterior	445	562	Feinstein et al. (1955)
Man	Med. gastrocnemius	579	1 934	Feinstein et al. (1955)
Baboon	Abductor pollicis brevis	43	220	Wray (1969)
Baboon	Med. gastrocnemius	292	790	Wray (1969)

* Average values

intrinsic muscles of the hand and foot (lumbrical, first dorsal interosseous) have fewer motor units than the larger muscles (brachioradialis, tibialis anterior and medial gastrocnemius) situated nearer the trunk. However, since the motor units in the distal muscles are relatively small, these muscles have greater numbers of units in relation to their mass. Table 6.1 also draws attention to the remarkable properties of the external ocular muscles (external rectus) and the superficial muscles of the face and neck (platysma) which contain large numbers of very small units.

Neurophysiological estimates of numbers of motor units

Until recently the only electrophysiological method available for estimating the degree of innervation of a human muscle has been that of interference-pattern electromyography. A concentric needle electrode is inserted into a muscle and the subject is instructed to make a maximum contraction. In a normal subject the potential inflections occur so frequently that no base-line can be distinguished between them on the oscilloscope (Figure 6.1, c). Although the density of the interference pattern can be analysed automatically (see, for example Rose and Willison, 1967 and Kopec et al., 1973) the techniques do not enable the number of motor units to be estimated in a normal subject. In a patient with severe denervation, however, the potentials generated by each surviving unit can be distinguished from those of other units by differences in amplitude, duration and configuration (Figure 6.1, d). Under these circumstances the number of functioning motor units in the vicinity of the recording electrode may be determined readily. If the electrode is of the concentric (coaxial) variety, however, it is unlikely to detect all the units within the muscle and so there are advantages in using an electrode with a much larger surface area.

Further drawbacks with interference-pattern electromyography are that it is relatively insensitive (Figure 6.1, e) and that it requires the full co-operation of the subject; this means that it cannot be used on very young children or on adults in confusional or comatose states.

An alternative approach which offers some advantages is the increment-counting technique devised by McComas et al. (1971a; see also Sica et al., 1974). As many of the results described in the sections on neuromuscular diseases have been obtained with this method, some of the experimental details may now be given. The nerve to a muscle is stimulated through electrodes attached to the overlying skin (Figure 6.2). A recording electrode, consisting of a thin strip of silver foil, is fixed to the skin over the end-plate zone of the muscle. A similar electrode is placed at a distance from the muscle and serves as a reference. The limb is grounded at some point between the recording electrodes and the nearest stimulating electrode (cathode). The stimuli are delivered at a low frequency (e.g. 0.5 Hz) and their intensity is gradually increased from a subthreshold value. Eventually an intensity is reached at which an amplified response appears on the oscilloscope screen. If the stimulus is now maintained at this threshold value, the response can be seen to have an 'all-or-nothing' character; that is, it is either present and reproducible or else completely absent. This type of behaviour indicates that the responses are arising from a single motor unit and that the stimuli are only strong enough to excite intermittently a single motor axon in the nerve trunk. The response can be made to occur consistently by increasing the stimulus intensity slightly; the axon is now being excited each time the stimulus is delivered. A further increase in stimulus intensity evokes a larger response—the increment is due to excitation of a second axon and motor unit. If the stimulus intensity is gradually raised the response can be seen to enlarge in discrete steps (Figure 6.3, top).

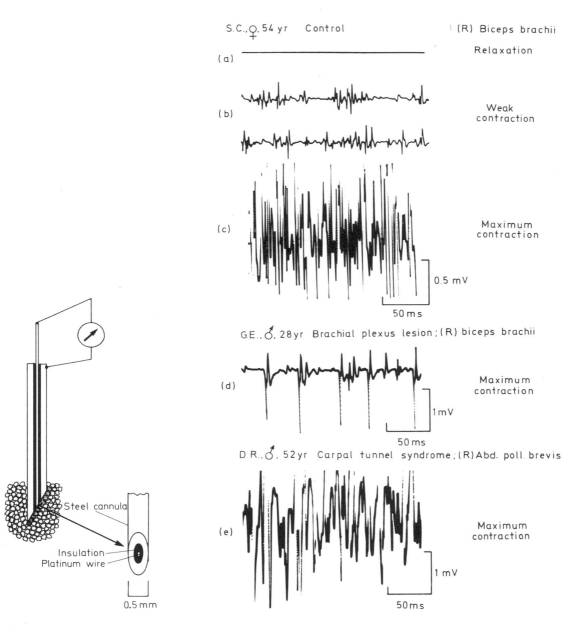

Figure 6.1. (Left) The coaxial type of recording electrode frequently employed in clinical electromyography. An insulated wire (copper, steel or platinum) is fixed within a stainless steel cannula and the end is sharpened; the internal wire forms the stigmatic electrode and the cannula becomes a reference electrode. In the figure the muscle fibres have been drawn to scale and it can be seen that 10 (shaded) are abutting the electrode tip. (Right) The recordings from the abductor pollicis brevis muscle of a normal subject at rest (a) and during increasingly strong voluntary contraction (b—c). Shown for contrast in (d) is the reduced interference pattern in a patient with very severe denervation. The insensitivity of the method is evident from record (e) in which the interference pattern of another patient appears full, even though the motor unit counting technique (see text) revealed that only 10 per cent of units were left (carpal tunnel syndrome)

Each step, or increment, is thought to signify the excitation of an additional motor unit and axon. After a number of increments have been evoked their mean size is calculated; this will correspond to the *mean motor unit potential amplitude*. A stimulus is now delivered to nerve which is large enough to excite all the motor axons (*Figure 6.3; second trace from top*). If the amplitude of this

cent). In addition, the mean amplitude might be biased if the motor axons with the lowest excitatory thresholds innervated motor units which were either larger or smaller than average. In practice this hazard can be discounted for the most important factor governing excitability in these experiments appears to be the accessibility of an axon to the

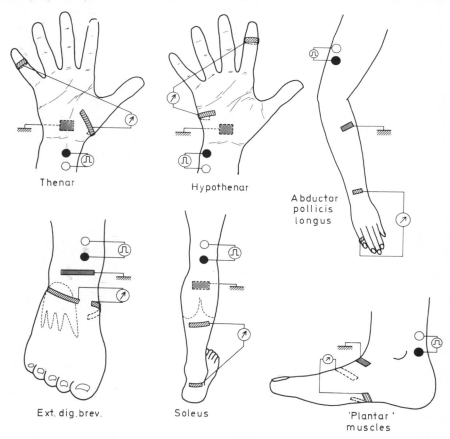

Thenar

Hypothenar

Abductor pollicis longus

Ext. dig. brev.

Soleus

'Plantar' muscles

Figure 6.2. experimental arrangements for estimating numbers of motor units in six human muscles (or muscle groups). ● = cathodal stimulating electrodes (see text for description)

maximal 'M' response is divided by the mean amplitude of the motor unit potentials, an estimate is obtained of the number of motor units in the muscle, and hence of motor axons in the nerve (Appendix 6.1).

A number of factors will combine to make this estimate a very approximate one. To begin with, the range of amplitudes of motor unit potential increments evoked in a single muscle is considerable, such that the mean amplitude has an appreciable coefficient of variation (typically 30–70 per

stimulating current rather than any intrinsic biophysical property of the axon itself. It can be shown, for example, that in the peroneal nerve the axons with the lowest thresholds to stimulation at the ankle have relatively high thresholds when the stimulating electrodes are moved to the head of the fibula (McComas *et al.*, 1971a). Also, within the pooled sample of incremental responses from many subjects, there is no significant difference between the mean motor unit potential amplitudes evoked by stimulation of the lowest and highest threshold axons respectively. Another factor affecting the accuracy of the estimate would be the existence of motor axons with identical thresholds. The possibility that two axons would be mistaken for one can be diminished, however, for the more often that the stimulation is repeated the less likely it is that the two axons will respond together on every occasion. A more serious problem presented by two

B.C.   Control EDB

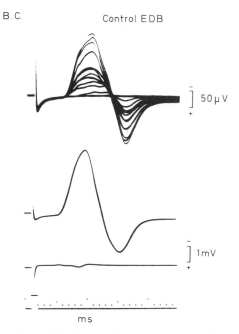

] 50 μV

] 1 mV

ms

Figure 6.3. Estimation of the numbers of functioning motor units in the left extensor digitorum brevis muscle of a 25-year-old healthy female subject. At top are shown the 11 increments recorded as the stimulus intensity was gradually increased from a subthreshold value; each of the first eight increments had been superimposed several times. The trace below shows the largest potential that could be recorded from the muscle when stronger stimuli were applied; this is referred to as the maximum M wave. The next trace shows that the dorsal interosseous muscles made very little contribution to the recorded potentials. In this subject the maximum M wave was 7.1 mV and the mean motor unit potential amplitude was 34 μV; by division, the number of motor units was estimated to be about 208. (From McComas et al (1974a), courtesy of the Editor and publishers of Annals of the New York Academy of Sciences)

axons with similar thresholds is that of *alternation*. If, on different occasions, either or both axons are excited, then the three types of response will be interpreted as arising from three motor units, rather

than two. If the thresholds of the motor axons approximate to a Gaussian distribution, then the likelihood of this phenomenon occurring will increase as the stimulus is raised. For this reason it is only possible to sample a relatively small number of motor unit potentials in any one patient, usually between 7 and 12. Another limitation of the sample size is the fact that, as more motor units are excited, the gain of the amplifier has to be reduced in order to accommodate the enlarging evoked response on the oscilloscope screen. At increasingly low amplification, however, it becomes progressively more difficult to distinguish each additional increment in the response. Another error, and one of uncertain magnitude, will be caused by the 'shunting' effect of inactive muscle fibres when only a small proportion of the fibre population is generating action potential currents.

In spite of these uncertainties the results in any one subject are sufficiently reproducible for the method to be acceptable. Furthermore, in the extensor digitorum brevis, the numbers of motor units estimated are in reasonable agreement with values obtained by counting axons in specimens of nerve obtained *post mortem* (McComas *et al.*, 1971a). In view of the importance of the results obtained with this method for an understanding of neuromuscular diseases, the validity of the technique is considered more extensively in Appendix 6.1.

Muscles investigated

The muscles studied with the evoked potential method have included the extensor digitorum brevis, the muscles of the thenar and hypothenar eminences, the soleus, the abductor pollicis longus and the plantar muscles. The essential feature possessed by each of these muscles is the existence of a single end-plate zone which can be spanned by the (stigmatic) recording electrode. Other muscles investigated, such as the brachioradialis and sartorius, have more than one end-plate zone and are therefore unsatisfactory. In the latter muscles a recording electrode over one end-plate zone frequently picks up muscle action potentials arising at another zone. These 'distant' potentials have an opposite polarity to those generated locally and the recorded evoked potential therefore diminishes instead of increasing. Rather surprisingly, it has proved feasible to obtain technically satisfactory recordings with a stigmatic electrode placed over the soleus, in spite of the fact that this muscle is multipennate in man and must therefore possess a spatially complex innervation. The results of the various studies in healthy control subjects may be summarized as follows (Table 6.2):

TABLE 6.2

Numbers of Motor Units Estimated in Various Human Muscles and Muscle Groups, using the Electrophysiological Technique Described in the Text

Muscle	No. of motor units (Mean ± S.D.)	Range	No. of observations
Extensor digitorum brevis	210 ± 65	120–414	151
Thenar*	342 ± 97	220–693	115
Hypothenar	390 ± 94	250–734	109
Abductor pollicis longus	421 ± 99	272–666	40
Soleus	957 ± 254	542–1579	41

* Units innervated by the median nerve

The *extensor digitorum brevis* muscle was studied in 151 muscles of controls aged between 7 months and 58 years; stimuli were delivered to the deep peroneal nerve at the ankle. The estimated numbers of motor units ranged from 120 to 414 with a mean value of 210 ± 65. The scatter of values in these and in older subjects is shown in *Figure 6.4.*

The *hypothenar muscles* (palmaris brevis, flexor digiti minimi, opponens digiti minimi and abductor digiti minimi) were investigated in 109 hands of

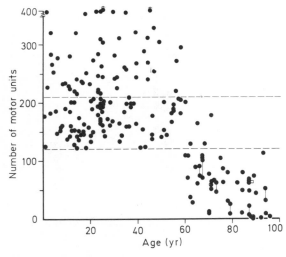

Figure 6.4. Estimated numbers of functioning motor units in the extensor digitorum brevis muscles of 207 healthy subjects between the ages of 7 months and 97 years. Bilateral observations on the same subject have been linked. The lower interrupted horizontal line indicates the bottom of the normal range (120 units) and the upper line shows the mean value (210 units) for those subjects below the age of 60

healthy subjects aged between 7 months and 58 years. The ulnar nerve was stimulated at the wrist and in most subjects both hands were examined; the mean number of units was 390 ± 94 with a range of 250 to 734 units.

The *thenar muscles* innervated by the median nerve (abductor pollicis brevis, opponens pollicis, and part of flexor pollicis brevis) were studied in 115 hands of healthy subjects aged between 7 months and 58 years; a mean value of 342 ± 97 units was obtained (range 220–693 units). In another series of experiments in which a small stigmatic electrode was placed over the abductor pollicis brevis, Brown (1972) found a mean value of 253 ± 34 units in subjects below the age of 40; the same author subsequently reported the same mean value for a rather larger series of controls below the age of 60 (Brown, 1973). In all these studies graded stimuli were applied to the median nerve at the wrist.

As yet the number of *soleus* muscles studied is small (41) and no values have been obtained for normal subjects outside the range of 5–50 years. In this restricted population the numbers of units have varied from 542 to 1579 with a mean of 957 ± 254. Some of this scatter may well have been due to the variable contributions of muscles other than soleus to the evoked responses.

The *abductor pollicis longus* muscle has been studied by De Faria (1976) in 40 arms of 26 healthy subjects aged between 16 and 43 years; a mean value of 421 ± 99 units was obtained.

The *plantar muscles* have yet to be studied systematically and the often complex configurations of the M-responses make the investigations difficult. Nevertheless, this test is extremely useful in the study of the lumbosacral root lesions and, rather empirically, we have come to regard fewer than 120 motor units as an abnormal result.

How well do the numbers of units estimated by the electrophysiological method compare with anatomical determinations? Unfortunately, there are no published figures for the numbers of axons in nerves to the thenar and hypothenar muscles in man. The most relevant observations are probably those on the first dorsal interosseous muscle of the hand in which Feinstein and colleagues (1955) estimated that there were 119 motor units; the corresponding value for the first lumbrical muscle was 96 units. For reasons already stated, these values are liable to considerable error.

If, in fact, each of the small muscles in the hand have approximately 100 motor units then the mean electrophysiological estimate of 380 would be appropriate for the four hypothenar muscles. Of the thenar muscles, the median nerve supplies only the abductor pollicis brevis, opponens pollicis and part of the flexor pollicis brevis. The abductor pollicis and the remainder of the flexor are innervated by the ulnar nerve. It might therefore be expected that the thenar count, as determined in these experiments, would be somewhat lower than the hypothenar one; again, the values of units 342 (present study) and 253 units (Brown, 1973) are probably not unreasonable.

In the case of the extensor digitorum brevis (EDB) specimens of nerve were obtained *post mortem* from two previously healthy young adults who had been killed in a road accident. In one patient the nerve diameters showed a bimodal distribution with a division at 7.0–7.9 μm; there were 729 fibres larger than this. In the second patient the distribution was unimodal and there were 560 fibres with diameters of 8 μm or more. It is not known what proportions of these larger fibres were motor; also, some of the fibres from the lateral terminal branch of the deep peroneal nerve do not end in EDB but run through to supply dorsal joints and dorsal interosseous muscles (Davies, 1967).

One criticism which might be levelled at the choice of EDB for experimental studies is that, in apparently normal subjects, the muscle shows morphological changes consistent with denervation and reinnervation (Jennekens, Tomlinson and Walton, 1972) and the possibility of repeated minor trauma to the peroneal nerve at the knee and ankle has been raised (Appendix 61). There is good

evidence, however, that although transient denervation may occur in this muscle, only a small number of axons are likely to be damaged irreparably. More extensive denervation would cause the estimated number of motor units to drop with age; instead no correlation between these two factors could be demonstrated in those subjects below the age of 60 (see *Figure 6.4*). In order to explain the discrepancies between the various observations in EDB, an alternative explanation is presented later (page 297), in which trauma plays a possible role. The significance of the changes in elderly subjects will be considered separately (page 102).

SIZES OF MOTOR UNITS

Various methods have been employed to determine the sizes of motor units, i.e. the number of muscle fibres innervated by individual motor axons. For a given muscle the average size of the motor units may be estimated simply by dividing the total number of muscle fibres by the number of motor axons. It has been found that a relatively large muscle, the human medial gastrocnemius, has an average of about 2000 fibres in each unit whereas the much smaller external rectus muscle has only 9 (Feinstein *et al.*, 1955; Table 6.1).

With the advent of electrophysiological studies, it became apparent that, even within the same muscle, the sizes of motor units varied so greatly

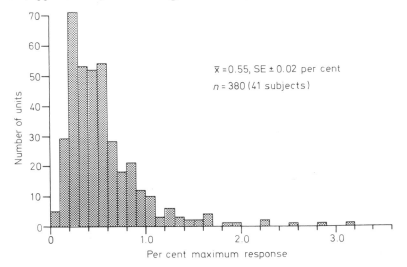

$\bar{x} = 0.55$, SE ± 0.02 per cent

$n = 380$ (41 subjects)

Figure 6.5. The sizes of 380 motor unit potentials in the EDB muscles of 41 control subjects below the age of 60. Each value has been expressed as a percentage of the maximum response in order to compensate for variations in electrode placement and in the thickness of the tissues overlying the muscle. Modified from McComas et al. (1971a) courtesy of the Editor and publishers of the Journal of Neurology, Neurosurgery and psychiatry

that the estimation of mean size had limited significance. For example, Burke (1967) stimulated single
motoneurones and measured the tensions produced in the cat triceps surae muscle. He found that
the twitch tensions ranged from 0.2 to 97 g and
noted that the scatter of results was much greater
in the gastrocnemius muscle than soleus (see
Figure 6.9). Although these results indicated that
the motor unit sizes varied considerably they did
not permit the absolute numbers of muscle fibres
to be determined. These determinations may now
be performed using a technique developed independently by Edström and Kugelberg (1968) and
Brandstater and Lambert (1969). In this method a
single motor axon is stimulated repetitively and
the muscle is then excised and stained with PAS
for glycogen. The glycogen depleted fibres are
those which will have been stimulated and will
therefore correspond to a single motor unit (*Figure
6.6a, upper*). In the rat tibialis muscle the sizes of
the motor units are within the 50–200 fibre range
(Brandstater and Lambert, 1973; Edström and
Kugelberg, 1968). As might have been expected,
the comparatively large tibialis anterior and
extensor digitorum longus muscle of the cat have
larger units, the range observed by Mayer and
Doyle (1970) being 43–1099 fibres. In the cat
triceps surae complex the sizes of the motor units
in soleus range from less than 50 to more than
400 fibres, while in the medial gastrocnemius an
'average' unit contains between 400 and 800 fibres
(Burke and Tsairis, 1973; Burke, *et al.*, 1974;
Figure 6.6b).

Direct studies of motor unit size have not yet
been undertaken in man, though it is certainly
possible, by using just-threshold stimuli, to selec-
tively excite a single motor unit (McComas *et al.*,
1971a; Bergmans, 1970). The nearest attempt so
far is the demonstration of glycogen depletion in
motor units of a patient with myokymia, a condition in which spontaneous repetitive firing is pronounced (Williamson and Brooke, 1972). An
alternative approach to the human situation is to
measure the twitch (or tetanic) tensions of single
motor units as has been done in other mammals
(see above). Although this method does not permit
the absolute numbers of muscle fibres to be determined, it does provide some indication of the
relative sizes of the units. So far few such studies
have been reported. In one of these Sica and
McComas (1971a) found that the twitch tensions
of 122 single units in the extensor hallucis brevis
varied from 2 to 14 g (mean 5.5 ± 2.2 g). In
another study, Milner-Brown, Stein and Yemm
(1973a) obtained a range of 0.1 to 10 g for units
in the first dorsal interosseous muscle of the hand.
Rather less satisfactory is to measure the sizes of
the motor unit potentials recorded with large surface electrodes. Although the size of each potential
will be proportional to the number of muscle fibres
in that unit, the potential will also be influenced by
the diameters of the fibres and their proximity to
the stigmatic recording electrode. *Figure 6.5* should
be viewed with these qualifications in mind; it
suggests that there is a greater than 30-fold variation in motor unit size in the extensor digitorum
brevis muscle but that the number of 'large' units
is small (the distribution of values is skewed to the
right).

UNIT ARCHITECTURE

Until fairly recently it was thought that the muscle
fibres supplied by a single axon were distributed
in clusters, or subunits, within the muscle belly.
The validity of this concept was questioned by
Ekstedt (1964) on the basis of recordings with a
special electrode which had small recording surfaces 180 degrees apart (the 'Janus' electrode).
He observed that, when a motor unit fired, usually
only one of the two surfaces was next to an active
fibre; had sub-units been present the electrode
should have been surrounded by discharging
fibres. It is now recognized that the sub-unit
arrangement is only true of motor units in partially
denervated muscles in which collateral reinnervation of muscle fibres has taken place (see page 224).

The correct architecture of the motor unit was
revealed by the glycogen-depletion method of
Edström and Kugelberg (1968) and Brandstater and
Lambert (1969). These authors have shown that,
within a given volume of muscle, the fibres in a
single motor unit appear to be arranged randomly
amongst those of other units and only a few fibres
in the same unit are contiguous (*Figure 6.6, upper*).
It was found that in the rat tibialis anterior muscle,
fibres belonging to the same motor unit could be
distributed over a surprisingly large volume of
muscle, typically 12–26 per cent of the cross-
sectional area (Edström and Kugelberg, 1968);
similar observations have been made in the cat
medial gastrocnemius muscle (Burke and Tsairis,
1973; *Figure 6.6b*). In the human brachial biceps
muscle Buchthal, Guld and Rosenfalck (1957),
using a multilead electrode, have electrophysiological evidence that the territories of individual
motor units have mean cross-sectional diameters
of 5 mm and that 10–25 motor units overlap with
each other in any region of the muscle. Even
greater degrees of overlap, comprising at least
40–50 motor units, were found by Burke and
Tsairis (1973) in the cat medial gastrocnemius
muscle.

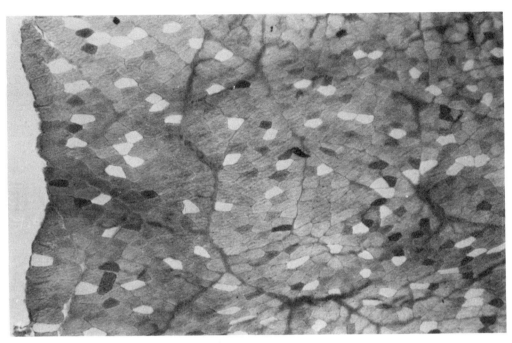

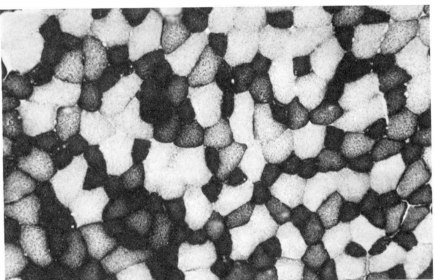

Figure 6.6a. (Upper) Part of a motor unit in the tibialis anterior muscle of a rat. A single motor axon had been stimulated repetitively; the activated muscle fibres became depleted of glycogen and failed to stain with PAS, appearing white in the photograph (courtesy of Dr M. E. Brandstater). (Lower) Transverse section of tibialis anterior muscle from a 3-month-old normal mouse stained for succinic dehydrogenase. Three types of fibre can easily be differentiated on the basis of their staining reaction (courtesy of Dr Ethel Cosmos). Magnifications 150 × (upper) and 320 × (lower)

TYPES OF MOTOR UNITS

Not only do motor units differ from each other in size but also in the biochemical and physiological properties of their muscle fibres. Early evidence that such differences existed was provided by Ranvier (1873) who noted, in a comparative study of several species, that some muscles were those which were used continuously in the maintenance of posture. In contrast, the fast-contracting pale muscles were only employed intermittently, being reserved for special movements of a non-repetitive nature. Denny-Brown pointed out that some mammalian muscles contain both pale and red parts; for example, the deeper region of the cat tibialis anterior is red

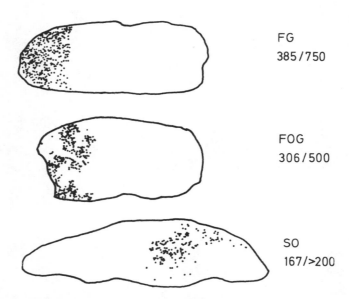

FG
385/750

FOG
306/500

SO
167/>200

Figure 6.6b. Territories of three different motor units in the cat medial gastrocnemius muscle, as determined by the glycogen-depletion method. Since, in this muscle, the fibres do not run the full length of the belly, only about half of the respective fibre populations can be seen in a single cross section. The numbers of fibres counted in these sections and the total numbers of fibres estimated to be present in the three units are given at the right, together with the designations of the motor units (FG, FOG or SO; see table 6.4). Redrawn from Burke and Tsairis (1973), courtesy of the authors, the Editor and publishers of the Journal of Physiology

muscles contracted more slowly than others and that these muscles had a more pronounced red coloration. It was shown later that the red colour of the muscle was due to the increased amounts of the oxygen-bearing pigment *myoglobin* in the muscle fibres and that these fibres also had a rich capillary network. More detailed comparisons between muscles were made by Denny-Brown (1929). He confirmed the earlier observations of Ranvier but demonstrated that in some muscles of animals the relationship between muscle colour and contraction speed did not always apply. Denny-Brown also noted that the slowly-contracting red while the superficial part is pale. In other muscles, and this is particularly true of man, red and pale muscle fibres are intermingled so as to form a mosaic.

With the development of methods for staining muscles histochemically, further differences between muscle fibres emerged. Some fibres were found to stain strongly for the enzymes phosphorylase and myosin ATPase. Other fibres, because of their numerous mitochondria, were shown to be rich in enzymes such as malic and succinic dehydrogenase which are associated with these organelles (*Figure 6.6a, lower*).

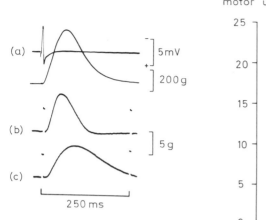

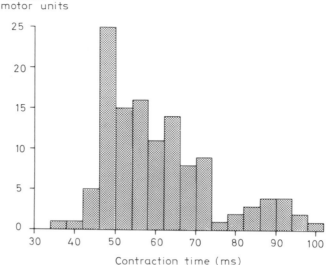

Figure 6.7. Isometric contractions recorded from the human EHB muscles of healthy adults below the age of 60. At left (a) is the maximum response of the muscle, with the M wave, in a 30-year-old male, (b) and (c), are single motor unit responses after averaging; (b) is a fast-contracting unit and (c) is slow-contracting. At right are the pooled contraction times of 122 motor units, recorded from 60 normal muscles. From McComas et al. (1973) courtesy of Plenum Press *and the Editors of* Control of Posture and Locomotion

Attempts have also been made to differentiate fibres on the basis of electronmicroscopy; it has been found that considerable variations exist in the structure of the myofibrils and mitochondria and in the amount and complexity of the sarcoplasmic reticulum. The feature which can be correlated best with other properties of the fibre is the thickness of the Z-line. In the guinea pig the line is more than twice as wide in the 'red' fibres of the soleus as in the 'white' fibres of the vastus muscle (Eisenberg, 1974; see also Padykula and Gauthier, 1967).

Muscle Twitch Studies in Man

Most studies in man have been restricted to analysis of either the contractile or else the histochemical properties of units but not both. In the extensor hallucis brevis (EHB) muscle Sica and McComas (1971a) found that some units had twitch contraction times as short as 35 ms while others had values as long as 96 ms. In their pooled data there was a suggestion of at least two types of unit being present (*Figure 6.7*). In the abductor digiti minimi and first dorsal interosseous muscle of the hand similar ranges of motor unit contraction times have been found but with no clear division between 'fast' and 'slow' units (Burke, Skuse and Lethlean, 1974; Milner-Brown, Stein and Yemm, 1973a).

In some human muscles the contributions of fast and slow twitch units can be distinguished in the maximal isometric twitch responses of the whole muscles. For example a recording from the gastrocnemius muscle shows an early inflexion which probably corresponds to the contraction of fast-twitch units (Marsden and Meadows, 1970). Similar inflexions are commonly seen in maximal EHB twitches (*Figure 6.7, a*). In the facial muscles the units are nearly all of the fast-twitch type since the mean contraction time is only 43 ms; in contrast, the relatively long contraction times reported for human calf muscles indicate the presence of a predominantly slow-twitch motor unit population (McComas and Thomas, 1968a; *Figure 6.8*). Unlike the situation in other mammals, there appears to be no difference between the twitch times of the human gastrocnemius and soleus muscles (Buller, *et al.*, 1959). Finally, in the small muscles of the hand and foot the contraction times are intermediate between those of the calf and facial muscles, indicating substantial proportions of both fast and slow twitch units (Table 6.3).

Histochemical studies in man

That there are histochemical differences between muscle fibres in man was clearly established by Wachstein and Meisel (1955) in an autopsy study of succinic dehydrogenase activity. Since then many different staining methods have been applied (see, for example, Dubowitz and Pearse, 1960) but the most useful one for clinical purposes is that for myosin ATPase (Engel, 1962). The fibres which stain strongly at pH 9.4 are referred to as type II, in contrast to the poorly-reacting type I fibres.

enzymatic reaction; hence the fibres have a slower twitch and stain less strongly.

The myosin ATPase staining reaction has been employed extensively in the study of diseased muscle and has proved a useful technique for detecting denervation. Until recently, however, little was known concerning the distributions of

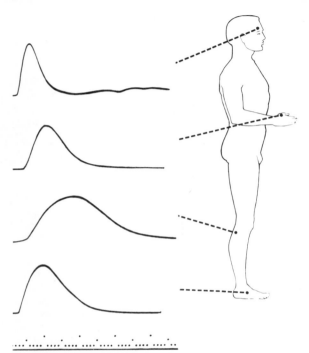

Figure 6.8. Isometric contractions recorded from various human muscles using a stiff piezo-electric bender which was pressed over the muscle belly. Note the marked variation in twitch speed. From McComas and Thomas (1968a) courtesy of the Editor and publishers of the Journal of Neurological Sciences. *Smallest time unit: 10 ms*

Brooke and Kaiser (1970) have divided the type II fibres into A, B and C subtypes on the basis of differences in staining which can be brought out by pre-incubating the tissue at various pH values. Brooke and Kaiser (1974) believe that the IIC fibres are precursors which have the ability to develop into type IIA or IIB fibres. It is now known that the myosin-ATPase activities of the fibres are related to their rates of shortening, as measured from isometric twitch and force-velocity studies (page 43). The reason for this is that the velocity with which the action and myosin filaments can slide over each other depends on the speed with which the myosin molecules can break down ATP. It is probable that in a type I fibre the myosin molecules lack one of the reactive sites for this

the fibre types in normal human muscles. In an autopsy study of 36 human muscles Johnson et al. (1973) have now shown that in most muscles there is a considerable variation in the relative proportions of type I and type II fibres. The two exceptions to this statement were the soleus, which was largely composed of type I fibres, and the orbicularis oculi, in which type II fibres predominated. Other histochemical studies make use of the fact that some of the fibres are specially equipped for anaerobic metabolism. These fibres are able to produce ATP by breaking glycogen down to glucose and thence to lactic acid; they contain correspondingly large amounts of glycogen phosphorylase and lactic dehydrogenase which can be detected histochemically.

TABLE 6.3
The Varying Twitch Speeds of Human Muscles*

	Muscle	Contraction time mean (ms)	Authors
Face	Frontalis/orbicularis oculi	43	McComas and Thomas (1968a)
Foot	Extensor hallucis brevis	63	Sica and McComas (1971a)
Hand	Adductor pollicis	70–80	Desmedt et al. (1968)
		56†	Marsden and Meadows (1970)
		65	Slomić et al. (1968)
		55–77	Takamori et al. (1971)
	Dorsal interosseous	65	McComas and Thomas (1968a)
	Abductor digiti V	63	Burke et al. (1974)
Calf	Gastrocnemius	110	Buller et al. (1959)
	Soleus	120	
	Lateral gastrocnemius	118	McComas and Thomas (1968a)
	Gastrocnemii and soleus	150	Lambert et al. (1951)
	Gastrocnemii and soleus	104†	Marsden and Meadows (1970)

* The values given are those of contraction time, i.e. the time elapsing between the start of the contraction and the moment of peak tension during an isometrically—recorded twitch. In two instances only the ranges of results were stated.
† Calculated from the published data.

Other fibres have numerous mitochondria and therefore react strongly in histochemical tests for reaction products of the various enzymes associated with these organelles, for example succinic and malic dehydrogenase. These fibres also have substantial amounts of myoglobin and possess rich capillary networks around their peripheries. All these properties make the fibres well suited for continuous work since they are able to maintain a supply of ATP through their oxidative reactions. Some authorities have combined the results from a battery of histochemical tests and in this way have been able to recognize many types of fibres. Romanul (1964), for example, has distinguished eight types. Increasingly, however, there has been a tendency to accept only three histochemical types—a 'glycolytic' fibre, an 'oxidative' fibre and a fibre which has strongly developed features of both. Some of the terminologies which have been suggested for the muscle fibre types are considered in the next section (see also Table 6.4).

CORRELATIVE STUDIES

Many attempts have been made to correlate the various differences between fibres and one of the most comprehensive studies is that of Burke et al. (1971; see also Burke et al., 1973). These authors stimulated spinal motoneurones through an intracellular microelectrode and recorded the twitch and tetanic contractions of the corresponding motor units. At the end of an experiment they demonstrated the architecture of the motor unit which they had been investigating, using the glycogen-depletion technique (see page 54). By staining consecutive sections for various enzymes, they

were able to establish other biochemical characteristics of the previously activated fibres. As part of this study, they were able to confirm that all the muscle fibres belonging to the same motor unit were histochemically similar in that they stained strongly for the same enzyme activities.

The conclusion of Burke and colleagues (1971) was that certain properties of the motor units were closely linked together and that three types of units could be recognized. One type had a slow twitch, developed relatively small tension and was resistant to fatigue (Figure 6.9); the muscle fibres had high contents of mitochondrial enzymes, were poor in glycogen, stained weakly for myosin ATPase and had rich capillary networks. These fibres appeared to be well equipped for aerobic metabolism and hence for prolonged activity.

A second type was a complete contrast. It had a fast twitch, commonly developed large tensions and was susceptible to fatigue; the fibres had low contents of mitochondrial enzymes, were rich in glycogen, stained strongly for myosin ATPase and had a poor capillary network. These fibres were suited for anaerobic metabolism and could engage in brief contractions.

A third type had intermediate properties. It had a fast twitch, developed moderate tensions, and was resistant to fatigue. The muscle fibres had high contents of glycogen and mitochondrial enzymes and had considerable myosin ATPase activity; they were well supplied with capillaries. These fibres would be expected to work under both aerobic and anaerobic conditions and were therefore likely to be involved in prolonged work as well as in intense effort.

Burke and colleagues termed the three types of motor unit S (slowly contracting), FF (fast contracting, fast fatigue) and FR (fast contracting, fatigue resistant) respectively. The recognition that there are two types of fast-twitch fibre, one of which is rich in most types of enzyme (and pre-

sumably myoglobin) may explain the discrepancies between muscle colour and contraction speed noted by Denny-Brown (1929; see above).

In a detailed biochemical investigation, involving

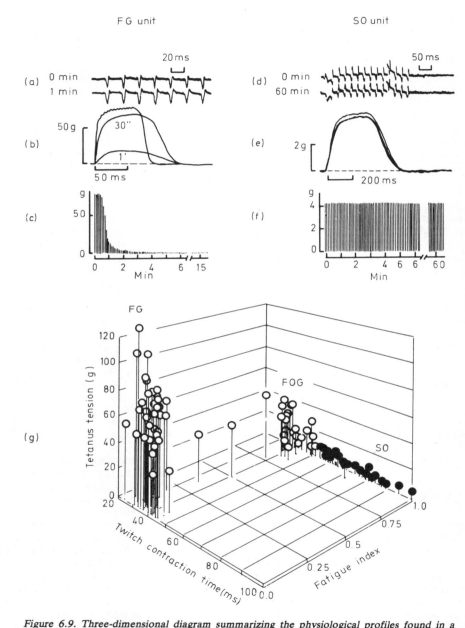

Figure 6.9. Three-dimensional diagram summarizing the physiological profiles found in a sample of 81 medial gastrocnemius muscle units studied in three cats. The motor units have been designated according to the scheme of Peter et al. (1972); see also page 61. The black circles denote type SO units. Modified from Burke et al. (1973), courtesy of the authors and the Editor and publishers of the Journal of Physiology

hind limb muscles of the rabbit and guinea pig, Peter *et al.* (1972) have also recognized three types of fibre. These authors have proposed a different classification and the FF, FR and S units become fast-glycolytic, fast-glycolytic-oxidative and slow-oxidative types respectively (Table 6.4).

In the case of human muscle only Buchthal and his colleagues have attempted to make a systematic correlation between histochemical properties and contractile behaviour. In their studies small bundles of muscle fibres were stimulated and the time-courses of the twitches were recorded by a needle-mounted strain gauge inserted into the tendon. This technique did not enable the responses of single motor units to be analysed but the results were nevertheless important. Buchthal and Schmalbruch (1970) found that long contraction times predominated in muscles which had a large proportion of fibres rich in mitochondria (soleus, gastrocnemius) while short contraction times were common in muscles which consisted mainly of motor units poor in mitochondrial enzymes (lateral head of brachial triceps and platysma).

Also of interest is an isolated observation by Sica and McComas (1971a) on a 44 year old patient with a neuropathy of the Guillain–Barré type (see page 234). A muscle biopsy showed denervation atrophy restricted to type II fibres (i.e. those with high myosin ATPase activity). The surviving motor units, presumably all type I, generated an abnormally slow twitch. Slow twitches have also been observed in patients with partial denervation by Buchthal, Schmalbruch and Kamieniecka (1971a) and in their cases type I muscle fibres tended to predominate.

CLASSIFICATIONS OF FIBRE TYPES

So far three classifications for mammalian striated muscle fibres have been mentioned, all of which feature three types of fibre. The scheme of Brooke and Kaiser (1970) was based solely on the myosin ATPase staining reaction and divided the fibres into types I, IIA and IIB. The advantage of this scheme is that it is unambiguous and makes no inferences about muscle fibre properties not tested directly; it suffers in that it is not descriptive and that it gives an incomplete specification of a muscle fibre. There is little doubt that clinicians will prefer to use this scheme for the interpretation of human biopsy material; it is simple and it is already widely used.

The FF, FR and S classification of Burke and colleagues (1971; page 59) is based on the most thorough examination of muscle fibre and motor unit properties yet undertaken. Although the scheme is descriptive, it does not utilize all the information available, being based only in the contractile behaviour of the fibres. Thus, it is necessary to remember that the FF fibres probably exhibit their 'fast-fatigue' property because their glycogen is quickly depleted during repetitive activity.

In the scheme of Peter and colleagues (1972) the fibres are termed 'fast-twitch-glycolytic', 'fast-twitch-oxidative-glycolytic' or 'slow-twitch-oxidative'. This classification has much to commend it. It has the advantages of completeness and flexibility; because it is open-ended it leaves room for any fresh type of fibre to be incorporated at a later date. The possible objection to its clumsiness can be overcome by making appropriate abbreviations (to FG, FOG and SO).

In addition to the three classifications described above, several others have been devised and have found substantial use in the past; these schemes are included in Table 6.4. Now that much more is understood about muscle fibre properties and the way in which some are interrelated, it is to be hoped that one scheme will eventually be selected as being the most appropriate and will find universal application. In the meantime we shall assume an ambivalent posture by making simultaneous use of the classification of Peter *et al.* (1972; the best?) and that of Brooke and Kaiser (1970; the most convenient?).

FIBRE TYPE CONVERSION

Before leaving the subject of motor unit types one very important and fascinating qualification must be made. It now appears that the contractile and histochemical properties of some of the fibres are not fixed but instead can be changed by the amount of use made of those units. For example, if a 'fast' muscle, such as the cat flexor digitorum longus, is made to undergo repetitive activity by prolonged electrical stimulation of its nerve at 10 Hz, there is a very marked slowing of its twitch (Salmons and Vrbová, 1969). An alternative approach has been to 'over-load' muscles by either tenotomizing or denervating their synergists. In this way Lesch *et al.* (1968) were able to induce acute hypertrophy of the rat soleus; considerable slowing of the twitch and maximal rate of tension development was observed. Paradoxically, although the muscle fibres were enlarged and contained additional myofibrils, they actually developed less tension per unit cross-sectional area than controls; the same phenomenon is observed transiently after denervation of the diaphragm. One problem in such hypertrophy experiments is that new muscle fibres may form by longitudinal fission (e.g. Hall-Craggs, 1970) and thereby alter the proportions of the various types present. In other recent studies using a similar strategy it has been shown that the histochemistry of the muscle fibres may also change. Thus, in the overloaded rat soleus muscle Guth and Yellin (1971) were able to demonstrate that

reduced the activity of a slow muscle and caused speeding of the twitch. In related experiments Guth and Wells (1972) showed that reducing the functional demand on a soleus muscle (by denervation of its antagonists) not only caused the twitch to quicken but increased the proportion of muscle fibres with strong myosin ATPase activity (i.e.

TABLE 6.4

Histochemistry, Contractile Properties and Structural Features of the Three Types of Mammalian Muscle Fibre

	Fast-twitch-* oxidative- glycolytic (FOG)	Fast-twitch-* glycolytic (FG)	Slow-twitch-* oxidative (SO)
General features			
Red coloration	Dark	Pale	Dark
Myoglobin	High	Low	High
Capillary network	Rich	Poor	Rich
Mitochondria	Many, large	Few, small	Many, small
Z-line	Wide	Narrow	Intermediate
Fatigue	Resistant	Sensitive	Very resistant
Staining intensity			
PAS (glycogen)	High	High	Low
Phosphorylase	High	High	Low
Myosin ATPase	High	High	Low
Malate dehydrogenase	High	Low	Intermediate
Succinic dehydrogenase	High	Low	Intermediate
Other terminologies			
Dubowitz and Pearse (1960) Engel (1962)	II	II	I
Brooke and Kaiser (1970)	IIA	IIB	I
Yellin and Guth (1970)	$\alpha\beta$	α	β
Stein and Padykula (1962)	C	A	B
Padykula and Gauthier (1966)	Red	White	Intermediate
Burke et al. (1971)	FR	FF	S

* Classification of Peter et al. (1972).

the small type II population had been changed to type I fibres. In the studies by Barnard, Edgerton and Peter (1970a, b) guinea pigs were made to undergo exercise of the 'endurance' type by causing them to run on a treadmill. After 18 weeks the twitch characteristics of fibres were unaltered but the fibres were less susceptible to fatigue; in keeping with these observations there was an increase in the proportion of fibres rich in mitochondria but no change had occurred in the myosin ATPase staining reaction of the muscle. In terms of the various muscle fibre classification schemes (Table 6.4) one type of fibre (IIB: FF; fast-twitch-glycolytic) had been converted to another (IIA; FR; fast-twitch-oxidative-glycolytic). As might be expected the converse experiment has also been performed; thus tenotomy (Vrbová, 1963) or joint immobilization (Fischbach and Robbins, 1969)

type II). These and other observations are discussed further in Chapter 9; their importance is that they provide a partial solution to a question which should have been asked before, namely: 'How is it that a single nerve fibre is connected only to muscle fibres with similar histochemical and contractile properties?' The surprising answer is that these special properties are ultimately imposed on the muscle fibres by the 'trophic' action of the motoneurones. The precise mechanism by which such trophic action is exerted will be pursued in the next two chapters; it will be shown that most experimental situations are more complex than they might appear to be and that multiple factors are usually operating. For the present, the important point is that the contractile and biochemical properties of a motor unit are not static but are always being modulated by the type and amount of use to which the muscle is subjected.

Chapter 7

EXERCISE AND FATIGUE

RECRUITMENT OF UNITS

How are the motor units used during voluntary or reflex contractions? The very fact that the units exhibit such striking differences amongst themselves in terms of size, speed of contraction and biochemistry, suggests that their involvement is unlikely to be random but suited to the task demanded of them. Indeed, as we have already seen, to some extent the task will shape the unit.

The earliest study in man appears to be that of Adrian and Bronk (1929) who were able to record the activity of single motor units by means of a fine wire positioned within, but insulated from, a hypodermic needle (*Figure 6.1*). This device was the first concentric EMG electrode and it is interesting that electrodes manufactured to the same simple design have been the mainstay of clinical electromyography ever since. Adrian and Bronk found that their subjects were able to increase the force of their muscle contractions by raising the firing frequency of the motoneurones and by calling additional motor units into activity ('recruitment'). Since this important study there have been many investigations of firing rate in which a variety of fine electrodes have been used to distinguish the activities of single motor units (see, for example, Lindsley, 1935; Bigland and Lippold, 1954; Petajan and Philip, 1969). Because of the large movements of the muscle fibres which take place during muscle contraction some workers have preferred to introduce the fine recording wires through a hypodermic needle and then to withdraw the latter, allowing the wires to flex with the distortions of the muscle belly. From all these

studies it is evident that the motor units have different thresholds for recruitment, with some units coming in during weak contractions and others only involved in more forceful effort. In addition, however, each unit has the ability to modulate its firing frequency. Two issues have been of particular interest to investigators. One of these is the range of impulse firing frequencies of which motoneurones (and hence motor units) are capable. The second is the relative importance of changes in impulse firing rate and of recruitment of fresh units during the development of increasingly large muscle forces. In relation to the first topic, most workers are agreed that the minimum firing frequency for a unit during a *steady* contraction is about 5–10 Hz (impulses/s; *Figure 7.1, upper*). It is over the maximum frequency that disagreement has been evident, with some investigations reporting rates as high as 140 Hz (Norris and Gasteiger, 1955) and others insisting on much lower values (Dasgupta and Simpson, 1962).

One of the factors which may have contributed to the differences in experimental results is the speed of contraction. Tanji and Kato (1972) have found that a motoneurone will discharge at a much higher rate if a given tension is to be reached rapidly rather than slowly; they observed many units which could fire initially at rates as high as 70–90 Hz. Similar high rates were also noted by Marsden, Meadows and Merton (1971) who made use of the anomalous innervation of some units within the adductor pollicis by median nerve fibres. On blocking the major innervation (ulnar nerve) with local anaesthesia, the activity of single (median nerve) units could be followed even during maximum contraction. From these last two studies it is clear that units can fire at rates of 100 Hz or more but only at the start of a voluntary contraction; by 30 s the rate has declined to 20 Hz or so.

A less convincing answer has been obtained concerning the relative importance of firing rate and

mined (*Figure 7.2, top*). The method is simple but effective; its drawbacks are that only repetitively discharging units can be analysed in this way and that, in the case of slowly contracting units, the twitches will be partially fused and therefore distorted. The authors concluded that only at

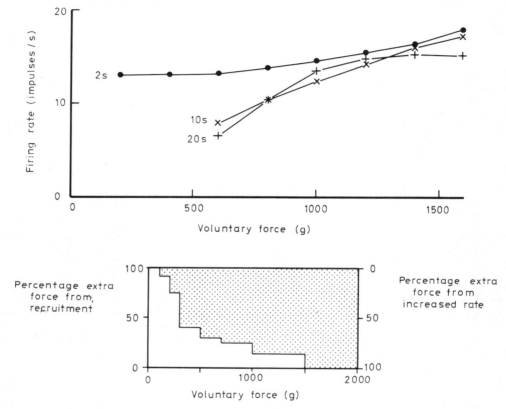

Figure 7.1. (Upper) The rise in firing rate of a motor unit in the human first dorsal interosseous muscle during increasingly forceful contraction. Note that the discharge frequency is also dependent on the speed of movement; in this experiment the highest initial firing rate was obtained during the most rapidly executed movement (lasting two seconds). (Lower) The relative importance of recruitment of additional motor units and of increase in firing frequency, during increasingly strong contractions. Same subject as for Figure 7.2 (lower). Modified from Milner-Brown et al. (1973b), courtesy of the authors and of the Editor and publishers of the Journal of Physiology

recruitment of units during graded contractions. Milner-Brown, Stein and Yemm (1973a, b) used fine electrodes to distinguish the activities of single motor units in the human first dorsal interosseous muscle during steady contractions of different intensities. On every occasion that the unit fired an action potential the tension developed by the muscle was recorded during the period immediately following and successive values were averaged. By improving the signal-to-noise ratio in this way the tension contributed by a single motor unit could be recognized and the time-course of its twitch deter-

low levels of force was recruitment the major mechanism. Increased firing rate became the more important mechanism at intermediate force levels and so contributed the large majority of force if the entire physiological range was considered (*Figure 7.1, lower*). The authors pointed out that this conclusion closely resembled Adrian and Bronk's original view. Milner-Brown and colleagues (1973a) also showed that recruitment was orderly with the smallest units having the lowest thresholds and the largest units the highest (*Figure 7.2, lower*); in addition the smallest units

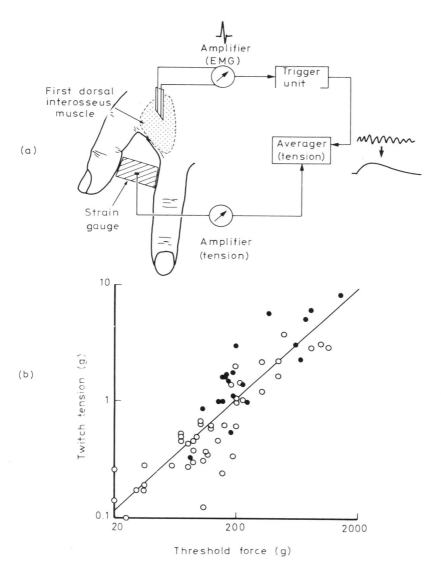

Figure 7.2 (Upper) Experimental arrangement used by Milner-Brown et al. (1973a, b) for detecting the force developed by a single motor unit during voluntary contraction. The action potential of the motor unit is distinguished and used to trigger an averager which then samples the muscle tension. By repeating the process many times the contribution of the unit can be recognized from among the activity of all the other units. (Lower) Proportional relationship between the force developed by a motor unit and its threshold for recruitment. From Milner-Brown et al. (1973a), courtesy of the authors and of the Editor and publishers of the Journal of Physiology

tended to have the slowest twitches. In the study by Clamann (1970) it was observed that the low-threshold units were situated deeply within the brachial biceps muscle belly whereas the higher-threshold units lay nearer the surface. In paraplegic patients Grimby and Hannerz (1970) have been able to show that in sustained ('tonic') reflexes there is also an orderly recruitment of motor units, irrespective of whether the stimulus is a cutaneous one or due to muscle stretch.

exposed for biopsy. The biopsy was then taken from the tissue surrounding the electrode. By using partially-denervated muscles with prominent collateral reinnervation it was possible to be sure of the identity of the previously active unit. It was found that the units firing briefly, and sometimes only during extreme effort (i.e. 'phasic' units), were of type II histochemically. In contrast, the units which could fire regularly for prolonged periods ('tonic' units) were invariably of type I.

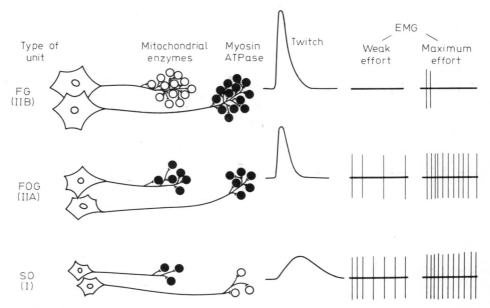

Figure 7.3. The three types of motor unit showing their differences in size, biochemical activity, twitch speed and ease of recruitment (see text)

The neurophysiological situation becomes more complex when brief movements, or the initial phases of contractions, are considered. Irrespective of whether the movement is volitional (Basmajian, 1963) or a phasic reflex (Grimby and Hannerz, 1970) the recruitment order may vary. Furthermore, there are a few units which will only fire on extreme effort, and even then may restrict their discharge to very short trains of impulses (Hannerz, 1974). Such units are well known to clinical electromyographers and their recognition during a full interference pattern is only possible because of their large action potentials. The sizes of their potentials suggests that these units belong to the FG (IIA) category and this has recently been confirmed by Warmolts and Engel (1972). These authors recorded motor unit activity from the superficial part of a muscle which had been

The finding of such contrasting behaviour suggested that the distinction between the two types of units was real, reflecting persisting differences in motoneurone excitability, and was not simply a result of the partial denervation. An interesting refinement of the discharge pattern of motoneurones has recently been described by Zajac and Young (1975) in decerebrate cats made to walk on a treadmill. The authors observed that during each step the flexor and extensor motoneurones commenced firing with 'doublets'; that is, the second impulse of each train followed quickly upon the first. A functional advantage of this manœuvre was that the first two twitches would make a good summation and bring the motor unit tension rapidly towards the tetanic level (see *Figure 5.10*) where it would stay for the remainder of the discharge.

Also of importance in the consideration of

motor unit activity are the studies by Gollnick, Piehl and Saltin (1974); and Gollnick *et al.* (1974); these authors exercised volunteers on a bicycle or else made them sustain isometric contractions of the quadriceps muscles. Specimens of muscle were taken at intervals using a needle biopsy technique (Bergstrom, 1962) and were stained histochemically. By correlating the presence of glycogen depletion with the staining reaction of the fibres for myosin ATPase, it was possible to determine whether type I or type II fibres had been employed in the exercise. Gollnick and colleagues referred to these as 'slow-twitch' and 'fast-twitch' fibres respectively, ignoring the fact that there are two types of fast-twitch fibre (i.e. FG and FOG fibres; see Table 6.4). In the cycling exercise it was found that slow-twitch (SO) fibres were the first to become depleted of glycogen at all workloads requiring less than the maximal oxygen consumption. At 'supramaximal' levels, when the oxygen uptake was insufficient and anaerobic metabolism also took place, the fast-twitch (FG and FOG) fibres were also involved. In the static exercise experiments the findings were similar. At isometric contractions of less than 20 per cent of maximum force, there was preferential use of the slow-twitch (SO) fibres. At higher forces, however, the fast-twitch (FG and FOG) fibres were the first to lose glycogen, suggesting that these had been most active. Thus, in both types of exercise—pedalling and sustained contraction—the slow-twitch (SO) fibres were used for weak contraction, the fast-twitch (FG, FOG) ones being reserved for greater effort.

In the bushbaby, *Galago senegalensis*, differential employment of motor units has been demonstrated in contrasting types of exercise also (Gillespie, Simpson and Edgerton, 1974). In steady exercise of moderate intensity (running) histochemical studies showed that greatest use had been made of the slow-twitch-oxidative (SO) fibres. Intermittent activity requiring maximal effort (jumping) made greatest demands on the fast-twitch-glycolytic (FG) fibres. The fast-twitch-oxidative-glycolytic (FOG) fibres were also used in both types of exercise, their levels of activity being intermediate to those of the FG and SO fibres.

Having now surveyed both the animal and the human studies it is possible to summarize the biochemical and functional properties of the three types of fibre diagrammatically. In *Figure 7.3* it can be seen that the SO units have slow twitches, are rich in mitochondria, stain poorly for myosin ATPase, and are recruited during weak effort. It should be noted that these units contain more fibres than their relatively small tensions would

indicate; the reason for this is that each SO fibre develops considerably less force in relation to its cross-sectional area than the fibres of the other two types (Burke and Tsairis, 1973). At the other extreme are the FG units which are large and have fast twitches, few mitochondria and strong myosin ATPase staining activity. These units are reserved for extreme effort and even then may be unable to sustain their discharges. In between these two types in their contractile and biochemical properties are the FOG units.

MECHANISM OF RECRUITMENT

It is, of course, functionally advantageous for the largest units to be reserved for extreme effort for they would impart marked unevenness to a weak contraction (as in an unfused tetanus). But how is the order of recruitment established? Henneman, Somjen and Carpenter (1965) have suggested a simple explanation which is based on a *size principle*. Thus, the smallest alpha-motoneurones in the ventral horn are likely to correspond to the smallest motor units since the metabolic activity of a motoneurone is probably proportional to the number of muscle fibres which it is required to maintain through its trophic action. Suppose that the motoneurone pool receives an excitatory input from the motor cortex and that roughly the same number of synapses are activated on all the motoneurones. The density of the synaptic current flowing between the excitatory synapses on a motoneurone and the axon hillock will differ among the motoneurones. The smallest cells will have the highest densities because the current is concentrated in a smaller membrane area. A large current density will, in turn, produce a correspondingly large depolarization, and so the smallest cells should have the lowest thresholds for excitation. The 'cell size' hypothesis can be tested experimentally by impaling motoneurones with microelectrodes and measuring their input resistances during a current pulse; the input resistance of a motoneurone will be inversely proportional to its size (page 19). It turns out that although the largest axons arise from the largest motoneurones, as predicted (Burke, 1967), they do not necessarily supply the largest colonies of muscle fibres, at least in the large muscles of the cat hind limb (Stephens and Stuart, 1975; but see Bagust, 1974); in the small distal muscles a better correlation exists. On the basis of these observations it would appear that motoneurone size cannot be the sole factor determining excitation threshold during voluntary or reflex contractions.

FATIGUE

Central or peripheral?

It is an everyday experience that the force developed during a maximum voluntary contraction cannot be maintained indefinitely but declines rather rapidly. In muscles of the human hand, for example, some 50 per cent of force is lost within the first minute (Merton, 1954). This reduction in strength is termed *fatigue* and the nature of the underlying mechanisms has attracted much attention.

As a first step, it is obviously important to distinguish between 'central' and 'peripheral' fatigue processes. Central fatigue would occur if the membranes of some of the alpha-motoneurones could no longer be depolarized to firing threshold by descending inputs from the brain. A central

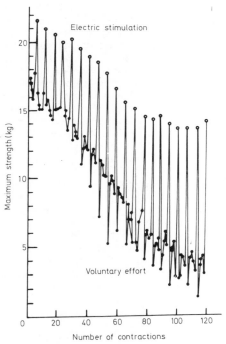

Figure 7.4. Maximal strength of the human adductor pollicis muscle measured during the course of 120 maximal voluntary contractions; note the progressive fatigue. When the muscle is activated by supramaximal stimulation of the ulnar nerve, much larger contractions are observed. This effect demonstrates that much of the fatigue 'process' is situated centrally (within the central nervous system). From Ikai et al. (1967), courtesy of the authors and of the Editor and publishers of Sportarzt Sportmed

mechanism seems plausible for two reasons. First, it is a common subjective experience that the mental 'effort' associated with a maximal contraction rapidly wanes. Secondly, motoneurones exhibit such a range in thresholds during voluntary contractions as to suggest that it might be difficult to maintain the excitability of the highest threshold units. It is therefore rather surprising that in the elegant study of Merton (1954) evidence for central fatigue was not found. This author made maximal contractions of the adductor pollicis muscle (usually his own) and, during this time, delivered a supramaximal stimulus to the ulnar nerve. If some of the motor units had been inactive due to quiescence of their motoneurones, they would have been excited nonetheless by the electrical stimulus to their axons and would have developed an increment of tension in the force recording. The fact that no extra tension could be detected led Merton to conclude that the entire motoneurone pool was participating in the contraction and that the site of the fatigue must lie peripherally. However, the matter cannot be considered settled since Ikai, Yabe and Ischii (1967) repeated Merton's experiments and were unable to confirm all his findings. In particular, they obtained evidence that some motoneurones had ceased firing during fatigue (*Figure 7.4*). In spite of this disagreement it would still appear that a large, and perhaps the major, contribution to fatigue comes from a failure of the peripheral neuromuscular apparatus.

Peripheral fatigue processes

In theory, the peripheral fatigue process demonstrated by Merton could involve any or all of the following factors:

(1) Presynaptic failure, due to an inability of the nerve impulse to invade the axon terminal.
(2) Synaptic failure, caused by insufficient depolarization of muscle receptors by acetylcholine.
(3) Muscle fibre action potential failure.
(4) Excitation–contraction uncoupling.
(5) Failure of the contractile machinery.

Since all of these factors have been incriminated in fatigue, the evidence for each will be reviewed critically.

Presynaptic failure

In an *in vitro* study Krnjević and Miledi (1958) made intracellular recordings of end-plate potentials in muscle fibres of the rat diaphragm following stimulation of the phrenic nerve. By stimulating single axons and recording with two microelectrodes they were able to compare the responses in two fibres belonging to the same motor unit. On some occasions they found that a normal sized end-plate potential in one fibre was not associated with any detectable response in the other fibre. This type of defect could best be explained by a failure of the impulse to invade the axon terminal. A similar defect is now known to occur in mice with hereditary motor end-plate disease (Duchen and Stefani, 1971). In Krnjević and Miledi's (1958) experiments it was found that the conduction failure was very sensitive to anoxia but it is difficult to escape the conclusion that this susceptibility may have been induced by the *in vitro* conditions of the experiment. Thus when single cat motoneurones were stimulated *in vivo* Burke et al. (1973) found that the summated muscle fibre action potentials showed no significant decrement, even after as many as 47 000 stimuli. Presumably the intact blood supply in the latter experiments was able to maintain the preterminal axon in satisfactory condition.

Synaptic failure

A number of investigators have shown that the liberation of acetylcholine from motor nerve terminals is markedly reduced during the course of repetitive stimulation. In the experiments of Brooks and Thies (1962), for example, the number of acetylcholine quanta (page 31) was depressed by about one third within seconds of starting stimulation at a frequency as low as 2 Hz. This experiment was carried out on the serratus anterior muscle of the guinea pig but, as in the case of the presynaptic failure considered above, the function of the neuromuscular junction may have been affected adversely by the *in vitro* nature of the experiment. The prolonged electrical responsiveness of the motor units studied by Burke and colleagues (1973) in the cat gastrocnemius muscle provides equally telling evidence against synaptic failure as against a presynaptic disorder.

Muscle fibre action potential failure

It is known that the giant axon of the squid can continue to propagate action potentials for long periods even when virtually all the axoplasm has been extruded (see page 23) and it would be surprising if the membrane of an intact muscle fibre were any less efficient. Yet there is strong evidence that, under certain circumstances, the muscle fibre membrane may no longer be excitable even though the fibre remains capable of twitching. Some of the relevant experiments are those of Lüttgau (1965) who isolated single fibres of the frog and stimulated them *in vitro*. Lüttgau found that, at a stimulation rate of 100 Hz, some action potentials began to drop out within 2 s (see also Ramsay and Street, 1942). Rather unexpectedly Lüttgau found that if stimulation was given at *lower* rates until the fibre became exhausted and could twitch no longer, the action potential mechanism recovered. Membrane excitability was also maintained if the contractile responses were abolished by metabolic inhibitors such as sodium cyanide and iodoacetate, or by immersing the fibre in a hypertonic bathing solution. Lüttgau concluded that the fatigue of the action potential mechanism was caused by reactions connected with contraction of the muscle fibre. Interesting though this phenomenon is, it may have little relevance to mammalian muscle *in vivo* since Burke and colleagues (1973) found no evidence of significant muscle action potential failure in their experiments involving prolonged stimulation.

Excitation–contraction coupling and the contractile machinery

A further possible cause of fatigue is failure of the excitation–contraction coupling or of the contractile machinery itself. In contrast to the other possibilities considered above, there is very good evidence from experiments on man and laboratory animals that one or the other does occur under natural, or relatively natural, conditions. In one of a meticulously-contrived series of experiments, Merton (1954) recorded the twitch and action-potential responses of the human adductor pollicis muscle immediately after a maximum voluntary contraction which had proceeded to fatigue. The crucial observation was that, at a time when the twitch was still greatly reduced, the evoked action potentials retained a normal amplitude. These important observations have now been extended at the level of the single motor unit by Burke and colleagues (1973). In the cat gastrocnemius muscle they found that the tensions developed by some motor units fell to about 20 per cent of the original value within one minute of intermittent tetanic stimulation at 200 Hz. They classified such units as 'fast twitch, fatigue sensitive' (types FF and FG in Table 6.4) and were able to show that the action potentials in the exhausted fibres were hardly altered. Neither of these experiments could distinguish between a failure of excitation–contraction coupling and one of the contractile machinery. To do so requires a different approach which has yet to be extended to mammalian muscle *in vivo*. In the frog, however, Eberstein and Sandow (1963) treated isolated muscle fibres which had been stimulated to exhaustion with either 0.1 M potassium chloride solution or with caffeine and found that under both circumstances contractures resulted and normal tension could be recorded; this result implicated a fault in the coupling system.

It is possible that faulty excitation–contraction coupling also underlies the early fatigue of the FG motor unit fibres studied by Burke *et al.* (1973) though neither ultrastructural nor biochemical investigations provide any indication as to why this should be so. Thus, Eisenberg (1974) has found that the T-tubular system actually has a greater surface area in fibres of the white vastus (FG) than of soleus (SO); the lateral sacs of the sarcoplasmic reticulum are also larger in the former type of fibre. In addition the FG fibres, although so easily fatigued, are much more efficient at pumping calcium ions back into the sarcoplasmic reticulum, exhibiting rates four times as high as those of the SO fibres (Fiehn and Peter, 1971). An alternative possibility is that the contractile machinery can no longer respond to the fibre action potential because the immediate sources of energy have been exhausted. The fact that the FG fibres are most readily depleted of glycogen by tetanic stimulation, as shown by PAS staining, may well be relevant since there are no alternative fuels available for the synthesis of ATP in these fibres.

depleted of glycogen, in keeping with the findings of Burke *et al.* (1973) in tetanically-stimulated single motor units (see Table 6.4 for correlation of fibre types).

It is likely for other reasons that the experimental results of Burke and colleagues (1973) on the cat gastrocnemius are relevant to the human situation. Using intermittent trains of stimuli at 40 Hz, these workers had found that the tetanic tension of an FG unit could fall by about 80 per cent within the first minute. Since these units produced the largest initial tensions, and since 40 Hz is within the physiological range of motoneurone discharge frequencies (see page 63), their failure could well account for much of the 50 per cent reduction in strength observed in the first minute during maximal voluntary contractions by Merton (1954) and Stephens and Taylor (1972).

Nevertheless, the presence of complete ischaemia in an isometrically contracted muscle does raise the possibility that other factors may be operating in addition to the fatigue susceptibility of the FG units. One such factor may be synaptic or presynaptic failure for Stephens and Taylor (1972) found an early decline in the maximal evoked muscle action potential of the human first dorsal interosseous muscle. This finding is at variance with that of Merton (1954) in the adductor pollicis, in which the action potential amplitude remained unchanged. Stephens and Taylor suggest that Merton may have been recording from muscles other than the fatigued adductor but the problem remains unsettled and further investigation appears warranted.

Effects of muscle ischaemia

The foregoing experiments provide much additional information about the nature of the steps linking the nerve fibre impulse to the contraction of the muscle fibre, but of those experiments quoted only Merton's (1954) were carried out on human muscles during maximum voluntary contraction. This is an important reservation for in real life the conditions may be considerably different from those in the laboratory. The most significant change is that, during isometric contraction of more than 20 per cent maximum power, the arterial blood supply to the exercising muscle is occluded by a rise in intramuscular pressure (Barcroft and Millen, 1939). In the experiments of Edwards, Hill and McDonnell (1972) a pressure as high as 692 mm Hg was recorded in the vastus lateralis muscle of one subject. Gollnick *et al.* (1974) have shown that in maximal isometric contractions the type II (FG, FOG) fibres are still the first to be

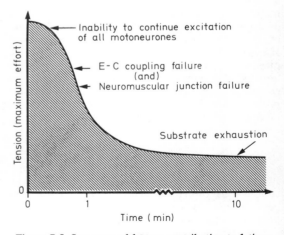

Figure 7.5. Summary of factors contributing to fatigue during maximum effort (see text)

Conclusions

At present the best summary of the results is to suggest that fatigue can occur as the result of several mechanisms and that their relative importance depends partly on the nature of the motor unit and partly on the stage which has been reached during the exercise (*Figure 7.5*). In the first few seconds of exercise loss of motoneurone recruitment appears important; subsequently, a failure of excitation–contraction or of the contractile machinery becomes the limiting factor in the fast-twitch glycolytic (FG) fibres. In isometric contractions, or in other circumstances in which the arterial blood supply is compromised, additional fatigue mechanisms may appear and cause a failure of neuromuscular transmission. Finally, in the late stages of exercise, exhaustion can result when supplies of energy are no longer available; that is when the muscle fibre glycogen has been depleted and reserve sources of fuel (blood glucose and free fatty acids) have been used up.

FATIGUE IN NEUROMUSCULAR DISEASES

Patients with neuromuscular disease invariably complain that they tire easily. Analysis of this important symptom is hampered by a dearth of detailed information, except perhaps for myasthenia gravis which has been considered separately (Chapter 18). Intuitively one would expect that the various types of disease process might affect the neuromuscular apparatus differently. For example, in 'dying-back' neuropathies the action potential might fail to invade the preterminal axon or else insufficient acetylcholine might be released by the impulse (presynaptic failure). In a microelectrode study of rats treated with acrylamide Swift and Lambert (1974) were able to show that, in fact, there was a reduced pool of acetylcholine quanta available for release from the axon terminal (see page 31). It is not surprising therefore that decremental muscle responses to repetitive nerve stimulation are observed in a proportion of patients with motoneurone disease (amyotrophic lateral sclerosis); as in myasthenia gravis, there is often an improvement with anticholinesterase therapy (Mudler, Lambert and Eaton, 1959). Similar decremental responses have been found in poliomyelitis (Hodes, 1948), peripheral neuropathies (Baginsky, 1968; Miglietta, 1971), and in hemiplegic atrophy (McComas et al., 1973b). In each of these disorders the lower motoneurone is affected and it is tempting to suppose that the electrophysiological findings reflect functional abnormalities in presynaptic neuromuscular function secondary to impaired axoplasmic flow (page 12). Although this explanation may be proved correct, the present findings do not exclude the presence of a postsynaptic defect as a cause of the observed abnormalities since decremental responses have also been seen in some patients with muscular dystrophy (McComas, Campbell and Sica, 1971; Sica and McComas, 1971b) and in myotonia congenita (Brown, 1974). Finally, although the mechanism is not known, neuromuscular failure has also been noted in multiple sclerosis (Patten, Hart and Lovelace, 1972).

In those neuromuscular diseases in which muscle fibre degeneration is the dominant feature, the muscle fibre action potential, coupling mechanism or contractile machinery might become the limiting factor responsible for fatigue. In the study by Desmedt et al. (1968), the contractile responses were disproportionately small in relation to the evoked muscle action potential in the adductor pollicis muscles of boys with Duchenne muscular dystrophy. These authors interpreted their data as indicating loss of contractile proteins or else interference with the activation of the myofilaments. Similar defects would account for Lenman's (1959) finding that, in patients with polymyositis or muscular dystrophy, isometric voluntary strength was small in comparison with the integrated EMG activity recorded with surface electrodes. Earlier reports that the muscles of dystrophic mice were unusually *resistant* to fatigue (Sandow and Brust, 1958; Eberstein and Sandow, 1963) now appear unfounded and the observed results have been dismissed as an *in vitro* artefact by Hofmann and Ruprecht (1973).

Chapter 8

TROPHIC INTERACTIONS OF NERVE AND MUSCLE: DENERVATION AND REINNERVATION

MUSCLE DENERVATION

If the nerve to a muscle is severed, the muscle will gradually waste over a period of weeks. This process is termed *denervation atrophy*; it is a demonstration that the muscle fibres are dependent upon the motoneurone for the maintenance of their normal structure. This sustaining action of nerve on muscle is described as *trophic*; it will be shown later that the trophic influence is mutual since the motoneurone is itself affected by the muscle fibres to which it is connected. Other sections of this chapter describe the characteristics of the denervated muscle fibre and the results of cross-innervation studies. In the next chapter descriptions are given of the changes induced in muscle fibres by excessive activity of moto-neurones or by disuse; the mechanism of this trophic influence will also be considered.

Gross structural changes

The gross changes which take place in a muscle following denervation have been studied on many occasions (see, for example, Tower, 1939; Sunderland and Ray, 1950; Adams, Denny-Brown and Pearson, 1962). The changes which take place probably involve every part of the muscle fibre.

Muscle fibre atrophy

The most obvious change in the muscle following denervation is its reduction in size. This atrophy can be first detected at about the third day and is most rapid in the ensuing 2 months. At the end of this period only 20–40 per cent of the original muscle mass remains (Sunderland and Ray, 1950); much of this will be connective tissue since this accounts for 10–25 per cent of the initial muscle weight. Although further atrophy may occur it is now a much slower process. According to Stonnington and Engel (1973) the denervation atrophy affects red and white fibres equally throughout. It is of interest that in the hemi-diaphragm denervation atrophy is preceded by a 1–2 week phase of hyper-trophy, in which the cross-sectional area of the fibres is almost doubled and new myofibrils are formed (Miledi and Slater, 1969). This curious response is apparently due to excessive stretch of the denervated half of the diaphragm by the con-tractions of the innervated remainder (see page 80).

Myonuclei

As early as the second day after denervation the myonuclei start to become rounded instead of narrow and elongated; at the same time the nucleoli become enlarged and more prominent. Many of the nuclei then move into the centres of the fibres where they may line up to form chains. There is dispute as to whether the number of nuclei actually increases; it is accepted that much of the apparent preponderance of the nuclei is due to their preservation within atrophying fibres but a true increase has also been reported (Bowden and Gutmann, 1944). In late atrophy (e.g. 6 months) all that remains of some fibres are chains or clumps of nuclei surrounded by thin cylinders of cytoplasm.

Degeneration

In addition to the changes described above, which are those of 'simple' atrophy, a variable proportion of the muscle fibres undergo degenerative changes after several months have elapsed. These changes are probably irreversible and may result in the death of the fibre; not uncommonly they are restricted to part of a fibre. The affected fibres swell; the nuclei also enlarge and then begin to fragment. Vacuoles appear in the cytoplasm of the fibre; elsewhere the sarcoplasm stains darkly because of increased basophilia. The cross-striations become less distinct and the sarcolemma thickens before disintegrating. Mononuclear cells appear at the site of necrosis and subject the accumulating fibre debris to phagocytosis. Complete destruction of the muscle fibre may eventually occur.

Connective tissue

As the muscle fibres atrophy or degenerate the connective tissue within the muscle becomes increasingly prominent with large fat cells occupying spaces between the surviving fibres and fibre bundles.

Ultrastructural changes

Several excellent studies have been published of the fine structure of the denervated muscle fibre, as examined with the electronmicroscope (Pellegrino and Franzini, 1963; Miledi and Slater, 1969; Stonnington and Engel, 1973); of these the account by Stonnington and Engel is notable for the measurements of cross-sectional areas of the various fibre organelles (*Figure 8.1*). In this last study the soleus and superficial medial gastrocnemius muscles of rats were studied between 1 and 84 days after section of the sciatic nerve. During the period of atrophy the change in fibre area was matched throughout by a fall in the mean area of the myofibrils. The atrophy began at the periphery of the myofibrils but after the first month degeneration was also visible in the interior of the myofibrils. During the first week the mitochondria in both red and white fibres enlarged in the longitudinal axis of the fibre. Subsequently these organelles shrank and formed clusters; some mitochondria underwent frank degeneration and inclusion in autophagic vacuoles. Similarly the sarcoplasmic reticulum at first enlarged and then diminished, though to a lesser extent than the fibre itself. Other changes observed with the electron-

microscope included abnormalities of the Z-disc, irregularities and small papillary projections of the sarcolemma, and focal dilatations of the transverse and sarcoplasmic tubules. Increased numbers of ribosomes were found in between the myofibrils and under the surface membrane.

Biochemical and histochemical changes

There have been several studies of the effect of denervation on the biochemical and histochemical properties of muscle and those of Romanul and Hogan (1965) and of Hogan, Dawson and Romanul (1965) are particularly thorough. These authors found that in rat calf muscles there was a rapid decrease in the high enzyme activities typical of a particular type of fibre; as a result fibre types could no longer be distinguished. In addition the red muscle fibres (as in soleus) became paler, partly due to a reduction in myoglobin concentration.

Contractile changes

Even though the nerve supply to a muscle may have been interrupted it is still possible to stimulate the muscle directly. As would be expected, the tensions developed during a single twitch or during a tetanus are reduced, for the muscle will be undergoing denervation atrophy and will have lost some of its

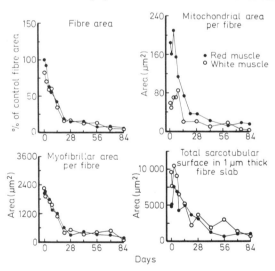

Figure 8.1. Quantitative changes in 'red' (soleus) and 'white' (superficial medial gastrocnemius) muscle fibres of the rat following denervation (see text). (From Stonnington and Engel (1973) courtesy of the authors; reprinted from Neurology by the New York Times Media Company, Inc.

myofibrils (see above). In addition, however, the twitch becomes significantly slower and this is true for a 'slow' muscle such as soleus as well as for 'fast' muscles like the flexor hallucis longus (FHL) and flexor digitorum longus. Lewis (1972) has shown that the slowing occurs relatively abruptly during the third week of denervation; even in chronically-denervated animals, however, the

Membrane changes

Following denervation important changes take place at the surface of the fibre in addition to those in the fibre interior. The irregularity of the sarcolemma and the development of small papillary projections have already been described; their relationship to the altered electrophysiological

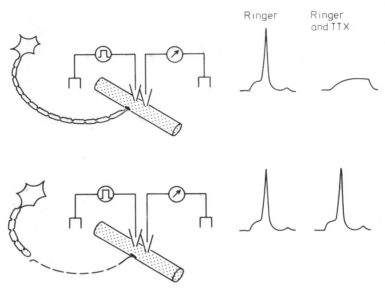

Figure 8.2. The development of tetrodotoxin (TTX) resistance following denervation. At top left is a still innervated muscle fibre which has been impaled by stimulating and recording microelectrodes. In a standard Ringer solution, the fibre responds to direct stimulation with an action potential but, after adding TTX, only an electrotonic potential is seen (top, right). Following denervation, however (lower part) an action potential can be elicited by direct stimulation in the presence of TTX

twitches of the 'fast' muscles remain considerably faster than those of 'slow' muscles studied in control animals. Lewis also found that in both types of muscle the tetanus : twitch ratio fell and that in the FHL, but not in the soleus, the maximum rate of rise of tetanic tension was somewhat diminished. Although some of the slowing of twitch might have been due to a reduction in impulse conduction velocity, the most satisfactory way of reconciling the various findings was to attribute them to an increase and prolongation of 'active state' following a single stimulus (page 41). This, in turn, could have been due to such factors as the increased duration of the muscle fibre action potential and the greater proportion of sarcoplasmic reticulum relative to the myofibril mass in the atrophied fibres.

properties of the sarcolemma described below is uncertain.

(1) The first electrophysiological change which can be detected following denervation is a fall in resting membrane potential at 2 hr. (Albuquerque, Schuh and Kauffman, 1971). This begins at the endplate and spreads outwards, eventually amounting to about 20 mV; it is caused by inhibition of the sodium pump (Bray *et al*, 1976; see also page 23).

(2) The *permeability* of the muscle fibre membrane alters, becoming smaller for both potassium and chloride (Klaus, Lüllmann and Muscholl, 1960; Thesleff, 1963).

(3) The *muscle action potential,* which can be initiated by direct stimulation of the muscle fibre, has a lower rate of rise and a longer duration.

Unlike the situation in a normal fibre, the action potential can still be elicited in the presence of tetrodotoxin (TTX; *Figure 8.2*); this resistance to TTX is first evident at about 36 hr (Harris and Thesleff, 1972). The impulse has a reduced propagation velocity and the refractory period which follows is prolonged.

(4) The sensitivity of the muscle fibre to acetylcholine (ACh), while remaining highest in the end-plate region, after about 24 hr begins to spread this region but not elsewhere. Intracellular recordings have shown that this region of the membrane is electrically unstable, developing spontaneous *oscillations* which may build up and become large enough to initiate action potentials (Purves and Sakmann, 1974; Thesleff and Ward, 1975; see *Figure 8.3, c*). A second type of generator activity consists of irregularly-occurring sudden depolarizations (*fibrillatory origin potentials* or f.o.p.s.). These last potentials are sometimes too

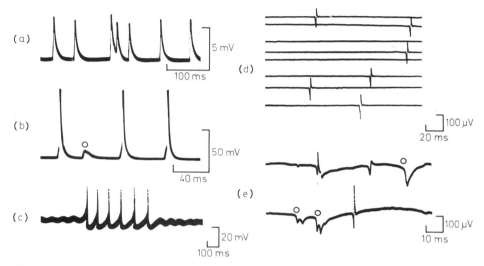

Figure 8.3 Spontaneous electrical activity in denervated muscle fibres (a), (b), and (c) show intra-cellular recordings from denervated rat diaphragm muscle maintained in organ culture. (a) subthreshold f.o.p.s (see text); in (b) the f.o.p.s are large enough to initiate action potentials except on one occasion (O); note that amplification is lower than in a; (c) shows spontaneous oscillation of muscle fibre membrane potential resulting in a burst of action potentials. (From Purves and Sakmann (1974) courtesy of the authors, and the Editor and publishers of Journal of Physiology). (d) and (e) depict recordings made with coaxial needle electrodes from 2 patients with severe denervation. Fibrillation potentials are evident in both records but in (e) there are also simple and complex positive sharp waves (O)

out to involve the remainder of the fibre membrane (Axelsson and Thesleff, 1959). This development results from the formation of new acetylcholine receptors in the previously inert membrane.

(5) After an interval of about 1 week the muscle fibre membrane becomes spontaneously excitable; the impulses are termed *fibrillation potentials* (*Figure 8.3, d*). These impulses are fully developed action potentials which recur with a frequency of 0.5–3 Hz. Belmar and Eyzaguirre (1966) analysed this activity using an extracellular electrode at different points along the fibre and, from the configuration of the potentials, argued that it must have arisen at the site of the original end-plate. Further evidence supporting this conclusion was that they could alter the frequency of the fibrillations by passing a current through the membrane in

small to trigger an action potential (*Figure 8.3, a, b*) and may possibly correspond to the *positive sharp waves* (*Figure 8.3, e*) which can be recorded with a coaxial EMG electrode from denervated muscle. This second type of activity is also encountered most commonly at the old end-plate zone but, like the oscillatory activity, can sometimes occur elsewhere. Since fibrillation potentials persist after curarization the underlying membrane depolarizations cannot have resulted from the action of circulating acetylcholine. The spontaneous depolarizations do, however, depend on transient increases in the sodium permeability of the membrane for they are abolished by removing sodium from the bathing solution or by applying tetrodotoxin.

(6) The concentration of *cholinesterase* in the

sole-plate falls by a variable amour t which, in the rat sternomastoid muscle, is as much as 50–70 per cent of the original value; this change takes place in the first few days following denervation (Guth, Albers and Brown, 1964).

(7) 'Fast' muscles become sensitive to *caffeine* and respond to this drug with a contracture (Gutmann and Sandow, 1965).

(8) Although the mechanism is completely

remaining sections of the present chapter the effects of allowing the muscle to become reinnervated are briefly presented in order to illustrate further the trophic action of the motoneurone on the muscle fibre. The first section briefly describes the changes brought about in the muscle fibre membrane when reinnervation is effected by the original muscle nerve ('self-reinnervation'). In the final section the reality of the neurotrophic

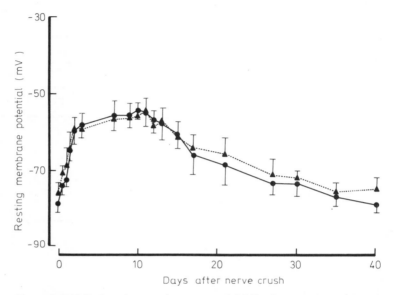

Figure 8.4. Fall of resting membrane potential following temporary denervation produced by nerve crush. After reinnervation has taken place the resting potential is eventually restored to its original level. (From McArdle and Albuquerque (1973) courtesy of the authors, and the Editor and publishers of Journal of General Physiology*)*

unknown, the denervated muscle fibre stimulates neighbouring intact motor axons to sprout. Unlike the situation in an innervated muscle fibre, the denervated muscle fibre membrane becomes receptive to the arrival of an axonal sprout and will permit a new neuromuscular junction to form. Usually the site of the original end-plate is chosen but, if this is prevented by mechanical factors, other regions of the fibre will engage in synaptogenesis. The matter is discussed further in Chapter 20.

MUSCLE REINNERVATION

The ability of the central ends of divided axons to grow back toward their muscle and to establish new synaptic connections with denervated muscle fibres will be considered later (Chapter 20). In the two

influence is emphasized by reference to 'cross-innervation' experiments in which certain biochemical properties of the muscle fibres are altered by permitting reinnervation by foreign motor axons.

Self-reinnervation experiments

As far as is known, all the effects of denervation on muscle fibres are potentially reversible provided the new nerve is introduced within a reasonable period of time. Exactly what constitutes a 'reasonable' period is not clear, for the requisite experiments do not appear to have been performed. From studies of chronically denervated muscle, however, it is apparent that a small proportion of muscle fibres will undergo frank degeneration rather than simple atrophy so that a loss of muscle fibres may result. In some of the other fibres the myonuclei may survive with only vestigal collars of cytoplasm and it is doubtful if these fibres can recover their function. Another reason why reinnervation is more likely to be successful when attempted early rather than late is that fewer moto-neurones will have undergone irreversible retro-grade degeneration. Also, with increasing time the peripheral nerve stump retracts, the endoneurial spaces decrease in size, and the Schwann cells become less active (Gutmann, 1971). With these qualifications in mind there is no doubt that an excellent return of muscle function can result if reinnervation is able to take place within a few months. Of the various self-reinnervation studies that of McArdle and Albuquerque (1973) is par-ticularly thorough, inasmuch as these authors investigated the temporal sequence of the events involved in the restoration of membrane normality. These authors produced temporary denervation in the hindleg of the rat by crushing selected nerves as close as possible to the muscles. They found that 9 days after a nerve crush there was a return of miniature end-plate potentials, initially with a low discharge frequency. At about this time the resting membrane potential started to rise and had reached normal values at 30 days (*Figure 8.4*). The ionic permeability of the membrane and the sensitivity of the latter to acetylcholine had also assumed normal levels by about 30 days.

It is of considerable interest that, in the early stages of reinnervation, the new neuromuscular junctions pass through a phase in which they are unable to excite the muscle fibres even though adequate supplies of transmitter are available in the axon terminals. This point was first demonstrated by Miledi (1960b) who found that miniature end-plate potentials were present at a time when no evoked response could be detected in the muscle fibre following nerve stimulation. Originally shown in the frog, the presence of non-transmitting synapses during reinnervation has since been established in the rat (Dennis and Miledi, 1974) and in the fowl (Bennett, Pettigrew and Taylor, 1973), though not in the mouse (Tonge, 1974b). Dennis and Miledi supposed that the trans-mission failure was caused by a block of impulse conduction in the distal motor axon since in some instances a second electric shock to the nerve, given 4 ms after the first, was able to elicit a muscle fibre response. In the frog the non-transmitting stage appears to last only a day or two and in the rat its duration is shorter still. Of great significance for an understanding of trophic mechanisms is the observation that, even before the synapse has be-come operational, some of the denervation phenomena are already beginning to disappear

from the muscle fibre. For example, the acetyl-choline sensitivity of the membrane starts to resume its normal pattern and a change can be detected in the contracture responses of frog 'slow' muscle fibres to potassium and acetylcholine (Elul, Miledi and Stefani, 1968). These findings can only be explained by postulating that some neural factor other than impulse-induced activity in the muscle fibre is exerting a trophic action on the muscle.

Effect of 'cross-innervation'

The reversal of denervation characteristics described in the previous section depend only upon the reappearance of a functioning neuromuscular junction and are not affected by the origin of the motor axon. Suppose that, instead of a motor axon, a cholinergic autonomic axon was presented to the denervated skeletal muscle fibre. Would the muscle fibre be able to accept the new axon because, like the original motor nerve, it was cholinergic—or would its autonomic origin in some way preclude it from establishing a functional synapse? These are fascinating questions, to which the answers were recently obtained by Landmesser. In an ingenious experiment she was able to introduce the (auto-nomic) preganlionic fibres of the frog vagus nerve to a denervated sartorius muscle transplant (Landmesser, 1971, 1972). It was found that the vagal fibres could make functional synaptic con-nections and usually did so at the site of the original end-plates. The vagal neurones were able to maintain the normal structure and electrical properties of the sartorius fibres but could not induce the formation of cholinesterase at the neuromuscular junction. Because of the dis-crepancy between the cholinesterase and other properties of the reinnervated muscle, Landmesser concluded that more than one nerve trophic factor must be involved. Remarkable though this experi-ment is, for a more detailed analysis of the effects of cross-innervation it is necessary to return to studies of mammalian skeletal muscles. What happens if muscle fibres capture axons from moto-neurones which normally supply a different type of fibre (e.g. type I as opposed to type II)? Until fairly recently it was assumed that a reinnervated muscle fibre would regain all its old characteristics (colour, enzyme profile, twitch speed, etc.). In an elegant experiment Buller, Eccles and Eccles (1960b) showed that this prediction was incorrect. They had taken two muscles in the cat, one with a fast twitch (the flexor digitorum longus; FDL), and one with a slow twitch (soleus). The nerves to these muscles were divided and then the central stump of one was sutured to the distal portion of the other. Following regeneration of the axons the soleus muscle became connected to FDL motoneurones while the FDL muscle was supplied by soleus motoneurones. On examining the twitch characteristics of the reinnervated muscles it was found that the behaviour of the muscles had changed. The flexor digitorum longus had acquired a slow twitch and the contraction of the soleus had speeded up (*Figure 8.5*).

berra to New York (Bárány and Close, 1971), and from Bristol (England) to Los Angeles (Buller, Mommaerts and Seraydarian 1969); a third team of investigators (Samaha, Guth and Albers, 1970) proved self-sufficient. All three studies showed quite clearly that the myosin did change in the cross-innervated muscle. Further, since the muscle had been required to manufacture a new type of protein, the appropriate gene in the muscle fibre must have been under neural control. This type of

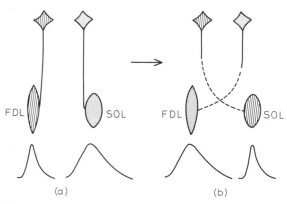

Figure 8.5. the now classic cross-innervation experiment of Buller et al. (1960), in which the twitch speeds of the cat soleus (SOL) and flexor digitorum longus (FDL) muscles were largely reversed (see text)

The basis of the induced change in twitch speed is of great interest. In the case of denervated muscle it was shown that the slowing probably resulted from a decrease in muscle impulse conduction velocity and a prolongation of the active state (Lewis, 1972). However, the difference between normally-innervated fast and slow muscles is due to the rate of sarcomere shortening, that is to the speed with which the actin filaments slide over the myosin rods during a contraction. Bárány (1967) showed that a strong correlation existed between the enzymatic properties of myosin and the speed of shortening of the muscle. Thus the actin-activated ATPase activity of myosin from a fast muscle was higher than that in a slow muscle, presumably because of a structural difference in the myosin molecule itself. In view of these observations one would naturally wish to know whether the molecular properties of myosin are changed in a cross-innervated muscle. To answer this point truly international experiments were performed in which muscle was flown from Can-

experiment and its attendant conclusion are obviously of great significance for an understanding of the mechanism of the neurotrophic influence (see Chapter 9).

Although the change in twitch speed affords the most striking illustration of an alteration in muscle fibre chemistry induced by cross-innervation, there are other biochemical and histochemical features of the muscle fibres which also deserve scrutiny in this type of study. It will be recalled from Chapter 6 that there are marked differences in the histochemical staining reactions of muscle fibres and that various schemes had been put forward for classifying the fibres into histochemical types. From the experimental results already presented it would be anticipated that at least one of the staining reactions—that for myosin ATPase—would alter following cross-innervation. Thus, in the type of experiment just described, the cross-innervated soleus should now stain heavily for myosin ATPase while a cross-innervated FHL or FDL muscle should stain poorly, thereby reversing their normal behaviour. Such is indeed the case and was first demonstrated by Romanul and Van Der Meulen (1966), Dubowitz (1967) and Yellin (1967). Do the mitochondrial enzymes also change? From the work of the above authors it appears that they do. Furthermore, by using whole soleus muscle for biochemical analysis, Drahota and Gutmann (1963) were able to show that the levels of potassium and glycogen in a 'slow-twitch' muscle rose following cross-innervation with a 'fast' nerve and that the electrophoretic protein patterns were also changed. These observations were subsequently confirmed and extended in similar studies on cross-innervated fast and slow muscles by Prewitt and Salafsky (1967) and by Guth, Watson and Brown (1968). Changes in myoglobin, though significant, were much smaller (McPherson and Tokunaga, 1967).

CONCLUSIONS

It has been seen that the denervation of a muscle sets in train a series of profound alterations in structure and function of the fibres. Extensions of this experiment have been, first, to allow the muscle to become reinnervated through its original nerve supply and, secondly, to introduce a 'foreign' nerve to the denervated fibres. Taken together, the results of these manipulations of muscle innervation have provided powerful evidence for the normal existence of a 'trophic' controlling influence passing from nerve to muscle. In the next chapter the effects of use and disuse on muscle are presented and examined in terms of the light which they shed on the nature of the neurotrophic mechanism.

Chapter 9

USE AND DISUSE

There are two possible ways in which the moto-neurone might exert a trophic influence on muscle. One is through the initiation of impulse activity in muscle fibres; abolition of this activity produces the effects of *disuse* in the muscle fibre. The other possibility is the secretion of special messenger molecules by the motoneurone and their subsequent transfer into the muscle fibre; this type of neural activity has already been considered under the heading of *axoplasmic flow* (Chapter 2). In relation to the nature of the trophic influence both types of activity have their protagonists and antagonists; the debate between the two schools has made trophic mechanisms one of the most fascinating topics in contemporary neurosciences. It is clear that the denervation and cross-innervation studies described in the last chapter cannot resolve this issue; the results of such experiments can be used to demonstrate a trophic effect but only under special circumstances (see below) can they give a clue as to the mechanism involved.

In an attempt to distinguish between the effects of impulse activity and axoplasmic flow additional investigations have been undertaken. One approach has been to subject the muscle to excessive use, either by employing exercise or else by electrical stimulation of the motor nerve. The opposite strategy has been to deprive the muscle of activity and for this purpose several ingenious experiments have also been conceived. Finally, there are other experiments which fall outside these two main categories and involve such observations as the effect of nerve stump length or the consequences of blocking axoplasmic flow. The results of these experiments will now be considered.

OVER-USE EXPERIMENTS

Exercise

It is common knowledge that muscle can be developed through exercise and quite remarkable results can be achieved in a matter of weeks by body-building courses. In such courses use is made of prolonged and repeated near-isometric contractions (DeLorme, 1945); isotonic contractions are relatively ineffective in increasing muscle bulk. This simple observation tells us much; clearly the extra muscle fibre action potentials cannot be the stimulus for hypertrophy themselves since these are common to both types of contraction. Instead it seems that it is the amount of sarcomere stretching which is responsible. In an isometric contraction the muscle belly undergoes a certain amount of shortening but the muscle attachments are not free to move. Although the tendons may lengthen slightly, most of the stretch must be taking place in some of the sarcomeres themselves. Thus while some sarcomeres are shortening, they can only do so at the expense of others in which the active contractile force is overcome by the passive tension imposed upon them. In keeping with the importance of stretch is the observation that passive lengthening of muscle will largely prevent the atrophy of disuse and denervation (Gutmann, Schiaffino and Hanzlikova, 1971). Goldspink (1965) has shown that in a muscle undergoing hypertrophy the myofibrils may thicken rapidly within 2 days and then split longitudinally into separate myofibrils. Eventually the muscle fibres themselves may split, a phenomenon originally described by Erb (1891) and recently re-examined by Hall–Craggs (1970). The initial step in this process seems to be a movement of myonuclei into the centre of the fibre, followed by the laying down of new membranes in the vicinity of the nuclei. The remarkably varied patterns in which hypertrophied fibres can split and sometimes re-unite has been demonstrated by Isaacs, Bradley and Henderson (1973) using cinematography of serial transverse sections of dystrophic mouse muscle (*Figure 16.23*).

In normal muscle the type of fibre which develops hypertrophy depends on the nature of the over-activity. Extremely strenuous bursts of effort, as in weightlifting, will cause hypertrophy of type II fibres; this would be expected since the high threshold type II (FG) units can only be recruited under such circumstances (page 66). Interestingly, type II fibre hypertrophy has now been demonstrated not only in human weightlifters (Edström and Ekblom, 1972) but also in rats trained to lift weights. These rats were required to climb a 16-in pole 50 times a day for many weeks with packs on their backs weighing up to 100 g (Gordon, 1967). In contrast, type I (SO) fibre hypertrophy can be made to occur if the experimental conditions are changed so that prolonged exercise of only moderate intensity is undertaken. For example, Guth and Yellin (1971) looked for changes in the plantaris and soleus muscles of rats in which synergistic muscles had been excised. They found that in the plantaris muscle the type I (SO) fibres were enlarged and that, in addition, the type IIA (FOG) fibres appeared to have been converted to type I (SO). Fibre conversion had also taken place in soleus where all the type IIB (FG) fibres had been transformed to type I (SO). Use has also been made of patients with chronic overuse of muscles; thus Edström (1970a) studied patients with upper motoneurone lesions or Parkinsonism. In both conditions type I (SO) fibre hypertrophy was observed; it was attributed to over-activity of type I units as part of the spasticity, rigidity or tremor manifested by these patients.

It can be seen that the results in hypertrophied muscles are variable and depend upon the type of activity undertaken. In contrast there is good agreement that in exercise of the endurance type there is little or no increase in contractile protein and no change in twitch speed; instead the fibres acquire more mitochondria and are thereby able to increase their capacity for aerobic metabolism (Barnard, Edgerton and Peter, 1970a, b). In effect this change causes a conversion of type IIB (FG) fibres to type IIA (FOG). In line with the increased metabolic activity of the exercised muscle, new capillaries form (Romanul and Pollock, 1969). It should be stressed, however, that in all these experiments purporting to show conversion of muscle fibres from one type to another, only a small number of fibre parameters have been studied and it is uncertain whether the conversion has been complete. With this qualification in mind, some of the results have been summarized in *Figure 9.1*.

Indirect stimulation experiments

In an interesting experiment Salmons and Vrbová (1969) explored the possibility that the pattern of impulse activity in a muscle determined its contractile properties. They based their experiments on the observation of Eccles, Eccles and Lundberg (1958) that motoneurones innervating soleus, a 'slow' muscle, discharge at a low frequency (10–20 Hz) whereas those supplying a 'fast' muscle fire at a higher frequency (30–60 Hz; see also Granit *et al.*, 1957). By stimulating the peroneal nerves of rabbits at 10 Hz, Salmons and Vrbová attempted to change the twitch speeds of tibialis anterior and extensor digitorum longus muscles from fast to slow. They employed a small stimulator which was embedded in epoxy resin and powered by a mercury cell; the device was implanted in the abdomen and connected to the stimulating electrodes around the peroneal nerve. After several weeks of continuous stimulation Salmons and Vrbová found that a conversion of contractile properties had indeed taken place. The same type of experiment' has since been repeated by Al-Almood, Buller and Pope (1973) who used a

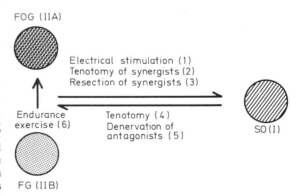

Figure 9.1. Possible examples of fibre type conversion. Some of the studies have been concerned with only one parameter (twitch speed or histochemistry) and other interpretations of data are conceivable. Fibre type classifications are as in Chapter 6 (page 61). References (numbers in brackets) are as follows: (1) Salmons and Vrbová, 1969; (2) Lesch et al., 1968; (3) Guth and Yellin, 1971; (4) Vrbová, 1963; (5) Guth and Wells, 1974; (6) Barnard et al., 1970a, b

miniature stimulator mounted on a vertebral spinous process to excite one of the ventral roots of the cat; these authors also found that slowing of contraction could be made to occur in a previously 'fast' muscle. In keeping with the altered contractile properties of chronically-stimulated muscles has been the demonstration, by Sréter and colleagues (1973), of a change in the structure of myosin. In the 'slowed' tibialis anterior muscle of the rabbit these workers were able to show by gel electrophoresis that the myosin had acquired the light chain pattern normally characteristic of slow muscle.

In an extension of her original work Vrbová has shown that the chronically-stimulated fast muscle acquires a greater capillary density at an early stage in its conversion, and that this precedes a rise in the activity of oxidative enzymes (Cotter, et al., 1972). One of the interpretive problems of the early stimulation studies was that the treated muscles showed clear evidence of deterioration; for example, in the experiments of Salmons and Vrbová (1969) the tetanic tensions of the 'converted' fast muscles fell to about one-half of the control values. Vrbová and her colleagues have since shown that the muscle degeneration can be prevented, and a satisfactory conversion of the fibres still obtained, if stimulation at 10 Hz is applied intermittently rather than continuously (Pette et al., 1973).

DISUSE EXPERIMENTS

So many types of experiment have been devised for studying the effects of disuse that it is necessary to consider them systematically, starting with the elimination of supraspinal excitation of the motoneurone and finishing with alterations to the mechanical properties of the muscle and tendon (*Figure 9.2*). One of the fascinating aspects of this work is that, no matter how elegant the experimental method might appear, the observations themselves, instead of proving definitive, can nearly always be negated by those of an equally impressive technique. Nevertheless, in view of the importance of the trophic influence for an understanding of normal physiology and its derangements in disease, a survey of the substantial but often conflicting evidence is justified.

Prolonged general anaesthesia

One method for obtaining an experimental state of disuse is to keep laboratory animals anaesthetized for prolonged periods. Although the approach is an obvious one, the nursing care of the experimental animals makes heavy demands on the investigator. Davis (1970) was able to keep cats anaesthetized with intravenous Nembutal for up to 3 weeks. At the end of this time he found that the 'fast' muscles were unchanged in their twitch speeds while the slow muscles showed only a slight speeding-up.

Isolated cord preparation

One of Sarah Tower's contributions to neurology was her analysis of the possible mechanisms involved in the effects of disuse and denervation.

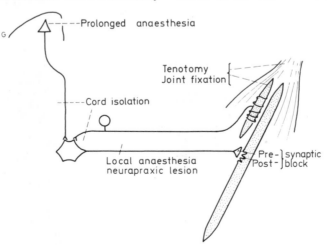

Figure 9.2. Experimental techniques employed for studying the effects of disuse on extrafusal muscle fibres (see text)

To produce disuse alone, she attempted to render motoneurones quiescent by depriving them of their normal synaptic bombardment; this was achieved by cutting through the spinal cord above and below and by also sectioning the dorsal root fibres. In three puppies treated in this way Tower observed a marked decrease in the diameters of the paralysed muscle fibres. The fibres failed to stain well and there was a reduction in the numbers and sizes of the myonuclei; the motor end-plate regions of the fibres were well preserved. Associated with the muscle fibre atrophy was considerable proliferation of connective tissue (Tower, 1937). Use of the isolated cord preparation was subsequently made by Johns and Thesleff (1961) who found only a small spread of acetylcholine sensitvity in the muscle fibres. Atrophy of muscle fibres was noted by Klinkerfuss and Haugh (1970) and by Karpati and Engel (1968); the last authors also observed features in the muscles which would normally be described as 'myopathic'. These features included necrosis of muscle fibres, proliferation of endomysial connective tissue, and the presence of muscles with obvious distortions of their myofibrillar architecture ('ringed' and 'snake-coil' fibres). It is interesting that cord isolation in very young animals causes a failure of the normal differentiation of 'slow' twitch muscles; instead the muscles become fast-contracting (Buller, Eccles and Eccles, 1960a) and contain an abnormally high proportion of type II fibres (Karpati and Engel, 1968). However, when the same operation is performed on older animals there is little effect on the contraction speeds of the muscles (Montgomery, 1972); the two observations indicate that the motoneurone and muscle fibre lose some of their 'plasticity' with advancing age.

Attractive though the concept of motoneurone quiescence is, the Tower approach suffers from one serious disadvantage which renders suspect any conclusions drawn from this type of experiment. The objection is that, following a rostral transection of the cord, the motoneurones will themselves undergo transynaptic degeneration due to deprivation of the trophic input which they normally receive from descending pathways. The evidence for this type of degeneration is summarized elsewhere (Chapter 27). Thus the muscle may be expected to show the effects of true denervation as well as any changes due to disuse.

Prolonged local anaesthesia

Robert and Oester (1970) introduced a technique for implanting a plastic cuff containing local anaesthetic around a muscle nerve. The local anaesthetic was gradually released from the cuff and was able to block impulse conduction from the motoneurones for a week or more. In rabbits treated in this way Robert and Oester found that there was no spread in the sensitivity of the muscle fibres to acetylcholine. In a repetition of this experiment in rats, Lømo and Rosenthal (1972) arrived at precisely the opposite conclusion. Not only was there a spread in the sensitivity but, in surgically-denervated fibres, the spread could be prevented by direct stimulation of the muscle fibres. In a later study Lømo and colleagues showed that following impulse blockade the affected muscle fibres would readily accept a fresh innervation, thereby resembling denervated fibres. This characteristic could also be repressed by direct electrical stimulation of the muscle fibres (Jansen et al., 1973). It is important to note that in this type of experiment the motor axons distal to the anaesthetic cuff remained excitable and there was no impairment of synaptic function at the neuromuscular junction. One criticism of this type of experiment is that the local anaesthetics used are now known to block axoplasmic flow as well as impulse propagation (Byers et al., 1973; Bisby, 1975). This complication can be avoided by the use of tetrodotoxin, given by intraneural injection every 48 hr; the toxin combines with the sodium carriers and inactivates them while leaving axoplasmic flow undisturbed (page 23). Pestronk, Drachman and Griffin (1976) found that within 4 days of this treatment there had been a spread of acetylcholine receptors outside the neuromuscular junction; however, even at 7 days the effect was still substantially smaller than that due to surgical denervation.

Neurapraxic lesions

Some of the most telling evidence against the unique importance of impulses in trophic phenomena comes from investigation of the neurapraxic type of lesion. In this condition nerve fibres are compressed to an extent which leaves their axis cylinders in continuity while temporarily depriving their membranes of excitability, and hence of the ability to conduct impulses. In muscles supplied by affected nerves there is a paralysis which may last hours, days or several weeks before spontaneous recovery ensues. In spite of the complete loss of function, the muscles show very little atrophy and there is no fibrillation activity. The significance of these observations for an understanding of trophic mechanisms was appreciated by Denny-Brown and Brenner (1944) who conducted a detailed study of neurapraxic lesions in cats. These authors pointed out that the prevention of atrophy and fibrillation in normal muscle could not depend on the continued receipt of impulses by the muscle fibres. The matter is discussed more thoroughly in Chapter 22, in which clinical illustrations of neurapraxic lesions are presented.

Neuromuscular transmission block

The effect of a prolonged blockade of neuromuscular transmission has been studied on muscle using agents which have either pre- or postsynaptic actions. Thesleff (1960) found that *botulinum toxin*, a substance which prevents the release of acetylcholine (page 214), caused the acetylcholine sensitivity of the muscle fibre membrane to spread outside the end-plate region; the same change occurs after denervation. *β-Bungarotoxin* also prevents acetylcholine release and causes similar changes to take place in the muscle fibre membrane (Hofmann and Thesleff, 1972). At first sight, it might appear that acetylcholine itself was one of the trophic factors affecting the muscle fibre but the possibility remains that botulinum toxin and β-bungarotoxin also interfere with the release of other substances, including neurotrophic ones, from the axon terminal (Bray and Harris, 1975). Indeed, there is good evidence that acetylcholine (ACh) is not the only trophic factor from two other studies, one of which involved mice with a hereditary disease of the motor end-plate ('*med*' mice). In these animals it appears that impulses fail to invade the nerve terminal but that the spontaneous release of ACh at the end-plate continues normally (Duchen and Stefani, 1971). In spite of the presence of ACh the muscle fibres show features of denervation—atrophy, fibrillations, slowing of the twitch and a spread of ACh sensitivity. The inability of ACh alone to prevent the development of denervation phenomena was also shown by Miledi (1960a) who added ACh to the nutrient medium of frog sartorius muscle fibres in *organ culture*.

By studying newly formed neuromuscular junctions during *reinnervation,* it has been possible to demonstrate that the return of normal muscle function can begin before synaptic transmission has been restored; these observations indicate the existence of a neurotrophic influence other than impulse-directed activity in the muscle fibre. For example, in both frog and mammalian muscle it has been found that the extrajunctional acetylcholine sensitivity decreases before transmission has been re-established at the neuromuscular junction (Miledi, 1960b; Dennis and Miledi, 1974); in rabbit muscle the resumption of transmission was

preceded by a change in the excitability of the muscle fibres to direct stimulation (Desmedt, 1959). Similarly, in cross-innervated muscles of frogs, Elul, Miledi and Stefani (1968) were able to demonstrate that the contracture responses changed before restoration of neuromuscular transmission.

It has already been observed that presynaptic blocking agents, in addition to depriving the muscle fibre of acetylcholine and impulse activity, may also be preventing the release of other neurotrophic substances. This interpretive hazard does not arise if postsynaptic blocking agents, such as *d-tubocurarine*, *succinylcholine* and *α-bungarotoxin*, are used instead. Berg and Hall (1975) used these substances to paralyse rats and maintained the animals for 3 days with artificial respiration. At the end of this time the muscle fibres showed such denervation features as a fall in resting potential, spread of acetylcholine sensitivity and resistance to tetrodotoxin.

Tenotomy and joint fixation

The purpose of *tenotomy* is to allow the muscle to shorten passively and thereby diminish any excitatory input to the motoneurones from the muscle spindle; the motoneurones should therefore become quiescent. Following tenotomy changes do take place in the muscles of the rabbit; the most marked of these is atrophy, particularly of red (type I) fibres. Associated with the atrophy is a speeding-up of the twitch (Vrbová, 1963). Again however, the experimental situation is not ideal. For one thing the motoneurones may sometimes be subjected to an increased, rather than a reduced, sensory bombardment (Hnik, 1972). Secondly, by depriving the muscle fibres of passive stretch, atrophic changes may be anticipated anyway (Gutmann, Schiaffino and Hanzliková, 1971).

So far as *joint fixation* is concerned, it is a common clinical observation that muscle atrophy follows treatment of a fracture by immobilization of the affected limb in a plaster cast; it is assumed that this atrophy is due to 'disuse'. Edström (1970b) has shown that, in patients with injuries of the anterior cruciate ligament of the knee, the atrophy which occurs in the quadriceps muscle is confined to type I (SO) fibres. Experimental immobilization, achieved by bone-pinning, has been applied to animals by Fischbach and Robbins (1969). A very considerable reduction in background impulse activity was produced in muscles and a marked speeding of the twitch was noted. At the single motor unit level it has been possible to confirm the susceptibility of SO units to immobilization but it appears that the FOG units are even more affected, as judged by reductions in their twitch and tetanic tensions. Although smaller changes in force generation were noted in the FG units, both these and the SO units exhibited a speeding-up of their twitches (Burke, Kanda and Mayer, 1975). As in the tenotomy experiments, however, the absence of passive stretch of the muscle may have produced some of the effects (Gutmann, Schiaffino and Hanzlíková, 1971), the remainder presumably resulting from a reduction in impulse activity in the immobilized muscles.

OTHER OBSERVATIONS

Lastly, we come to three observations which cannot be fitted into the 'over-use' and 'disuse' categories, but which are important nevertheless.

Block of axoplasmic flow

Using an implanted cuff technique it is possible to block axoplasmic flow with colchicine without interrupting impulse propagation (Hofmann and Thesleff, 1972; Albuquerque *et al.*, 1972; Cangiano, 1973). The deprived muscle fibres will then acquire the features of denervation—a fall in resting membrane potential, a spread of ACh sensitivity and the development of TTX-resistant action potentials. Possible concerns in this type of experiment are (*a*) the occurrence of true axonal degeneration in some fibres as an effect of colchicine, (*b*) pressure effects of the cuff on axons and (*c*) remote effects of colchicine on muscle following its absorption into the circulation from the vicinity of the cuff (Cangiano, 1973).

Effect of nerve stump length

Several groups of workers have demonstrated that the onset of denervation phenomena can be delayed if a nerve is cut proximally so as to leave an appreciable 'stump' attached to the muscle (*Figure 9.3*). The importance of this type of observation is that it cannot be explained by an absence of impulse activity since the latter will occur as soon as the nerve is cut and will be independent of the site of section. An explanation can be provided in terms of axoplasmic flow, however, by suggesting that, following nerve section, the muscle fibre is able to use up the trophic material in the distal nerve stump. A longer stump will contain a greater amount of material and the onset of denervation phenomena would be delayed correspondingly.

Partial denervation of single fibres

The muscle fibres of the frog sartorius muscle receive a double innervation from the obturator nerve. In theory, division of one nerve branch should not affect the activity of the muscle appreciably since the fibres would still be excited through the remaining nerve branch. In such fibres, however, there is a definite increase in acetylcholine sensitivity around the denervated end-plates (Miledi, 1960a), suggesting that some factor other than muscle fibre activity was normally controlling the distribution of acetylcholine receptors.

CONCLUSIONS

For reasons already given, the results of experiments involving tenotomy or isolation of the cord should be interpreted with caution. Similarly the use of pharmacological agents introduces a degree of uncertainty since the full action of a drug on a preparation may not be known; botulinum toxin and local anaesthetics are good illustrations. A more convincing type of experiment would appear to be that involving direct stimulation of denervated muscle fibres (Lømo and Rosenthal, 1972). But are the experiments as convincing as they seem? For example, why are the effects of denervation not overcome by the impulses associated with fibrillation activity? It could be argued that the fibrillation impulse frequency is too low (0.5–3 Hz)

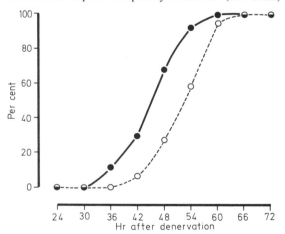

Figure 9.3. The development of resistance of tetrodotoxin (TTX) in mammalian muscle fibres which had been denervated by nerve section either close to the muscle (●) or else well away from the muscle (○). The ordinate shows the percentage of TTX-resistant fibres. (From Harris and Thesleff (1972); sciatic nerve–EDL preparation. Reproduced by courtesy of the authors, and the Editor and publishers of Nature)

but against this is the fact that the fibrillations are remarkably persistent and may still be present several months after the denervating episode. It is also pertinent to point out that, although the experimental excitation of a muscle continuously at 10 Hz may simulate the background impulse activity in the soleus muscle of the rabbit (Vrbová, 1963), it bears little relationship to the activities of most other mammalian muscles. For example, clinical electromyographers study many normal muscles as well as diseased ones in the course of their work. Such normal muscles have no fibrillation activity to suggest functional denervation and yet during complete relaxation the motor units are silent. Even during the course of everyday activities (walking, sitting, writing, eating, etc.) only a small proportion of the motor unit population will be involved and these will always be the same units with the lowest thresholds. In contrast the largest units will only be recruited during maximal voluntary contractions, but there are probably few occasions during the course of a week when the ordinary person makes such extreme efforts.

Arguing along similar lines, one would expect the muscle fibres of infrequently-used motor units to have low resting membrane potentials since depolarization can be detected as early as 2 hr after denervation (Albuquerque, Schuh and Kaufman, 1971). In fact it has been found that in the mouse the soleus, a postural muscle, has a slightly *lower* fibre resting potential than FDL, a phasic muscle (Harris and Luff, 1970). In human studies too, the measurements of resting membrane potential give no hint of the presence of a functionally denervated muscle fibre population (McComas *et al.*, 1968). It will also be recalled from studies on patients and animals with neurapraxic lesions (see above and Chapter 22) that impulse activity is not a necessary condition for the prevention of several signs of denervation—the disruption of the motor end-plate, the fall in resting membrane potential, the onset of fibrillation activity and the initiation of collateral reinnervation. It follows that the motoneurone must be able to exert its influence on the muscle fibre membrane through the only other controlling mechanism available to it—axoplasmic flow. This, of course, would be in keeping with the nerve stump experiments (page 85) in which the delay in denervation was proportional to the length of nerve attached to the muscle. These experiments strongly suggest that, after the nerve section, the muscle is able to make use of the trophic material in the stump and so maintain its normal properties for a little while longer. These considerations do not imply that muscle impulses or the resultant mechanical activity have no trophic action at all; on the contrary there is good evidence that activity

is important for the suppression of extrajunctional acetylcholine receptors and of tetrodotoxin sensitivity; the relevant experiments are those involving block of neuromuscular transmission and those in which denervated muscle was stimulated directly (see above). Similarly, muscle fibre activity does appear to promote continued synthesis of myofibrillar proteins; in some way the stretching of the sarcomere acts as an essential link in this regulatory mechanism (Gutmann, Schiaffino and Hanzlíková, 1971). Perhaps the most sensible point of view is to accept that muscle activity and axoplasmically-conveyed messenger molecules are both important trophic mechanisms and that some properties of the muscle fibre are more dependent on one than on the other.

In Chapter 2 the phenomenon of axoplasmic transport was considered in some detail. It was shown that the transported material travelled at different rates and Harris and Thesleff (1972) have established that the factor responsible for preventing TTX-resistant action potentials moves with the fast fraction. This fraction also includes the trophic factor necessary for maintaining the integrity of the neuromuscular junction (Miledi and Slater, 1970). It is probable that several chemically distinct trophic factors are involved. Although their identities have not yet been established several types of substance have already been shown to be released from motor nerve endings and are therefore possible candidates; they include amino acids, phosphorus compounds, proteins, polypeptides and prostaglandins (page 14). In some instances impulse activity has been observed to enhance the release of these substances (Musick and Hubbard, 1972); indeed it would not be unexpected if impulse modulation of the transfer of trophic material were eventually shown to occur. A further speculation, though also unproven, is that acetylcholine may facilitate the entry of trophic material into the muscle fibre.

Once the trophic factors have passed into the muscle fibre they must produce their effects. But how? The nature of the trophic effects provide a clue for in a number of instances it is evident that new proteins are being formed—examples are myosin, cholinesterase, and the various glycolytic and oxidative enzymes which are known to be under neural control (see above). However, it is equally clear that synthesis of other proteins is being inhibited. A good example is myosin since a muscle fibre will manufacture either 'fast'- or 'slow'-twitch myosin, depending on its innervation, but not both types simultaneously (Samaha, Guth and Albers, 1970). Other examples are the membrane proteins responsible for the various electrophysiological features of denervation. Thus Miledi

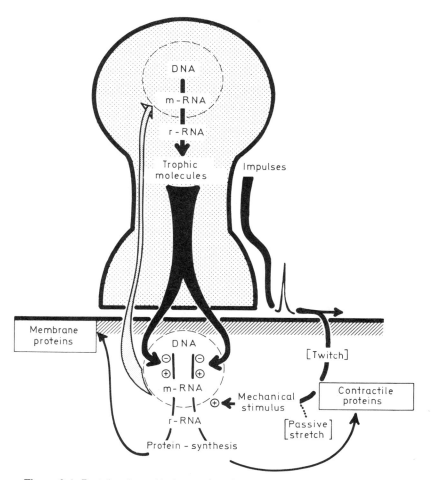

Figure 9.4. Postulated trophic interactions between motoneurone (at top) and muscle fibre (at bottom); respective nuclei shown by interrupted circles. Much of the trophic control exerted by neurone is through special molecules transported down axon. These may either stimulate or repress transcription of myonuclear DNA. Thus the neurone normally represses synthesis of membrane proteins required for (i) TTX-resistant sodium channels, (ii) extra-junctional ACh receptors, (iii) resting ionic permeability channels and (iv) stimulation of axonal sprouting. Similarly myonuclear DNA will be stimulated for synthesis of one type of myosin but not of the other (i.e. for 'fast' or 'slow' twitches). Impulses are conceived as having an important supplementary trophic role which is mediated through the mechanical effects of the ensuing twitches; these could ultimately affect the translation step (m-RNA—r-RNA) as suggested by Thesleff (1975). The feed back action of the muscle fibres on the motoneurone is also shown. The evidence on which the diagram is based is given in the text

(1960a) found that if a frog sartorius muscle was transected, acetylcholine receptors developed in the part of the fibre which had been separated from the end-plate. This experiment showed that in the intact fibre some trophic factor must move along the fibre from the end-plate and prevent the membrane from displaying its inherent denervation characteristics.

All the examples cited demonstrate that the motoneurone can either stimulate or inhibit protein synthesis; in doing so, the trophic factors must ultimately be modifying expression of the genes within the muscle fibre. In theory there are many ways in which this could be achieved including the use of relatively indirect mechanisms, such as the control of enzyme reaction rates through alterations in local factors (pH, co-factor availability, etc.). However, experiments by Fambrough (1970) and by Grampp, Harris and Thesleff (1972) suggest that the trophic action is a direct one on the transcription of DNA to messenger (m)-RNA. Both groups treated animals either with actinomycin-D to prevent transcription or with puromycin to prevent translation of m-RNA. It was found that in such animals denervation phenomena could be suppressed; in Fambrough's experiment ACh-sensitivity was examined while Grampp, Harris and Thesleff (1972) also studied the membrane potential and TTX-resistant action potentials. In addition to the effect on transcription, the neurotrophic factors also control the DNA level within the muscle fibre since a rise can be observed after denervation (Gutmann and Žák, 1961).

By exerting its influence on the DNA of the fibre the motoneurone makes use of an error-free system and takes advantage of its chemical amplification features; the concentration of myonuclei in the end-plate region probably ensures that the trophic factors have ready access to muscle fibre DNA. *Figure 9.4* summarizes these views; it includes a trophic pathway from muscle fibre to motoneurone, for which evidence is presented in the next session. The figure also gives a role to nerve and muscle fibre impulses. With the accumulation of further information it should be possible to modify this diagram by showing precisely which, if any, muscle fibre properties are governed solely by activity or axoplasmic transport; such a figure should also indicate how the two controlling systems are functionally related to each other.

Chapter 10

TROPHIC INFLUENCE OF MUSCLE ON NERVE

Can muscle influence nerve? In view of the extensive use made by the body of feedback systems, the expected answer would be 'yes'. Indeed, it would be unnecessarily wasteful if, following a peripheral nerve injury, a motoneurone continued to manufacture trophic material for a colony of muscle fibres to which it was no longer connected. Nor could a motoneurone gear its metabolic activity to a higher level, in order to support an enlarged muscle fibre colony, in the absence of a message from the periphery informing the cell that collateral reinnervation was taking place (see page 224). The very existence of a system of neurotubules within the axon suggests that there might be a centripetal, as well as a centrifugal, flow of information between the motoneurone and the muscle fibres. Thus, if only centrifugal signals were required the cell could achieve this simply by bulk movement of axoplasm, though this would be a rather slow process.

MORPHOLOGICAL ASPECTS

The possible existence of a two-way traffic in trophic effects between the cord and periphery has exercised a number of investigators, amongst whom pride of place must surely rest with Nissl (1892)—and not for historical reasons alone. Nissl avulsed the facial nerve in rabbits and studied the changes visible in neurones of the facial nucleus under the light microscope (*Figure 10.1*). He noticed especially striking alterations in the granular material situated in the region of the axon hillock. This material, since called Nissl substance, is now known to consist of RNA. Following axotomy the granules became smaller and were dispersed to the periphery of the motoneurone soma (*chromatolysis*). At the same time the neurone became swollen and rounded in outline. The nucleus was usually pushed to the edge of the soma opposite the axon hillock; within the nucleus the nucleoli were enlarged. These changes were complete at 7–10 days and were sufficiently prominent for the affected neurones to be readily distinguished from the other cells. Subsequent workers have confirmed Nissl's observations and have described additional features. For example, the glial cells in the vicinity of the affected motoneurones swell (see Watson, 1972) and lysosomes may appear in the neuronal cytoplasm. In addition, there is retraction of the dendrites and loss of the synaptic connections which they normally make with the axon terminals (boutons) of other neurones; these changes probably underlie the longer latencies and increased temporal dispersion of reflex discharges. Microelectrode recordings from axotomized motoneurones have revealed little change in resting potential although the overshoot of the action potential becomes larger and there is a considerable reduction in impulse conduction velocity along the axon stump (Eccles, Libet and Young, 1958; Kuno, Miyata and Muñoz-Martinez, 1974a). Normally the motoneurones supplying the

89

fast and slow twitch muscles can be differentiated on the basis of the hyperpolarization which follows the action potential; after axotomy this difference becomes less marked but it is restored as soon as reinnervation takes place (Kuno, Miyata and Muñoz-Martinez, 1974b).

In a series of elegant experiments on the hypoglossal nerve and tongue muscles of the rat,

RNA could be detected in these animals also the phenomenon could not have been due to axonal injury but rather to a loss of functional contact between the nerve ending and muscle fibre. Thus it seems probable, but has not yet been proved, that the toxin prevents not only the centrifugal, but also the centripetal, transfer of trophic material at the neuromuscular junction. Gutmann

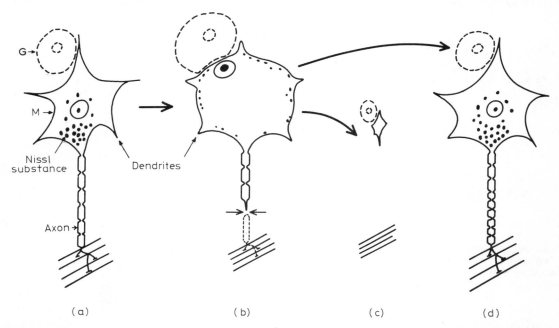

Figure 10.1 Changes in motoneurone (M) following interruption of its axon. (a) shows a normal motoneurone (M) innervating several muscle fibres. (b) represents situation about 7 days after axotomy (at arrows) ; note swollen motoneurone soma with displaced nucleus and enlarged nucleolus. Nissl substance is dispersed and dendrites have retracted. Distal axon stump is degenerating and muscle fibres have started to atrophy. The glial cell (G) close to the motoneurone is also enlarged. If reinnervation of muscle is successful normal neuronal architecture is restored (d), though the axon now has shorter internodal segments. Failure to innervate is associated with progressive atrophy of motoneurone (c) and, in some instances, leads to its eventual disappearance

Watson has analysed the nature and course of some of the biochemical events taking place within the motoneurone following axotomy. He has shown that the first detectable change within the motoneurone is an increase in the formation of ribosomal RNA within the nucleolus (Watson, 1968a). It is probable that this RNA is required for the synthesis of proteins as part of the forthcoming repair process in the axon. The latency of this change in RNA depends on the site of nerve injury, being least following a lesion close to the hypoglossal nucleus. In another type of experiment Watson (1969) injected botulinum toxin, a substance which is known to interfere with the release of acetylcholine (and probably other trophic factors) at the end-plate. Since a rise in nucleolar

(1971) has pointed out that the vigorous metabolic response of the motoneurone to disconnection from its target organ hardly deserves the term 'retrograde degeneration' and that Nissl's own description 'primare Zellreizung' (primary cell excitation) is more appropriate. Watson (1970) was also able to show that if the motoneurone was allowed to reinnervate muscle fibres through axonal sprouting a second rise in its metabolic activity took place. During this phase the dendrites expanded to their original lengths and acquired fresh synaptic connections. Successful reinnervation enables the motoneurone to resume its normal appearance in other respects (*Figure 10.1*)—the cell size becomes normal, the nucleus regains its central position and the Nissl substance reforms at the axon hillock; at the same time the regenerating axon enlarges its diameter (Sanders and Young, 1946). In contrast, if reinnervation of muscle is prevented many motoneurones will disintegrate or else gradually atrophy, particularly in young animals.

AXOPLASMIC FLOW

Experimental data has now accumulated to show that several different types of substance can be transported from muscle to nerve but the nature of the naturally-occurring trophic messengers is unknown. For example, Watson (1968b) has shown that the injection of [^{3}H]-lysine into muscle is followed after a short interval by its appearance and proximally-directed movement in motor nerves. More recently it has been possible to demonstrate that material injected into the muscle belly may eventually reach the cell bodies of the motoneurones. In the experiments of Glatt and Honegger (1973) the fluorescent dye, Evans Blue, was coupled with albumin and used as a marker. Within 12 hr of injection of this marker into the rat triceps muscle, motoneurones in the cervical cord could be seen to fluoresce; the length of the neural pathway was 30 mm. In the study of Kristensson and Olsson (1971) horseradish peroxidase (HRP) was injected into the gastrocnemius muscles of mice. It is known that this electrondense material is taken up by pinocytosis at the neuromuscular junction and can then be seen with the electronmicroscope to be contained in coated vesicles within the axon terminal (Zacks and Saito, 1969). Kristensson and Olsson found that HRP, after being transported centripetally in the axons, was distributed in small cytoplasmic granules around the nucleus within 24 hr of injection. With suitable control experiments the authors were able to exclude the possibility that the HRP had been conveyed to the cord by the bloodstream.

In conclusion, the demonstration that an axon can take up exogenous proteins and transport them to the neurone soma has important implications. It provides a possible mechanism for the trophic influence of muscle on nerve, in the absence of which chromatolysis occurs. The process also sheds light on the way in which certain toxins and neurovirulent viruses may spread from the periphery to the central nervous system.

Chapter 11

MUSCLE GROWTH

The growth of muscle has been studied in many ways, ranging from observations on normal fetal development to those on muscle fibres in tissue culture. In addition, the regenerative processes set in train following injury to the muscle are reasonably assumed to resemble those occurring naturally during development. In the section which follows the main results of these investigations are given, together with varying amounts of detail regarding the particular techniques employed. More extensive reviews of muscle development have been given elsewhere (Holtzer, 1970; Fischman, 1972; Goldspink, 1972).

EMBRYONIC DEVELOPMENT OF MUSCLE

Following fertilization of the ovum the newly formed cell, or *zygote,* undergoes mitotic division. This process is repeated by successive generations of cells with the formation first of the multicellular *morula,* and then of the *blastula.* Within the blastula three types of tissue start to differentiate: (*a*) *ectoderm,* which will eventually form the skin and nervous system; (*b*) *mesoderm,* giving rise to bone, muscle, heart and blood vessels, and (*c*) *entoderm,* forming the alimentary canal and associated viscera.

The mesodermal (mesenchymal) cells, following mitosis, can develop into either *myogenic* (muscle forming) or *chondrogenic* (cartilage forming) lineages. In the myogenic lineage the first generation of cells ('stem' cells, *Figure 11.1*) has the potential to produce connective tissue progeny (*fibroblasts*)

as an alternative to muscle-forming cells (*myoblasts*). The myoblasts themselves continue to multiply but eventually mitotic activity ceases and the cells fuse with each other to form *myotubes.* These stages will now be considered more fully.

Myoblast stage

The myoblast is a spindle-shaped cell with a single nucleus (*Figure 11.2*). The nucleus is ovoid and has a prominent nucleolus, indicating that the cell is actively synthesizing RNA. The cytoplasm of the cell is also packed with RNA, this being in the form of ribosomes. Scattered mitochondria are present and a small Golgi apparatus is evident; the endoplasmic reticulum is poorly developed. Electromicroscopy also reveals some thin (60 Å) filaments lying in the periphery of the cell under the plasma membrane. Some of these filaments are actin (page 38) and are probably involved in movements of the myoblast and its appendages. Thick filaments are not to be seen in mammalian myoblasts except just prior to cell fusion and there is therefore no evidence of myofibrils in most of the cells. From microelectrode studies of muscle developing in tissue culture it appears that the resting membrane potential of the myoblast is low (around -20 mV; Fambrough *et al.,* 1974). Since the internal potassium concentration is normal the low potential presumably results from 'leakiness' of the plasma membrane for sodium; the fact that a basement membrane has not yet developed may also be relevant in the control of permeability. Functional acetylcholine receptors do not appear to

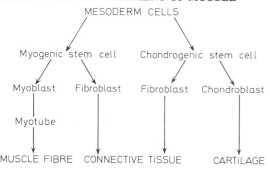

MESODERM CELLS

Myogenic stem cell   Chondrogenic stem cell

Myoblast   Fibroblast   Fibroblast   Chondroblast

Myotube

MUSCLE FIBRE   CONNECTIVE TISSUE   CARTILAGE

Figure 11.1. Stages in the differentiation of mesoderm into muscle fibres, connective tissue and cartilage

be present in the plasma membranes of most myoblasts (Fambrough *et al.*, 1974).

The myoblasts divide repeatedly by mitosis and, both in tissue culture and in regenerating muscle, are seen to be mobile. After these *'proliferative' mitoses,* the cell undergoes a final division, the *'quantal' mitosis,* and then prepares for fusion. In culture the cells now extend cytoplasmic processes which explore the surfaces of other myoblasts and of myotubes (see below) lying alongside. After a relatively long period of mutual contact which, in culture, may amount to 5 hrs (Bischoff and Holtzer, 1969) a myoblast may, or may not, fuse with its neighbour. If fusion does follow, the necessary steps are taken relatively swiftly, usually within 8–10 minutes. The contiguous cell membranes break down and the nuclei of the myoblasts come into apposition in the centre of the cell. The new cell which has been created is termed a *myotube.* The factors which determine whether or not two cells will eventually fuse are not known, nor is the nature of the molecular changes which take place in the adjacent membranes. Bischoff and Lowe (1974) have shown that a surface factor containing glucosamine is likely to be necessary for fusion and that this can be removed by treatment with EDTA; it is also known that calcium ions must be available (Shainberg, Yagil and Yaffe, 1969). Experiments using cycloheximide to block protein synthesis have shown that the formation of new protein is not involved in the fusion process (Bischoff and Lowe, 1974).

Myotube stage

Once a myotube has been formed further myoblasts will add themselves to it, as described above (*Figure 11.2*). The *nuclei* of the new cells continue to line up with pre-existing nuclei in the centre of the myotube so as to form a chain; at the same time

they become somewhat larger and rounded. These nuclei will not partake in any further mitoses. Meanwhile the cytoplasm of the myotube increases in amount and contains increasing numbers of thick and thin *filaments* (myosin and actin) which have been synthesized by polysomes. The myofilaments are grouped in bundles; these become thicker and form *myofibrils.* Soon the A- and I-bands of the myofibrils can be distinguished, indicating that the component myosin and actin filaments are now in register, the Z-lines appear subsequently. Other changes are evident. *Mitochondria* become more numerous and are elongated with densely packed cristae. A rudimentary *T (transverse tubular)-system* forms from an invagination of the plasma membrane; similarly *sarcoplasmic reticulum* is derived from the outer nuclear envelope. A fuzziness on the surface of the myotube denotes the development of a *basement membrane.* Intracellular microelectrode studies of cultured cells show that the properties of the surface membrane, or *sarcolemma,* are changing. The resting membrane potential rises as the myotube becomes larger and reaches maximum values of about -60 mV (Fischbach, Nameroff and Nelson, 1971); this change is probably caused by a rise in the relative permeability of the membrane for potassium as opposed to sodium. The membrane is now capable of firing action potentials both spontaneously or following direct stimulation. In tissue culture the myotubes can be seen to twitch spontaneously and synchronously. It is possible that the cells are electrically coupled to each other; the presence of 'tight' junctions between adjacent myotubes, visible upon electronmicroscopy, would provide a possible mechanism. By iontophoretic application of acetylcholine or the use of ^{125}I-labelled α-bungarotoxin it can be shown that the membrane now contains *acetylcholine receptors,* some of which are formed internally and then transported to the surface of the myotube. Although the whole surface of the cell is sensitive to acetylcholine there are certain 'hot spots' corresponding to particularly high receptor densities. Fambrough *et al.* (1974) have estimated that in 1 hr roughly 100 ACh receptors may be formed per $μm^2$ of membrane (see their Figure 5). The myotubes also contain *cholinesterase* and, like the ACh-receptors, much of this appears to be manufactured in the vicinity of the nuclei and carried to the surface.

Muscle fibre stage

As the myotube enlarges it forms more myofilaments and both the sarcoplasmic and transverse tubular systems become better differentiated. At

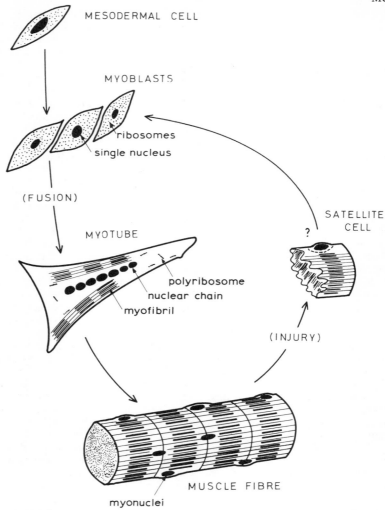

MESODERMAL CELL

MYOBLASTS

ribosomes
single nucleus

(FUSION)

MYOTUBE

SATELLITE
CELL

?

polyribosome
nuclear chain
myofibril

(INJURY)

MUSCLE FIBRE

myonuclei

Figure 11.2. Stages in the development of the muscle fibre. Also shown are events following injury in which the myonuclei are transformed into satellite cells; these, in turn, become myoblasts and enable regeneration to take place (see page 99)

the same time the nuclei move from the centre of the cell to take up new positions under the sarcolemma. The myotube has now completed its transition into a muscle fibre.

Development of the neuromuscular junction

When the developing muscle is still at the myoblast stage it is invaded by unmyelinated axons which have grown toward it from motoneurones in the ventral part of the fetal spinal cord. The work of Landmesser and Morris (1975) in the chick

embryo suggests that there is nothing haphazard about this outgrowth and that 'the motoneurones are . . . initially specified with respect to their peripheral destination, and that they synapse with appropriate muscles from the start'. The first axons are 'exploring' ones; they form a neuromuscular junction on each of the myotubes which have developed by fusion of the myoblasts. Subsequently other axons may arrive and establish neuromuscular junctions in the same regions of the myotubes (Bennett and Pettigrew, 1974a). In the human embryo the neuromuscular junctions are first seen in the intercostal muscles at the age of

8.6 weeks (corresponding to a crown-rump length of 3.2 cm); their appearance in the tibialis anterior occurs rather later, at 10 weeks (4.3 cm; Juntunen and Teravainen, 1972). Initially, newly-formed junctions have a primitive appearance, consisting of a simple (primary) *cleft* between the apposed nerve and locally-thickened muscle fibre membranes (Kelly and Zacks, 1969). At about 19 weeks of human fetal development folding of the muscle membrane starts to take place, with the formation of the secondary clefts. The density of *acetylcholine receptors* is high on the postsynaptic membrane and, by a series of ingenious experiments, Steinbach and Heinemann (1974) have shown that this feature does not depend on the release or uptake of acetylcholine at the junction although it is probably dependent on some other factor released by nerve. In contrast, *acetylcholinesterase* appears relatively late at the neuromuscular junction, usually one or more days after successful synaptic function has been established.

As the neuromuscular junction continues to develop the myonuclei migrate into its vicinity and begin to heap up on each other, increasing the complexity of the *sole-plate*. Meanwhile in the axon terminal increasing numbers of synaptic vesicles are to be seen, though initially very few of these (e.g. 1–4) are available for release following a single impulse (Robbins and Yonezawa, 1971); hence the resulting depolarization is too small to initiate an action potential. With time, however, the quantal release increases and successful transmission becomes established. Some of the vesicles in the miniature axon terminal are relatively large and have dense cores; possibly these vesicles have a special trophic function. As these changes are taking place at the neuromuscular junction the motor axon is also developing. It becomes thicker and it acquires a myelin sheath from the Schwann cells which have followed the axon outwards from the meninges. Both in the fetus and in tissue culture multiple neuronal innervation of single muscle fibres is common. That these multiple synapses are functional is evident from microelectrode studies of rat muscle (Redfern, 1970; Bennett and Pettigrew, 1974a) and also from the measurements of muscle twitch and tetanic tensions in newborn kittens by Bagust, Lewis and Westerman (1973). Within the first few weeks of life the surplus innervation in these species is relinquished; the nature of the signal which is responsible for this change is unknown. In the human embryo the results of cholinesterase staining suggest that the regression of the 'extra' neuromuscular junctions takes place before birth, probably between 25 weeks of gestation and term (Toop, 1975).

POST-NATAL DEVELOPMENT

At birth the muscle fibres are still relatively small and mostly no larger than 20 μm in diameter. In human muscle, however, a 20-fold enlargement of the muscle belly must take place during childhood and puberty, assuming that the proportional contribution of muscle to the total body weight is roughly the same. Obviously much of this increase will take place in an axial direction through the formation of new sarcomeres and this process has been demonstrated at the ends of growing fibres by Williams and Goldspink (1971). The nature of the stimulus for this longitudinal expansion is not known for sure, though *growth hormone* is certainly involved. Thus when a deficiency of growth hormone occurs, as in panhypopituitarism of childhood, there is a failure of all tissues to develop, including the somatic musculature. In experimental animals, in which the pituitary glands have been ablated, it can be shown that muscle growth is restored by the injection of growth hormone (Goldberg and Goodman, 1969). *Insulin* is another hormone necessary for muscle growth; at the level of the muscle fibre it has been shown to stimulate amino acid transport, enhance protein synthesis and inhibit protein degradation (Goldberg, 1968; Fulks, Li and Goldberg, 1975). This is not the complete explanation, however, for it now appears that local mechanical factors are also of major importance in determining muscle length and may be partly responsible for the effects of growth hormone. It is certainly intriguing that the number of sarcomeres, i.e. the true length of the muscle, always appears to remain appropriate for the distance separating the attachments of the muscle, irrespective of whether the subject is a dwarf or a giant. The explanation for this relationship has come from recent work by Tabary and colleagues (1972). They have shown that if a cat soleus muscle is maintained in a shortened position, by fixing the leg in a plaster cast, there is a 40 per cent loss of sarcomeres within 3 weeks. Conversely prolonged extension results in the formation of new sarcomeres. The functional advantage of an adjustable fibre length is clear since the muscle will always be able to work at, or below, the optimal region of the length-tension curve (page 44); over stretching of the muscle and damage to the crossbridges will not occur.

At the same time that the fibres are growing longitudinally, their diameters will be increasing so that, in man, mean values of about 50 μm will eventually be achieved (Brooke and Engel, 1969). It is this change in muscle growth which is responsible for the increased muscle strength during development. McComas, Sica and Petito (1973) have recently measured isometric twitch tensions in the extensor digitorum brevis muscle in boys of different ages. It was found that muscle strength increased in two phases (*Figure 11.3*). The first phase lasted until puberty and during this time there

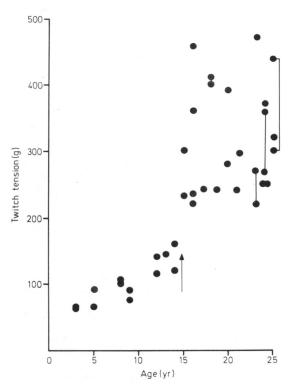

Figure 11.3. *Maximal isometric twitch tensions of exterior hallucis brevis muscles of males at different ages. Bilateral observations have been linked together. Arrow denotes usual time of puberty, as judged by development of sexual characteristics—deepening of voice, coarsening of skin, facial hirsutes etc.; note the increase in strength subsequently. (From McComas, Sica and Petito (1973), courtesy of the Editor and publishers of* Journal of Neurology, Neurosurgery and Psychiatry)

was a gradual increase in strength, such that an approximately linear relationship could be demonstrated between maximum twitch tension and age:

i.e. $F = 38 + 7.3t$,

where F = twitch tension (g) and t = time (yr).

The second phase occurred at puberty and was more dramatic in that a doubling of contractile force took place within a comparatively short time,

certainly no longer than 2 years. It is probable that this spurt in muscle strength is due to the direct action of *testosterone* on muscle fibres for the serum levels of this hormone are raised at puberty and it is known that testosterone has a direct anabolic effect on muscle fibres. This anabolic effect has been demonstrated by experiments on the levator ani muscle of the rat which is particularly hormone dependent. If an animal is castrated marked atrophy of this muscle occurs; the atrophy can then be reversed by the administration of testosterone (Wainman and Shipounoff, 1941). In man, synthetic steroid substances closely related to testosterone, the 'anabolic steroids', have been found to increase muscle bulk and strength. These substances have been used therapeutically and have also been taken by athletes anxious to improve their performance in such 'heavy' field sports as shot-putting and discus-throwing.

According to MacCallum (1898) the number of muscle fibres does not increase in a human muscle (sartorius) after birth. If this is true of all human muscles then the increased strength at puberty can only have resulted from the synthesis of new myofibrils in existing muscle fibres. This last process has been studied in mice during the vigorous postnatal growth phase by Goldspink (1970). He found that in some fibres the number of myofibrils increased by as much as 15-fold. On the basis of electronmicroscopical observations on individual myofibrils, Goldspink suggested that the myofibrils first enlarged and then split in two, with the rupture commencing in the Z-discs. Myofibril enlargement and splitting also occurs during induced work hypertrophy and in recovery from the atrophy induced by starvation; the cycle may be completed in the remarkably short time of 1.5–2 days (Goldspink, 1965). From observations on 'body-building' courses and weightlifting exercises in man, it is clear that muscle contraction is a far more potent stimulus for muscle fibre hypertrophy if it is isometric rather than isotonic. Since the action potential is common to both types of contraction the difference must be related to the degree of muscle stretch. In an isotonic contraction all the sarcomeres are allowed to shorten; in an isometric contraction, however, some sarcomeres will shorten but others must be stretched, since the two ends of the muscle remain almost the same distance apart. Hence stretch has two anabolic effects on muscle. Maintained stretch, as in the plaster cast experiments by Tabary and colleagues (1972), induces the formation of new sarcomeres, including fresh myofilaments, at the extremities of the fibre. Severe intermittent stretch, as in forceful isometric contraction, results in the synthesis of new myo-

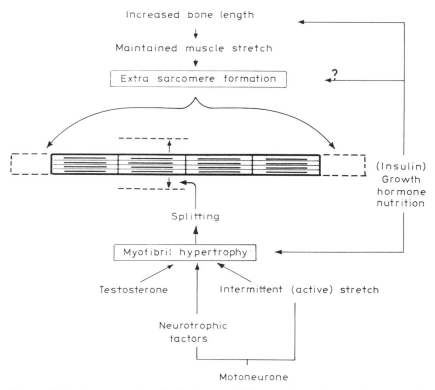

Increased bone length

Maintained muscle stretch

Extra sarcomere formation

?

(Insulin)
Growth
hormone
nutrition

Splitting

Myofibril hypertrophy

Testosterone   Intermittent (active) stretch

Neurotrophic
factors

Motoneurone

Figure 11.4. Summary of extrinsic factors which stimulate the growth of muscle (see text)

filaments around existing myofibrils, but there is no increase in sarcomeres.

Since protein is being formed during myofibrillar enlargement one might expect some change in the number or disposition of the ribosomes to become evident. Galavazi and Szirmai (1971) were able to demonstrate an increase in intermyofibrillar poly-ribosomes in electronmicrographs of levator ani muscle from castrated rats treated with testo-sterone. Surprisingly, however, the increase in myofilaments occurred rather earlier than that of the polyribosomes. That the ribosomes in such animals are being driven by myonuclear DNA is suggested by the rise in DNA, increased incor-

poration of [³H]-thymidine, and proliferation of nuclei within the fibres.

It is of interest to consider what the advantage might be of myofibrillar splitting as opposed to having thicker myofibrils, since the contractile force should be no different in the two situations. One possibility is that the biochemical 'support systems' for the myofibrils, operating through the mitochondria and sarcoplasmic reticulum, may be relatively ineffective in nourishing large cylinders of contractile material and that the myofibrils have an optimal surface:volume ratio. *Figure 11.4* sum-marizes the factors which are known to influence muscle growth; they are both hormonal (growth hormone, insulin and testosterone) and mechanical (muscle stretch). The ability to produce muscle atrophy by either denervation or starvation at any age indicates that an intact nerve supply and adequate nutrition must be considered as additional factors necessary for normal growth.

The isometric twitch studies of McComas, Sica and Petito (1973) were of interest for another reason in that they enabled the speed of the muscle twitch to be measured. In newborn kittens all muscles have 'slow' twitches but in those destined to become 'fast' a speeding-up occurs during the next few weeks under the controlling influence of the motoneurone (Buller, Eccles and Eccles, 1960a). In the human extensor digitorum brevis muscle the contraction time has already reached adult values by the age of 3 years but the relaxation phase remains slow for a rather longer time. The motoneurone also controls the enzyme concentrations of the muscle fibres and these can, of course, be studied histochemically. From the work of Dubowitz (1965) it appears that differentiation of fibres on the basis of myosin ATPase or mitochondrial enzyme staining commences in the fetus at about 20 weeks and is complete at 30 weeks.

Finally, the electrical properties of the muscle fibre membranes also change during growth. In the 1-week old mouse the resting potentials of the fibres are still well below those of the adult. Subsequently the potentials rise in both 'fast' and 'slow' muscles, with the former achieving rather higher values (Harris and Luff, 1970).

STUDIES OF MUSCLE REGENERATION

Muscle transplanation experiments

The pioneer studies in muscle transplantation were undertaken in Russia by Studitsky and reported in 1952. Possibly because this work was published in journals which were not freely available in the West, a long delay ensued before this important experimental approach became generally known. Subsequently, Carlson (1970) and others were able to confirm the main findings of Studitsky by demonstrating the remarkable capacity of mammalian muscle to regenerate after transplantation. The technique, as practised by Studitsky and Carlson, commonly consists of removing a muscle such as the gastrocnemius or tibialis anterior, resecting the tendon, and then cutting the muscle with scissors into fragments roughly 1 mm³ in size (*Figure 11.5*). The minced tissue is then replaced

into the bed from which the muscle was removed (*autograft*) or, in the case of dystrophy experiments (page 175), transferred into a similarly prepared bed in another animal (*homograft*). In normal studies the replaced tissue assumes the contours of the original muscle belly due to pressure of surrounding tissues; gradually, however, the mass shrinks until it occupies only 15–25 per cent of the original volume. During the first few days the sarcoplasm of the minced transplant degenerates but the nuclei appear more resistant and are able to initiate the regenerative mechanism by developing into myoblasts

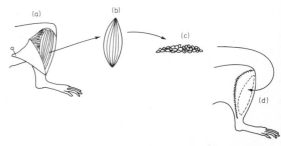

Figure 11.5. The transplantation of minced skeletal muscle (tibialis anterior) using the techniques of Studitsky (1952) and Carlson (1970). The muscle is exposed (a), removed (b), cut into small pieces (c) and packed into the tissue bed left by the same or a different muscle (d) (see text)

(page 92). Regeneration starts at the periphery of the transplant and proceeds inwards; it is associated with an invasion of the tissue by newly-formed blood vessels. Macrophages, brought into the regenerating region by these vessels, assist in the destruction of the sarcoplasmic material. In grafts into a second animal (homografts) there is also a marked influx of lymphocytes which cause considerable tissue rejection as part of an immunological response to foreign antigens. Within the regenerating tissue the myoblasts derived from the original nuclei multiply and, by the third day, are already fusing to form myotubes; these in turn develop into muscle fibres (page 93). Contractile activity can be detected 7–8 days after transplantation; at first the evoked muscle twitches are slow but by 30–40 days considerable speeding up has taken place (Carlson and Gutmann, 1972). At the completion of regeneration the new muscle is smaller than the original but contains many normal fibres and an increased proportion of connective tissue. As would be anticipated from the results of experiments on nerve trophic factors (Chapters 8 and 9), it appears that reinnervation is a prerequisite for optimal maintenance of the newly-formed tissue. In muscle tissue transplanted for more than 30 days the newly-established neuro-muscular junctions have a normal appearance, with both primary and secondary clefts being present, and synaptic transmission is fully effective (Bennett, Florin and Woog, 1974).

In a variation of this work, an *intact* muscle may be transplanted into its original bed, into another site in the same animal, or into a second animal. Under these circumstances some regeneration may also occur but it is not usually as marked as after mincing.

One problem in these experiments is to ensure that the regenerated muscle does not arise from myoblasts which have migrated into the graft from the muscle bed of the host animal. Control experiments, using Gelfoam in place of the muscle graft, suggest that this possibility is unlikely. Also Neerunjun and Dubowitz (1975), having labelled the myonuclei in the donor animal with isotope, showed that radioactivity remained confined to the nuclei of the transplant during the first few weeks of regeneration.

Limb amputation experiments

In this experimental model advantage is taken of the fact that certain amphibia, for example the newt and the salamander, are able to grow a new limb following amputation of the original one (*Figure 11.6*). The first stage in this regenerative process is the disappearance of the cartilaginous skeleton in the limb stump and the release of undifferentiated cells. These cells multiply and form a growing limb-bud, or *blastema.* Other mononucleated blastema cells are derived from the nuclei of degenerating muscle fibres in the limb stump. The blastema continues to grow and eventually forms cartilage, connective tissue and muscle, thereby producing a nearly perfect replica of the original limb. There is suggestive evidence that the capacity of a blastema cell to differentiate into cartilage or muscle is quite independent of its immediate tissue ancestry. Thus a blastema cell derived from cartilage may ultimately produce a

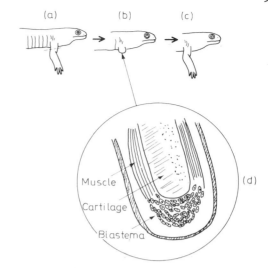

Figure 11.6. Muscle regeneration in the newt or salamander. A forelimb is amputated above the elbow (— — —, a). A blastema develops at the end of the growing stump (d); it is composed of undifferentiated cells which are released by cartilage and muscle and then multiply (see text). Eventually the limb is completely reformed

muscle, connective tissue or cartilaginous cell progeny (Hay, 1970).

Muscle injury experiments

There are many ways of injuring muscle and all have been used for the study of muscle regeneration; examples are crushing, heat, ischaemia, cold, X-irradiation and viral infection. The changes which take place in the muscle are common to all forms of injury though their magnitude will obviously depend on the intensity and spatial extent of the damage. Within 2 or 3 days of the injury three zones can be distinguished in the muscle (Reznik, 1970): (a) a necrotic region, (b) a normal region, and (c) an intermediate area (*Figure 11.7*).

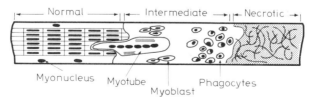

Figure 11.7. Stages in regeneration following damage to a muscle fibre (see text)

In the necrotic part of a fibre the cell components disintegrate. The mitochondria swell, lose their cristae and disappear; myofibrils break up into clumps and the sarcoplasmic and transverse tubular systems disintegrate. Many of the nuclei are also lost but others seem able to survive; the basement membrane of the fibre may also persist.

In the *intermediate part* of a muscle fibre there is a great increase in the number of nuclei, due to the presence of mononuclear cells. Some of these are phagocytes and leucocytes which have invaded the fibre and are concerned with the dissolution of the adjoining necrotic region. Other cells are *myoblasts* which have formed from pre-existing satellite cells or myonuclei within the muscle fibre (page 92). Finally, regeneration proceeds, the myoblasts fuse with each other to form myotubes and these, in turn, attract further myoblasts. As the myotubes enlarge they form buds at the regenerating end of the injured fibre. Finally the interface between the newly-constituted segment of fibre and the undamaged region becomes indistinguishable.

THE SATELLITE CELL CONTROVERSY

In the fetal muscle the myoblasts are obviously descendants of the mesenchymal (mesodermal) cells (see *Figure 11.1*). But from where do the myoblasts arise in regenerating adult muscle? The most favoured explanation is that they are identical with satellite cells. These interesting cells were not recognized until 1961 when Mauro, using the electronmicroscope, pointed out that some of the nuclei lying under the basement membrane of the

muscle fibre were separated from the remainder of the fibre by a plasma membrane (see *Figure 1.1*). In other words these nuclei were not the ordinary myonuclei but were part of individual cells lying within the muscle fibre itself. Subsequently MacConnachie, Enesco and LeBlond (1964) postulated that these cells were the source of the myoblasts responsible for muscle regeneration. There is extremely good evidence that the satellite cells are able to divide mitotically; they contain centrioles, mitotic figures have been seen after colchicine and, unlike the myonuclei, they will take up thymidine required for DNA synthesis. Unfortunately, as pointed out by Reznik (1970), there is one serious flaw in this argument; some muscles, for example the mouse gastrocnemius, have no demonstrable satellite cells and yet can regenerate perfectly well. Reznik agrees that the satellite cells are the source of myoblasts but postulates that the satellite cells themselves are derived from the myonuclei. In support of this conclusion he has published electronmicrographs of developing cells at a transitional stage between the myonucleus and the satellite cell. In these cells the forming plasma membrane has not yet fully separated the myonucleus from the sarcoplasm of the muscle fibre. Notwithstanding the curious inability to demonstrate tritiated thymidine in the myonuclei of regenerating muscle, Reznik's hypothesis seems plausible and has been included in *Figure 11.2*. It is important to appreciate that the incidence of satellite cells will be increased whenever the muscle fibre has been damaged or if denervation has occurred. It is the increased satellite cell population which is responsible for the so-called 'plastic state' of muscle, such that specimens of tissue taken for culture or grafting display optimal growth.

Chapter 12

AGEING

In old age, muscles become thinner and strength declines. For example, Burke and colleagues (1953) tested maximum grip strength and found that this fell by almost half between the ages of 25 and 79 years. In a different type of study, Campbell, McComas and Petito (1973), were able to exclude 'volitional' factors by measuring the isometric twitch tension of a muscle (the extensor hallucis brevis). They found that the maximum tension declined from a mean of 310 ± 88 g for subjects below the age of 59 to 210 ± 131 g for an elderly population aged 60–96 years, a reduction of 32 per cent. The maximum evoked action potentials recorded from the same muscles fell by a mean of 53 per cent (*Figure 12.1*). The fact that the mechanical response was reduced to a lesser extent than the electrical one may have been due to an alteration in the length–tension curve of human muscle with age (page 45).

What are the changes in the muscle which are responsible for this weakness and wasting? It is not altogether surprising that there have been few adequate studies in man. Obviously one cannot obtain biopsy specimens from elderly subjects who are otherwise well. On the other hand, unselected *post-mortem* specimens of muscle are not acceptable since almost any terminal illness may be expected to affect the neuromuscular system—whether as a result of disuse (through rest in bed), malnutrition, chronic infection or ischaemia. Similarly the neuromuscular system may be involved as a remote effect of carcinoma, or as a consequence of metabolic disturbances such as renal failure and diabetes. Even elderly patients

killed in accidents may have been harbouring serious chronic illness beforehand.

PATHOLOGICAL STUDIES IN MAN

Muscle fibres

Subject to reservations regarding adequacy of material (above), the following pathological changes have been described in muscles of the elderly (Rubinstein, 1960; Serratrice, Roux and Aquaron, 1968; Tomlinson, Walton and Rebeiz, 1969):

(1) *Loss of muscle fibres,* particularly those of type II (page 58). In the surviving fibres there are,

(2) *Variations in fibre size* due to the presence of (*a*) hypertrophied fibres, some of which contain central nuclei and are splitting longitudinally, and (*b*) atrophied fibres with pyknotic (dense) nuclei.

(3) *Degenerative changes,* such as hyaline degeneration, vacuoles at ends of fibres, lipofuchsin pigmentation, and loss of the remaining myofibrils so as to form spirals (Ringbinden) or central masses surrounded by sarcoplasm.

(4) *Necrotic changes,* with infiltrations of macrophage cells in and around the degenerating fibres.

An increase in the amount of endomysial connective tissue is also to be found. It should be added that the changes in the senile muscle are often patchy and, in addition, Tomlinson and colleagues (1969) have drawn attention to the presence of groups of atrophied fibres, suggestive

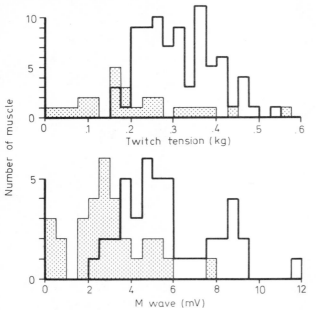

Figure 12.1. (Upper) Comparison of twitch tensions in 26 legs of elderly subjects and in 81 legs of controls (means 210 ± 131 g and 310 ± 88 g respectively; P = < 0.001. (Lower) Comparison of M wave amplitudes in 34 legs of elderly subjects and in 43 legs of controls (means 2.7 ± 1.7 mV and 5.7 ± 2.1 mV respectively; P = < 0.001). Observations in elderly subjects shown by stippling. (From Campbell, McComas and Petito (1973), courtesy of the Editor and publishers of Journal of Neurology, Neurosurgery and Psychiatry)

of denervation (see below). It is of interest that the periphery of the muscle fibre is not only the last part to form during growth (Williams and Goldspink, 1971) but is also the first to suffer from the effects of ageing. One possible, and not unlikely, reason for the earlier degeneration of the fibre periphery is that the trophic factors spreading from the end-plate zone become no longer sufficient to supply the whole fibre and are completely used up in the central region.

Intramuscular motor axons

A question which now arises is whether the changes described are due to intrinsic degeneration of the muscle fibres (i.e. 'myopathic') or to muscle fibre atrophy following denervation. The pathological study of muscle itself by conventional methods is of limited value for any of the features described above can occur as part of the so-called secondary myopathic complications of a chronic neuropathy (see Drachman et al., 1967) as well

as in a primary myopathy (see Chapter 13). While accepting that the presence of groups of atrophied muscle fibres (Tomlinson, Walton and Rubeiz, 1969) or of fibre-type grouping (Jennekens, Tomlinson and Walton, 1971) are suggestive of denervation, the relevant studies are still subject to criticism over the source of material (see above).

A second, and more acceptable, approach to the problem of denervation in old age has been to study the innervation of muscle directly using a variety of staining techniques, including the intravital methylene blue method. In the latter, the dye is first applied to the surface of the muscle over the innervation zone and the specimen is excised 5 minutes afterwards; the nerve fibres are stained blue (Cöers and Woolf, 1959). This technique has revealed that the neuromuscular junctions are often complex due to the presence of additional nerve twigs from the original motor axons (Harriman, Taverner and Woolf, 1970). In the pre-terminal axons spherical swellings are evident and there is an increased incidence of axon sprouting, suggesting that denervation of muscle fibres may be occurring with subsequent reinnervation by surviving motor axons ('collateral' reinnervation, see page 224).

Ventral roots

Finally, there are important studies on the ventral roots in man which are also relevant to the question of denervation (Corbin and Gardner, 1937; Gardner, 1940). The content of Table 12.1 is taken from Table 2 of Gardner (1940); it shows the numbers of fibres counted in the 8th and 9th

TABLE 12.1

Numbers of Axons in 8th and 9th Thoracic Ventral Roots in Post-mortem Specimens from 60 Subjects of Varying Ages

Age	Mean no. of axons	
	(T8)	(T9)
10–19	5968	6081
20–29	6205*	6204*
30–39	5816	5648
40–49	5495	5506
50–59	5361	5293
60–69	4805	4845
70–79	4420*	4628*
80–89	4923	5086
Max loss (%)	28.8	25.4

Results for each decade have been averaged
* Maximum axons losses calculated from highest and lowest values observed for each root.
Reproduced from Gardner (1940), courtesy of the Editor and publishers of the *Anatomical Record*

thoracic ventral roots of human cadavers and averaged for each decade. Two conclusions seem evident; there is a modest (about 27 per cent) loss of ventral root fibres with age and this loss is progressive beyond the age of 30. But are these conclusions really valid? In the first place there was an unfortunate choice of *post-mortem* material for many of the patients had died from illnesses likely to be complicated by a generalized neuropathy—for example, tuberculosis, carcinoma, cirrhosis of the liver and chronic nephritis. Secondly, there are only four values for each root below the age of 30, so that the mean values for the first decades are extremely approximate. Unfortunately, studies on peripheral nerve, as opposed to ventral roots, are unlikely to prove helpful for the percentage of alpha-motor axons in the nerve to a muscle is unknown (page 47).

Sensory nerve studies

It could be argued that any changes in motoneurones as part of the ageing process will be mirrored by the sensory neurones; if so, there is no difficulty in obtaining specimens, either at biopsy or *post-mortem*, of purely sensory nerve.

One of the first sensory studies was that of Swallow (1966) who counted the number of axons in the medial terminal branch of the deep peroneal nerve. This branch is not altogether satisfactory for this type of study since it receives a communicating twig of varying size from the musculocutaneous nerve on the dorsum of the foot. In a subsequent study with O'Sullivan (O'Sullivan and Swallow, 1968) *post-mortem* specimens of the radial and sural nerves were examined instead. The numbers of fibres in selected fascicles of these nerves were counted and the fibre density per unit cross-sectional area was calculated. Table III of O'Sullivan and Swallow's study has been reproduced and is shown below (Table 12.2), with

the addition of significance levels. It can be seen that there was hardly any difference between the mean fibre densities in sural nerves of subjects aged 17–39 and those aged 40–59 (p = 0.5). In contrast, there was a barely significant difference between the means for subjects aged 17–59 and those aged 60–80 (p = 0.05). The results for the radial nerve were less clear cut since there was a greater, though still insignificant, difference between the mean values for subjects aged 17–39 and those aged 40–59. Inspection of Figure 2a in O'Sullivan and Swallow's paper shows that this difference was largely due to relatively high fibre densities in both radial nerves of the youngest patient studied (aged 17).

Other studies on the sural nerve, by Arnold and Harriman (1970) and by Ochoa and Mair (1969), have also shown a decline in the number of apparently viable axons with age. In keeping with a loss of sensory nerve fibres in old age is a reduction in amplitude of the compound action potential (Buchthal and Rosenfalck, 1966), although increased temporal dispension of the component nerve fibre potentials will also have been a contributory factor.

NEUROPHYSIOLOGICAL STUDIES

A quite different experimental approach to the study of ageing changes was adopted by Campbell and McComas (1970; see also Campbell, McComas and Petito, 1973) who employed the electrophysiological motor unit estimating technique of McComas, *et al.* (1971a). These authors were careful to study only those subjects considered to be in good physical condition for their age and without any evidence of neurological and other organic disease, or of significant ischaemia of their limbs. The results in these subjects were compared with those in a large number of younger volunteers. In the initial studies, the extensor digitorum brevis

TABLE 12.2

Mean Fibre Densities in Sural and Radial Nerves of Subjects of Different Ages

Age	Radial nerve			Sural nerve		
	Nerves (no.)	Fibre density* (Mean + S.D.)	P	Nerves (no.)	Fibre density (Mean + S.D.)	P
17–39	11	7.44 ± 1.34		9	6.13 ± 1.11	
40–59	7	6.34 ± 1.05	0.10	10	5.78 ± 0.90	9.5
60–80	9	5.98 ± 1.07	0.02	8	4.78 ± 1.09	0.05

* Densities expressed as thousand fibres/mm
Probability values refer to differences from results in youngest age group (i.e. 17–39)
Modified from O'Sullivan and Swallow (1968) by courtesy of the authors and the Editor and publishers of *Journal of Neurology, Neurosurgery and Psychiatry*

104

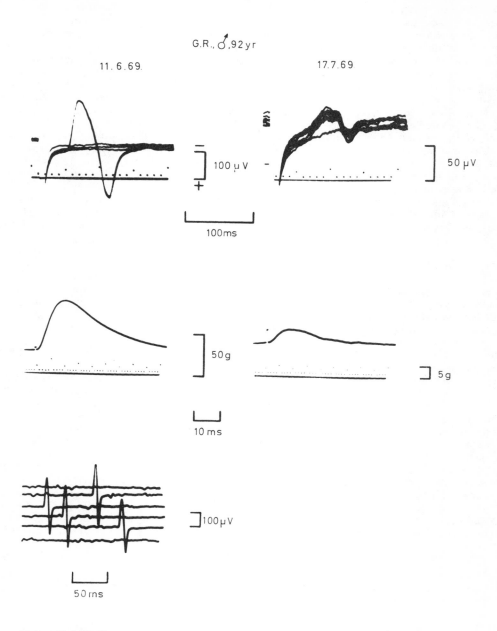

Figure 12.2. *Studies on the sole surviving motor unit in the EDB muscle of a 92-year-old man. The left column shows observations made at initial examination; all-or-nothing responses on indirect stimulation (top), isometric twitch (middle) and electromyogram during maximum effort (bottom). The right column displays the results obtained 5 weeks later, showing much smaller electrical and mechanical responses. Electrical recordings made with surface electrodes. (From Campbell, McComas and Petito (1973), courtesy of the Editor and publishers of* Journal of Neurology, Neurosurgery and Psychiatry)

muscle was used; with additional results a total of 207 muscles have now been studied and the values have already been presented in Chapter 6 (see *Figure 6.4*). As would be expected of such an approximate technique, the results for any one age exhibit considerable scatter. Nevertheless when the results for different ages are compared a striking feature emerges. Until the age of 60 the number of functioning motor units shows little change; beyond the age of 60, there is a progressive fall in the number of functioning units such that, by the age of 70, the population of units is reduced to less than half its original size. In some of the oldest subjects only a very small number of motor units remained and *Figure 12.2* shows the functional properties of the sole surviving EDB unit in a man of 92. Subsequently the function of this unit was shown to deteriorate (*Figure 12.2, right*). Recently, the same electrophysiological method has been applied to the median-innervated thenar muscles (page 50) and the hypothenar group (Sica, *et al.*, 1974). *Figure 12.3* shows the numbers of motor units in a total of 518 thenar, hypothenar and EDB muscles of healthy subjects of different ages; the values have been expressed as means for each decade. It can be seen that in the small muscles of the hand also there is a pronounced loss of motor units beyond the age of 60; before this time only a slight decrease is observed. It is of some interest that the thenar and EDB motor unit populations are affected more severely by the ageing process than the hypothenar muscle group; this difference is well seen in *Figure 12.3* and is also a feature of other neuropathic disorders (see Chapter 25). In a recent study by Brown (1972) the electrophysiological motor unit estimating technique was applied quite independently to the thenar muscles. Here again a loss with age was demonstrable and in a subsequent study (Brown, 1973) it was apparent that this was especially marked beyond the age of 60.

Before considering the significance of the motor unit findings it is important to recognize that the true loss of functioning units with age is actually more marked than *Figures 6.4* and *12.3* would indicate. Thus, at ages beyond the mean life expectancy (approximately 68 and 73 years for males and females respectively), the population of subjects sampled becomes increasingly biased in favour of those with particularly favourable physical endowments. One 'endowment' which might well enable ageing subjects to keep fit through physical activity is the number of functioning motor units available for use. For this reason a better indication of the severity of the ageing phenomenon in an *unselected* population would be given by an extrapolation of the results for the

sixth, seventh and eighth decades in *Figure 12.3*.

The finding of a reduced number of motor units in old age is not sufficient evidence in itself for denervation. For example, the reduction could have arisen by a gradual paring away of muscle

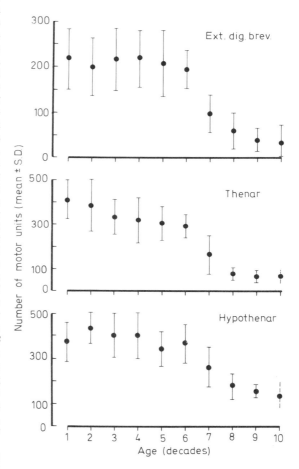

Figure 12.3. Numbers of functioning motor units in 207 EDB, 154 hypothenar and 157 thenar muscles of control subjects. The values shown are means for each decade (± S.D.)

fibres within motor units, as part of a 'myopathic' process, until some units had ceased to exist; a 'destitute' motoneurone would be left. Had this been the case, one would have expected the surviving motor units, because of their reduced fibre populations, to have generated smaller potentials than normal in the study by Campbell, McComas and Petito (1973; see also page 112). In fact the mean amplitude of the motor unit potentials was significantly larger in the elderly than in the controls. Considered together, these observations strongly suggested that, while some motoneurones (or axons) had completely ceased to function, others had successfully adopted denervated muscle fibres by sending out new axonal branches. In old age the capacity of the surviving motoneurones to reinnervate is limited, however, for it is found that the motor unit potentials are not as large as those in younger subjects with a similar amount of denervation. Further information about the properties of the surviving units has come from isometric twitch measurements which indicate that most of the units are of the slow-twitch type; a corresponding increase in the incidence of type I fibres in aged human muscles has been noted by Jennekens, Tomlinson and Walton (1971). While it is likely that the ageing process affects fast-twitch units most severely, there is also the possibility that surviving motor units develop slow twitches through excessive use as part of a compensatory mechanism (Salmons and Vrbová, 1969; Olson and Swett, 1969). This reduction in twitch speed may be advantageous in old age if neuromuscular transmission is at all critical. Thus the occurrence of occasional sub-threshold end-plate potentials may have little effect on strength since fewer impulses are necessary to produce a tetanic contraction in a slow-twitch muscle fibre.

What is the nature of the process responsible for the impaired neural function of old age? One ready explanation is that the neural degeneration results from an extraneous factor, such as ischaemia of the peripheral nerve or of the spinal cord due to obliterative arterial disease. Because of the first possibility Campbell and colleagues (1973) paid particular attention to the examination of arterial pulses in the limbs of their elderly subjects. Results were only considered acceptable if either or both of the dorsal pedal and medial plantar arterial pulses were palpable. Although this procedure did not entirely exclude the possibility of an ischaemic neuropathy, the alternative view favoured by Campbell and colleagues was that the reduction in functioning motor units resulted from an ageing process in the parent motoneurones. This interpretation would be in accord with the loss of ventral root fibres demonstrated by Gardner (1940) and by Corbin and Gardner (1937), though it is important to note that the depletion of functioning motor units far exceeds that of ventral root fibres (compare *Figure 12.3* and Table 12.1). The inference is that many of the motor axons persisting in old age have been unable to maintain functional synaptic connections to muscle fibres; in addition, it is possible that the axon membranes become inexcitable.

NEUROMUSCULAR STUDIES OF AGEING IN ANIMALS

It is interesting to inquire whether decreasing neural function in old age is a general property of the animal kingdom. In a comprehensive series of investigations, the answer obtained by Gutmann and his colleagues in the rat is by no means as definite as that in man (for review, see Gutmann and Hanzlíková, 1972). These authors counted motor axons and were able to show that there was no reduction in those supplying the soleus muscles of aged rats (Gutmann and Hanzlíková, 1966). In contrast the number of muscle fibres was considerably reduced, suggesting that there was a normal number of motor units but that each unit contained fewer fibres. Nevertheless, evidence for abnormal neuromuscular function was present, for recordings with microelectrodes in the levator ani muscle revealed a marked reduction in the discharge frequency of miniature end-plate potentials (Gutmann, Hanzlíková and Vyskočil, 1971). This did not appear to be due to an inability of the end-plate to form transmitter vesicles for normal or increased numbers of these were visible on electronmicroscopy. The impairment of transmitter release did not seem to progress to frank denervation, however, for fibrillation potentials were absent and the resting membrane potentials and acetylcholine sensitivities of the fibres were normal. Other animal data suggestive of impaired neuromuscular function in old age have been obtained by Tuffery (1971) in the cat. Using teased silver preparations from the soleus and peroneus digiti quinti (PDG) muscles, Tuffery observed that with advancing age the motor end-plate became more complex due to the receipt of one or more axonal sprouts from a node of the parent motor nerve fibre. It is tempting to suppose that these sprouts, by opening up new synaptic areas for the transfer of trophic material (page 14), are able to boost the declining influence of the motoneurone on its muscle fibre colony. Even the ability of the axon to sprout is limited, however, for Drahota and Gutmann (1961) found that axonal regeneration after a crush injury was considerably delayed and much less vigorous in older animals. In contrast to the absence of muscle fibre denervation on electrophysiological examination, neuropathological studies in animals have revealed evidence that at least some of the motoneurones are undergoing degeneration. In rats aged between 300–800 days, a mean loss of 10 per cent of ventral root axons was demonstrated by Duncan (1934). In still older rats, aged 900–1100 days, Bari and Andrew (1964) found that there was 18–38 per cent loss of ventral horn neurones.

Furthermore obvious degenerative changes were present in a high proportion of the surviving neurones; cell bodies were smaller and had accumulated pigment, the Nissl substance was reduced in amount and the nuclei were paler and vacuolated. Other morphological evidence in favour of a loss of neurones has come from Wright and Spink (1959) who used squash preparations of single segments of mouse spinal cord. After staining, the cells were counted under the microscope; the authors found that the total number of large ventral horn neurones (presumably mainly motoneurones) was unchanged up to 50 weeks of age but fell by 15–20 per cent during the next 60 weeks.

An important consideration is that, even if a normal number of motor axons remains in a given muscle nerve, this finding does not necessarily mean that all the axons are still functional. There is some support for this argument from the unpublished experiments of Caccia who has employed an incremental evoked potential technique to estimate numbers of functioning motor units in the soleus muscles of aged mice. In the soleus muscles of mice of two different strains approximately one-third of the motor units ceased to function after the first year of life. Thus, although abnormal findings are not as prominent in the animal studies as in the human ones, they nevertheless lend some support to the concept of declining motoneurone function during ageing.

Summary

It is postulated that the underlying defect in the neuromuscular system during ageing is progressive motoneurone dysfunction. In man this is first manifested after the age of 60 by an increasing inability of the motoneurone to maintain its colony of muscle fibres in a fully viable condition. During this phase the motoneurone may temporarily compensate for its declining trophic action by opening up a fresh synaptic connection with the muscle fibre by means of an accessory nodal sprout. In these ageing axon terminals the amount of acetylcholine released by impulses progressively declines and eventually becomes too small to initiate an action potential in the muscle fibre. The fibre is now functionally denervated; if the receipt of axoplasmically-conveyed material is also diminished the muscle fibre will begin to atrophy and to show other denervation phenomena. At this stage some of the motoneurones will be less affected than others by the ageing process and will remain able to adopt some of the denervated muscle fibres by axonal sprouting. Meanwhile most of the dysfunctional motoneurones, having relinquished their muscle fibre colonies, will persist in the spinal cord; relatively few cells will die or cause their motor axons to undergo Wallerian degeneration (page 221).

SPECULATIONS ON MOTONEURONE AGEING

An intriguing question may now be asked. What is it that causes the motoneurone to die with advancing age? One possibility is that some factor outside the motoneurone may be responsible. For example, there might be ischaemia of the ventral horn or perhaps the body might accumulate a neurotoxin; alternatively, a deficiency might develop of some undiscovered humoral factor necessary to sustain the motoneurone. A different type of explanation is that some intrinsic factor within the motoneurone is involved.

With increasingly successful methods available for maintaining neurones in tissue culture, these rival hypotheses could be tested by determining the life-spans of motoneurones removed from animals of the same species but of different ages (e.g. mouse). This approach has already been used to study fibroblasts and it does appear that these cells are only able to undergo a certain number of mitotic divisions before dying (Hayflick, 1965). Whether the 'intrinsic factor' is DNA and whether the life-span of the motoneurone is genetically programmed are other matters beyond the scope of this book (see, however, Gutmann and Hanzlíková, 1972).

Another equally fundamental question arises. Do the changes in motoneurones reflect a more widespread loss of neural function with advancing age? On the basis of frequently quoted studies on cerebellar Purkinje cells, cerebral cortex, olfactory bulb and optic nerve, it is generally believed that there is a steady loss of neurones throughout adult life. Wright and Spink (1959) have argued that, in the mouse cord, the loss of motoneurones is delayed until relatively late in life. The recent and ingeniously simple experiments on whole brains of mice by Johnson and Erner (1972) have shed new light on this controversy. After fixation in formalin, the brains were mashed in water and then further broken up into a fine suspension by ultrasonic vibration. Using a standard dilution, the suspension was stained with thionin and samples were examined in a standard haemocytometer chamber. The somata of the neurones were well preserved and could be identified and counted; the total brain neurone content was determined by a multiplication factor appropriate

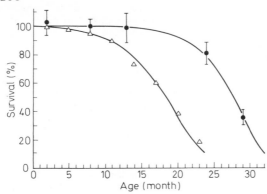

Figure 12.4. Per cent survival of mice (△) and their neurones (●) as a function of age. Smooth curves are survival curves derived from the Gompertz relationship; see Johnson and Erner (1972). (Modified and reproduced by courtesy of the authors, and the Editor and publishers of Experimental Gerontology)

for the dilution of the suspension. Johnson and Erner found that a marked loss of neurones did take place during ageing but that this only occurred relatively late. Allowing for differences in the life-spans of the species, these results are remarkably similar to those of Campbell and associates (1973) for human motor units (compare *Figures 12.3* and *12.4*). It seems reasonable to conclude that results obtained by the motor unit counting technique do indeed mirror more general ageing changes within the central nervous system.

Finally, how important are the neural events to ageing in other tissues? From the investigations presented in this chapter it seems probable that the motoneurones dictate the tempo of the ageing process in muscles. But observations on wasted limbs following infantile poliomyelitis show that neurones exert a trophic influence which ultimately affects such diverse tissues as skin, connective tissue and bone. This conclusion is not necessarily in conflict with that drawn from experiments on fibroblasts in tissue culture (see above) for the life history of these cells and their progeny may have depended on the 'intensity' of neurotrophic influences received by the original cells prior to the initial explantation. The intriguing possibility remains that the nervous system acts as a master clock which, by withdrawal of its trophic influence, determines the onset and speed of the ageing process throughout much of the remainder of the body.

PART 2

DISORDERS OF MUSCLE AND NERVE

Chapter 13

NEUROPATHIC AND MYOPATHIC DISORDERS: SICK MOTONEURONE HYPOTHESIS

We come now to a consideration of those diseases which affect the muscle fibre and its nerve supply. In doing so, one is struck by the rich variety of these disorders—some genetically determined and others acquired, some mainly affecting proximal muscles and others involving distal ones, some diseases rapidly progressing and others running insidious courses or even resolving spontaneously, some associated with gross derangements of muscle architecture and others manifesting little structural change. It has been customary to classify these diseases according to the site of greatest functional or structural abnormality. In muscular dystrophy, for example, the primary lesion has been thought to involve the muscle fibre since, at a stage when most of the fibres show evidence of severe degeneration, the motoneurones and their axons appear normal. Muscular dystrophy has accordingly been designated a *muscle fibre disorder* (or 'primary myopathy'; *Figure 13.1*). In the case of myasthenia gravis the motoneurone and most muscle fibres appear normal; in contrast, electrophysiological and pharmacological investigations reveal defective excitation at the motor endplate; the disease is therefore regarded as a *neuromuscular junction disorder*. In another group of diseases the development of muscle weakness and wasting is associated with degeneration of motor nerve cells in the spinal cord; motoneurone disease (amyotrophic lateral sclerosis) and the spinal muscular atrophies are examples of these *motoneurone disorders* (or 'motoneuronopathies', *Figure 13.1*). The last category of diseases is that in which the axon of the motoneurone, including its myelin covering, appears to be primarily affected; of particular interest among these *nerve fibre disorders* ('peripheral neuropathies') are those conditions caused by injury. As already stated, this system of classification is conventional and it is still convenient to think of neuromuscular diseases in this way; it has been employed in the following sections of the book. There is, however, a danger in this approach for it discourages thought as to the pathogenetic mechanisms underlying each of the neuromuscular disorders. For more than a century it has been known that the muscle fibre and the motoneurone normally exert a sustaining or 'trophic' influence on each other; the evidence has already been given in Chapters 9–11. In view of this interdependence the possibility exists that a subtle metabolic defect of a motoneurone, producing little outward effect in the cell itself, might result in a profound disturbance of the muscle fibre. Conversely, muscle fibre dysfunction could initiate major aberrations in the motoneurone. In regard to some of the primary myopathies, and to muscular dystrophy in particular, there has long been a body of evidence pointing to abnormalities in the peripheral and central nervous systems; the relevant findings will be presented subsequently in relation to the various disorders.

QUANTITATIVE MOTOR UNIT STUDIES IN DISEASE

Perhaps the strongest evidence for involvement of the nervous system in certain 'primary myopathies' has come from estimations of the numbers and sizes of motor units made by the method of McComas *et al.* (1971a; see pages 48–53). In the hands of McComas and colleagues this test has shown that there are losses of functioning motor units in a high proportion of patients with dystrophy. Such losses cannot be explained on the basis of inadvertent trauma to peripheral nerves

is important to recognize that the mean sizes of the remaining units should be appreciably smaller (*Figure 13.2, c*). Further advancement of the disease leads to further loss of motor units and even smaller survivors (*Figure 13.2, d*). *Figure 13.3* shows how the same results can be expressed in another way, by plotting the numbers of functioning motor units against the mean sizes of the survivors. By 'size' is meant the number of excitable muscle fibres still connected to a parent motoneurone through its multiply branched axon. Unfortunately, the size of a motor unit cannot be determined directly in a human muscle, although an ingeniously simple technique, combing both electrophysiology and histochemistry, has been devised for this purpose in experimental animals (Brandstater and Lambert, 1969;

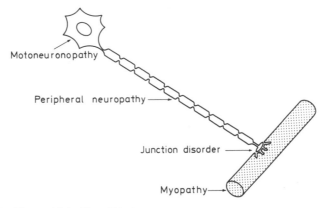

Figure 13.1. The different types of disorder which can affect a skeletal muscle fibre and its innervation (see text)

since they can affect a muscle such as soleus which is supplied by a relatively unexposed nerve; also, the denervation can sometimes be detected at a very early stage in the illness before the patient is disabled and likely to suffer nerve trauma. Could a loss of units be accounted for by a primary myopathic process? After all, there might come a certain point in a myopathic disorder when all the muscle fibres in an individual motor unit had degenerated or otherwise become inexcitable. This explanation seems unlikely for the reasons set out by McComas *et al.* (1974b):

If dystrophy really were a myopathy, then one would anticipate that the fibres within a muscle would be affected in a random manner. In some units more muscle fibres would be destroyed than in others but, at least in the early stages of the disease, there would still be a full complement of motor units within a muscle although their mean size would be reduced. This situation has been represented by the curve (*b*) in *Figure 13.2*, where (*a*) represents the motor unit population in health. As the disease progresses, more muscle fibres will degenerate; eventually some motor units would have lost all their muscle fibres. At this stage the number of functioning motor units would start to decrease, but it

Edström and Kugelberg, 1968). It is, however, possible to measure the amplitudes of the action potentials generated by single motor units in a human muscle; the values obtained will be directly proportional to the number of muscle fibres comprising those units. Obviously, the amplitudes of the unit responses will also be affected by other factors, such as the presence of muscle fibre atrophy or hypertrophy, the amount and disposition of intramuscular connective tissue, and the impulse-generating properties of the muscle fibre membranes. Of these factors the only one that will enlarge the motor unit potentials is muscle fibre hypertrophy, for the reduced internal resistance of an hypertrophied fibre will allow a larger than normal action current to flow during an impulse. Yet, although hypertrophied fibres may be found in all types of dystrophy, the arguments to be developed later would not be seriously weakened by their presence, as will be shown. For simplicity, however, we still regard a large motor unit potential as indicative of a large population of muscle fibres; conversely, an unusually small motor unit potential will be interpreted as muscle fibre depletion (McComas *et al.*, 1974b).

McComas and associates (1974b) showed that a different type of relationship between numbers and sizes of motor units would be expected to hold

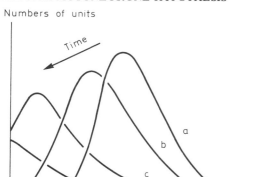

Numbers of units

Time

Sizes of motor units

Figure 13.2. Numbers and sizes of motor units in a healthy muscle (a) and those that would be expected to be present at various times in the course of a myopathic illness (b, c, d; see text). (From McComas et al. (1974b) courtesy of the Editor and publishers of Annals of the New York Academy of Sciences)

in a chronic neuropathic disorder, due to the ability of surviving motoneurones to enlarge their motor units by giving off axonal sprouts and thereby 'adopting' denervated muscle fibres (see page 224).

If this mechanism were completely successful, the relationship between the numbers of motor units and their mean potential size should follow the upper curve in *Figure 13.3.* For example, when the number of motor units is reduced to half, the mean sizes of the survivors should be doubled through collateral reinnervation. Similarly, if only a quarter of the units remained, their mean size should be quadrupled. In reality there are probably several factors which prevent attainment of the ideal relationship. One is the fact that not all the surviving motoneurones will be healthy; another is the presence within the muscle belly of fibrous septa that appear to impede the growth of the new axonal branches (Kugelberg, Edström and Abbruzzese, 1970). Even so the capacity and success of healthy motoneurones in undertaking reinnervation are remarkable.

On the basis of considerations such as these McComas and colleagues reported that there was a neural defect in myotonic dystrophy (Campbell, McComas and Sica, 1970), limb-girdle and facioscapulohumeral dystrophies (McComas and Sica, 1970) and Duchenne dystrophy (McComas, Sica and Currie, 1970). Elsewhere they pointed out (McComas, Campbell and Sica, 1971):

'if the denervation is not secondary to a myopathy then only two possibilities remain. Either it is an independent phenomenon occurring in association with the primary myopathy responsible for dystrophy or alternatively

muscular dystrophy is the result of a neuropathy. It is sufficient at the present time to state that, while the first possibility cannot be excluded, the second hypothesis has the merit of simplicity and is compatible with all the observed features of dystrophic muscle.'

THE SICK MOTONEURONE HYPOTHESIS

McComas and associates developed their line of thought into the 'sick motoneurone hypothesis'; they based their arguments on electrophysiological observations made on the various types of muscular dystrophy as well as on myasthenia gravis, motoneurone disease and spinal muscular atrophy (McComas, Sica and Campbell, 1971). It was suggested that muscular dystrophy and myasthenia gravis might arise from dysfunction of motoneurones; in some cases the motoneurones went on to lose all influence on the muscle fibre and could be considered as 'dead'. The appearance of the muscle on histological, histochemical and electrophysiological examination would depend largely on the proportions of healthy, dysfunctional ('sick') and dead motoneurones in the spinal cord.

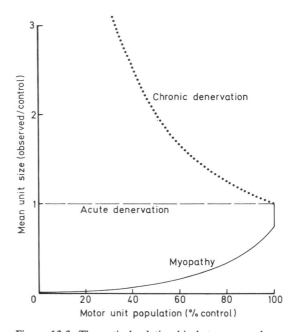

Figure 13.3. Theoretical relationship between numbers and sizes of motor units in acute and chronic denervation and in a myopathy (see text). (From McComas et al., 1974b, courtesy of the Editor and Publishers of Annals of the New York Academy of Sciences)

Employing the motor unit counting technique, the authors showed that the proportion of moto-neurones in each of these categories could be calculated for a given muscle, and they were able to estimate the average duration of the postulated 'sick' phase. In view of the controversy which has come to surround the hypothesis, it is perhaps best to consider it as originally presented (courtesy of the Editor of the *Lancet*).

'SICK' MOTONEURONES: A UNIFYING CONCEPT OF MUSCLE DISEASE

Summary

New electrophysiological techniques have demonstrated a loss of motor units in muscular dystrophy and myasthenia gravis; the sizes of the surviving motor units suggest that both diseases result from disordered function of motoneurones. Estimates have been made of the incidence of healthy, sick, and dead moto-neurones in these conditions and, for comparison, in recognized denervating processes such as motorneurone disease and the Kugelberg–Welander syndrome.

THE HYPOTHESIS

The present hypothesis is concerned with a number of disorders of the peripheral nervous system, each of which is characterized by weakness or wasting of muscles. Some of the diseases to be considered (motor-neurone disease, Kugelberg–Welander syndrome) are known to affect the lower motoneurone directly; in others the primary pathological attack is thought to fall upon the neuromuscular junction (myasthenia gravis) or upon the muscle fibre (muscular dystrophy). The hypo-thesis says nothing about the nature of the aetiological agents responsible for these various conditions. Instead it seeks to reconcile all these disorders, hitherto regarded as widely disparate, in terms of a common patho-physiological mechanism. In short, each condition is regarded as resulting from disordered motoneurone function.

Our starting-point is that, until now, it has been customary to consider motoneurones as existing in one of only two states—healthy or dead. Nevertheless, it seems reasonable to assume that, just as with other cells in the body, there must be an intermediate phase between these two extremes when the neurone is dysfunctional, or expressed more simply, 'sick'. We shall suggest that in some conditions the sick period is transitory and reversible, that in others it swiftly culminates in death, while in yet others, it may persist for years. We further postulate that, whenever a neurone enters a sick phase, degenerative changes inevitably ensue in the muscle fibres which it innervates. To make the hypothesis as explicit as possible we shall now define the functional attributes of motoneurones classed as 'healthy', 'sick', or 'dead'.

Healthy motoneurones

A motoneurone can continue to be regarded as healthy as long as it conducts impulses at normal rates down the axon, transmits excitation effectively across neuro-muscular junctions, and, by its 'trophic' influence [see below], maintains all the muscle fibres of the motor unit in a healthy condition. (A motor unit, as defined by Sherring-ton[1], is the population of muscle-fibres innervated by a single motoneurone.) An important property of a healthy motoneurone is that it can grow new axonal branches which will successfully establish synaptic connections with previously denervated muscle fibres. That is, a healthy motoneurone has an inherent potentiality for enlarging the size of its motor unit.

Sick motoneurones

The most important characteristic of a sick moto-neurone is that it has difficulty in maintaining satis-factory synaptic connections with muscle fibres. This difficulty is manifested in two ways. Firstly, when tested by maximum volitional effort or by repetitive nerve stimulation, neuromuscular transmission is impaired. Secondly, although the motoneurone may still command a normal, or slightly reduced, number of muscle fibres, it is quite unable to acquire previously denervated muscle fibres. If axonal sprouting does occur, it is ineffective. Impulse conduction down the axon generally occurs at normal velocities but may be slowed in terminal regions.

Dead motoneurones

Dead motoneurones are those which have ceased to exert any excitatory or trophic influence on muscle fibres.

The three types of motoneurone have been defined in purely functional terms with no mention of neurone morphology. The significance of loss of cells from the anterior horn of the spinal cord is evident; similarly, severe chromatolytic changes in neurones must surely denote impending death. On the other hand, there is no reason for assuming that the normal appearance of a motoneurone signifies normal function. A good example of the lack of correlation between appearance and function in the nervous system may be found in the work of Thesleff[2] on the neuromuscular junction in the frog. He has shown that over a period of several days following the administration of botulinum toxin no changes in the nerve terminal can be detected, even with the electronmicroscope. Yet in spite of this, marked denervation changes are already taking place in the under-lying muscle fibres. The studies of Miledi and Slater[3] provide a second example, which is especially pertinent to the present discussion. These workers have found evidence that there is normally a centrifugal flow of (trophic) substance along the axon which is necessary for the normal structure and function of the neuromuscular junction. Within a relatively short period following nerve section the neuromuscular junction undergoes complete

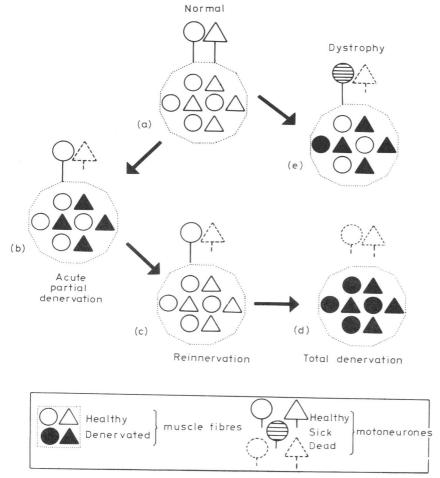

Figure 13.4. Muscle changes induced either by death or by 'sickness' of motoneurones. Only two motoneurones are represented, each of which is normally supposed to innervate four muscle-fibres (in reality, several hundred) (see text)

disruption and ceases to function: yet for several hours the nerve axon appears normal and continues to conduct impulses at normal velocities.

Effects of motoneurone dysfunction on muscle

Figure 1 [*Figure 13.4*] depicts, in a very simplified diagrammatic form, the different pathological types of motoneurone together with the associated findings in the muscle. In the normal situation (a) two motoneurones are shown connected to their motor units, each of which consists of four muscle fibres and overlaps with fibres belonging to the other unit. The succeeding stages (b–d) in Figure 1 [*Figure 13.4*] set out the changes which take place in a muscle during a 'classical' denervating process, such as motoneurone disease; this part of the figure is based largely on the recent motor unit

study of Kugelberg *et al*[4]. It can be seen that death of one motoneurone (b) causes acute denervation of the corresponding muscle fibres. As the surviving motoneurone is healthy, however, it successfully reinnervates the denervated fibres to form an enlarged unit (c) in which fibres are grouped together. It is this clustering of fibres which is responsible for the large muscle action-potentials found during electromyographic examination of partially denervated muscles with concentric needle electrodes. If death of the second motoneurone supervenes (d) all the muscle fibres will be denervated and will degenerate; there is now 'grouped' atrophy. In (e) a different situation obtains. Once again a motoneurone has died; but this time, according to the present hypothesis, the surviving motoneurone is sick and cannot annex the denervated fibres. Indeed the sick motoneurone has lost one of its own muscle fibres. In this situation histological examination would not reveal any grouping of muscle fibres; accordingly, the specimen would be labelled myopathic. If the present considerations are extended to whole populations of motoneurones, as in Figure 2 [*Figure 13.5*] two further conclusions can be drawn. Firstly, in a chronic partially denervated muscle, the 'myopathic' quality will be greater the more sick motoneurones there are amongst the survivors. Secondly, a 'neuropathic' appearance results from the presence of healthy motoneurones; in such a muscle the sizes of the muscle fibre groups will depend on the ratio of dead to healthy motoneurones.

EVIDENCE FOR HYPOTHESIS

The sick motoneurone hypothesis is based on well-established evidence concerning the 'trophic' influence of motoneurones. The need for the hypothesis arose from the results of recent electrophysiological studies in diseased muscles.

Trophic influence of motoneurones

Several types of experiment indicate that the motoneurone normally controls not only the excitation but also the basic metabolic processes of muscle fibres. The experimental techniques and results have been reviewed elsewhere[5]; at present it seems that the trophic effects cannot be accounted for solely in terms of use or disuse and that specific messenger substances(s) are probably transmitted from nerve to muscle. The importance of the trophic action lies in its hypothetical corollary—namely, that dysfunction of the motoneurone will result in the altered metabolism characteristic of the degenerating muscle fibre. The next step in the conceptual argument is critical and demonstrates the unifying nature of the present hypothesis. Thus, if evidence of primary motoneurone dysfunction can be adduced in a disease state then it is no longer necessary to invoke the additional existence of a primary myopathic process. Accordingly, a disease such as muscular dystrophy is considered to represent part of a spectrum of motoneurone disorders rather than a pathological entity [see below].

Electrophysiological studies

A method has now been devised for estimating the numbers of motor units in human extensor digitorum brevis muscles. The method involves comparison of the potentials evoked by stimulation of single motor units and of the whole muscle. Examples of the use of this technique have already been briefly reported[6-8], pending publication of a full account in which the inherent assumptions are critically analysed[9]. All control subjects below the age of 60 have been found to have more than 120 units, the mean estimate being 199 S.D. ± 60 (*n* = 41). The method also enables the sizes of the motor units to be assessed, since these are proportional to the amplitudes of the individual motor unit potentials. The mean unit size can be further checked by measuring the isometric twitch tension of the whole muscle and dividing it by the estimated number of units in the muscle.

The accompanying table and Figure 2 [*Figure 13.5*] summarize the results of the motor-unit investigations in control subjects and in each of the disease states (motorneurone disease; Kugelberg–Welander syndrome; myotonic, Duchenne, limb-girdle, and facioscapulohumeral dystrophies; myasthenia gravis). In Figure 2 [*Figure 13.5*] the average number of units present in each disease is shown and the sizes of the motor units have been indicated in terms of their evoked potential amplitudes.

TABLE 13.1

Numbers of Surviving Extensor Digitorum Brevis Motoneurones in Patients with Various Neurological Disorders*

Patients (no.)	Age mean (range) (yr)	Mean duration illness (yr)	Total surviving cells (mean ± S.D.)	Healthy cells (no.)	Yearly cell loss (bo.)	Duration sick phase
Myotonic dystrophy (17)	43 (17–63)	43	75 ± 47	5	3	24 yr
Duchenne dystrophy (19)	11 (2–16)	11	53 ± 38	4	13	4 yr
Limb-girdle, Facioscapulohumeral dystrophies (11)	49 (36–60)	49	65 ± 41	31	3	12 yr
Kugelberg–Welander (11)	28 (8–56)	28	77 ± 50	48	4	7 yr
Motor neurone disease (15)	52	2	11 ± 11	9	94	8 days
Myasthenia gravis (10)	43	7	121 ± 47	48	(11)	(7 yr)
Controls (41)	28 (3–58)	—	199 ± 60	—	—	—

* Motoneurones were arbitrarily designated 'sick' if, in a chronic partially denervated muscle, the amplitudes of their motor-unit potentials were less than 40μV. Duration of 'sick phase' calculated as in text assuming that, in inherited disorders, spinal cord is already affected at birth

INTERPRETATION OF RESULTS IN TERMS OF HYPOTHESIS

In all the diseases studied there was evidence of loss of motor units. This result would have been expected in motorneurone disease and the Kugelberg–Welander syndrome, but such a finding in muscular dystrophy and myasthenia gravis was of great interest and demanded careful consideration.

although some of the surviving motor units were reduced in size, the majority were within the normal range (Figure 2 [*Figure 13.5*]). In *Duchenne dystrophy,* nearly all the units were within the normal range. These findings indicated that these conditions could not have been affecting muscle fibres randomly but must have been destroying individual motor units in their entirety,

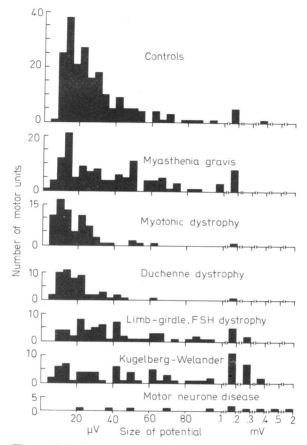

Figure 13.5. Sizes of motor units in various disorders, as indicated by amplitudes of evoked potentials. For each condition the results have been expressed in terms of the mean number of surviving motor units

Firstly, it might be argued that, in any disease process thought to affect either muscle fibres or neuromuscular junctions randomly, a stage might eventually be reached when all the fibres in a motor unit had become involved, thereby leading to the destruction of that unit. Yet the sizes of the surviving motor units in these conditions suggested that this could not have been the correct explanation. Thus, in a random process, the surviving motor units should all be affected to various extents; in particular, there should have been many abnormally small units. In *myotonic dystrophy,* however, it was found that,

presumably by acting at the level of the motoneurone. These diseases should therefore be classed as neuropathies and not myopathies; further evidence in favour of a neurogenic mechanism has been marshalled elsewhere[8]. In these two dystrophies the surviving motoneurones could not be regarded as healthy, however, for the relatively normal sizes of their units indicated that the cells had failed to innervate muscle fibres relinquished by the dead motoneurones. It appeared that, until the terminal episode, the surviving motoneurones could maintain the *status quo* but were quite unable to take on fresh commitments. These observations, allied to the finding of impaired neuromuscular transmission (myotonic dystrophy[6]) and of slowed impulse conduction in terminal nerve regions (Duchenne dystrophy[10]), suggested that virtually all the remaining motoneurones were sick. In the *limb-girdle* and *facioscapulohumeral dystrophies* the evidence for a neurogenic process was even stronger, since enlarged motor units were commonly found. This result could only have meant that potentially healthy muscle fibres had lost their original (defective)

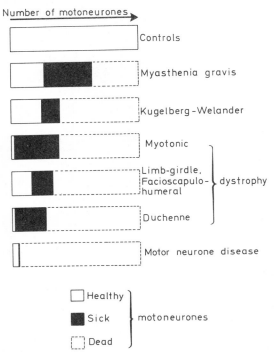

Figure 13.6. Estimated proportions of healthy, sick and dead motoneurones in the different neurological disorders, using data of table

nerve-supply and had been reinnervated by healthy motoneurones. On the other hand, the occurrence of relatively normal-sized motor units, together with decremental muscle responses to repetitive nerve stimulation, indicated the presence of sick as well as healthy motoneurones among the surviving population.

The results in the *Kugelberg–Welander syndrome* and *motorneurone disease* differed only in degree from those in the limb-girdle and facioscapulohumeral dystrophies. In *motorneurone disease* the denervation was greatest, but the large sizes of most remaining units suggested that the motoneurones remained healthy until they underwent relatively sudden destruction. In *myasthenia gravis* there is already considerable evidence that the disease results from a presynaptic defect of the neuromuscular junction—i.e. that it is neurogenic[11]. In the present study only four out of the ten patients examined had decremental responses in the extensor digitorum

brevis muscle following repetitive nerve stimulation. However, in each of these and in one further patient an abnormally small population of motor units could be demonstrated. This finding of a loss of whole motor units suggested that the disease was not involving neuromuscular junctions randomly but, as in dystrophy, was operating at the level of the motoneurone.

In Figure 3 [*Figure 13.6*] a pictorial attempt has been made to summarize the experimental findings in terms of the present hypothesis. This figure shows the average numbers of dead and surviving motoneurones at the time when patients with each type of disease were investigated. On the basis of the sizes of the surviving motor units, estimates have been made of the numbers of motoneurones falling into the sick and healthy categories. In a severely denervated muscle any motoneurone with a motor-unit potential amplitude of less than 40 μV was arbitrarily regarded as sick. We judged that such a motoneurone had either been unable to take over denervated fibres or, having previously enlarged its territory, had now begun to lose muscle fibres. It has already been seen that the relative incidence of each type of motoneurone will determine whether a muscle specimen appears myopathic or neuropathic. However, Figure 3 [*Figure 13.6*] is of value in another respect, for it reflects the tempo of the dysfunctional process in each cell. Thus the duration of the sick phase in any one cell will be equal to the number of sick cells present at a given moment divided by the rate of cell loss. Let us consider two extreme examples, using the average values in the table. In motorneurone disease 188 cells have died in two years, this being the average duration of the clinical symptoms prior to investigation. Of the 11 cells remaining, suppose that only two are sick. Then the duration of the sick phase for each motoneurone will be $\frac{2}{188} \times 2$ years = 8 days. This value may be contrasted with that for myotonic dystrophy where, assuming that the disease is active at birth, it takes 43 years to lose 124 cells. If 70 of the remaining 75 cells are sick then the duration of the dysfunctional phase in each motoneurone will be $\frac{70}{124} \times 43$ = 24 years. These two estimates and the corresponding values for the other conditions are given in the last column of the table. The figure for myasthenia gravis is tentative, since it assumes that the disease is steadily progressive. In the absence of serial motoneurone counts in the same patient, it is doubtful whether this assumption is valid. Indeed the acute onset of the illness and the not infrequent spontaneous remissions suggest that cell death occurs early and that many sick cells subsequently recover.

CONCLUSIONS

Perhaps the most remarkable aspect of a normal human motoneurone is that, for more than sixty years, it can successfully supervise the excitatory and metabolic behaviour of several hundred muscle-fibres. Considered in this light, the present hypothesis in favour of a neurogenic explanation for 'myopathic' and 'neuromuscular' disease does not seem unreasonable, particularly if the supporting experimental evidence is taken into account. Unfortunately hardly anything is known at present about the nature of the substance(s) responsible for the trophic effects of neurones. Nevertheless it seems almost certain that trophic mechanisms will prove to be as much a feature of synaptic organisation in the central nervous system as in the motor unit. If that is so, then one may safely predict that many neurological disorders, other than those considered in this article, will also eventually be shown to involve the breakdown of trophic relationships.

REFERENCES

1. Sherrington, C. S. *Proc. R. Soc.* B. 1929, 105, 332.
2. Thesleff, S. J. Physiol. Lond., 1960, 151, 598.
3. Miledi, R., Slater, C. R. ibid. 1970, 207, 507.
4. Kugelberg, E., Edström, L., Abbruzzese, M. *J. Neurol. Neurosurg., Psychiat.* 1970, 33, 319.
5. Guth, L., *Physiol. Rev.* 1868, 48, 645.
6. Campbell, M. J., McComas, A. J., Sica, R. E. P. *J. Physiol., Lond.* 1970, 209, 28P.
7. McComas, A. J., Sica,. R. E. P. *Lancet,* 1970, i, 1119.
8. McComas, A. J., Sica, R. E. P., Currie, S. *Nature, Lond.,* 1970, 226, 1263.
9. McComas, A. J., Fawcett, P. R. W., Campbell, M. J., Sica, R. E. P. *J. Neurol. Neurosurg. Psychiat.* (in the press).
10. McComas, A. J., Sica, R. E. P., Currie, S. Unpublished.
11. Elmqvist, D., Hofmann, W. W., Kugelberg, J., Quastel, D. M. J. *J. Physiol., Lond.* 1964, 174, 417.

It should be added that the possibility of a neural aetiology for dystrophy had been raised independently by Dubowitz (1969) on the basis of histological similarities between muscle fibres in this condition and in denervated muscle. Somewhat later Engel proposed a similar basis for myotonic muscular dystrophy (Engel, 1971a) and myasthenia gravis (Engel and Warmolts, 1971) while invoking a vascular aetiology for Duchenne dystrophy (Engel, 1971b). In Engel's case as in Dubowitz's, the evidence for a neural mechanism was indirect, being based on the histological and histochemical appearances of muscle. In a subsequent article, Engel and Warmolts (1973) drew an interesting analogy between motor units and trees; they pointed out that in both a central dying-off process could be incomplete, resulting in a patchy loss of muscle fibres (leaves), or total, causing complete denervation. The former type of disorder they termed 'in portio' while the latter was described as 'in toto'. It is clear that the *in portio* lesion is the same as the 'sick motoneurone' of McComas, Sica and Campbell (1971) for the latter was described as commanding 'a normal, or *slightly reduced,* number of muscle fibres' (italics added). The inability of the sick motoneurone sometimes to maintain a full complement of muscle fibres was emphasized in Figure 1 (*e*) of McComas, Sica and Campbell (1971) which showed part of a motor unit missing. The main differences between the neural hypotheses of Engel and Warmolts (1973) and of McComas, Sica and Campbell (1971) may be summarized as follows:

(1) The McComas group had more direct evidence of neural involvement (though some of their electrophysiological findings have been disputed; see Appendix 6.1).

(2) Among the major neuromuscular disorders, Engel and Warmolts applied the neural hypothesis to myotonic dystrophy and myasthenia gravis whereas McComas and colleagues extended it to other forms of dystrophy as well.

(3) In muscular dystrophy and in myasthenia gravis the McComas group recognized an additional category of motoneurone, the 'dead' cell. Such a cell could no longer influence the muscle, having lost both excitatory and trophic connections with its population of muscle fibres.

(4) The electrophysiological approach of McComas and colleagues enabled them to quantitate the proportions of healthy, sick and dead motoneurones, as well as the average duration of the sick phase.

Since its formulation the sick motoneurone hypothesis has been subjected to vigorous attacks from a number of directions; criticisms have been levelled at the choice of muscle, the electrophysiological technique used, and the clinical diagnosis of some of the patients. Apparently conflicting results from pathological studies of muscle, peripheral nerve and spinal cord have also been brought forward. These criticisms are considered in detail in Appendix 6.1. For the present it is fair to say that the concept of sick motoneurones continues to provide a valid basis for a hypothesis of certain neuromuscular diseases and that, through a study of motoneurone disorders, it has been possible to define the stages of motoneurone dysfunction with more precision (see Chapter 25). From a practical standpoint, however, it is still easiest to consider neuromuscular diseases in terms of the sites of maximum observed abnormality. This philosophy has been pursued in the chapters which follow, each disease being categorized in terms of its presentation as a muscle fibre, neuromuscular junction, nerve fibre or motoneurone disorder. At the end of the book the question of a neural pathogenesis is taken up once more, this time drawing upon observations cited in each of the chapters.

DISORDERS OF MUSCLE FIBRE MEMBRANES

The membrane of the muscle fibre, as described in Chapters 1, 3 and 5, was seen to be a highly complex structure which not only surrounds the fibre (the sarcolemma) but also comprises a complex interlacing network of tubules within the fibre (the transverse tubular system). Another system of tubules, the sarcoplasmic reticulum, runs in the long axis of the muscle fibre and is connected to the transverse system at the triads. The functional inter-relationship of the membrane systems is an important feature of the normal fibre while in certain diseases an abnormality in one type of membrane system may produce effects in another. For example, in the next chapter it will be shown that if the sarcolemma exhibits a reduction in chloride permeability, as in certain types of myotonia, it will also become hyperexcitable through the effects of potassium released into the transverse tubular system. The subsequent chapter deals with a contrasting situation in which paralysis is caused by inexcitability of the sarcolemma; by bringing about changes in ionic concentration, the internal tubular systems are likely to play an important role in this type of disorder also.

Chapter 14

MYOTONIA

CONDITIONS AFFECTING MEMBRANE EXCITABILITY

In certain diseases the excitability of muscle fibre membranes can undergo striking alteration. In *myotonia* and *tetany* the excitability is increased, so that the fibres fire impulses spontaneously or after mechanical or electrical stimuli which are normally ineffective. In contrast, in *familial periodic paralysis* the fibre excitability is depressed so that impulses can no longer be initiated at the neuromuscular junction or by electrical stimulation at other points along the surface of the fibre. In some conditions the changes in excitability are more complex. For instance, in the *hyperkalaemic* form of familial periodic paralysis there is often an initial increase in membrane excitability, the myotonic phase, followed by a depression. All the conditions mentioned above are clearly of great neurophysiological interest and for this reason they have now been studied with intracellular recording techniques in a number of laboratories. It should not be assumed, however, that these are the only conditions in which responsiveness of muscle fibres is disturbed. For example, it is known that the permeability of the muscle fibre membrane is extremely sensitive to *anoxia* since the latter causes the sodium permeability to increase and the resting potential to decline (Creese, Scholes and Whalen, 1958). The membrane potential is also affected by *protein molecules* in the interstitial fluid; if these are absent the membrane depolarizes by 10–15 mV (Kernan, 1963; McComas and Mossawy, 1965). Part of this protein effect is due to insulin

since Zierler (1959) has shown that insulin causes potassium to enter muscle fibres and the membrane potential to rise. It now appears that the primary action of the hormone is to stimulate the sodium pump, thereby producing hyperpolarization by electrogenic extrusion of sodium; potassium ions are then attracted into the fibre interior by the increased negativity (see Creese, 1968). The protiens of the interstitial fluid, and the globulin fraction in particular, have a further action in limiting the sodium permeability of the fibre(Creese and Northover, 1961); it is possible that the proteins exert this effect by forming a layer on the outer surface of the membrane. Even a brief immersion of an excised muscle in a protein-free medium is sufficient to produce a substantial sodium entry into the fibres (Krnjević and Miledi, 1958). In addition, as we have already seen, the resting membrane potential depends not only on the high permeability of the membrane for potassium relative to sodium, but also on the concentrations of potassium on both sides of the membrane. Taking all these factors into account, one might expect to find the membrane potential altered in any condition characterized by tissue anoxia, reduced plasma proteins, abnormal insulin secretion and electrolyte imbalance. Finally it is important to remember that the high internal concentration of potassium is itself a consequence of the electrical force exerted by the internal anions (page 16). Therefore in any condition in which there is a loss of anions due to destructive changes within the sarcoplasm, a depolarization of the muscle fibre membrane may also be predicted. A prolonged fall in resting potential will, of course, inactivate a proportion of the sodium carriers and make them no longer available for impulse initiation, as in the phenomenon of accommodation (page 24). Whether this process is sufficient, in any of the conditions considered, to block impulse propagation or excitation–contraction coupling, is another matter. Certainly the weakness and fatiguability of which patients with various metabolic disorders often complain make the possibility worth exploring. With the exception of thyrotoxicosis, which is considered in Chapter 26, there is a lack of experimental observations in most of these systemic conditions; for this reason attention will be directed instead to relatively specific disorders of the muscle fibre membrane.

THE PHENOMENON OF MYOTONIA

In myotonia the muscle fibres undergo prolonged contraction due to repetitive firing of action potentials. These discharges are abnormal in that they prevent the muscles from relaxing promptly after a willed contraction. In most patients the small muscles of the hand and the long flexors of the fingers seem to be especially vulnerable to this type of disorder but in some individuals virtually every muscle may be affected. Patients may often complain that they have difficulty in releasing their grip after unscrewing bottle tops or that they cannot let go of hand tools immediately after using them. Most subjects find that the stiffness

TABLE 14.1
Classification of the Myotonias (References in text)

Hereditary myotonias
  (A) In man
        (i) Myotonia congenita
        (ii) Myotonic dystrophy
        (iii) Hyperkalaemic familial periodic paralysis
        (iv) Paramyotonia
        (v) Chondrodystrophic myotonia
  (B) In animals
        (i) Goat
        (ii) Horse (Stringhalt)
        (iii) Dystrophic mouse
        (iv) Dystrophic chicken
Acquired Myotonias
        (i) Drug-induced
              Triparanol
              Clofibrate
              2.4-dichlorphenoxyacetate
              Diazacholesterols
              Monocarboxylic acids
        (ii) Low external chloride
        (iii) Vitamin E deficiency
        (iv) Denervation
        (v) Hypothyroidism

can be worked off by repeated contractions though weakness sometimes ensues (the 'warm up phenomenon). Often the disability is aggravated by cold weather and in some patients washing the face and hands in cold water may provoke local myotonia. The myotonia may also be induced by tapping a muscle sharply; the thenar eminence and the tongue are usually used to demonstrate this sign. On clinical grounds a number of naturally-occurring myotonic conditions can be distinguished, most of which are inherited (Table 14.1).

Myotonia congenita (Thomsen's disease)

This disorder is usually transmitted by an autosomal dominant gene but sometimes by a recessive one. The myotonia tends to be more severe than in the conditions mentioned below and in affected infants may cause difficulty in feeding. The muscles in this disorder are often conspicuously enlarged and histological examination shows that there is a true hypertrophy of the fibres with the presence of additional myofibrils. Myotonia congenita is readily differentiated from myotonic dystrophy by the absence of weakness and of other somatic abnormalities. Interestingly, there are mild reductions of motor unit populations in about half of the patients (McComas and Upton, unpublished observations).

Dystrophia myotonica (Myotonic dystrophy)

In this condition the muscles are both myotonic and dystrophic. In addition the patients may suffer from the following abnormalities—cataracts, mental deficiency, frontal baldness (males), gonadal atrophy, and various skeletal and endocrine disorders. The disease is considered more fully in Chapter 16.

Hyperkalaemic familial periodic paralysis

Patients with this disorder undergo attacks of paralysis preceded by a myotonic phase (see Chapter 15).

Paramyotonia congentia

This is recognized by some as a separate entity. In this condition the otherwise normal muscle fibres exhibit myotonia which is particularly dependent on temperature, being readily brought out by cooling; attacks of weakness also occur. However, myotonia in any of the other conditions is nearly always made worse by cooling and, in view of the episodic weakness, it is doubtful if patients with 'paramyotonia' are qualitatively different from those with familial periodic paralysis (see Chapter 15).

Chondrodystrophic myotonia and other myotonias

Myotonia associated with dwarfism and diffuse bone disease was reported in a 10-year-old boy and his 6-year-old sister by Aberfeld, Hinterbuchner and Schneider (1965). Each patient showed an unusual facies with narrowing of the palpebral fissures, long eyelashes, a depressed bridge of the nose, a high-arched palate and receding chin. The children were undersized with 'pigeon-breasts' and had limited mobility of many joints, particularly the hips. The muscles were 'myopathic' and exhibited myotonia on electromyography. An earlier but less complete account of chondrodystrophy was given by Schwartz and Jampel (1962), after whom the syndrome is sometimes eponymously referred to.

It is of interest that myotonic discharges have recently been reported in *glycogen* storage diseases (Isch, Isch-Truessard and Jesel, 1972; Engel *et al.*, 1973). Myotonia can also occur in animals and is a prominent feature of the Bar Harbour 129 strain of dystrophic mice (McIntyre, Bennett and Brodkey, 1959) and has also been reported in the horse (Steinberg and Botelho, 1962) and dystrophic chicken (Holliday *et al.*, 1965). The most florid example of animal myotonia, however, is that which occurs in a certain type of goat. These goats have been a valuable experimental model for the investigation of myotonia; the discovery of these very useful animals makes a fascinating story which is told in Appendix 14.1.

Myotonia may also be acquired. For example, it may complicate *hypothyroidism* (Humphrey and Richardson, 1962) and disappears completely following adequate treatment of the endocrine disorder. Of great interest is the observation that recovery from various types of *polyneuritis* may be associated with true muscle hypertrophy and myotonia (Krabbe, 1934); this phenomenon is apparently an over-compensation by the neuro-muscular system. Myotonia has also been reported in the *vitamin E deficiency* neuromyopathy of the Rottnest quokka (Durack, Gubbay and Kakulas, 1969). Finally a number of compounds will induce myotonia in man and experimental animals; these include 20,25-diazacholesterol, mono-carboxylic aromatic acids, 2,4-dichlorphenoxy-acetate, clofibrate and triparanol. In addition to myotonia, the first of these drugs also produces cataracts; this observation is of interest since cataracts are a naturally-occurring feature of human myotonic dystrophy.

Central and peripheral components in hereditary myotonia

When a concentric needle electrode is inserted into a myotonic muscle it is possible to record two types of spontaneous activity. One type has been largely ignored in experimental studies. It consists of irregular discharges of large complex potentials and for this reason is likely to originate in a group of muscle fibres belonging to the same motor unit. It can be demonstrated in dystrophic mice that some of these discharges originate in the motoneurones for their frequency is reduced by nerve section (McComas and Mossawy, 1965). Similarly, in an important and earlier study of human myotonia by Denny-Brown and Nevin (1941), it was argued that these potentials were produced by motoneurone activity; the authors described this activity as 'after-spasm'.

One observation by Denny-Brown and Nevin was particularly intriguing. They found that if they anaesthetized the ulnar nerve at the elbow and the median nerve at the wrist, the (still-innervated) long flexor muscles in the forearm of a patient with dystrophia myotonica were now able to relax completely and without delay following

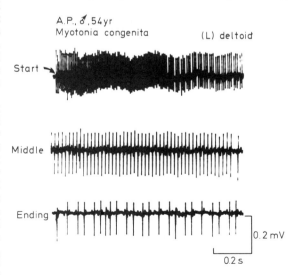

Figure 14.1. Myotonic activity of the peripheral type, recorded with a coaxial needle electrode from the left deltoid muscle of a 54-year-old man with myotonia congenita

maximal voluntary contraction. This experiment suggested that the after-spasm arose because the long flexor motoneurones were responding to a proprioceptive input from the intrinsic muscles of the hand. In the dystrophic mouse the central component may also be reflex in origin for these animals can be shown to respond to various stimuli in unusual ways. For example, when the animals are lifted by their tails, their hindlegs flex at the hips and knees; in a normal mouse the appropriate response is extension of the limbs. Recent unpublished studies by Douglas and Law have shed further light on this type of activity; they have found that the spontaneous spasms persist after the spinal cord has been transected rostrally but that they are abolished by division of the dorsal roots. These observations could indicate that normal motoneurones were being excited by abnormal inputs

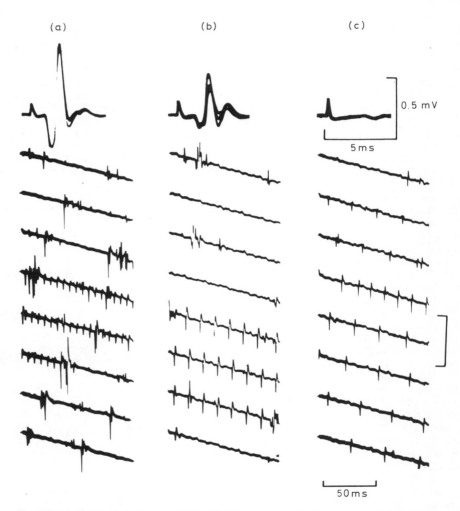

Figure 14.2. Recordings made with a coaxial needle electrode from the tibialis anterior muscle of a dystrophic mouse; the sciatic nerve had been sectioned. At top are superimposed responses to nerve stimulation before (a) and following the injection of d-tubocurarine (b, c); (below) high-frequency trains of spontaneous muscle fibre impulses which withstand complete neuromuscular block (c). The occasional complex and rather larger potentials which are present in (a) are eventually abolished by curarization (c); they probably correspond to 'central myotonia' (after-spasm). (From McComas and Mossawy (1965) courtesy of the Muscular Dystrophy Group of Great Britain and Pitman Medical Publishing Company)

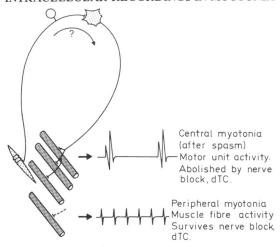

Central myotonia
(after spasm)
Motor unit activity.
Abolished by nerve
block, dTC.

Peripheral myotonia
Muscle fibre activity
Survives nerve block,
dTC.

Figure 14.3. The contrasting features of central myotonia (after-spasm) and peripheral myotonia; dTC, d-tubo-curarine (see text)

arising in the periphery; alternatively the moto-neurones could be abnormal but still require a certain amount of normal synaptic bombardment from the periphery in order for them to discharge. It is of interest that spontaneous spasms can be induced in previously normal mouse muscle following cross-innervation from a dystrophic animal, as in the parabiotic experiments described in Chapter 16.

In contrast to after-spasm, the second type of myotonic discharge, *'peripheral' myotonia,* is much better known. It consists of high frequency discharges of potentials which, because of their small sizes and brief durations, are likely to have originated in single muscle fibres. These discharges can be triggered by very slight movements of the recording electrode within the muscle belly. They have a sudden onset and the initial frequency of 100–200 impulses/s slowly declines over the next few seconds (*Figure 14.1*). The declining frequency and amplitude of these potentials give rise to the characteristic 'dive-bomber' sound over the loud-speaker. Further information concerning the origin of these discharges was obtained by Brown and Harvey (1939) in myotonic goats; they found that the activity could still be elicited after nerve section and after curarization. This last observation excluded the possibility that the discharges could have arisen at the end-plate following spontaneous release of acetylcholine. The ability of the high frequency myotonic discharges to withstand curarization has been confirmed in man (Lanari, 1947; Floyd, Kent and Page, 1955) and in the dystrophic mouse (McComas and Mossawy, 1965; see *Figure 14·2*). The curare experiments have firmly established hyperexcita-bility of the muscle fibre membrane as being the cause of the peripheral myotonic phenomenon. The contrasting features of central and peripheral myotonia have been summarized in *Figure 14·3* and in Table 14·2 which has been reproduced, with slight modification, from the paper by Denny-Brown and Nevin (1941).

INTRACELLULAR RECORDINGS IN MYOTONIA

Further information concerning the properties of the muscle fibre membrane in peripheral myotonia will now be considered. The first microelectrode study of myotonia was that of Norris (1962) who investigated one patient with dystrophia myotonica and one with myotonia congenita. Norris reported that the muscle fibres underwent spontaneous slow depolarizing pre-potentials which eventually triggered off action potentials. Although he

TABLE 14.2

The Differences between After-spasm and Peripheral Myotonia, as Noted by Denny-Brown and Nevin (1941)

After-spasm	*Peripheral (muscular) myotonia*
(*a*) Large action currents	Very small action currents
(*b*) Increase of intensity compared with the preceding contraction	Only a small percentage of the preceding contraction
(*c*) Easily fatigued	Difficult to fatigue
(*d*) Not necessarily related to previous contraction in the same muscle	Determined by, and proportional to, the intensity of previous contraction in the same muscle
(*e*) Not elicited by percussion	Elicited by percussion
(*f*) Onset delayed by as much as 0.4 seconds when in weak or moderate degree	Is maximal immediately the eliciting contraction ceases and thereafter wanes
(*g*) Impedes the action of opposing muscles	Very weak opposition to antagonistic muscles
(*h*) In early dystrophia myotonica may appear in fixators of wrist only when synergic with grasp movements and not when used as prime movers	In early dystrophia myotonica may be elicited only in the small muscles of the hand, and in the tongue

considered the resting potentials to be normal his values were low in comparison with others reported for human muscle. Furthermore three of his four control subjects had conditions in which the resting membrane potential might well have been reduced (benign congenital hypotonia, dermatomyositis and familial periodic paralysis). Riecker and colleagues (1964) used the *in vivo* cannula technique (Appendix 3.1) to study 50 fibres in five patients, all of whom had myotonia congenita. These authors were not able to detect the depolarizing pre-potentials noted by Norris but they did find that the resting potentials were normal. The next microelectrode study in myotonia was that of Hofmann, Alston and Rowe (1966), who studied

---

TABLE 14.3

Resting Membrane Potential and Critical Membrane Depolarizations of Muscle Fibres from Two Patients with Myotonia Congenita and Two with Myotonic Dystrophy

	Resting potential (mV)	Critical membrane depolarization* (mV)
Controls	−83.6 ± 0.5 (134)	11.8 ± 0.4 (37)
Myotonic dystrophy	−71.4 ± 1.1† (94)	11.3 ± 0.8 (14)
Myotonia congenita	−82.0 ± 0.8 (42)	8.8 ± 0.8† (17)

* The critical membrane depolarization is the amount of depolarization necessary to bring the membrane from the resting level to the firing threshold.
† Values significantly different from those of controls (P = <0.01). Mean values have been given with their standard errors. From McComas and Mrożek (1968).

---

intercostal muscles from 10 patients. Nine of these patients had myotonic dystrophy while the tenth, and youngest, was thought to have myotonia congenita; since there was no histological evidence of dystrophy in a muscle biopsy, however, this seems a questionable diagnosis. Hofmann and colleagues found that the resting membrane potentials were reduced in specimens from all the patients and they were also able to confirm the membrane oscillations reported previously by Norris. In 1968 McComas and Mrózek published observations on two patients with myotonic dystrophy and two with myotonia congenita. As shown in Table 14·3 the resting membrane potentials differed in the two conditions, being normal in myotonia congenita and reduced in myotonic dystrophy. In contrast, slightly increased resting potentials were found in myotonia congenita by Lipicky, Bryant and Salmon (1971).

POSSIBLE MEMBRANE DEFECTS RESPONSIBLE FOR PERIPHERAL MYOTONIA

Reduced chloride permeability

In myotonic goats Bryant (1969) found that the muscle fibres were also slightly hyperpolarized. By passing current through intercostal muscle fibres *in vitro* and measuring the induced change in membrane potential (page 19), the same author then showed that the specific membrane resistance was increased. Since the membrane of a resting muscle fibre is only permeable to potassium and chloride, the increased resistance must have resulted from decreased permeability to either or both of these ions (see page 19). In another series of experiments the resistance measurements were repeated after chloride had been replaced by methylsulphate in the bathing fluid, so as to abolish the contribution of chloride to the total membrane conductance. It was then found that whereas the fibre membrane resistances of normal goats increased by an average of 6.9-fold, that of the myotonic goats rose by a much smaller amount (1.5-fold). From this Bryant and Morales-Aguilera (1971) deduced that it was the chloride permeability of the membrane which was reduced in myotonic goats. Lipicky and Bryant (1973) have also made observations on human myotonia. In four of six patients with myotonia congenita and in a solitary patient with dystrophia myotonica there was evidence of a reduction in chloride permeability.

The chloride permeability hypothesis has been strengthened by two other observations. First, it was shown by Bryant (1962) that myotonic features developed in the muscle fibres of normal goats after the chloride conductance had been abolished by substituting methylsulphate for chloride. Secondly, there are a number of chemical agents which can induce myotonia in normal muscle fibres and these appear to reduce the chloride permeability of the resting membrane. One group of substances is the *monocarboxylic aromatic acids;* four of these were recently studied by Bryant and Morales-Aguilera (1971) and a fifth by Rüdel and Senges (1972). Another myotonia-inducing drug is *20,25-diazacholesterol,* also investigated by Rüdel and Senges (1972). These drugs are effective both *in vitro* and *in vivo;* for example, Bryant and Morales-Aguilera (1971) were able to produce stiffness and percussion myotonia in goats within 1–2 minutes of injecting anthracene-9-carboxylic acid into the external jugular vein. Bryant and Morales-Aguilera (1971) suppose that the aromatic acid molecule reacts with the chloride permeability channel in the membrane at two points. They suggest that the hyperphobic end of the molecule attaches itself to the outer lipid rim of the channel while the carboxyl group combines with the active site within the channel, so as to cause a steric reduction in permeability. Curiously, these compounds do not induce myotonia in frog muscle even though the muscle fibres in this species have a high chloride permeability at rest (Hutter and Noble, 1960; Hodgkin and Horowicz, 1959). It is also puzzling that myotonia does not occur in normal human intercostal muscle even though the membrane resistance is as high as that in the myotonic goat. It should be added that there are other drugs such as *veratrine* and *aconitine* which can produce repetitive discharges in muscle fibres without appearing to reduce the chloride permeability. In spite of these last considerations, the chloride permeability hypothesis appears very attractive for most, but not all, cases of myotonia congenita and also for goat myotonia. In view of the clinical observations that myotonia is often made worse by cold it is interesting that Rüdel and Senges (1972) found that the membrane resistance increased on cooling normal muscle fibres. It seems possible that this effect may be an important contributory factor in the induction of myotonia in affected fibres.

As a result of recent work by Adrian and Bryant (1974) it is now possible to suggest the way in which the reduced chloride permeability of the myotonic muscle fibre leads to instability of the membrane (*Figure 14.4*). These authors used an intracellular microelectrode to pass depolarizing currents through intercostal muscle fibres of myotonic goats. They noted that, unlike normal fibres, the myotonic ones could be excited by very small currents and would often continue to fire repetitively after the stimulating current had stopped. The repetitive activity appeared to rise from unusually large negative after-potentials which followed the spike potentials; the after-potentials and the repetitive activity were abolished by treating the muscle with glycerol. It has already been shown (page 19) that this substance disrupts the connections of the transverse (T)-tubules to the surface membrane of the muscle fibre. Adrian and Bryant linked their observations together by suggesting that, as in a normal fibre, the myotonic fibre conducts an action potential down the T-tubule (page 39). During the phase of high potassium permeability which terminates the action potential some potassium ions will leave the fibre and enter the T-tubule (page 20). The reduction in the potassium concentration gradient across the tubular membrane will cause the

membrane to stay slightly depolarized; the depolarization is terminated when the excess potassium has been lost by diffusion from the mouth of the T-tubule into the interstitial fluid surrounding the fibre. However, successive action potentials will cause the after-depolarizations to add; eventually they will be large enough to activate the regenerative sodium permeability mechanism and cause an action potential themselves. Thus the action potentials become self-perpetuating and give rise to the typical myotonic

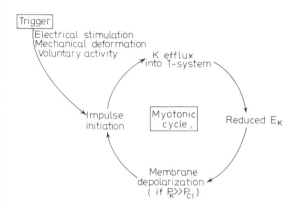

Figure 14.4. Mechanism proposed to account for peripheral myotonia, based on the findings of Adrian and Bryant (1974) (see text)

discharge. In a *normal* fibre the after-potentials are much smaller because the *high chloride* permeability of the surface membrane acts as a stabilizing influence; that is, the membrane potential of the fibre will be intermediate between the equilibrium potentials for chloride (at the sarcolemma) and that for pottassium (at the tubular membrane). Reference to *Figures 3.2, 3.3* and the Goldman equation (page 18) makes this point clear. Adrian and Bryant conclude 'that the high chloride permeability of normal skeletal muscle fibres appears to be a specialization to stabilize the surface membrane, by making the potential across it relatively independent of ionic concentration changes in the tubular lumen which result from propagating a radial signal in the tubules'.

As a result of the loss of chloride permeability the myotonic membrane will also become hyperexcitable in any circumstance in which the sodium permeability is increased. Transient stretching of the fibre is one such situation and is then responsible for the sign of 'percussion myotonia'.

Reduced critical membrane depolarization

Although the chloride permeability hypothesis provides a plausible explanation for goat myotonia and myotonia congenita, it does not necessarily follow that myotonia in other conditions has a similar basis. Hyperexcitability of the membrane could arise in a number of ways, in which activation of the regenerative sodium permeability mechanism was the common end-stage. One such possibility would be a fall in the resting membrane potential so that only relatively small depolarizations would be required to bring the membrane to the firing level. The normal or increased values of resting membrane potential described above show that this could not be an explanation for myotonia congenita or goat myotonia. In contrast, in dystrophia myotonica the resting membrane is decreased in a substantial fraction of the muscle fibres (*Figure 16.20*). Possibly because of the accommodation phenomenon (page 24) the excitability of these fibres to applied currents is not increased (Table 14.3). Suppose that, instead of a persisting depolarization, the membrane potential were to fall relatively rapidly from a normal level. In these circumstances accommodation might not be sufficient to prevent spontaneous activity from occurring. This seems a reasonable explanation for the myotonia which occurs in *hyperkalaemic familial periodic paralysis* for it has now been convincingly shown that the membrane spontaneously depolarizes during an attack of paralysis. The myotonic phase begins as the membrane reaches the critical potential for impulse initiation; paralysis follows because the potential goes beyond this critical level (Brooks, 1969; *Figure 15.1*).

Another possible myotonic mechanism would be for the resting membrane potential to be unchanged but for the critical membrane potential to be altered so that, once again, very little depolarization was required for excitation. Such an abnormality does occur in a proportion of the fibres in dystrophic mice but there is no evidence that it is involved in any of the human forms of dystrophy. Thus, although McComas and Mrożek (1968) observed that the resting membrane potential was normal in myotonia congenita, they found that normal-sized depolarizations were still required to trigger-off the myotonic action potentials. An example is given in *Figure 14.5* (*lower*), which shows a single potential during the early stages of a myotonic discharge. It can be seen that the myotonic impulse was preceded by a pre-potential of some 13 mV; the resting membrane potential itself was −92 mV and was at the upper part of the normal range. However, during the remainder of a myotonic discharge the membrane does under-

go progressive depolarization between impulses and less critical depolarization is needed for excitation. An example is the fibre discharge shown at the top of *Figure 14.5* where the resting potential has fallen to −74 mV and the critical membrane depolarization was only 5 mV. It is difficult to discount the possibility that this progressive fall in resting potential had resulted from tearing of the membrane around the microelectrode during the myotonic twitching; for this reason one should hesitate to attach significance to such observations.

Calcium ion depletion

Another possible explanation for the myotonic phenomenon is that the membrane becomes hyperexcitable due to lack of calcium ions, as in tetany. It is known, for example, that removal of ionizable calcium by the application of citrate or oxalate to a muscle will produce long-lasting spontaneous runs of action potentials which resemble myotonia (Adrian and Gelfan, 1933). In

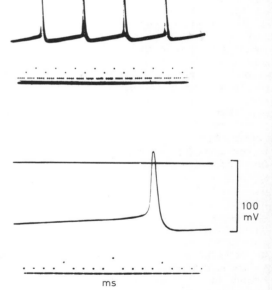

100
mV

ms

Figure 14.5. Myotonic activity recorded in situ with an intracellular microelectrode from two fibres of a patient with myotonia congenita. Note that the upper recording was made with a slower sweep of the oscilloscope time-base (see text). (From McComas and Mrozek (1968), courtesy of the Editor and publishers of Journal of Neurology, Neurosurgery and Psychiatry)

naturally-occuring myotonia, however, there is no evidence that the concentration of calcium is reduced in the serum (and presumably in the interstitial fluid). It could be argued that local abberations in calcium concentration might occur on either side of the fibre membrane which would not be reflected in serum levels. While the calcium-handling properties of the sarcolemma in myotonic fibres do not appear to have been studied, the membrane of the sarcoplasmic reticulum has normal pumping activity (Samaha *et al.*, 1967); this observation suggests that a generalized membrane defect involving calcium transport is unlikely to be present. Also against the possibility of a low calcium ion mechanism is the observation of Hofmann, Alston and Rowe (1966) that myotonic activity persists in excised human muscle fibres immersed in solutions containing normal or raised calcium concentrations.

'Fragile' membrane

McComas and Mossawy (1965) postulated that myotonia might arise if the muscle fibre membranes were abnormally 'fragile', such that they could tear and reseal following relatively minor mechanical stresses (e.g. following percussion or during voluntary contraction and relaxation). At the site of the tear the absence of membrane would abolish the resting potential; this zone would act as a 'sink' for current, initiating action potentials in surrounding areas of membrane (see *figure 3.8*). Interesting though this possibility is, there is at present no supporting evidence for its existence.

BIOCHEMICAL PROPERTIES OF THE MYOTONIC MEMBRANE

Since peripheral myotonia is a membrane abnormality the phospholipids of muscle from affected patients have been investigated by means of gas chromatography. Kuhn (1973), summarizing work carried out in collaboration with Seiler, has reported that there are differences in the relative amounts of fatty acids between myotonic patients and controls. The most striking abnormality was the finding of appreciable amounts of *docasadienoic acid* in the dominant form of myotonia congenita; in control muscles this acid was absent or only present in very small amounts. The fatty acid abnormalities found may have been peculiar to muscle membranes for they were not detectable in red cells. Furthermore the changes demonstrated were not common to all forms of myotonia since there were differences between the results for the

dominant and recessive forms of myotonia congenita and between these and the values for paramyotonia. In the experimental myotonia induced by diazacholesterol there is a change in the lipid composition of the sarcolemma due to the substitution of *desmesterol* for cholesterol (Peter and Fiehn, 1973) but there is no evidence for the abnormal accumulation of desmesterol in the human forms of myotonia (Peter *et al.*, 1974).

Studies have also been made of the enzymatic activity of cell membranes in myotonic dystrophy. In both muscle fibres and red cell 'ghosts' there appears to be reduced phosphorylating ability of the protein kinases (Roses and Appel, 1973, 1974). In addition Hull and Roses (1976) have demonstrated an alteration in the stoichiometry of the sodium pump such that 2 Na ions are exchanged for 2 K ions; in normal cells the ratio is 3 Na for 2 K ions. It is possible that the decreased enzymatic activity results from the loss of one Na binding site on each of the membrane ATPase molecules responsible for pumping these ions. The altered kinase activity could also be explained in terms of reduced numbers of molecules; alternatively the enzyme could be normal but its activity diminished by some change in the physical properties of the membrane. This last possibility deserves special consideration in view of the demonstration, using electron spin resonance, of increased fluidity in red cell membranes of patients with myotonia congenita and myotonic dystrophy (Butterfield *et al.*, 1074).

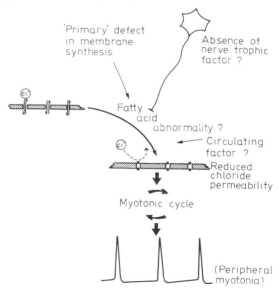

Figure 14.6. Factors which may ultimately result in the formation of an abnormal muscle fibre membrane and so lead to the development of myotonia (see text)

INDUCTION OF THE MYOTONIC MEMBRANE

It has been shown, in the peripheral myotonia of goats and patients with myotonia congenita, that the defect resides in the muscle fibre membrane, that it involves a reduction in chloride permeability and that the fatty acids composing the membrane may be abnormal. The question which now arises is whether the myotonic membrane is formed because one of the genes for membrane synthesis is defective or whether the gene expression in the muscle is modified by the presence or absence of some external factor. Of such factors the neurotrophic messenger molecules would be obvious candidates (page 12). Alternatively the myotonic membrane could develop through the direct action of some circulating agent on the muscle fibre. There is some evidence for both these last possibilities (*Figure 14.6*).

Neural influence

One of the trophic actions exerted by the motoneurone is the maintenance of potassium and chloride channels in the resting muscle membrane. If the fibre loses its nerve supply the permeability to both these ions falls (page 74). The possibility therefore exists that the reduced membrane chloride permeability in myotonia congenita and goat myotonia could result from selective absence of the appropriate neurotrophic factor. As yet there is no convincing answer to this possibility though two observations suggests that it deserves further exploration.

(1) In some cases of myotonia congenita, as in most patients with dystrophia myotonica (page 165), there is evidence for a neurotrophic lesion from the finding of a loss of functioning motor units (McComas and Upton, unpublished observations).

(2) In patients with 'true' denervation of muscle, myotonic discharges may occasionally be encountered. Brumlik and Cuetter (1969) described five patients with radiculopathies in whom this phenomenon was present and we have noted profuse myotonia in the brachial biceps and deltoid muscles of a 54-year-old man with severe denervation resulting from cervical spondylosis. In addition, the denervation resulting from polyneuritis may be associated with myotonia during the recovery phase, as already mentioned (page 125).

An understanding of the role of the nervous system in myotonia is complicated by the fact that denervated muscle is resistant to the induction of myotonia by drugs, as Caccia *et al.* (1975) have shown.

Humoral agent

Evidence for a circulating agent capable of inducing myotonia has come from a study by Krull and colleagues (1966) on a 33-year-old woman with *hyperkalaemic familial periodic paralysis*. They used a cuff to prevent venous return during exercise of forearm muscles and found that generalized myotonia occurred when the cuff was released. In another experiment some of the pooled venous blood was withdrawn and stored; myotonia could be produced in rabbits and rats if a sample of this blood was injected intravenously.

Treatment of hereditary human myotonia

In the past, various drugs have been found useful in the treatment of myotonia congenita and, to a lesser extent, of the myotonia associated with myotonic dystrophy. The three most commonly employed drugs are quinine (e.g. quinine sulphate, 200 mg twice daily), procaineamide (e.g. procaineamide hydrochloride, 0.5 g four times daily) and diphenylhydantoin (e.g. 100 mg three times daily), all administered orally. In a controlled trial Leyburn and Walton (1959) found procaineamide to be superior to quinine. Potassium depletion by ion-exchange resins is rather less effective but beneficial results have been achieved with corticosteroids (Leyburn and Walton, 1959). Unfortunately all these medications have potential side-effects, some of a serious nature, and for this reason the myotonia should only be treated if it causes major interference in daily living.

Chapter 15

FAMILIAL PERIODIC PARALYSIS

INTRODUCTION AND CLINICAL FEATURES

Of all the neurological syndromes which have been recognized to date, one of the most fascinating is undoubtedly familial periodic paralysis. Underlying this fascination is the intriguing combination of muscular paralysis and well-marked serum electrolyte disturbances; the challenge to the experimenter of relating these two events is obvious but, strangely, has yet to be met satisfactorily.

Historically, the first definite account of this unusual syndrome was given by Hartwig in 1874. His patient was a 23-year-old man in whom the attacks were associated with disturbances of speech, respiration and swallowing. Hartwig mistakenly thought that the underlying lesion was hyperaemia of the spinal cord but he demonstrated correctly the unresponsiveness of the paralysed muscle fibres to electrical stimulation. Another outstanding early contribution was that of Goldflam (1895) who discovered and drew the dilated vacuoles within the affected muscle fibres. The first description of the disease in the English scientific literature was by Singer and Goodbody (1901) who gave the following account of the onset and progression of an attack. Their patient was a 16-year-old boy who had been admitted to hospital for prolonged observation.

This attack is chosen because it was observed practically from the onset, which took place in the afternoon, the patient having been kept in bed for purposes of observation. He had been feeling perfectly well, and, as usual, had no warning whatsoever; he was lying talking to some friends about *3 p.m.* when he noticed a 'dull aching' about his knees, and found, on moving them, that his legs were weak; the aching was at once relieved by change of position. He also found, on trying to sit up, that he had great difficulty in doing so. His hands and arms were at this time quite strong.

At *4 p.m.* The weakness in the legs had very considerably increased, but he could still draw them up in bed, while extension of hips and knees was distinctly weak in the proximal joints, but the change was not nearly so marked as in the legs.

At *4.30 p.m.* The legs much in the same condition, but grasp as tested with dynamometer was distinctly less.

At *5.30 p.m. Upper extremities.* All movements present, with the exception of flexion of the elbow on the right side, but all are feeble. The best movements are those of the fingers and wrists, the left a little stronger than the right. *Lower extremities.* Flexion of hip and knee and adduction of the thighs are now impossible; all other movements are still present, but are very feeble, the best of all being those of the toes. Neck muscles are also weak, although the the head can be still raised off the pillow, but not against the slightest resistance, while extension of the neck is more powerfully performed. Trunk muscles can all be voluntarily contracted, but all are feeble.

The muscles supplied by cranial nerves are quite normal. . . .

Mentally he is perfectly natural, talks normally, and complains of nothing except the discomfort of being unable to change his position.

No change in objective sensibility to any form of stimulus could be detected.

At *7 p.m.* he managed to eat a little food, but was unable to feed himself.

At *7.30 p.m.* He is quite unable to move the head or shoulders; on sitting him up he simply doubles up and his head falls either forward or backward without his being able to control it in the least. Respiration is almost entirely diaphragmatic; coughing is almost impossible as the abdominal muscles only just contract in the attempt and only the very feeblest movement is perceptible in the latissimus dorsi on either side. All arm movements are very small, flexion of the elbow and extension of the wrist being quite absent on the right, but just present on the left side where extension of elbow and flexion of wrist are quite absent. The fingers on both sides can still be flexed, extended, adducted or abducted though with small power, and the grasp is practically nil. In the lower extremities slight extension and external rotation of hips is still possible and the quadriceps can just support the weight of the lower leg. Feeble movements of ankles and toes are present.

Reflexes. Knee-jerks are present but only a very feeble contraction is obtained, though it is noticeable that this is very ready and is not reinforceable. All other deep reflexes are unobtainable. Abdominal and cremasteric skin reflexes absent. Plantars still ready but the movement of the toes is small and flexor in type.

The muscles supplied by the cranial nerves are still normal.

11.30 p.m. Some improvement in arms; can now flex fingers and wrists slightly and also pronate and supinate faintly; there is also a very feeble contraction in left triceps humeri with faint triceps-jerk. Right leg completely paralysed with absent reflexes; slight power in left quadriceps femoris and big toe with very faint knee-jerk and plantar reflex.

Coughing and deep breathing are impossible.

The paralysed muscles, although the palsy is of the flaccid type, do not show any degree of hypotonicity and feel firm and solid to the touch; none of them contract to direct percussion. . . .

12.45 a.m. Arms are steadily improving and the biceps and triceps on both sides contract feebly, while their tendon-jerks have returned. Shoulder girdle muscles and those of extraordinary inspiration are still paralysed. Slight movement of toes on right side now present, with return of right plantar reflex (flexor), otherwise legs much as before. . . .

3.15 a.m. Some power now in all muscles, best in periphery of all limbs. All reflexes are present, but still feeble.

4.30 a.m. Much improved; he can now move all limbs and head, but not yet able to sit up. Feels well but rather stiff and sore, as if he had done some hard exercise.

10.30 a.m. Power now everywhere good, though still some feeling of stiffness.

The paper by Singer and Goodbody is also notable in that these authors were the first to draw attention to the therapeutic effect of potassium salts. The next landmark was the observation by Biemond and Daniels (1934) that the serum potassium level fell during the paralytic episodes and this was subsequently confirmed by Aitken *et al.* (1937). Subsequently another form of familial periodic paralysis was discovered in which the serum potassium level rose, rather than fell, and a large population of patients with this condition were studied by Gamstorp (1956) after whom the syndrome is sometimes called. Finally a third form of the disease was

encountered in which there was no significant change in serum potassium concentration (Tyler *et al.,* 1951; Poskanzer and Kerr, 1961). On the basis of the serum potassium level it is therefore possible to distinguish three types of familial periodic paralysis—hyper-, hypo- and normokalaemic. Each type is inherited as an autosomal dominant trait and tends to breed true; in most patients the types can be distinguished on the basis of differences in clinical characteristics and precipitating features. For example, hyperkalaemic attacks tend to be brief and may occur during exercise; they may be precipitated by the administration of potassium but not by heavy meals. In contrast, hypokalaemic paralytic episodes usually last longer and may be provoked by carbohydrate meals or by glucose and insulin; they can sometimes be aborted by exercise (or, in individual muscles, by indirect stimulation; see Campa and Sanders, 1974). These and other differences are listed in Table 15.1. However, the functional similarity between the three types is indicated by the observations of Pearson (1963) on a patient in whom 80 per cent of spontaneous attacks were associated with an elevation of serum potassium, 15 per cent with no change and 5 per cent with a decline.

One interesting feature of the syndrome is that patients may develop permanent weakness of proximal muscles between attacks and that this may be associated with muscle wasting, the combination being attributed to a myopathy (Biemond and Daniels, 1934; McArdle, 1962). The most likely explanation is that vacuolar dilatation is responsible for these features; in the early stages of the disease the vacuoles disappear between attacks of paralysis but later they may persist and so permanently disrupt the structure and function of the fibres (Pearson, 1963).

Treatment

In the *hypokalaemic* disorder a paralytic episode can be curtailed by the administration of potassium chloride (10 g) by mouth. In most patients attacks can be prevented by diuretics such as acetazolamide (125 mg twice daily, up to 250 mg three times daily) or dichlorphenamide (50 g daily). McArdle (1974) has found even better results can be achieved by combining a diuretic with a slow-release oral potassium preparation (e.g. 2.4–4.8 g Slow-K [Ciba] daily).

In the *hyperkalaemic* form a useful prophylactic effect can be gained from the same diuretics (acetazolamide and dichlorphenamide) and also from chlorthiazide or hydrochlorthiazide. The beneficial action of these diuretics is possibly due to the fact that potassium, as well as sodium, is excreted in

TABLE 15.1
Typical Features of the Three Types of Periodic Paralysis

	Hypokalaemic	Normokalaemic	Hyperkalaemic
Age of onset (yr)	10–20	0–10	0–10
Intervals between attacks	Weeks or months	Weeks or months	Days
Duration of attacks (hr)	6–24	24	1–3
Time	Night	Night	Day
Carbohydrate meals	+	—	—
During heavy exercise	—	—	+
After heavy exercise	+	+	—
Iatrogenic provocation	Glucose + insulin	Potassium	Potassium
Prophylactic treatment	Potassiun chloride Low salt diet Spironolactone	High salt diet 9-alpha-fluoro- -hydrocortisone	Chlorthiazide Hydrochlorthiazide Acetazolamide
Treat of attack	Potassium chloride	Sodium chloride	Calcium gluconate, glucose and insulin

Modified from Pearson (1963)

increased amounts. Since the paralytic episodes are comparatively brief and mild in this type of disorder, the attacks will require treatment only occasionally; McArdle (1974) advocates 1–2 g of calcium gluconate intravenously.

Attacks of *normokalaemic* paralysis are improved by giving sodium chloride and may be prevented by a combination of acetazolamide and 9-α-fluoro-hydrocortisone (0.1 mg daily; see Poskanzer and Kerr, 1961).

SPECIAL INVESTIGATIONS

Each type of periodic paralysis will now be considered separately with particular attention being paid to measurements of resting membrane potential. Subsequently the laboratory findings in the three types will be reviewed and a number of possible aetiologies for the disorders will be examined.

HYPERKALAEMIC TYPE

(Adynamia episodica hereditaria: Gamstorp's syndrome)

Biochemistry

In this condition the episodes of paralysis are accompanied by a rise in the serum potassium concentration, for example from 4–5 mM to 6–8 mM. Since there is no reduction in the urinary excretion of potassium (Gamstorp, 1956) the elevated serum level must have resulted from a loss of this cation from the cells. This supposition has been confirmed by measurements of the total body exchangeable potassium (McArdle, 1962); at the same time a rise in intracellular sodium can sometimes be demonstrated (Carson and Pearson, 1964).

Microelectrode recordings

Creutzfeldt, Abbott, Fowler and Pearson (1963) observed a fall in resting potential to a mean value of −51.5 mV in a patient during a spontaneous episode of paralysis and to −44.3 mV in an induced

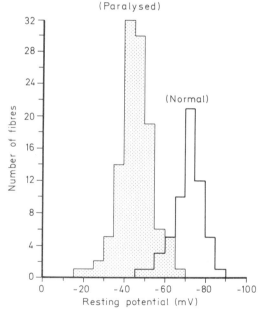

Figure 15.1. Measurements of resting membrane potentials in a patient with the hyperkalaemic type of familial periodic paralysis. In between attacks of paralysis the values were normal (open histogram) but during an episode of weakness depolarization occurred (hatched histogram) and the fibres became inexcitable on direct stimulation. (From Brooks (1969) courtesy of the author, and the Editor and publishers of the Archives of Neurology)

attack; in between attacks the mean value was −68.5 mV. In this study the muscle fibres were examined by the *in situ open* method (see Appendix 3.1) but in a more recent investigation of a patient by Brooks (1969) the *in situ cannula* technique was employed instead. In this last study the mean membrane potential during an attack was −45 ± 8.5 mV, compared with a value of −72 ± 9 mV in the preceding control period; the results have been reproduced in *Figure 15.1*. This last study was important for another reason since Brooks tested the excitability of the muscle fibre membranes directly, by passing current through the intracellular electrode, and observed that during the paralytic

phase all the muscle fibres sampled were inexcitable.

As stated earlier, not all the patients with this condition have complete recovery of function following the paralytic episodes and this observation can be correlated with the measurements of resting membrane potential. In the patient studied by Creutzfeldt and associates the mean resting potential of −68.5 mV, observed between attacks, was low in comparison with values obtained in normal subjects. Low resting potentials in between attacks of paralysis were also observed by McComas, Mrožek and Bradley (1968) in four patients with hyperkalaemic periodic paralysis. In *Figure 15.2* the individual fibre potentials from these four patients have been pooled and compared with those of three control subjects. It can be seen that not only did the mean values differ significantly, being −66.3 ± 10.0 mV and −83.6 ± 5.5 mV for the patients and controls respectively (p = <0.001), but almost half of the fibres in the patients had potentials below the lower limit of the normal range (−64 mV). McComas and colleagues, like Brooks (1969), used a Wheatstone bridge to simultaneously stimulate and record from the impaled fibres. Although none of their patients was paralysed at the time of study, McComas and colleagues were unable to evoke action potentials with depolarizing currents which would have been effective in normal subjects. In contrast, action potentials could be elicited readily at the conclusion of hyperpolarizing pulses, as *Figure 15.3* shows.

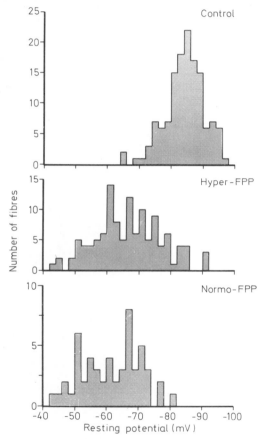

Figure 15.2. Measurements of resting membrane potential in three normal subjects (top), four patients with hyperkalaemic type of paralysis (middle) and in one patient with the normo-kalaemic form. Mean values (± S.D.) were −83.6 ± 5.5 mV, −66.3 ± 10.0 mV and −61.3 ± 10.5 mV respectively. (From McComas et al. (1968) courtesy of the Editor and the publishers of Journal of Neurology, Neurosurgery and Psychiatry*)*

HYPOKALAEMIC TYPE

Biochemistry

In this type of paralysis there is a fall in the serum potassium concentration, often to 2 mM or even lower. As in the hyperkalaemic form of paralysis, there is no evidence of an alteration in the renal excretion of potassium and for this reason it was assumed that the biochemical changes signified a net flux of potassium into cells. In keeping with this assumption was the finding of a significant arterio-venous difference in potassium concentration by Zierler and Andres (1957) and by Grob, Johns and Liljestrand (1957).

Microelectrode recordings

In the first microelectrode investigation of a patient with this condition, Shy and colleagues (1961) were unable to detect any change of membrane potential during the paretic phase. In a study by Creutzfeldt et al. (1961) mild weakness was induced by glucose and insulin and the mean membrane potential decreased from -85 ± 6.1 mV to -77.1 ± 8.2 mV; during this time the serum potassium level fell from 4.25 mM to 3.17 mM. Creutzfeldt and colleagues thought it probable that at least some of the depolarization had resulted from damage to superficial fibres caused by drying or cooling. In a third patient to be studied with hypokalaemic paralysis the results were less equivocal for Riecker and Bolte (1966) observed a reduced membrane potential of -49.1 mV at a time when paralysis was present and the serum potassium concentration had fallen from 4.5 mM to 2.0 mM.

Of particular interest has been the *in vitro* study by Hofmann and Smith (1970) on specimens of external intercostal muscle obtained from three patients. These authors confirmed that a substantial depolarization was present even when the muscles had been equilibrated in a solution with a normal

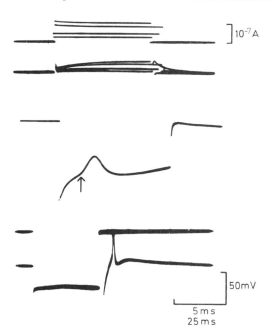

Figure 15.3. Responses of three muscle fibres in hyperkalaemic periodic paralysis to intracellular stimulation. (Top) This fibre yielded electrotonic potentials only and had a resting potential of -50 mV. (Middle) In this fibre an 'abortive' action potential is indicated by the arrow. (Bottom) A fibre which could not be excited by depolarization fired an impulse at the end of a hyperpolarizing current pulse ('break excitation'; see text). The horizontal bar represents 5 ms for top and middle sections and 25 ms for lower one. (From McComas et al. (1968) courtesy of the Editor and publishers of Journal of Neurology, Neurosurgery, and Psychiatry)

potassium concentration (5 mM); the mean values ($\pm$S.E.) for fibres from the controls and patients were -75.8 ± 1.2 mV and -54.0 ± 1.3 mV respectively. In keeping with clinical observations on the provocative effects of carbohydrate meals or of glucose and insulin was the finding that insulin depolarized the fibres further. In contrast, repolarization of the fibres to normal levels was achieved by replacing most of the external sodium with choline or by substituting nitrate for chloride. Procaine, a drug which normally stabilizes the membrane by inactivating the sodium channels, also increased the resting potential.

NORMOKALAEMIC TYPE

Biochemistry

No change in the serum sodium or potassium concentrations can be detected in association with the paralysis.

Microelectrode recordings

The only study reported to date appears to be that of McComas, Mrożek and Bradley (1968), who found a reduced mean resting potential of -61.3 ± 9.5 mV in one patient observed between attacks.

EFFECT OF THE DEPOLARIZATION ON MEMBRANE EXCITABILITY

Before analysing the ionic mechanism responsible for the membrane depolarization in familial periodic paralysis it is instructive to consider the ways in which the change in potential might affect membrane excitability. From Chapter 3 it will be recalled that *rapid* depolarization of a muscle fibre causes it to fire an impulse when the critical membrane potential is reached; it is therefore significant that, in some patients with hyperkalaemic periodic paralysis, the weakness is preceded by myotonia (page 125). *Slow* depolarizations may not cause excitation because activation of the sodium carrier population over a longer period of time is less efficient than near-synchronous activation. This inexcitability of the membrane is termed *accommodation* (page 24) and may underlie the absence of myotonia in hypo- and normokalaemic paralysis, if indeed the depolarizations are slower than in the hyperkalaemic type. As long as the membrane remains depolarized the sodium carriers will be unavailable for further impulse activity (*depolarization block*). That adequate numbers of sodium carriers are present in the membrane is shown by the ability of the 'paralysed' fibres to fire at the end of a hyperpolarizing current pulse (*Figure 15.3, bottom*). The intracellular stimulation studies are of importance for another reason since the absence of excitability following random electrode penetration suggests that the membranes are affected throughout their lengths rather than solely at regions subjected to stretching by dilated internal vacuoles.

It is of interest to inquire whether, in addition to membrane inexcitability, there is any interference with excitation–contraction coupling or with the contractile system itself. This aspect has now been tested by Engel and Lambert (1969) who delivered calcium ions iontophoretically from a micropipette on to the surfaces of desheathed muscle fibres. In muscle biopsy samples from the arms of three patients with hypokalaemic paralysis they found that calcium induced normal muscle contractions. From this study the sole factor responsible for the paralytic attacks would still appear to be membrane inexcitability.

PATHOGENESIS OF THE MEMBRANE DEPOLARIZATION

The various studies have shown that in the three types of familial periodic paralysis there is a fall in the resting membrane potential during the paralytic episodes and that a smaller depolarization is sometimes present between the attacks. In each of the conditions the paralytic phase is associated with swelling of the muscle fibres due to the presence of dilated central vacuoles. How can these observations be fitted together? An acceptable approach would be to concentrate on the finding of membrane depolarization and to consider the alterations in permeability or ionic concentration which could have been responsible.

In Chapter 3, it was shown that the membrane potential depended on the concentrations of sodium, potassium and chloride on either side of the membrane and on the relative permeabilities of the membrane for these ions. In normal circumstances the resting permeability was high for potassium and chloride but very low for sodium; the effect of an increase in sodium permeability was to depolarize the fibre. A depolarization could also be produced by reducing the transmembrane concentration gradient for potassium (see *Figure 3.1, right*). It was also shown that changes in membrane chloride permeability or in chloride concentration were less important since potassium, chloride and water were rapidly redistributed so as to restore to previous transmembrane concentration gradient for chloride. In effect, then, the depolarization observed in familial periodic paralysis could result only from an increase in the sodium permeability of the membrane or from a reduction in the potassium transmembrane concentration gradient. Consideration will now be given to this first possibility as a mechanism for the induction of the paralytic attacks.

First hypothesis: increased sodium permeability

If the permeability of the membrane for sodium were to increase, with no change taking place in the potassium and chloride permeabilities, the net membrane permeability would be increased and, conversely, the electrical resistance of the membrane would fall (see page 18 and *Figure 3.2*). Because of this last event, a smaller than normal potential would be developed when current was passed across the membrane from an intracellular stimulating microelectrode (page 19). Experimentally, this is so in familial periodic paralysis; furthermore, the membrane time constant is reduced, as would also be expected (McComas, Mrożek and Bradley, 1968). Support for the sodium hypothesis has come from the study of Hofmann and Smith (1970; see above). These authors showed that in hypokalaemic periodic paralysis there was an increase in the *internal* sodium concentration of the muscle fibres and that the abnormal depolarization could be reversed if 90 per cent of the *external* sodium was replaced with choline. On the basis of these two observations it is difficult to avoid the conclusion that the sodium permeability of the membrane was increased, thereby allowing sodium ions to enter the fibre and also causing the resting potential to fall.

There is, however, a problem in a simple sodium permeability hypothesis and this concerns the movements of potassium. If, in a normal fibre, the sodium permeability increases, sodium will enter the fibre down its concentration and electrical gradients; the entry of this cation allows potassium to leave since the admitted sodium can now help to balance the internal anions. One would therefore expect the internal concentration of potassium to decrease and the external concentration to rise. This is exactly what does happen in the hyperkalaemic form of periodic paralysis, but in the hypokalaemic variety the potassium *enters* the fibres while, in the normokalaemic type, there is no net movement of potassium at all. The only 'normal' mechanism which could either preserve or increase the sarcoplasmic potassium concentration, in the face of a rise in sodium permeability, is active transport by means of the sodium–potassium coupled pump (page 21); it would therefore be necessary to postulate that the activity of the pump became extremely high.

Second hypothesis: internal potassium sequestration

An alternative hypothesis is that the concentration of potassium on the inside of the membrane is reduced in each type of familial periodic paralysis. In the hyperkalaemic form this is likely to take place anyway, since biochemical studies reveal a net movement of potassium from the fibres into the extracellular fluid compartment. Even so, the observed depolarization is much larger than would have been anticipated from the Nernst equation. Suppose that the extracellular potassium concentration rose from 5 mM to 8 mM; the intracellular concentration would be hardly changed, since the total muscle mass in the body is much larger than the volume of extracellular fluid volume, and therefore a depolarization of only about 12 mV would be expected. It is therefore necessary to postulate that, in this and the other types of periodic paralysis, much of the internal potassium is held within some intracellular compartment and is no longer available to the sarcoplasm bordering the sarcolemma. The obvious candidate for such an internal compartment would be the dilated vacuoles; according to Shy *et al* (1961) these swellings develop from the sarcoplasmic reticulum though the T-tubules are also involved (Engel, 1970).

Two explanations may now be advanced for the entry of potassium into the vacuoles. One is that as a result of abnormal intermediary carbohydrate metabolism an excess of organic anions is secreted into the reticulum together with hydrogen ions and that the latter are then replaced by potassium ions (Aitken *et al.*, 1937; *Figure 15.4*). Because of the osmotic pressure exerted by these ions, water would be taken into the vacuoles and swelling would result. This explanation has the double attraction of explaining the precipitation of attacks by carbohydrate meals (or by the administration of glucose and insulin) as well as the ability of the vacuolar contents to stain with PAS in all three types of periodic paralysis. For hyperkalaemic paralysis the relationship of the naturally-occurring attacks to carbohydrate metabolism is less obvious but they could conceivably result from the synthesis of glycogen following depletion of the latter during heavy exercise. If the carbohydrate explanation is correct the excess anions have yet to be identified; for example, Engel, Potter and Rosevear (1967) were unable to detect abnormal amounts of glucose, hexose-6-phosphate, fructose-1:6-diphosphate, pyruvate or lactate in specimens of paralysed muscle from a patient with the hypokalaemic disorder.

A second possible cause for the vacuolar dilatation is that the sarcoplasmic reticulum may normally be one of the pathways for the efflux of ions and water from the sarcoplasm and that this route may become temporarily obstructed. By immersing muscle fibres in hypertonic sucrose solutions Birks and Davey (1969) have recently shown that the sarcoplasmic reticulum communicates with the interstitial fluid, presumably through the transverse tubular system. In the later stages of paralysis, however, any obstruction disappears for Engel (1970), using HRP as a marker, has been able to demonstrate free communication between the vacuoles, T-system and extracellular fluid. Indeed the rupture of the vacuoles may conceivably initiate the recovery mechanism. Engel was also able to

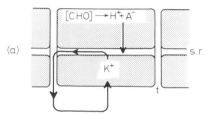

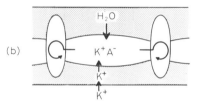

Figure 15.4. 'Carbohydrate' hypothesis for familial periodic paralysis. In (a) there is excessive formation of H^+ and anions from abnormal intermediary metabolism. In (b) K^+ substitute for H^+; the osmotic effect of the metabolites draws water into the fibres and dilates the sarcoplasmic reticulum and T-system (see text)

show that, in the earliest stages of the disorder, the vacuoles arose from dilated vesicles of the sarcoplasmic reticulum and from proliferations of the T-tubules. It is interesting that swelling of the T-tubules can be readily produced in normal fibres by immersing the latter in solutions containing glycerol or lacking in chloride (page 19).

Intuitively the concept of potassium retention in obstructed sarcoplasmic reticulum is an attractive explanation for familial periodic paralysis and one which is not incompatible with the carbohydrate hypothesis presented above. It would still be necessary to determine why, in the hyperkalaemic form, potassium leaks out of the fibres as well as entering the sarcoplasmic reticulum. Also, the potassium sequestration hypothesis does not exclude the co-existence of an increase in membrane permeability to sodium (first hypothesis) during the paralytic episodes; thus the two mechanisms may operate together.

POSSIBLE EXTRAMUSCULAR PRECIPITATING FACTORS

Aldosterone

The relationship of hypokalaemic periodic paralysis to primary aldosteronism is one which has attracted considerable attention. Aldosterone, a hormone released from the adrenal cortex, is known to pro-mote renal excretion of potassium and to cause hypokalaemia, often associated with episodes of muscle weakness. From the investigation of Conn and colleagues (1957), it appeared that hypersecre-tion of aldosterone might indeed be responsible for some instances of 'true' hypokalaemic periodic paralysis: however, in other studies no abnormality of aldosterone secretion has been detected.

Other humoral agents

Krull et al. (1966) obtained evidence for a circulat-ing agent which could precipitate myotonia in one patient with hyperkalaemic periodic paralysis (see page 132). Conceivably the same substance could have caused paralysis if larger amounts had been administered in their experiments. Barium is another example of an external agent able to pro-duce episodes of weakness which resemble those of familial periodic paralysis. In the Szechwan province of China an endemic illness, Pa Ping, was eventually traced to barium poisoning; the clinical features closely resembled those of sporadic periodic para-lysis (Huang, 1943). Another striking similarity was the occurrence of hypokalaemia in barium poisoning due to the uptake of potassium by cells (Diengott et al., 1964). Schott and McArdle (1974) have recently drawn attention to the use of barium administration in mammals as a possible model for hypokalaemic periodic paralysis and have confirmed that the muscle fibres become inexcitable during the paralytic phase.

Thyroid hormones

A definite association exists between thyrotoxi-cosis and hypokalaemic periodic paralysis and this is particularly striking in male inhabitants of Japan and China (Okinaka et al., 1957). The existence of this association offers an approach towards the understanding of familial periodic paralysis for it is possible that the thyroid hormones, through their metabolic stimulating action, accelerate the bio-chemical reactions leading to formation of the vacuoles. A more specific abnormality which has been reported during the paralytic episodes is a reduction of calcium pumping by the sarcoplasmic reticulum (Au and Yeung, 1972). While this defect could be a primary event in the development of the paralytic phase it is equally likely that dilatation of the sarcoplasmic reticulum resulting from some other cause could lead to temporary failure of any enzymic mechanisms involving the membrane. It is of interest that the paralytic episodes cease once the thyrotoxicosis has been brought under control.

Potassium depletion

Offerijns, Westerink and Willibrands (1958) investi-gated rats fed on a low potassium diet. They found that the diaphragm muscles of these animals, when mounted in vitro, became paralysed following the administration of insulin to the bath fluid, while the muscles of control animals did not show this response. These results suggest that, in terms of membrane excitability, insulin may have an adverse effect in conditions in which potassium dynamics are disturbed (see also Otsuka and Ohtsuki, 1965).

Neural factors

In a study by Sica and Aguilera (1972) the numbers of functioning motor units were estimated in the extensor digitorum brevis muscles of two patients with hyperkalaemic familial periodic paralysis. Between attacks of paralysis there was evidence of a selective involvement of motor units suggesting the presence of a neutral factor. During an attack the numbers of functioning units declined further and the sizes of individual units became smaller, reflecting the presence of increasing numbers of inexcitable fibres.

CONCLUSION

Of all the disease syndromes in the neurology, familial periodic paralysis, because of its dramatic association of paralysis with potassium shifts, might have been thought most amenable to a neuro-physiological solution. Yet it is evident that the neurophysiological findings, far from clarifying the nature of the disease mechanism, have only served to draw attention to the complexity of electrolyte dynamics within the muscle fibre.

DISORDERS OF MUSCLE FIBRE CONTENTS

The next disorders to be considered are those in which there are obvious pathological abnormalities in the interior of the muscle fibre. In muscular dystrophy and polymyositis the tubular systems, myofibrils and myonuclei—often the entire fibre—are affected and may ultimately be destroyed. In the mitochondrial myopathies fibre destruction may also be present but in this instance the earliest changes in the muscle can be assigned to one type of organelle. In the glycogen storage diseases it is possible to be even more precise for it is now known that a single enzyme is deficient in each of the sub-types of this condition. So far as the other diseases are concerned the designation 'disorders of muscle fibre contents' does not imply that the muscle fibre membranes and motoneurones have no role to play in pathogenesis. Indeed two of the current hypotheses concerning muscular dystrophy suggest that this condition may result from a defect of the cell membrane or from motoneurone dysfunction.

Chapter 16

THE MUSCULAR DYSTROPHIES

INTRODUCTION

If the muscular dystrophies appear to have had an inordinately long chapter devoted to them, it is for three reasons; first, the genuine fascination which these diseases exert upon the clinician and scientist; secondly, their central place in the present debate concerning the neural hypothesis of muscle disease, and thirdly, the mass of information which has become available from experiments on animal models of dystrophy.

The controversies which have surrounded these disorders were present almost from their first recognition in the last century. Credit for the first description of a patient with dystrophy is given to the Scottish surgeon, Charles Bell, who published a report in 1830 (see Ogg, 1971). It is generally considered that the next advances in knowledge came from the studies of the French school of neurologists. Among these neurologists was Duchenne; not only was he an astute clinical observer but he was also a pioneer in the application of electrical methods to the diagnosis of neurological disorders. Duchenne's other contribution was the invention of a 'harpoon' which enabled him to obtain specimens of muscle without the need to incise the skin and expose the muscle. In the second edition of his book *De l'électrisation localisée et son application a la pathologie et a la thérapeutique*, published in 1861, Duchenne clearly described the type of dystrophy which now bears his name. He drew attention to the pseudohypertrophy of the calf muscles and also noted that his first patient was mentally retarded. This last observation together with the fact that, until then, it had been customary to ascribe all muscle weakness and wasting to disease of the peripheral nerves or spinal cord, prompted Duchenne to term the disorder 'paraplégie hypertrophique de l'enfance de cause cérébrale'.

In recognizing the importance of Duchenne's work there has been a tendency to overlook the equally significant studies of Edward Meryon. This London physician anticipated Duchenne by reporting four affected brothers in 1852, upon one of whom he had performed a *post-mortem* examination. Meryon observed that the disease was hereditary with a predilection for males; he found no evidence of abnormality in the nervous system and believed that the disease reflected a primary defect of the muscle fibres. The normal appearance of the nervous system was subsequently confirmed by Duchenne (1872) who went on to describe another type of dystrophy now referred to as the *facioscapulohumeral type*. In this form also it was shown that the severe destructive changes in the muscles were unaccompanied by similar abnormalities in their innervation (Landouzy and Déjérine, 1886). At about this time similar hereditary wasting diseases were shown to affect the muscles of the pelvic and shoulder girdles (limb-girdle dystrophy; Leyden, 1876; Mobius, 1879) and the shoulder muscles (*scapulohumeral dystrophy*; Erb, 1884).

It was Erb who did most to define and contrast the newly-described syndromes while grouping them together as primary diseases of muscle or 'dystrophia muscularis progressiva'; he postulated that they were due to 'a complex nutritional

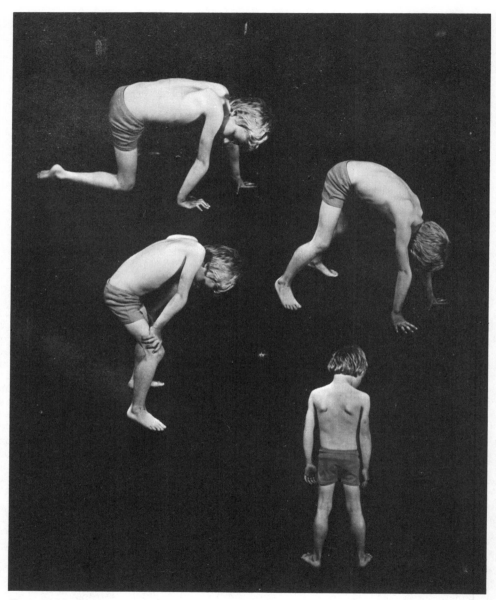

Figure 16.1. Duchenne muscular dystrophy in a 6-year-old boy. Note the enlargement of the calf muscles and the atrophy of the shoulder muscles; there is already 'winging' of the scapulae. The patient 'climbs' up his body in order to stand upright (Gower's sign: see text)

disturbance' of the muscle fibres (Erb, 1891). Other types of dystrophy also came to be recognized including those involving the external *ocular* muscles (Hutchinson, 1879) and the *distal* muscles of the limbs (Gowers, 1902). Possibly the most bizarre of all the dystrophies, the *myotonic* form, was not described until 1909, by Steinert; the unusual nature of the disorder stems from its association with striking somatic abnormalities and with disabling stiffness of the muscles on effort (see below).

CLASSIFICATION

Classification of the muscular dystrophies is not easy, being complicated by similarities as well as differences in mode of inheritance, age of onset, rapidity of progression, distribution of affected muscles and the presence or absence of abnormalities outside the muscles themselves. In a recent review Walton and Gardner-Medwin (1974) have separated progressive muscular dystrophy into 'pure' forms and that associated with myotonia. According to these authors the following types of disorder can be differentiated.

I. *'Pure' Muscular Dystrophies*
   (*a*) X-linked muscular dystrophy
   Severe (Duchenne type)
   Benign (Becker type)
   (*b*) Autosomal recessive muscular dystrophy
   Limb-girdle types
   Childhood muscular dystrophy (except congenital muscular dystrophy)
   (*c*) Facioscapulohumeral muscular dystrophy
   (*d*) Distal muscular dystrophy
   (*e*) Ocular muscular dystrophy
   (*f*) Oculopharyngeal muscular dystrophy
II. *Muscular dystrophy with myotonia* (myotonic muscular dystrophy)

Of these disorders, only the Duchenne, limb-girdle, facioscapulohumeral and myotonic forms of dystrophy will be considered; they are the commonest dystrophies and also those which have been investigated most thoroughly. The other types have been reviewed by Walton and Gardner-Medwin (1974).

DUCHENNE MUSCULAR DYSTROPHY

Clinical features

In both the Duchenne and Becker types of

muscular dystrophy only males are affected, the disease being transmitted as a sex-linked recessive trait. The Duchenne form of the disease is the more common of the two and unfortunately, the more severe also. Estimates of its incidence range from 13 to 33 per 100 000 males; of these one-third arise from new mutations. The first sign of the disease is usually difficulty in walking. The boy may be late in starting to walk or, having started at a normal age, is noticed to fall frequently and to be unable to run or climb. When rising from the floor the patient does so in a characteristic manner, by pushing down on to his thighs and levering his trunk upwards (Gowers's sign; *Figure 16.1*). Walking is performed on a wide base, with the abdomen thrust forward and the spine curved inwardly (lordosis). Even in infancy some of the proximal muscles are noticeably enlarged due to the deposition of fatty connective tissue in the muscle bellies (pseudohypertrophy), though sometimes the muscle fibres themselves are hypertrophied. The large muscles in the calves are especially striking (*Figure 16.1*); the gluteal muscles and deltoids are often conspicuously bulky too. With advancing age the enlargement of the muscles is succeeded by a generalized and progressive wasting; at the same time the muscle bellies harden and they undergo a permanent shortening (contracture), causing deformities to develop at some of the joints. Thus the ankles become plantar-flexed and inverted while the hips, knees and elbows assume flexion deformities; later a severe scoliosis appears. By the time the patient is aged 10 or so, he is unable to walk and is dependent upon a wheelchair for mobilization. He remains able to do things with his hands, to speak and to swallow. Eventually respiratory movements become weaker and the patient is liable to succumb to a chest infection; more commonly, death results from cardiac failure since the heart also participates in the generalized muscle degeneration. With the advent of antibiotics for the treatment of infection, the life expectancy in Duchenne dystrophy has risen to about 20 years.

Many *treatments* have been tried for Duchenne dystrophy, including glycine, corticosteroids, anabolic steroids, vitamin E, and a combination of nucleotides, nucleosides and their precursors. In every case the initial enthusiasm has been dissipated by the absence of confirmatory results. Currently under investigation are corticosteroids (Drachman, Toyka and Myer, 1974; Siegel, Miller and Ray, 1974), dielthylstilbestrol (Cohen and Morgan, 1976) and penicillamine (Park *et al.*, 1974). Orthopaedic procedures have a role in treatment since surgical lengthening of the Achilles tendon will compensate for the contracture in the calf muscles by allowing the patient to place his foot flat upon the ground and so walk for a little longer. Passive movements are useful in delaying the development of contracture deformities in other joints. Perhaps most important of all are the psychological attitudes of the patient's family and friends, which should be encouraging and enthusiastic whenever possible, reserving sympathy for the inevitable occasions of disappointment and frustration.

Of all the diseases in neurology none is more disheartening for patient, parent and doctor than Duchenne dystrophy, for in no other condition is there the same relentless enfeeblement, leading to the eventual imprisonment of an often normal young mind within the confines of a cruelly distorted body.

'Carriers' and their detection

Mary Lyon (1961) suggested that in females a random inactivation of either of the two X-chromosomes would take place in all the body cells. This concept, which is now generally accepted, has important consequences for any disease inherited as a sex-linked recessive trait and for Duchenne dystrophy in particular. If dystrophy were indeed a primary disorder of the muscle fibre, the Lyon hypothesis would predict that a proportion of the myonuclei in female carriers would be abnormal. Whether or not the dystrophic process would be expressed in a muscle fibre might then depend on the relative proportions of normal and 'dystrophic' nuclei in that fibre. In practice, the predictions of the Lyon hypothesis seem to be borne out, for between half and two-thirds of the female carriers of the Duchenne gene can be detected by laboratory investigations (see Gardner-Medwin and Walton, 1974, for review). Of these the most useful is the serum creatine phosphokinase (CPK) estimation, though it is most important that more than one specimen of blood be sampled and that the subject should not have been exercising beforehand (otherwise spuriously high values may result). Examination of muscle biopsy specimens with the light and electron microscopes also has a role, as has measurement of muscle action potential parameters (duration and complexity) following recordings with a coaxial needle electrode. If the last analysis is to be performed manually, it becomes extremely time-consuming and for this reason has not been pursued. A recently-described biochemical method seems highly promising; it measures the *in vitro* synthesis of proteins by polyribosomes obtained from muscle biopsy (Ionasescu, Zellweger and Conway, 1971). Another new advance is to examine the red blood cells of suspected carriers; in most cases an unduly high incidence of cup-shaped cells (stomatocytes) can be found using scanning electronmicroscopy. Also, phosphorylation by a certain type of protein kinase (spectrin II) is commonly increased (Roses *et al.*, 1975). Finally, a small proportion of carriers appear abnormal on physical examination, exhibiting muscular hypertrophy (Emery, 1963) or weakness (Chung, Morton and Peters, 1960).

There is argument concerning the genetic status of a mother with an affected son in whom the carrier detection tests are negative. The usual interpretation is that in some such instances the results will have been 'falsely' negative and that the remainder will be 'true' negatives, the disease having arisen in the offspring as the consequence of a mutation in a maternal ovum. In fact it is thought that approximately one-third of all new cases are the result of a fresh mutation. This explanation has now been challenged by Roses and colleagues (1976) who examined suspected carriers clinically and studied the morphological and biochemical properties of their red blood cells. In view of the high incidence of detectable abnormalities in their population, these authors claim that the mutation rate is much lower than that previously thought to obtain.

SPECIAL INVESTIGATIONS IN DUCHENNE DYSTROPHY

Serum enzymes

Particularly in the early stages of Duchenne dystrophy, the blood levels of certain muscle enzymes are abnormally high, suggesting that the enzymes are able to leak through the membranes of the degenerating fibres. In support of this explanation Zierler (1961) has been able to demonstrate directly that the resting efflux of aldolase is abnormally high in isolated muscles from dystrophic mice. In human muscle disease, however, the most useful enzyme assay is that for creatine phosphokinase (CPK) since the elevation in serum titre is higher than that of other muscle enzymes studied to date. In Duchenne dystrophy the greatest increase occurs at about 1 year of age, when it may exceed the normal by 30–300 fold. The test is therefore invaluable for making a diagnosis at an early stage before clinical abnormalities are present. As the patient grows older the serum titres gradually fall, possibly reflecting reductions in the mass of available muscle as well as in the intensity of the degenerative process.

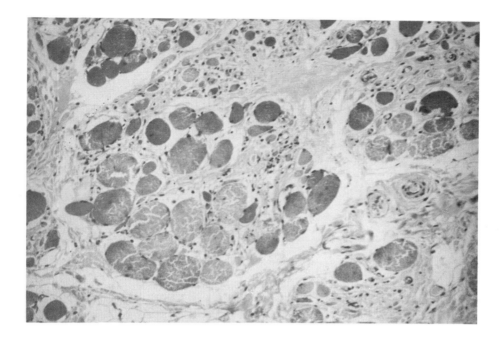

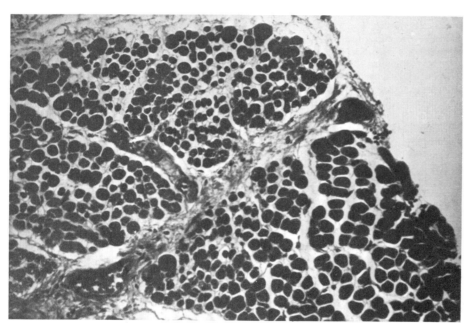

Figure 16.2. Transverse sections of gastrocnemius muscles, stained with haematoxylin and eosin, and taken from a 9-year-boy with Duchenne dystrophy (upper) and a 3-year-old one (lower). Note how the muscle fibres appear abnormally rounded and differ greatly in size. Although there is already an increase in fatty connective tissue in the specimen from the younger patient (lower) this change is more marked in the older boy, in whom there has been considerable loss of muscle fibres. (× 120 (upper) and × 60(lower))

Erythrocytes

Speculating that muscular dystrophy might prove to be a membrane disorder, a number of workers have searched for evidence of membrane dysfunction in tissues other than muscle. In the case of red blood cells it has now been shown that such iregularities exist; they include the presence of abnormal-shaped cells, either stomatocytes (Miller, Roses and Appel, 1976) or echinocytes (Matheson and Howland, 1974). There is also evidence of increased membrane fluidity and of increased phosphorylation by membrane kinases of the spectrin II moiety (Sha'afi *et al.*, 1975; Roses, Herbstreith and Appel, 1975) (see also Appendix 16.3).

Morphological studies

Muscle fibres

In the late stages of Duchenne dystrophy, specimens of muscle appear grossly abnormal on *light microscopy*. The most obvious abnormality is the paucity of muscle fibres, the muscle being largely composed of fatty connective tissue (*Figure 16.2*). Those fibres which remain are unusually rounded, may have central nuclei, and differ from each other considerably in size. It is probable that the fibres with largest diameters are those which have undergone work hypertrophy (see page 80) in an attempt to compensate for the drop-out of functionally effective fibres. In the earliest stages of the disease the muscle fibre hypertrophy may have a different basis, reflecting either an intrinsic abnormality of the fibre itself or conceivably one imposed upon it by a failing neurone (see also page 125). The unusually small fibres seen in dystrophy may arise in a variety of ways; some are atrophic fibres, others are regenerating ones and some, perhaps the majority, develop by the splitting of large parent fibres (see page 172). Further inspection of the fibres reveals some which show abnormal staining reactions and a loss of cross-striations, indicating that these fibres are undergoing hyaline degeneration. Other fibres may display regions of obvious necrosis in which complete destruction of cellular architecture is combined with the presence of many phagocytic cells. In muscles from younger subjects there is microscopic evidence of attempts at muscle fibre regeneration, the high levels of RNA in the sarcoplasm producing a basophilic staining reaction (bluish coloration with haematoxylin and eosin). In a small but significant proportion of biopsies groups of atrophied muscle fibres can be seen, raising the possibility that some denervation may have occurred (Dastur and Razzak, 1973; Nakao *et al.*, 1968).

With the *electronmicroscope* a bewildering amount of detail can be added including degenerating myofibrils, dilated sarcoplasmic reticulum, autophagic vacuoles, and abnormal mitochondria. Mokri and Engel (1975) suggest that the initial lesion is a defect of the sarcolemma; with the electronmicroscope they observed the membrane to be absent or disrupted in regions of fibres which had not yet undergone necrosis. Using horseradish peroxidase as a marker they showed that extracellular fluid could penetrate the fibres at these sites; they further suggested that the entry of extracellular calcium ions could cause the overcontraction of myofibrils often observed in dystrophic fibres. The formation of these overcontracted regions has been analysed by Cullen and Fulthorpe (1975) who believe that they ultimately result in destruction of the fibres; they divided the latter process into five stages.

In *stage 1* the muscle fibre appeared normal (though presumably with a developing membrane defect).

In *stage 2* widening and blurring of the Z-disc was evident, giving a 'streaming' appearance; the myofilaments were no longer in accurate register within the myofibrils. The changes at the Z-disc were due to 'overcontraction' of parts of the myofibril so as to form 'contracture knots'. In these regions the I-bands disappeared and the A-bands were forced up against the Z-discs; the strong contraction had the effect of overstretching the myofibril elsewhere and the actin filaments were pulled so strongly that they no longer overlapped with the myosin rods. Such myofibrils obviously could not have generated tension at these points and this was therefore one factor contributing to the muscle weakness. In the region of overcontraction the sarcolemma was bunched into folds.

In *stage 3* the overcontraction was more marked with little or no connection remaining between segments of contracted myofibrils. Within the resulting spaces could be found degenerating mitochondria, swollen sarcoplasmic reticulum, empty vesicles, glycogen particles and lipid droplets.

In *stage 4* further condensation of contractile material had occurred and the isolated segments of myofibril underwent homogenization with a loss of striations; this stage corresponded to the appearance of 'hyaline' degeneration in stained sections of muscle viewed with the light microscope.

In *stage 5* the fibre was invaded by macrophages and now consisted of largely structureless cytoplasm containing no contractile material.

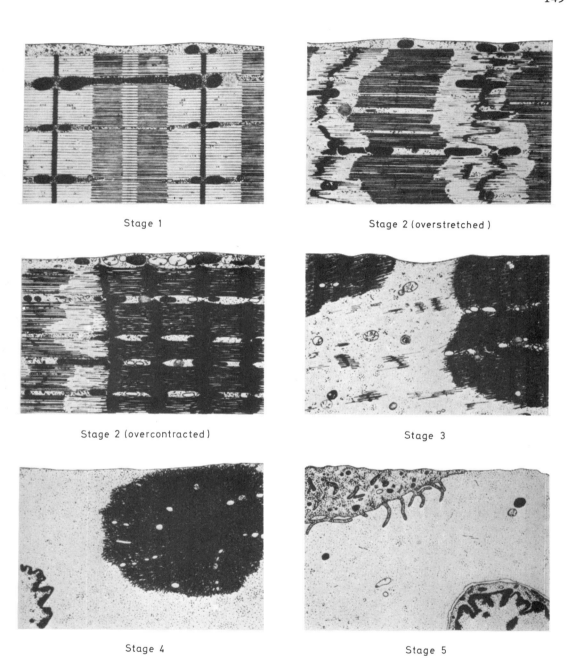

Stage 1

Stage 2 (overstretched)

Stage 2 (overcontracted)

Stage 3

Stage 4

Stage 5

Figure 16.3. Successive stages in the destruction of muscle fibres in Duchenne dystrophy as postulated by Cullen and Fulthorpe (1975) (see text). (Courtesy of the authors, and the Editor and publishers of Journal of Neurological Sciences)

Occasional regenerating fibres were to be found in the neighbourhood.

The possible significance of these changes in relation to a generalized defect of cell membranes is considered in Appendix 16.3.

When investigated histochemically, the dystrophic muscle fibres still show differences among themselves, though the fibre typing is not as definite as in normal muscles. The largest fibres are rich in phosphorylase but poor in oxidative enzymes (Dubowitz, 1974), suggesting that they belong to the type II category (page 58). If so, this is interesting for it is the same type of fibre which shows greatest enlargement when normal muscles are made to undergo work hypertrophy.

Neuromuscular junctions

Intravital staining with methylene blue has been employed to study muscle innervation in Duchenne dystrophy. Jędrezejowska, Johnson and Woolf (1965) noted that some terminal axon expansions were swollen, fused and simplified. With the electronmicroscope the same authors found that the axon terminals contained normal looking synaptic vesicles whereas the secondary synaptic clefts were widened and irregular. Essentially similar ultra-

structural findings were reported more recently by Jerusalem, Engel and Gomez (1974b) following a careful morphometric analysis. The implication from these studies is that any presynaptic change is likely to be secondary to muscle fibre degeneration; however, the former may sometimes occur without the latter being evident (Jędrejowska, 1968) and there is at least one report of axonal swelling and demyelination occurring in the sciatic nerve (Nakao et al., 1968).

Motoneurones

Following Erb (1891) the spinal cord has always been considered as normal in Duchenne dystrophy but, until the study by Tomlinson, Walton and Irving (1974), no quantitative data were available. These authors counted the numbers of presumptive motoneurones in transverse sections of cord in six post-mortem specimens. In five of these cords normal numbers were estimated; in the remaining cord a loss of neurones was found but was attributed to an attack of poliomyelitis in early childhood (see Appendix 16.1). In view of the tedious nature of the task and the difficulty in sometimes differentiating motoneurones from other cells in the ventral horns, it is curious that

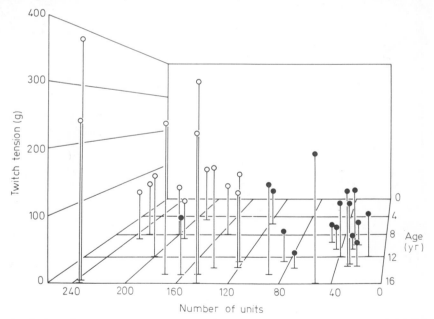

Figure 16.4. Relationship between the maximum isometric twitch tension of the extensor hallucis brevis muscle, the estimated number of functioning motor units in the extensor digitorum brevis muscle, and the age of the patient. ● *= values in patients; and* O *= controls.*
(From McComas, Sica and Currie, 1971 courtesy of the Editor and publishers of Journal of Neurology, Neurosurgery and Psychiatry)

measurements have not been made of the numbers of large (alpha-motor) axons in the ventral roots instead. Leaving aside the issue of cell numbers, it would appear that relatively subtle changes in the myelination of ventral root fibres can be detected in Duchenne dystrophy when comparisons are made of internodal distances and fibre diameters (Mukoyama and Sobue, 1975).

Physiological studies

Coaxial electrode recordings

The EMG findings in Duchenne dystrophy are quite typical of those termed 'myopathic'. On moderate effort there is a full interference pattern while individual muscle action potentials tend to be small, brief and often complex (as in *Figure 16.13*). Fibrillation activity can sometimes be detected, the incidence of this abnormality depending to a considerable extent on the obsessiveness of the examiner.

Microelectrode recordings

In the only microelectrode study reported to date, Gruener (1977) found that in many intercostal fibres there was a reduction in resting membrane potential and a loss of excitability to intracellular stimulation; tetrodotoxin-resistance (page 74) was not observed. Since the refractoriness of the fibres could be overcome by hyperpolarizing their membranes prior to stimulation, it appeared that the sodium and potassium carrier systems were intact.

Multielectrode recordings (page 200)

These yield evidence of increased neuromuscular 'jitter', occasional impulse blocking in axon twigs and increased density of muscle fibres within motor units (Stålberg, 1977).

Muscle twitch studies

Surprisingly few studies have been concerned with muscle strength in Duchenne dystrophy. McComas, Sica and Currie (1973) found that, in patients of similar ages, the isometric twitch tensions of extensor hallucis brevis muscles varied considerably; this variability is evident in *Figure 16.4,* which shows twitch tension as functions of age and of the number of surviving motor units. A conclusion from this study would be that most dystrophic muscle fibres are unable to respond to the pubertal growth stimulus or, alternatively, that any response is masked by increased destruction of other fibres. Un-responsiveness of the fibres to hormonal stimulation

would also be in keeping with the lack of clinical improvement following treatment with anabolic steroids (Barwick, Newell and Walton, 1963). As in any muscle disease, it is not sufficient merely to document the presence of weakness; an attempt should be made to determine its origin. Is it due simply to loss of muscle fibres or to a more subtle derangement such as inexcitability of the sarcolemma, abolition of excitation–contraction coupling, or to failure of the contractile machinery itself? Histological examination of muscle confirms that loss of fibres is certainly one factor. Similarly the presence of necrotic areas in some of the persisting fibres raises the possibility that impulses will not be able to propagate the full distance so that effectively some regions of the fibres will be 'functionally denervated' (page 171). In addition, local refractoriness to membrane depolarization was found by Gruener (1977; see above). In the study by Desmedt and colleagues (1968), there were two observations which pointed to an abnormality of the coupling mechanism or of the contractile machinery in fibres which were still normally excitable. First, in minimally affected muscles, maximal nerve stimulation evoked a diminished twitch but a normal-sized compound action potential. Secondly, in severely-involved muscles, repetitive stimulation of the motor nerve at 2 Hz caused a decline in twitch tension even though the electrical response of the muscle was unchanged. The rupture of myofibrils due to localized overcontraction (contracture), as demonstrated by Cullen and Fulthorpe (1975), would constitute one mechanism for a failure of the contractile machinery (see page 148). A final factor to take into consideration would be the possibility of impaired neuro-muscular transmission; from the ultrastructural studies of Jerusalem, Engel and Gomez (1974b) this possibility appears unlikely but, on the other hand, abnormalities have been seen in the motor nerve terminals after intravital staining with methylene blue (Jędrzejowska, Johnson and Woolf, 1965; Jędrzejowska, 1968). Microelectrode recordings from intercostal muscle fibres would provide the opportunity for resolving this problem.

In addition to its small size, the isometric twitch in Duchenne dystrophy is abnormal in having prolonged contraction and half-relaxation times (McComas and Thomas, 1968b); the difference in twitch speed is obvious in *Figure 16.5* which compares the responses in the extensor hallucis brevis muscles of a 16-year-old patient and a control of the same age. This difference is also evident when bundles of muscle fibres are stimulated through an intramuscular electrode; the proportion of bundles having slow contractions is increased and can be

E.H., 16 yr control

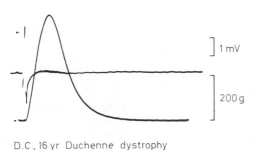

D.C., 16 yr Duchenne dystrophy

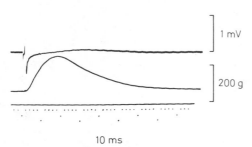

10 ms

Figure 16.5. Maximum isometric twitches and evoked muscle action potentials in the extensor hallucis brevis muscles of two 16-year-old boys, of whom one was normal (upper) and the other dystrophic (lower). Contraction times were 65 and 84 ms respectively. (From McComas, Sica and Currie (1971) courtesy of the Editor and publishers of Journal of Neurology, Neurosurgery and Psychiatry*)*

correlated with an abnormal preponderance of type I (SO) muscle fibres (Buchthal, Schmalbruch and Kamieniecka, 1971b). This last finding would suggest that type II fibres are preferentially involved in Duchenne dystrophy, though this conclusion is not generally accepted. It is important to remember that an increased amount of connective tissue within the muscle belly is likely to 'damp' the twitch and will also cause it to become slower.

Nerve conduction studies

There is argument as to whether or not the maximal impulse conduction velocities are reduced in motor axons of patients with Duchenne muscular dystrophy. According to Henricksen (1956) normal velocities are to be expected but statistically significant reductions in mean value have been found by Nakao *et al.* (1968) and by Jayam *et al.* (1970). In the peroneal nerves of 18 patients

McComas, Sica and Currie (1971) determined a mean value of 51.1 ± 6.0 m/s, which was not significantly different from their control mean (52.1 ± 5.0 m/s); in two of their patients, however, the velocities lay outside the normal range. Of considerable interest was the finding of an increased terminal latency by these authors; this was measured as the time elapsing between stimulation of the peroneal nerve at the ankle and the onset of evoked activity in the end-plate region of the extensor digitorum brevis. The difference between the mean values for the patients and controls (4.4 ± 1.1 ms and 3.5 ± 0.7 ms respectively) was significant at the p = 0·01 level. In contrast to the findings in motor axons, sensory nerve fibre function appears normal both in terms of impulse conduction velocity and amplitude of the compound action potential (McComas, Sica and Upton, 1974).

Motor unit counting studies

When the electrophysiological method for counting functioning motor units was first applied to Duchenne dystrophy, only one of 16 patients was observed to have a normal value for the extensor digitorum brevis muscle (McComas, Sica and Currie, 1971). There was no correlation between the ages of the patients and the sizes of the motor unit populations for the one normal value was obtained in one of the oldest boys (aged 15) whereas the two youngest boys, aged two and three, had considerable reductions (42 and 27 units respectively; see *Figure 16.4*). These findings have since been disputed, normal motor unit populations being reported by Panayiotopoulos, Scarpalezos and Papapetropoulos (1974) and by Ballantyne and Hansen (1974b); the disagreement has been analysed elsewhere (Appendix 6.1).

McComas, Sica and Currie (1971) pointed out that part of the 'denervation' in older patients might have been caused by nerve trauma since these boys were grossly disabled, usually with equinovarus deformities of the ankles, and some of them wore calipers; they also stated that such an explanation could not be applied to the younger patients in whom the denervation appeared to be a primary event. Since the choice of the extensor digitorum brevis (EDB) muscle had been criticized following the initial study (Appendix 6.1), the McComas group extended their investigations to the thenar, hypothenar and soleus muscles. In these muscles losses of functioning motor units were also observed, the change being least for the hypothenar group (*Figure 16.6* and McComas, Sica and Upton, 1974). Examples of electrophysiological recordings from the EDB, thenar and soleus muscles are given in *Figure 16.7*. A comparison of the numbers of motor units with the sizes of the survivors, measured as the mean amplitude of their evoked potentials in each patient, is presented in *Figure 16.8*. It can be seen that the mean sizes are approximately normal except in those patients with severe losses of units, in whom the mean values are reduced. Nevertheless

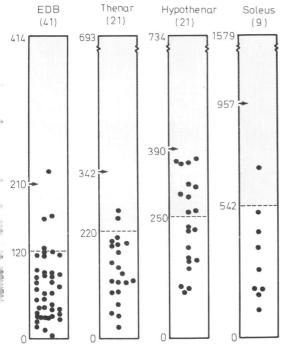

Figure 16.6. Numbers of functioning motor units in the extensor digitorum brevis, thenar, hypothenar and soleus muscles of 41 boys with Duchenne dystrophy. The corresponding ranges of values in control subjects are indicated by hatching; arrows show means

the distribution of points is unlike that anticipated for a primary myopathic process (see *Figure 13.3*).

Measurements of maximum isometric twitch tension also indicate that many of the surviving motor units are of approximately normal size (McComas, Sica and Currie, 1971). However, when the same patient is studied after an interval of a year or more, it is found that the number of motor units is unchanged while the surviving units have become smaller, suggesting that additional muscle fibres have been destroyed (McComas, unpublished observations; see also Chapter 28).

Having dealt at some length with the special laboratory investigations, the case for a neural pathogenesis in Duchenne dystrophy can now be made.

THE NEURAL HYPOTHESIS OF DUCHENNE DYSTROPHY

In marshalling the data which would support a neural hypotehesis it is essential to weigh the evidence carefully. In doing so, it is possible to recognize four classes of observation, each differing from the others in its degree of objectivity (see also McComas, 1975).

Class I observations are those yielding direct evidence that motoneurone dysfunction causes dystrophy. In animal models of dystrophy this type of observation can be sought from experiments involving such techniques as muscle or spinal cord transplantation, tissue culture, cross-innervation and parabiosis (see page 173). In Duchenne dystrophy, as in the other human forms of the disease, there are no observations in this category; apart from muscle transplantation, the necessary techniques would be considered both impracticable and unethical. Yet, if there is no direct evidence that Duchenne dystrophy is a neuropathic disorder, it is equally true that there is no incontestable proof that it is a primary myopathy either.

Class II observations are those comprising indirect evidence that at least some of the degenerative changes seen in dystrophic muscle result from motoneurone dysfunction. In this category the strongest evidence is considered to be the *loss of functioning motor units* described above; the conflicting observations of Panayiotopoulos and colleagues (1974) and of Ballantyne and Hansen (1974b) are dealt with in Appendix 6.1. A second observation is the occurrence of *grouped muscle fibre atrophy* which was found in 15 per cent of the muscles examined by Dastur and Razzak (1973); similar atrophy has also been reported by Nakao and associates (1968) and by Jedrzejowska *et al.* (1968). The third observation in this category is the presence of *fibrillation activity* in an appreciable proportion of dystrophic muscles (Buchthal and Rosenfalck, 1966). This finding has caused some authorities to reject fibrillation potentials as a reliable sign of denervation; others have suggested that they might arise in a segment of muscle fibre sequestered from the end-plate region by a necrotic plaque, the motor axon remaining intact. Split fibres (see *Figure 16.23*) or regenerating fibres might also temporarily lack an innervation and generate fibrillation activity as a consequence. Some or all of these factors may pertain in the same muscle, though it is worth noting that the sharp appearance of the fibrillation potential suggests that the active region of the fibre is still in good condition.

Class III observations describe motoneuronal or

antigens of peripheral and central nervous system origin (Caspary, Currie and Field, 1971).

Class IV observations indicate abnormalities in the central nervous system elsewhere than in the motoneurones. As with the previous class, it is

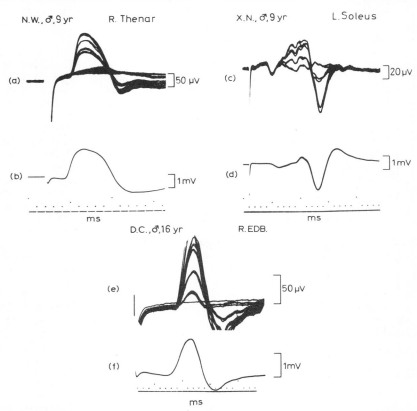

Figure 16.7. Estimations of numbers of functioning motor units in muscles of three boys with Duchenne muscular dystrophy. (a), (c) and (e) show the superimposed responses of the motor units which were stimulated by the weakest nerve stimuli; (b), (d) and (f) show the corresponding maximum evoked muscle responses. Based on slightly larger samples of motor unit responses it was calculated that the motor unit populations were roughly 74 (patient N.W.) 152 (X.N) and 52 (D.C.). These values correspond to 22, 16 and 25 per cent of the respective mean values for controls

axonal abnormalities which, by themselves, do not necessarily imply any related changes in the muscle. Within this class is the *slowing of impulse conduction velocity* found by Nakao and colleagues (1968) and by Jayam and associates (1970), together with the *increased terminal latency* noted by McComas, Sica and Currie (1971). Evidence of a different kind is the finding of *degenerating or demyelinated sciatic nerve fibres* in the patient studied by Nakao and colleagues (1968), the presence of ventral root fibres with abnormal myelination (Mukoyama and Sobue, 1975) and the demonstration of *lymphocytes* sensitized to

evidence by association and is therefore relatively weak. Prominent in this category is the increased incidence of *mental retardation* which was first observed by Duchenne himself and has since been confirmed by Allen and Rodgin (1960), Zellweger and Niedermeyer (1965), Nakao and associates (1968) and by Prosser, Murphy and Thompson (1969). Previously it had been suspected that the reduction in mean intelligence quotient might have been secondary to the intellectual and social deprivation which many patients with Duchenne dystrophy undoubtedly suffer. That this is not the correct explanation is suggested by the fact that

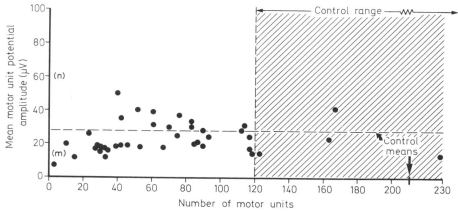

Figure 16.8. *Relationship between numbers and sizes of functioning motor units in 41 extensor digitorum brevis muscles of patients with Duchenne dystrophy. The mean values for control subjects are indicated by arrows; the hatched area indicates the lower part of the control range for the number of units. With reference to Figure 13.3, values above and below the horizontal interrupted line would suggest neuropathy (n) and myopathy (m) respectively*

children with spinal muscular atrophy have a significantly higher mean I.Q. even though the same environmental factors are present (Kozicka, Prot and Wasilewski, 1971). In keeping with the presence of a cerebral defect are reports of *abnormal EEGs* in patients with Duchenne dystrophy, the irregularities consisting of increased

slow wave activity and, in some cases, spikes and slow waves (Zellweger and Niedermeyer, 1965; Nakao *et al.*, 1968); in contrast, no abnormalities were noted in the study by Barwick, Osselton and Walton (1965). There is also argument over the presence of *macroscopic malformations* in the brain for while Rosman and Kakulas (1966) found neuronal heterotopias and pachygyria at autopsy, Dubowitz and Crome (1969) were unable to detect these abnormalities in their own series of 21 autopsied cases.

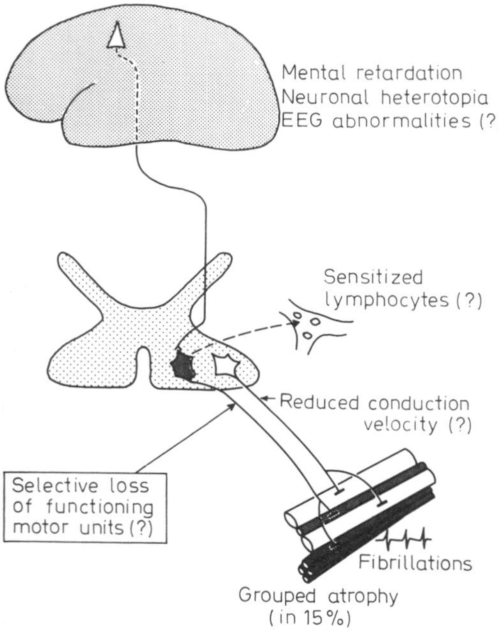

THE CASE AGAINST A NEURAL HYPOTHESIS

The 'myopathic' muscle biopsy

Many of the findings cited in the earlier sections have been used in arguments contradicting the neural hypothesis but, in assessing their significance, it is important to recall the terms of the neural hypothesis. For example, the diffusely abnormal appearance of a dystrophic muscle on light microscopy is pointed out as being different to the picture usually seen in chronic denervation in which regions of apparently normal muscle fibres can be seen alongside groups of atrophied fibres (see *Figure 20.5* and page 230 for explanation). One of the aims of the sick motoneurone hypothesis of McComas, Sica and Campbell (1971) was to suggest a mechanism whereby apparently 'myopathic' features might arise in the course of neuropathic disorder. It was postulated that a sick motoneurone might lose part of its colony of

Mental retardation
Neuronal heterotopia (?)
EEG abnormalities (?)

Sensitized
lymphocytes (?)

Reduced conduction
velocity (?)

Selective loss
of functioning
motor units (?)

Fibrillations

Grouped atrophy
(in 15%)

Figure 16.9. *Diagrammatic summary of evidence supporting a neural pathogenesis of Duchenne dystrophy (see text)*

muscle fibres and that these denervated fibres would continue to degenerate since they could not be reinnervated by other sick motoneurones. In this way the random pattern of degenerating muscle fibres would be produced; a similar mechanism, termed an *'in portio'* disorder, has been proposed by Engel and Warmolts (1973). The validity of this concept is enhanced by the not infrequent finding of 'myopathic' regions in muscles which have been chronically denervated (Drachman *et al.*, 1967).

The 'Myopathic' EMG

The differences between the 'myopathic' and 'neuropathic' electromyograms are also used as evidence favouring the existence of two sites of abnormality, that is, muscle and nerve. Once again, the sick motoneurone concept (*in portio* lesion of Engel and Warmolts, 1973) provided an explanation for the generation of small brief potentials during volition, since some of the motor units would contain fewer active fibres than normal around the tip of the coaxial recording electrode. Further, if the motor unit territory had previously been enlarged by collateral reinnervation (during a healthy phase of the motoneurone), the loss of muscle fibres during the sick phase might temporarily result in a motor unit with a

normal number of fibres but with a reduced density. Such a unit would be expected to yield a small brief spike on recording with a coaxial electrode but a normal-sized potential when a large surface electrode was used instead, as in the motor unit counting technique of McComas and colleagues (1971a). The fact that 'myopathic'-appearing potentials can often be recorded in chronic neuropathic disorders with an intra-muscular electrode is in keeping with these suggestions.

Another electromyographic observation which has been used against the neural hypothesis, is the full *interference pattern* which can be recorded from a patient with dystrophy or other myopathy. The problem with this argument is that the density of the pattern is poorly related to the number of functioning motor units. As Stålberg, Trontelj and Janko (1972) have shown, some of the EMG potentials in Duchenne dystrophy are abnormally complex and prolonged, especially when recorded with a multi-lead electrode (see also Desmedt and Borenstein, 1973). Thus a single unit firing at a physiological frequency could give a misleadingly 'full' look to the EMG. This concern is reinforced by the results of motor unit counting in neuro-pathic disorders for McComas *et al.* (1971a) pointed out '. . . up to 70 per cent denervation could be detected in . . . patients in whom the electromyographic interference pattern appeared normal' (see also *Figure 6.1, E*).

Normal numbers of motoneurones in spinal cords

As already stated, Tomlinson, Walton and Irving (1974) found normal numbers of moto-neurones in five spinal cords from patients with Duchenne dystrophy. This observation is not opposed to the sick motoneurone hypothesis, how-ever, for this stated 'The significance of a loss of cells from the anterior horn of the spinal cord is evident; similarly, severe chromatolytic changes in neurones must surely denote impending death. On the other hand, there is no reason for assuming that the normal appearance of a motoneurone signifies normal function.' If dystrophy was a motoneurone disorder, it would behave in a 'dying-back manner' (see Chapter 25) with the distal region of the axons being most affected and the cell bodies of the motoneurones showing least change. In fact, the motoneurones *may* appear abnormal in Duchenne dystrophy for Tomlinson, Walton and Irving (1974) found cells which stained poorly and showed evidence of chroma-tolysis.

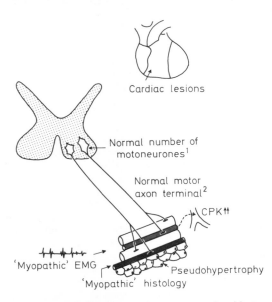

Figure 16.10. Diagrammatic summary of evidence cited as being incompatible with a neural patho-genesis of Duchenne dystrophy (see text). References: (1) Tomlinson, Walton and Irving (1974); (2) Jerusalem, Engel and Gomez (1974)

Normal motor nerve terminals

The careful morphometric investigations of Jerusalem, Engel and Gomez (1974b) failed to disclose any significant presynaptic abnormality in the neuromuscular junctions of dystrophic fibres in Duchenne dystrophy, even though the muscle fibres themselves often showed degenerative features in the end-plate region. The authors pointed out that these negative observations did not necessarily exclude a neural pathogenesis since a deficient trophic mechanism might be present without its morphological counterpart being visible in the nerve terminal. Both in the Eaton–Lambert syndrome and in botulinum poisoning, for example, synaptic transmission can be completely blocked by presynaptic mechanisms at a stage when the axon terminal still appears normal with the electron-microscope. Jerusalem and colleagues also observed that there might be little chance of encountering a

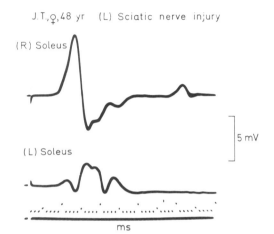

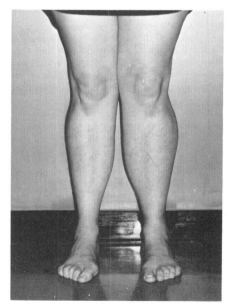
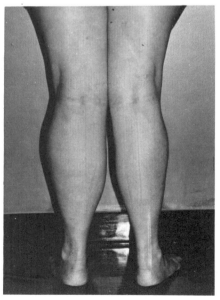

Figure 16.11. Gross pseudohypertrophy of the muscles below the knee in the left leg of a patient following injury to the sciatic nerve. The upper section shows the maximum potentials evoked from the two soleus muscles; note the smaller response from the left (pseudohypertrophied) muscle

degenerating axon terminal if this phase was short-lived in relation to the duration of the disease. Furthermore, the normal ultrastructural appearance of the terminal reported by these workers has to be balanced against the changes seen in the gross structure of the distal axon, as revealed by Jędrzejowska, Johnson and Woolf (1965) and Jędrzejowska (1968).

Serum enzyme levels

In the past the finding of high serum levels of muscle enzymes in Duchenne dystrophy has been used to differentiate this condition from neuropathic disorders in which normal or mildly elevated titres were considered the rule. With increasing experience, however, the diagnostic value of these tests diminished with the recognition that high titres could sometimes be encountered in denervating conditions also (Williams and Bruford, 1970). In one patient with typical motoneurone disease, confirmed by electromyography, a 60-fold rise in serum CPK was noted by the author.

Pseudohypertrophy

At first sight it seems improbable that the muscular pseudohypertrophy of Duchenne dystrophy could result from a neural abnormality, for how could a failing motoneurone promote an overgrowth of fatty connective tissue? Yet the fact that equally prominent pseudohypertrophy occurs in a proportion of patients with 'spinal muscular atrophy' (Namba, Aberfeld and Grob, 1970) is surely relevant, although in this instance it could be argued that the same gene was simultaneously influencing both nerve and connective tissue (that is, exerting a *pleiotropic* effect). Rather better evidence that partial denervation can unleash connective tissue hyperplasia has come from occasional clinical observations on the results of mechanical injuries to axons. Lapresle, Fardeau and Said (1973) reported pseudohypertrophy of calf muscles following lumbosacral root lesions. In our experience, it has been observed in the pronator quadratus muscle after a neurapraxic lesion of the anterior interosseous nerve (McComas, Jorgensen and Upton, 1974), disappearing as the palsy improved. *Figure 16.11* shows another striking example, this time in the calf muscles of a 42-year-old woman in whom an analgesic (nature unknown) had been injected inadvertently into the left sciatic nerve three years previously. The patient had felt sudden severe pain radiating down the leg during the injection and was left with moderate weakness of ankle movement together with patchy numbness. Over this three-year-period she had noticed that the calf muscles were enlarging in this leg, although remaining weak; a muscle biopsy was refused but electromyography confirmed that the excitable muscle fibre bulk was reduced (*Figure 16.11*). On the basis of observations such as these, it must be accepted that in certain circumstances muscle pseudohypertrophy can complicate a neuropathic lesion.

Cardiomyopathy

The existence of a severe cardiomyopathy in Duchenne dystrophy has also been cited as evidence against a neural disorder. It is difficult to discuss this issue at a cellular level for little is known concerning the origin of the trophic influence necessary to sustain cardiac muscle. Although the heart does receive an autonomic innervation it is possible that the cardiac muscle fibres are less dependent on external sources than skeletal fibres. The best defence for the neural hypothesis over this issue is the observation that a cardiomyopathy may complicate Freidreich's ataxia, a known neuropathic disorder. More pertinent still is the presence of a cardiac lesion in some patients with 'spinal muscular atrophy', as Tomlinson, Walton and Irving (1974) have recently described. These last authors have suggested that, instead of reflecting a direct action of the defective gene, the cardiac lesion may result from the development of circulating antibodies which have been induced by skeletal muscle antigen and are capable of attacking the myocardium.

Conclusions

The case for a neural hypothesis in Duchenne dystrophy remains unproven and, indeed, may forever be incapable of satisfactory resolution. Nevertheless the preceding sections have shown that sufficient evidence is available to justify the formulation of a hypothesis of this nature. It should be added that the neural hypothesis is not the only alternative to the tradional myopathic concept of the disease; in Appendix 16.2 a putative vascular aetiology is considered. Leaving aside the question as to whether or not the disease is caused by an intrinsic abnormality of the muscle, the possible nature of the induced muscle fibre defect is discussed in Appendix 16.3.

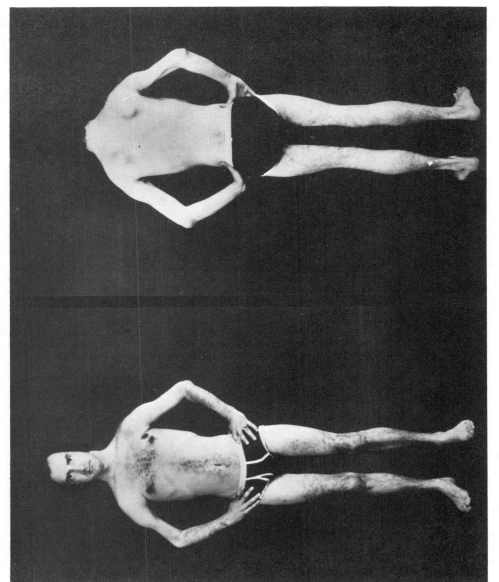

Figure 16.12. 35-year-old man with limb-girdle muscular dystrophy. Note the marked wasting of the right biceps and triceps muscles; the pectoral muscles are also atrophied and the weakness of the posterior shoulder girdle muscles has caused winging and elevation of the scapulae. In the legs the calf muscles appear to have a normal bulk but there is some atrophy of the thighs

LIMB-GIRDLE AND FACIOSCAPULOHUMERAL MUSCULAR DYSTROPHY

It is convenient to consider these two types of dystrophy together for both are slowly progressive and both usually have their clinical onsets in adolescence or early adult life, although this is not invariable. The slow courses of the diseases enable most patients to live to normal ages, although with increasing disability. Transmission in both conditions is by autosomal genes, the one for limb-girdle dystrophy usually being recessive and that for the facioscapulohumeral variety being dominant.

In *limb-girdle dystrophy* the most severely affected muscles are those of the pelvic and shoulder girdles, together with the trunk musculature (*Figure 16.12*). Initially the patient notices weakness in raising the arms above the head and consequently has difficulty in such tasks as combing the hair and putting objects on shelves. Weakness of hip muscles makes rising from chairs or climbing the stairs awkward; later, walking on level ground becomes difficult. The involvement of trunk musculature adds to the problems in locomotion; as in Duchenne dystrophy the patient walks with a lordotic gait, the abdomen protruding forwards and the shoulders being thrust backwards to preserve balance. As the disease advances weakness spreads to involve limb muscles situated more distally; movements involving the knee and elbow are affected first, followed by those of the wrist and ankle. As in Duchenne dystrophy the tendon reflexes are depressed, and about one-third of patients exhibit pseudohypertrophy of their muscles before atrophy sets in; intelligence is normal, however, and cardiac involvement is said to be unusual (Perloff, DeLeon and O'Doherty, 1966). It is probable, however, that careful autopsy studies will show a higher incidence of cardiac abnormality, in line with recent studies of patients with spinal muscular atrophy (see Tomlinson, Walton and Irving, 1974).

In *facioscapulohumeral dystrophy* the muscles of the pelvic and shoulder girdles are affected, as in limb-girdle dystrophy, but in addition there is weakness of the facial musculature. The patients become unable to close their eyes properly and to whistle; labial sounds are pronounced with difficulty. The mouth takes on a characteristic pouting appearance and the face is notable for the absence of wrinkles. Muscular pseudohypertrophy is considered to be very uncommon (Walton and Gardner-Medwin, 1974) and cardiac involvement is unusual; intelligence is normal.

Special investigations

In both types of muscular dystrophy the serum titres of muscle enzymes are usually mildly elevated but may be normal. Muscle biopsy shows the same sort of myopathic features as in Duchenne dystrophy (Page 148) except that there is less acute muscle fibre degeneration and necrosis while regenerating muscle fibres are less evident. In typical cases the EMG will show 'myopathic' features (page 151). In an *in vitro* microelectrode study of external intercostal muscle, Ludin (1970) found that the muscle fibre resting potentials were reduced in two cases of limb-girdle dystrophy and in one patient with the facioscapulohumeral variety.

The problem: are these two dystrophies myopathies, neuropathies or both?

A case has already been made for considering Duchenne dystrophy as a neural disorder (page 153). Many of the arguments concerning that dystrophy are also pertinent to the limb-girdle and facioscapulohumeral forms. In the latter dystrophies a further uncertainty arises for many patients have an illness which is indistinguishable on clinical grounds from a benign form of *spinal muscular atrophy*—a degenerative disorder of motoneurones (page 272). The credit for first recognizing the presence of a denervating process in some patients thought to have dystrophy rests with Wohlfart (1942). This author noted fasciculations and subsequently Kugelberg and Welander (1956), in an electromyographic study, were able to demonstrate other features of chronic denervation. It has since been customary to consider the Kugelberg–Welander form of spinal muscular atrophy as a disease entity which, in its pathogenesis, is quite distinct from the limb-girdle and facioscapulohumeral dystrophies. To Sica and McComas (1971b) this distinction appeared illogical for their electrophysiological studies showed similar losses of functioning motor units in both dystrophies and in spinal muscular atrophy (see below). Although the presence of fasciculations, Babinski responses or unusually prominent weakness of distal muscles would suggest a diagnosis of spinal muscular atrophy, in most patients these features are absent and, as already stated, it is impossible to make a diagnosis on clinical grounds alone. Since the serum enzyme titres are similar in all these conditions, the only remaining resources are muscle biopsy and electromyography. Whereas the finding of grouped muscle fibre atrophy or of fibre type grouping in the biopsy would correctly indicate a diagnosis of spinal muscular atrophy, the presence of myopathic features would have only limited diagnostic value since this picture is also known to occur in chronic neuropathic disorders (Drachman *et al.*, 1967).

Criticisms of a smilar type also apply to the results of electromyography but with this test it is at least possible to sample many muscles and to make a comprehensive survey of the skeletal musculature. Unfortunately for the purists, the results give little support to the concept of two types of disorder with discrete pathogenetic mechanisms. In an unpublished study conducted in 1971 Petito and Upton investigated a large series

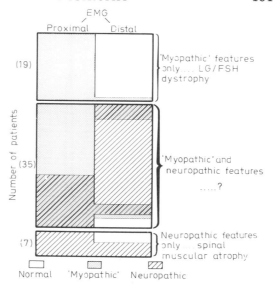

Figure 16.14. Analysis of 61 patients with muscle weakness suggestive of either limb-girdle or facioscapulohumeral dystrophy, or else spinal muscular atrophy. Examinations of proximal and distal muscles were performed with coaxial needle recording electrodes; each muscle was judged to be normal, 'myopathic' or 'neuropathic'. It can be seen that the findings were inconsistent in most patients (see text)

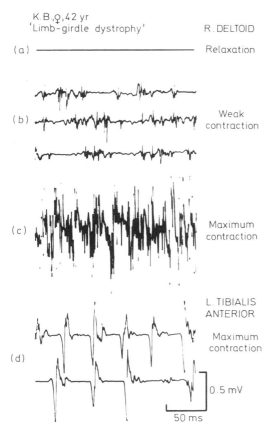

Figure 16.13. Recordings made with a coaxial needle electrode from two muscles of a patient with hereditary chronic proximal muscular atrophy, previously diagnosed as limb-girdle dystrophy. In the right deltoid the small brief potentials (b) and the full interference pattern (c) suggested a 'myopathic' disorder. However, in tibialis anterior (d) a very poor interference pattern comprising rather prolonged potentials was obtained on maximum effort, suggesting the presence of a 'neuropathic' process

of patients with chronic and slowly progressive atrophy of proximal muscles in whom a diagnosis of limb-girdle and facioscapulohumeral dystrophy had been entertained. Some of these patients had been examined previously by Sica and McComas (1971b) and the series was subsequently extended by the inclusion of patients from the Hamilton region in Ontario. On the basis of coaxial electrode recordings in a combination of proximal and distal muscles of the arm and leg only a minority of patients yielded patterns of results which were uniformly myopathic or neuropathic. A common finding was that some proximal muscles yielded 'myopathic' results while in the same patient other proximal muscles appeared 'neuropathic'; the results in distal muscles were usually normal or 'neuropathic' (*Figure 16.13*). Not uncommonly the same muscle might yield a 'myopathic' EMG picture in one part and a 'neuropathic' one in another; further, in one Hamilton family a sister is 'myopathic' and her brother 'neuropathic'. These results are in conflict with other studies which have yielded good correlation between the various laboratory findings (Humphrey and Shy, 1962; Schwartz, Archibald and Hagstron, 1966; Hausmanowa-Petrusewicz and Jędrzedowska, 1971; Black *et al.*, 1974). However, in the detailed study by Hausmanowa-Petrusewicz and Jędrzedowska, the EMG findings in some of the dystrophic patients were stated to include features normally indicative of neuropathy— enlargement of motor unit territory, large potentials and pseudomyotonic volleys. The same

some healthy motoneurones capable of under- taking collateral reinnervation of denervated *muscle fibres (see page 115 and Figure 13.4).* In the proximal muscles the weakness would be greater because the neuropathic process was more advanced. If previously healthy motoneurones had

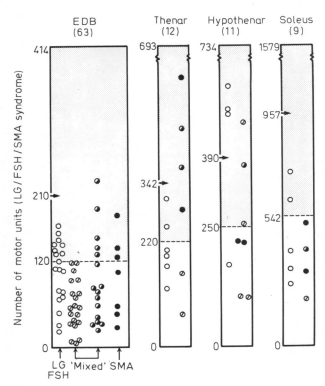

Figure 16.15. Numbers of functioning motor units in the extensor digitorum brevis (EDB), thenar, hypothenar and soleus muscles of patients thought to have either limb-girdle (LG) or facioscapulohumeral (FSH) dystrophy, or else spinal muscular atrophy (SMA). Symbols can be identified from base of EDB column. The corresponding ranges of results in control subjects are indicated by hatching; arrows show means

authors drew attention to the fact that, during histological examination in 'chronic cases of spinal neurogenic atrophy (e.g. the Kugelberg–Welander disease) . . . occasionally the entire section may show so-called myopathic changes'.

One interpretation of these various findings would be that these patients exhibit a continuum of pathological changes resulting from denervation. In the least affected muscles, the distal ones in the limbs, the changes seen are those typical of chronic denervation; in terms of the sick motoneurone hypothesis, they occur because the corresponding motoneurone pools in the spinal cord still retain

become 'sick' or 'dead', the proximal muscles would assume falsely myopathic complexions, as predicted by the sick motoneurone hypothesis.

On the basis of the coaxial electrode record- ings alone, the case for a neural pathogenesis of limb-girdle and facioscapulohumeral dystrophy appears strong. Further support for a neural origin has come for estimations of numbers and sizes of motor units, using the electrophysiological method of McComas and colleagues (1971a). Sica and McComas (1971b) found that 9 of 11 patients with limb-girdle or facioscapulohumeral dystrophy had reduced numbers of functioning motor units in the extensor digitorum brevis (EDB) muscle. This initial investigation was repeated and extended to the EDB muscles of other patients by Petito and Upton in 1971 with similar results. Finally, patients in the Hamilton (Ontario) region were studied with similar techniques and observations were made on the thenar, hypothenar and soleus muscles in addition to the extensor digitorum brevis. At the present time results are available for a total of 61 patients with clinical features suggestive of either limb-girdle or facioscapulo-humeral dystrophy. Within this population 39 patients had 'myopathic' EMGs in proximal muscles but in only 19 of these were the results in distal muscles compatible with a myopathic process (*Figure 16.14*). In 35 of the 61 patients the patterns of results among the various muscles were inconsistent and it was impossible to determine whether the disease processes had been myopathic or neuropathic. Finally in seven patients the EMG findings indicated a diagnosis of spinal muscular atrophy. *Figure 16.15* shows the numbers of functioning motor units in these three groups, and an example of the evoked responses in the EDB muscle of a 36-year-old woman with limb-girdle dystrophy is given in *Figure 16.16*. It can be seen from *Figure 16.15* that some of the muscles in these patients do have numbers of motor units within the control range, especially the hypothenar muscles. This finding is to be expected for, in a more detailed analysis, McComas *et al.* (1974b) showed that in such instances the function of these muscles also appeared normal, as judged by the maximum evoked action potentials and twitches.

In the limb-girdle and facioscapulohumeral dystrophies the sizes of the evoked motor unit potentials are significantly increased in most of the partially denervated muscles. This finding distinguishes these dystrophies electrophysiologic-ally from the Duchenne type in which the surviving motor units generate normal or diminished potentials. Comparison of *Figures 16.17* and *13.3* shows that the results in the limb-girdle and facio-scapulohumeral dystrophies resemble those predicted for, and found in, patients with chronic denervation (see *Figure 20.6*); they reflect the enlargement of the surviving motor units through collateral reinnervation. This type of observation is of particular significance in relation to the pathogenesis of dystrophy for it strongly suggests that dystrophic muscle fibres may be able to function properly if their innervation is changed. In other words, it is not the muscle fibre which is intrinsically defective but the 'original' moto-neurone innervating it.

Other physiological observations may be also mentioned for the sake of completeness (see Table 16.1 and Sica and McComas, 1971b). *Isometric twitch tension* studies show that in most muscles the contraction and half relaxation times are abnormally prolonged, affording another similarity to chronic partially denervated muscles. In keeping with their large potentials, the surviving motor units develop disproportionately large tensions. Maximal *impulse conduction velocities* and *terminal latencies* are normal in the deep peroneal nerve-extensor digitorum brevis prepara-tion but *repetitive nerve stimulation* produces

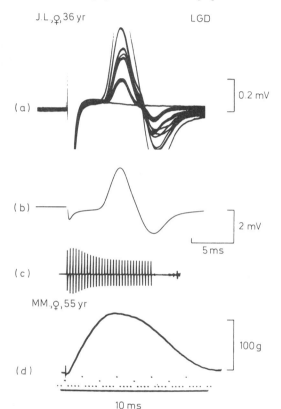

Figure 16.16. *Electrophysiological findings in two female patients thought to have limb-girdle muscular dystrophy and in whom EMG examination of proximal muscles yielded 'myopathic' activity. (a), (b), (c) are results from a 36-year-old woman; (d) is taken from a 55-year-old patient. (a) shows EDB responses to juxtathreshold nerve stimulation and (b) displays maximum muscle response. Repetitive stimulation of the peroneal nerve evoked decre-mental muscle responses (c). A maximum isometric twitch of the extensor hallucis brevis muscle is shown in (d); note the prolonged contraction time (130 ms; compare with Figure 16.5, upper). (From Sica and McComas (1971b) courtesy of the Editor and pub-lishers of Journal of Neurology, Neurosurgery and Psychiatry)*

TABLE 16.1

Mean Values ($\pm$ S.D.) of Pooled Electrophysiological Data from Control Subjects and 11 Patients with **Limb-girdle** or Facioscapulohumeral Dystrophy studied in detail by Sica and McComas (1971)*

	EDB motor units		Isometric twitch			Nerve stimulation	
	No.	Potential amplitude (μV)	Active tension (g)	Contraction time (ms)	$\frac{1}{2}$ Relaxation time (ms)	Conduction velocity (m/s)	Terminal latency (ms)
Patients	65 $\pm$ 41	59.5 $\pm$ 73.0	209 $\pm$ 111	85 $\pm$ 9.7	81 $\pm$ 16	48.1 $\pm$ 3.5	4.3 $\pm$ 0.6
Controls	199 $\pm$ 60	28 9 $\pm$ 27.1	313 $\pm$ 90	63 $\pm$ 7.3	53 $\pm$ 9.7	49.0 $\pm$ 4.0	4.0 $\pm$ 0.6
P	<0.001	<0.001	<0.01	<0.001	<0.001	>0.6	>0.2

* By courtesy of the Editor and publishers of *Journal of Neurology, Neurosurgery and Psychiatry*

decremental responses in about half of the muscles. This last finding suggests that synaptic transmission is impaired at some of the neuromuscular junctions within the surviving motor units; if so, the corresponding motoneurones would be in an early dysfunctional stage (Stage II, *Figure 25.5*) in terms of the sick motoneurone hypothesis.

Conclusions

Even without the results from motor unit counting studies, a strong case can be made for the presence of a major neural component in the limb-girdle and facioscapulohumeral dystrophies. The motor unit counting results themselves are so abnormal in some patients that they could not possibly be due to

methodological error, especially since the individual motor unit potentials are increased rather than decreased. Consequently the discrepancy between the present results and those of Ballantyne and Hansen (1974b) and Panayiotopoulos and Scarpalezos (1975) must have some other explanation, possibly the selection of patients considered to have 'dystrophy' as opposed to 'spinal muscular atrophy' (see Appendix 6.1). Even when all possible factors are taken into account, there will be some patients who, in life, manifest the clinical, histological and electromyographic features of limb-girdle or facioscapulohumeral dystrophy and yet can be shown to have reduced numbers of motoneurones in their spinal cords at autopsy, as in the patient (Case 9) studied by Tomlinson, Walton and Irving (1974). The argument put forward by these last authors, that the correct

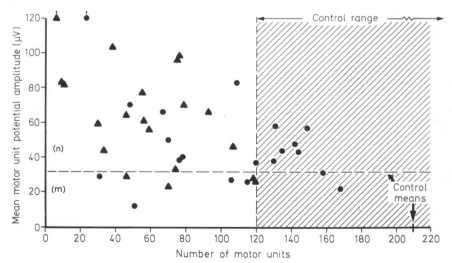

Figure 16.17. Relationship between numbers and sizes of functioning motor units in 40 extensor digitorum brevis muscles of patients thought to have limb-girdle or facioscapulohumeral dystrophy. The mean values for control subjects are indicated by arrows; the hatched area indicated the lower part of the control range for the number of units. With reference to Figure 13.3, values above and below the horizontal interrupted line would suggest neuropathy (n) and myopathy (m) respectively

diagnosis during life should have been spinal muscular atrophy, might be construed as circular reasoning when set against the original purpose of their inquiry.

MYOTONIC DYSTROPHY
(Dystrophia myotonica: Steinert's disease)

Clinical features

Myotonic muscular dystrophy is undoubtedly the most fascinating of the dystrophies for it combines degeneration of the muscle fibres with an array of other somatic abnormalities. These include a characteristic intermittent stiffness of the muscles, or *myotonia*, which has been discussed in detail in Chapter 14. There is a resemblance to the Duchenne type of dystrophy in the presence of a cardiomyopathy and of mental retardation. Unlike Duchenne dystrophy the degree of mental defect is proportional to the severity of the muscle weakness and progressive dementia may occur. In a male frontal baldness is common and in both sexes there is a high incidence of cataracts. The cataracts can be seen at an early stage by slit-lamp examination; they commence as small particles which later coalesce into a stellate form. Other, more variable, abnormalities in myotonic dystrophy include gonadal atrophy, mild hyper-insulinism and hyperostosis of the skull vault. Inheritance is by an autosomal dominant gene and the disease may manifest itself at any age. Thus a child with myotonic dystrophy may be weak and floppy at birth and have difficulty in breathing; it is usual for the weakness to improve. At the other extreme is the elderly adult patient without detectable weakness but in whom there is EMG evidence of myotonia; the characteristic cataracts may also be present. A common presentation is in middle age when the patient seeks advice for increasing weakness or for muscle stiffness (i.e. myotonia). The weakness is associated with atrophy and never with hypertrophy (unlike Duchenne dystrophy and some of the other types). The most severely affected muscles are the distal ones in the arms and legs together with those of the head and neck. As the disease advances, the facial appearance becomes characteristic—there is ptosis, the mouth sags open and the atrophy of the facial and neck muscles gives the patient a haggard look (*Figure 16.18, upper*). Walking is affected, mild cases showing foot drop and more severe ones being confined to wheelchairs. Mildly affected patients have a normal life expectancy; at the other extreme is death in infancy from cardiac or respiratory failure. A most intriguing aspect of the disease is

the phenomenon of *anticipation*, discussed in Appendix 16.4.

Special investigations

Blood tests

The *serum CPK* is usually only mildly elevated. One Hamilton infant who was slow to develop had myotonia on electromyography; however, a 300-fold rise in CPK raised the possibility of Duchenne dystrophy rather than the myotonic type and this was subsequently confirmed. In myotonic dystrophy the *immunoglobulins* may be abnormal and there is evidence of excessive catabolism of immunoglobulin G (Wochner *et al.*, 1966). In some patients a glucose tolerance test provokes hypersecretion of *insulin*. There is a close genetic linkage between myotonic dystrophy, the ABH secretor status and the Lutheran blood group. The newly-recognized abnormalities of red cell membranes are described on page 313.

Morphological studies

Muscle The muscles show the characteristic features of dystrophy described on page 148; there is variation in fibre size, central positioning of the myonuclei and increased connective tissue. A characteristic finding in myotonic dystrophy are chains of myonuclei in the interiors of the fibres (*Figure 16.18, lower*). Also typical of the condition are fibres with sarcoplasmic masses lying under the sarcolemma; these masses are composed of disorganized myofilaments, mitochondria and other organelles. In about half of the patients there appears to be selective involvement of type I muscle fibres during the early stages of the disease (Engel and Brooke, 1966).

Motor innervation (Coërs and Woolf, 1959; Coërs, Telerman-Toppet and Gerard, 1973) Intravital staining with methylene blue reveals a very abnormal motor innervation in myotonic dystrophy. The end-plate regions are elongated with the axon terminals being somewhat enlarged and increased in number. There is obvious axonal sprouting so that a single fibre may have several end-plates and, conversely, a single axon may supply an increased number of muscle fibres (collateral reinnervation, page 224). These findings are suggestive of a denervating process; stronger evidence in this direction has been provided by MacDermot (1961) who noticed that in the intramuscular nerve bundles

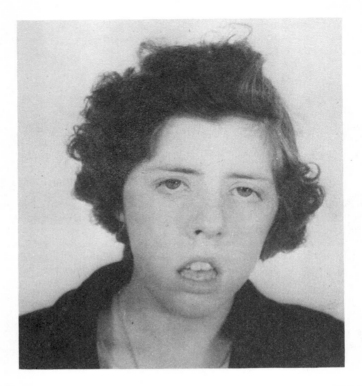

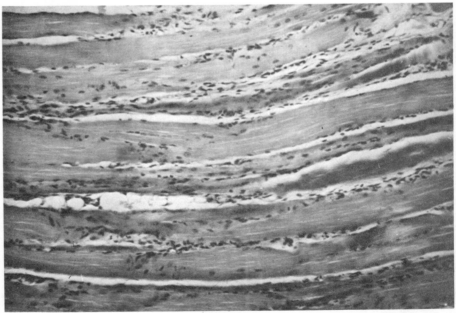

Figure 16.18. (Upper) Typical facial appearance of patient with myotonic muscular dystrophy (see text). (Lower) Longitudinal section of deltoid muscle from patient with myotonic dystrophy, stained with haematoxylin and eosin. Notice how some of the nuclei line up to form chains with the fibres (×150)

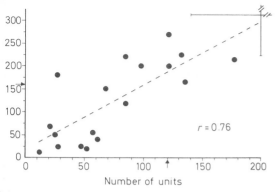

Figure 16.19. Relationship between numbers of functioning motor units and maximum isometric twitch tensions of EDB muscles in patients with myotonic dystrophy. The mean control values are also shown, together with one standard deviation. (From McComas, Campbell and Sica (1971), courtesy of the Editor and the publishers of Journal of Neurology, Neurosurgery and Psychiatry)

some of the axons exhibited 'a complete breakdown of nerve fibre substance'. Against the possibility of denervation is the normal distribution of muscle ACh receptors (Fambrough and Drachman, 1976) and the absence of nerve fibre loss or of ultrastructural abnormalities of axons (Pollock and Dyck, 1976).

Electrophysiological studies

Coaxial electrode recordings   Careful exploration of muscles with coaxial recording electrodes may yield myotonic activity (page 125) as the only abnormality in mildly affected patients with myotonic dystrophy. Usually the myotonia is more prominent in a distal muscle, such as the abductor pollicis brevis, than in a proximal one, but there is great variation between patients as well as in the same patient at different times. The myotonic activity is often greatest if the extremity is cold; repeated contraction diminishes the myotonia ('warm-up' phenomenon). In more severe cases the recordings will yield abnormal muscle action potentials during effort; commonly they are small, brief and complex ('myopathic') but they may be mixed with complex potentials of increased duration suggestive of neuropathic involvement. Fibrillation potentials may also occur.

Nerve conduction studies   Maximal impulse conduction velocities are usually normal in motor and sensory axons of patients with myotonic dystrophy (Table 16.2) but occasionally slightly reduced values are noted. Terminal motor latencies and sensory nerve responses are also normal. There are, however, reports of families with myotonic dystrophy in association with polyneuropathy (see below).

Repetitive nerve stimulation   Repetitive nerve stimulation, even at low frequencies, may evoke muscle responses which decrease in amplitude (McComas, Campbell and Sica, 1971). Although this observation is suggestive of impaired neuromuscular transmission and is presumably related to the abnormal appearances of the motor end-plates in myotonic dystrophy, no EMG or clinical evidence of improvement was found in two patients treated with anticholinesterase drugs by the author.

Muscle twitch   As would be expected in a dystrophic disorder, the isometric twitch tension is reduced and can be correlated with the amount of weakness apparent on clinical examination and with the numbers of surviving motor units (Figure 16.19). In view of the finding of selective atrophy

TABLE 16.2

Mean Values ($\pm$ S.D.) of Pooled Electrophysiological Data from Control Subjects and 17 Patients with Myotonic Dystrophy studied in detail by McComas, Campbell and Sica, (1971).

	EDB motor units		Isometric twitch			Nerve stimulation	
	No.	Potential amplitude* (μV)	Active tension (g)	Contraction time (ms)	$\frac{1}{2}$ Relaxation time (ms)	Conduction velocity (m/s)	Terminal latency (ms)
Patients	75 ± 47	18.6 ± 2.13	123 ± 89	71 ± 10	82 ± 19	45.1 ± 5.2	3.9 ± 0.8
Controls	199 ± 60	28.9 ± 27.1	313 ± 90	63 ± 7.3	53 ± 9.7	49.0 ± 4.0	4.0 ± 0.6
P	<0.001	<0.001	<0.001	<0.001	<0.001	>0.1	>0.5

* In more recent studies the mean motor unit potential amplitudes of patients with this disorder have been closer to the control values, as shown in Figure 16.22

of type I fibres in some patients (Engel and Brooke, 1966) and the known relationship between fibre type and twitch speed (page 59), it might be thought that the twitch would be abnormally brisk. In fact, such twitches are not seen; most contraction times lie within the normal range but a few are slowed. When the mean values are pooled there is a statistically significant increase in both the contraction and half-relaxation times in myotonic dystrophy (Table 16.2).

Intracellular recordings Microelectrode recordings have been made from single muscle fibres in myotonic dystrophy (Hofmann, Alston and Rowe, 1966; McComas and Mrožek, 1968). In their *in situ* study of two patients McComas and Mrožek found that the resting membrane potentials showed considerable scatter due to the presence of fibres with low potentials; the mean value was significantly reduced (*Figure 16.20*). It is reasonable to presume that the partially depolarized fibres were those with most evidence of degeneration

but this point has yet to be proven with fibre marking techniques. In terms of the factors known to influence the resting membrane potential (page 16), the depolarization could have resulted from an increased sodium permeability of the membrane or from a loss of anions (and potassium) from the interior of the fibre; both factors might be expected to be part of the dystrophic process.

Motor unit estimates McComas, Campbell and Sica (1971) found that in 12 out of 17 patients studied with myotonic dystrophy the numbers of functioning motor units were diminished in the extensor digitorum brevis (EDB) muscles. Although the greatest reductions were found in the weakest patients, abnormal values were sometimes encountered in early cases. An example was an 11-year-old girl who was regarded as 'rather slow' by her father, himself affected; on clinical examination she appeared normal but the presence of myotonic dystrophy was confirmed by a coaxial electrode recording, subsequent to completion of the motor unit studies. In another series of cases, Polgar *et al.* (1972) found reduced EDB motor unit counts in 14 of 17 patients; similar findings have since been reported by Ballantyne and Hansen (1974b) and by Panayiotopoulos and Scarpalezos (1976). In another study McComas, Sica and Upton (1974) were able to show that some patients with myotonic dystrophy had also lost functioning motor units in the thenar and hypothenar muscles, the reduction being greater in the former group (*Figure 16.21*).

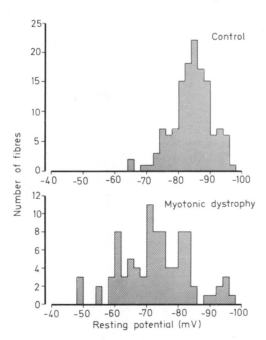

Figure 16.20. Measurements of resting membrane potential made in situ from 94 fibres in proximal muscles of two patients with myotonic dystrophy. Control values shown at top for comparison. Mean values −71.4 ± 10.7 mV (dystrophic) and −83.6 ± 5.8 (control); p = < 0.001. (From McComas and Mrožek (1968) courtesy of the Editor and publishers of Journal of Neurology, Neurosurgery and Psychiatry)

EVIDENCE FOR A NEURAL MECHANISM IN MYOTONIC DYSTROPHY

The case for a neural pathogenesis in myotonic dystrophy is an impressive one and, as with Duchenne dystrophy, it is appropriate to consider the evidence in four categories (see page 153).

Class I observations, comprising direct evidence, are absent.

In contrast there are several *Class II* observations. Regarding morphology, there is MacDermot's (1961) description of *axon degeneration* in intramuscular nerve bundles, and the finding of *collateral reinnervation* as revealed by increased axonal branching (Coërs and Woolf, 1959; Coërs, Telerman-Toppet and Gerard, 1973). There are also the case reports of myotonic dystrophy combined with features of neuropathy (Caccia, Negri and Preto Parvis, 1972; Pilz, Prill and Volles, 1974), peroneal muscular atrophy

(Wald, Loesch and Wochnik, 1962; Kalyanaraman, Smith and Chadha, 1973) and Friedreich's ataxia (Chaco and Taustein, 1969). Electrophysiological evidence of a neuropathic disorder includes the presence of *fibrillation activity* in some muscles although, as in any dystrophy, several interpretations of this abnormality are possible (see motor units (see *Figure 13.3*) the results in myotonic dystrophy are unlike those anticipated in a myopathy.

Class III observations comprise the *bizarre motor end-plates* seen on some of the dystrophic fibres, the *decremental muscles responses* on repetitive nerve stimulation in some patients, and the

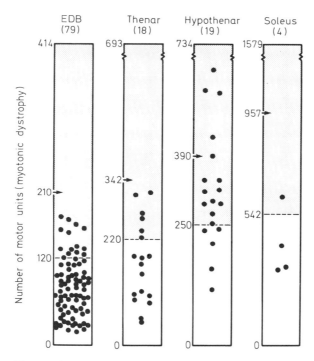

Figure 16.21. Numbers of functioning motor units in the extensor digitorum brevis (EDB), thenar, hypothenar, and soleus muscles of patients with myotonic dystrophy. Numbers of muscles studied given in parentheses at top. Hatched areas indicate control ranges and arrows denote respective control means

page 153). Rather stronger evidence for a neural mechanism comes from the *motor unit counting studies* described in the previous section, which revealed a loss of functioning units. Furthermore, when the results for EDB are pooled, it can be seen that there is no relationship between the numbers of motor units remaining and their sizes, as reflected in the amplitudes of their evoked potentials (*Figure 16.22*). In this type of dystrophy, then, there appears to be selective involvement of motor units, some being completely non-functional and others retaining their full complements of muscle fibres. In terms of the theoretical curves relating numbers and sizes of

occasional finding of *reduced impulse conduction velocities* in motor axons.

Class IV observations include the occurrence of *mental retardation, dementia, EEG abnormalities* (Barwick, Osselton and Walton, 1965) and *cerebral malformation* (Rosman and Kakulas, 1966).

EVIDENCE AGAINST A NEURAL PATHOGENESIS

Most of the counter-arguments which applied to Duchenne dystrophy (see page 155) are also relevant to the myotonic variety and can be met

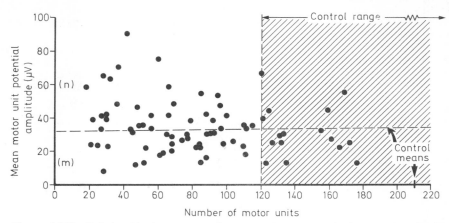

Figure 16.22. Relationship between numbers and sizes of functioning motor units in 79 extensor digitorum brevis (EDB) muscles of patients with myotonic dystrophy. Hatched area indicates lower part of control range for number of units. With reference to Figure 13.3, values above and below the horizontal interrupted line would suggest neuropathy (n) and myopathy (m) respectively

in a similar way. In myotonic dystrophy, however, the presence of so many defects in tissues other than nerve and muscle indicates that the abnormal gene is exerting a pleiotropic effect. If so, it could be reasoned that the nervous system and musculature were also being affected independently. It is difficult to rebut this argument conclusively though the selective involvement of motor units, as determined by the motor unit counting studies, makes it possible that an intrinsic myopathy is not an important factor.

MUSCULAR DYSTROPHY IN ANIMALS

A surprisingly large number of animal species are susceptible to genetically-determined degenerative disease of muscle. The list includes the mouse, Syrian hamster, chicken, Peking duck and the mink. In every instance the disease appears to be transmitted by an autosomal recessive gene but the severity and extent of the disorders vary considerably. In the *hamster,* for example, the disease runs a very slow course and produces little weakness; it is the associated cardiomyopathy which is responsible for death. At the other extreme is the rapid progression characteristic of dystrophy in the *Bar Harbor 129 Re¹ strain of mice.* Sometimes the affected mice can be detected at birth, being small in comparison with their littermates. In other instances diagnosis is possible at 2 weeks; the dystrophic animal then appears slow in moving its hindlegs and, when suspended by its tail, withdraws its hindlegs instead of giving the extension response

characteristic of the normal animal. This last aberration probably results from disordered reflex activity; the animals also exhibit myotonia with both peripheral and central features. The resemblance to human dystrophy is strengthened by the presence of prominent nuclear chains inside some of the muscle fibres (Pearce and Walton, 1963). The disease causes the mice to die prematurely; in the later stages of the disease they propel themselves with their forelimbs and drag their useless hindlegs. In the *chicken* the disease is largely restricted to the pectoral muscles and the birds have difficulty in righting themselves when laid on their backs. At least in the early phase of the disease this difficulty is probably due more to muscle stiffness than to weakness, for these animals also exhibit myotonia (Holliday *et al.,* 1965).

A brief survey of some of the more important investigations in these animal models of dystrophy will now be given; probably because of its convenience to the experimenter the most completely studied animal has been the mouse. At the conclusion of the chapter several remarkable experiments are described in detail; their importance lies in the fact that, for the first time, they yield direct (Class I) evidence concerning the pathogenesis of muscular dystrophy.

Electrophysiological studies

Microelectrode recordings show that the *resting membrane potentials* are often reduced in muscle fibres of dystrophic muscles; this is true both of he mouse) see review by McComas and Mossawy, 1965) and of the hamster (Harris and Ward, 1975). n both species *spontaneous muscle fibre potentials* can be found and in the hamster Harris and Ward have attributed this activity to small muscle fibres. Like the fibrillations recorded in human dystrophy, the activity could conceivably have arisen in fibres which were totally or focally denervated as well as n fibres which had split or were regenerating (see, or example, Harris and Montgomery, 1975). In an attempt to clarify this situation McComas and Mrožek (1967) found that about a quarter of the muscle fibres in dystrophic mice could not be excited through their motor innervation and were therefore *'functionally denervated'*. Law and Atwood (1972, 1974) were able to confirm these results and showed that in some fibres the defect was presynaptic since evoked potentials could not be recorded at the end-plate regions; in other muscle fibres the action potentials appeared unable to propagate fully. In contrast Harris and Marshall 1973) were unable to detect denervation and, in keeping with this result, did not find evidence of any spread of acetylcholine sensitivity; with a different technique, however, an increased sensitivity was found by Marshall, Moore and Wilson 1974) in older animals. Hironaka and Miyata 1975) have also made observations relevant to this problem; by comparing the tensions developed following direct and indirect stimulation of dystrophic muscles, they found results suggestive of the development of functional denervation in older animals. In the mouse *miniature end-plate potentials* have been reported as having diminutions in amplitude (McComas and Mossawy, 1965) and in frequency (Conrad and Glaser, 1964) but no significant alterations are present in the hamster Harris and Ward, 1975). As would be expected in a degenerative disorder, both the maximum isometric twitch and tetanic tensions are reduced in the mouse. When the twitches are compared with the maximum muscle response it appears that there is a loss of functioning motor units, though the results also suggest that the surviving units are much smaller than normal and have probably lost a proportion of their fibres (Harris and Wilson, 1971).

Morphological studies

In the dystrophic Bar Harbor mice Goldspink and Rowe (1968) carried out an exhaustive quantitative study by counting all the *muscle fibres* in the sternomastoid, biceps brachii, soleus, tibialis anterior and extensor digitorium longus muscles in animals of different ages. They were able to show

that, of these muscles, the soleus was affected least rapidly by the dystrophic process. Since the soleus is composed predominantly of type I (SO) fibres, this finding might suggest that these fibres are more resistant to degeneration and so explain the rather slower isometric twitches found in dystrophy. A notable contribution to the morphological study of dystrophic muscle fibres has been made by Isaacs, Bradley and Henderson (1973). These authors examined the ways in which hypertrophied fibres would sometimes split to form daughter fibres. Their technique was to cut transverse sections of muscle 10 μm thick. After each cut the surface of the remaining block of muscle tissue was stained with toluidine blue and photographed through a microscope with a ciné camera. When the developed film was projected in slow motion individual muscle fibres could be followed and seen to divide (*Figure 16.23*).

Ultrastructural studies of the *neuromuscular junction* are of interest for they reveal obvious abnormalities in the motor axon terminals, sometimes on fibres which have yet to show obvious morphological evidence of dystrophy. These presynaptic changes included reductions in the numbers and sizes of synaptic vesicles, increased neurofilamentous material and retraction of the axolemma from the sarcolemma (Gilbert, Steinberg and Banker, 1973; Ragab, 1971). There is disagreement as to whether or not there is a reduction in the *numbers of motor axons* in mouse dystrophy since the abnormal findings of Harris, Wallace and Wing (1972) in the nerve to tibialis anterior were not confirmed by Bradley and Jenkinson (1973). These last authors did observe a most interesting abnormality, however, in that many axons of the ventral and dorsal roots were without *myelin sheaths* and were clumped together; this change was most striking in the region where the oligodendroglia give place to the Schwann cells. In spite of their absent myelin sheaths, the motor axons in the ventral roots remain able to conduct action potentials, albeit with very low velocities (Huizar, Kuno and Miyata, 1975). One would expect that, without myelination, impulses would be conducted in a continuous, rather than a saltatory, manner and this has now been demonstrated (Rasminsky and Kearney, 1976). One important consequence of the loss of myelin insulation is that impulse activity may spread between adjacent fibres ('cross-talk'; see Huizar, Kuno and Miyata, 1975). It is interesting that although the myelin sheath appears normal in distal regions of the peripheral nerves, impulse conduction is still rather slow; it is possible that an abnormality of the axolemma is present (Rasminsky, Bray and Aguayo, 1975).

The abnormal structure of the roots appears to

be a developmental defect of myelination rather than a progressive demyelinating process; this point is emphasized by crushing the roots, after which partially successful attempts at remyelination can be shown to take place (Stirling, 1975). It has not been possible to demonstrate similar amyelination in other dystrophic species or in man.

So far as the *motoneurones* are concerned, the cells in the mouse appear normal on light microscopy and are not reduced in number (Papapetro-poulos and Bradley, 1972); furthermore, they have normal resting and action potentials (Huizar, Kuno and Miyata, 1975).

Axoplasmic transport

Several groups of investigators have described abnormalities of *axoplasmic flow* in motor fibres of dystrophic mice. In the first such study Bradley

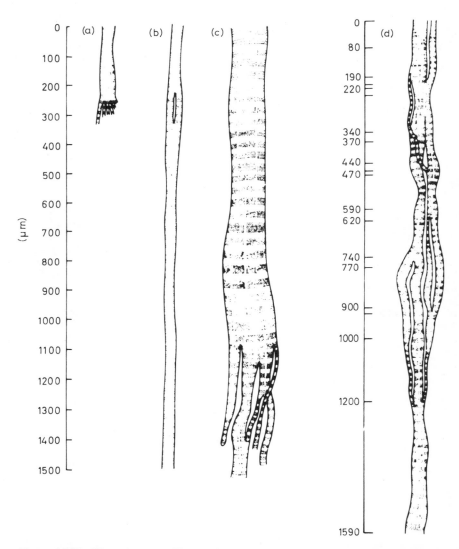

Figure 16.23. Fibres from gracilis muscles of dystrophic mice which have been reconstructed diagrammatically following study of serial transverse sections (see text). (From Isaacs, Bradley and Henderson (1973), courtesy of the authors, and Editor and publishers of Journal of Neurology, Neurosurgery and Psychiatry)

and Jaros (1973) noted that there was a reduction in the amount of material flowing at slower rates and an increase in the amount moving at faster rates. Since then Jablecki and Brimijoin (1974) have reported decreased axoplasmic transport of choline acetyltransferase enzyme and Austin and his associates have found abnormalities in the flow of proteins and lipids (Tang, Komiya and Austin, 1974; Komiya and Austin, 1974).

DIRECT EXPERIMENTAL APPROACHES TO THE PATHOGENESIS OF ANIMAL DYSTROPHY

Several types of experiment will now be described, all of which bear directly on the problem of the pathogenesis of muscular dystrophy and some of which are remarkable both for their originality and for the technical difficulties which had to be surmounted. Yet it will be seen that, far from providing an unequivocal answer regarding pathogenesis, the results and interpretations of the investigations appear to show striking differences. With further thought, however, some of these disagreements can be reconciled; the picture which then emerges is a fascinating one which may well have relevance for the various types of human dystrophy.

Hyperinnervation studies

At McMaster University Law (personal communication) has carried out a series of experiments in mice in which various attempts were made to modify the dystrophic process by altering the quantitative relationship between the muscle fibre and its innervation. The experiments involved the following stratagems (a) leaving the nerve supply intact and diminishing the volume of the muscle fibres by ablations on either side of the endplate zone; (b) increasing the number of endplates on the dystrophic fibres by encouraging hyperinnervation either from the 'original' pool of motoneurones alone or from 'foreign' motoneurones; (c) chronic electrical stimulation of motor axons; and (d) chronic electrical stimulation of muscle fibres. Although any one of these experiments might have been expected to improve the dystrophic process if the disease was a neural disorder, in the event all the results have proved negative.

Parabiosis with cross-innervation

Instead of attempting to maximize any remaining trophic action of the putatively 'dystrophic' motoneurones, an alternative experimental strategy is to observe the effects of introducing a normal innervation to the dystrophic muscles. One way of doing this is to join the adjacent hindlimbs of normal and dystrophic mice and to cross over the sciatic nerves, so that the normal leg is now

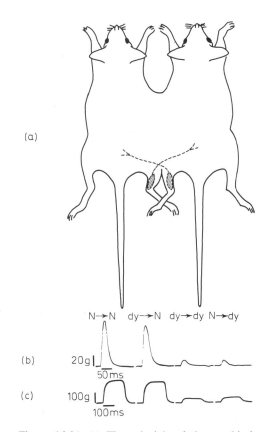

Figure 16.24. (a) The principle of the parabiotic cross-innervation experiment. A normal and a dystrophic mouse, each about 21–25 days old, are joined together by extensive suturing of the skin along the flanks. The sciatic nerves are cut close to the spinal cords and then the central stump in one animal is joined to the distal stump in the other. Either a single or a reciprocal cross (as shown) can be carried out. Alternatively the cross union can be performed distally between branches of the sciatic nerve. (b, c) twitch and tetanic responses of crossreinnervated triceps surae muscles; the arrows indicate direction of cross-innervation in normal (N) and dystrophic (dy) mice. (From Douglas (1975) courtesy of the author, and the Editor and publishers of Experimental Neurology)

innervated by a 'dystrophic' nerve and vice versa. This interesting approach was devised independently by Montgomery (Montgomery, 1975; Johnson and Montgomery, 1975, 1976) and by Douglas (Douglas, 1972, 1975; Douglas and Cosmos, 1975); in addition it has recently been exploited and modified by Law and colleagues (1976). In the hands of all three investigators and their teams, the dystrophic muscles failed to become normal and showed little or no improvement in strength (*Figure 16.24*; but see Appendix 16.5). However, even though the number of active muscle fibres remained depleted in the dystrophic muscles, Law and colleagues have observed that the survivors often appear better than before—they show stronger histochemical reactions and their resting membrane potentials are normal. In addition the muscle twitches are faster, indicating that the fibres are capable of responding to the trophic influence from fast motoneurones. These results might have been construed as providing limited support for the neural hypothesis. Unfortunately for the latter, however, the normal muscles remain in good condition in spite of receiving an innervation from the dystrophic animal.

Tissue culture experiments

The influence of normal nerve on diseased muscle may also be investigated by the technique of tissue culture. This has the advantage that fine nerve twigs can be distinguished following transillumination and inspection under the microscope; individual muscle cells can be recognized during repeated examinations and their unique life-histories established; the times of cell contact and cell fusion can be determined; microelectrode impalements of muscle fibres can be made for the investigation of electrophysiological properties of the membranes; finally, the influence of the composition of the nutrient medium and of various drugs on muscle growth can be examined.

A particularly elegant technique is that practised by Bornstein and colleagues (1968). Mice are killed 10–16 days after impregnation and the embryos taken out and dissected under sterile conditions. After the head and ventral tissues have been removed the dorsal region of the trunk is cut into a number of cross-sections of 0.5 mm thickness. Each slice will contain spinal cord, dorsal root ganglia, a developing vertebra with adjacent masses of myoblasts, subcutaneous tissue and skin. A slice is then placed on a coverslip coated with collagen and a single drop of nutrient medium added; the coverslip is then sealed into a Maximow slide

assembly and incubated in the 'lying-drop' position at 34–35 °C; the nutrient medium is changed twice a week.

Under the microscope a radial outgrowth of cell can be seen to form from the paravertebral muscle masses within the first day; some of these cells will be *myoblasts* and others *fibroblasts*. Similarly nerve cell processes (*neurites*) grow from the dorsal root ganglia and spinal cord. By the end of the first week many of the primitive muscle cells (*myoblasts*) have fused to form *myotubes*. Within the nervous tissue the cell bodies of the neurones can be distinguished and motor axons grow outward towards the muscle mass where they establish neuromuscular junction with the myotubes and muscle fibres. When tissue from normal animals is used some of the muscle fibres appear to become innervated by several motor axons.

All workers who have studied dystrophic muscle in culture agree that the initial outgrowth is at least as vigorous as that from a normal explant and may even be enhanced (Paul and Powell, 1974). Beyond this point, however, there is disagreement. On the one hand Paul and Powell (1974) claim that unlike normal mouse muscle in culture, the majority of dystrophic myotubes remain flat and unstriated with no spontaneous contractions irrespective of whether they are coupled to normal or 'dystrophic' spinal cord. On the other hand Hamburgh and associates (1973) achieved much better maturation of dystrophic fibres and were able to demonstrate that successful innervation could be achieved by normal or 'dystrophic' cords. Similar results to these, but obtained in the chicken, have been reported by Peacock and Nelson (1973). The only investigators who claim that a 'dystrophic' cord is incapable of supporting the proper development of normal muscle are Gallup and Dubowitz (1973). Thus the majority viewpoint is that, within the rather limited confines of muscle growth which are permissible in culture there is no convincing evidence that the 'dystrophic' spinal cord is defective.

Transplantation experiments

Several types of transplantation experiment have been devised of which the most simple is the transfer of muscle between normal and dystrophic animals. More complex experiments have involved the transfer of a limb-bud or of the developing neural tube. In a sense, the embryo fusion study of Peterson (see below) may also be considered as a transplant.

Muscle transplantation studies

Dr A. N. Studitsky, a Russian neurobiologist, was the first to develop a technique for successfully transplanting muscles (see Studitsky, 1952). The muscle was denervated *in situ* beforehand, excised and cut into small pieces about 1 mm^3 in size; the 'mince' was then placed into the bed left by the excised muscle of the same, or a different, animal. At first the sarcoplasm of the mince degenerated but the surviving myonuclei were able to form myoblasts which subsequently fused to become myotubes and eventually mature fibres. At the end of the first week nerve fibres began to enter the graft and, by the end of 3 weeks, the transplanted muscle ('regenerate') responded to nerve stimulation (see also Chapter 11 and *Figure 11.5*).

The technique was first applied to mouse dystrophy by Laird and Timmer (1965) who found that the regenerated muscle retained its original properties, normal or dystrophic. Salafsky (1971) repeated this work, using the tibialis anterior muscle, and measured the contractile properties of the regenerates. In contrast to Laird and Timmer, he found that the dystrophic regenerates in normal hosts fared much better than grafts of normal muscle in dystrophic hosts, most of which were inexcitable to nerve stimulation. Results rather similar to these have been reported for the hamster (Jasmin and Bokdawala, 1970; Neerunjun and Dubowitz, 1974a, b). In a variant of this experiment, Hironaka and Miyata (1973) transplanted whole muscles rather than minces and also found that the dystrophic muscles were considerably improved by being placed in a normal environment. Against these results must be set the findings of Cosmos (1973) and Cosmos and Butler (1972) who were unable to detect any improvement in dystrophic muscle minces transplanted into normal hosts whereas normal minces survived reasonably well in dystrophic environments; their experiments were conducted on chickens as well as on mice. It is interesting, nevertheless, that in the mouse some of the transplanted dystrophic muscles developed considerable hyperplasia of fatty connective tissue so that their weights matched those of normal grafts (Cosmos, 1973).

One hazard in this type of experiment is that some of the myoblasts in the regenerate may have migrated from neighbouring muscles of the host. In rodents it is not possible to differentiate between donor and host tissue using a nuclear sexing technique but experiments in which donor myonuclei were labelled with [^{3}H]-thymidine appear to confirm that the new muscle is formed from the transplant (Neerunjun and Dubowitz, 1975).

Limb-bud transplantation

It is possible to remove a limb-bud in a chicken embryo and to replace it with one taken from another embryo. Linkhart, Yee and Wilson (1975) have performed this type of transplantation between normal and dystrophic embryos at 3½ days of incubation, at which time the embryos were in stages 19 or 20 of development. The authors stressed that, at these stages, the motor nerve axons had yet to reach the primordial limb tissue; later the muscles of the transplanted wings became innervated by the motoneurones of the host and subjected to the 'host's systemic regulation'. The biceps muscles of the chickens were studied at 5–14 weeks after hatching and examined for acetylcholinesterase and for fibre diameter. Muscles of adult dystrophic birds normally differ in that the fibres are hypertrophied and have high levels of anticholinesterase, the isoenzyme pattern being characteristic of the embryo. Linkhart, Yee and Wilson (1975) found that these dystrophic features persisted in limb-buds transplanted from dystrophic to normal animals. They therefore concluded that dystrophy in the chicken was due to a defect in neurally-mediated muscle maturation.

Neural tube transplantation

A transplantation experiment at an even earlier stage has been devised and carried out on dystrophic chickens by Rathbone, Dimond and Vetrano (1975). Their technique has been to remove the region of neural tube destined to innervate the pectoral muscles and to replace it with neural tube from another animal (Le Douarin, 1973). The operation can be carried out at about 2 days of incubation; before this time no differentiation of muscle tissue from mesoderm has taken place and, of course, there has been no innervation either. Although the transplanted segment of neural tube establishes anatomical and functional continuity with the remainder of the central nervous system, the viability of the animal is affected inasmuch as it cannot usually proceed through hatching. For this reason Rathbone and his colleagues were dependent on a sensitive biochemical test capable of detecting the presence of dystrophy in late embryonic life. The test chosen was the estimation of thymidine kinase activity; the level of activity remains considerably higher in the dystrophic embryo than in the normal one (Weinstock and Dju, 1971). Rathbone and colleagues found that higher levels also occurred in the pectoral muscles of a normal embryo which had

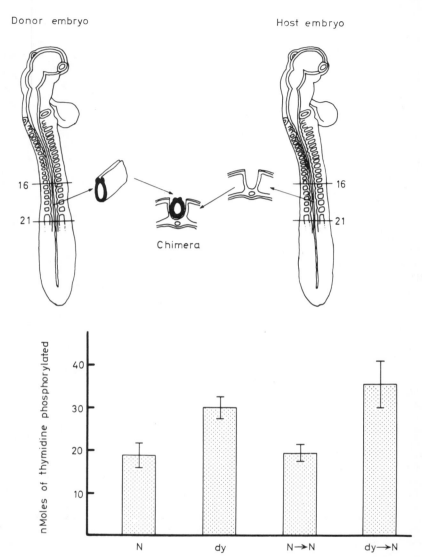

Figure 16.25. (Upper) Procedure used for transplanting neural tubes. The donor embryo was taken from its egg and the spinal cord between somites 16–21 was removed. The host embryo was exposed by drilling a small window in the egg shell, the vitelline membrane above the brachial region was removed and the spinal cord was cut out with a fine steel knife. The donor cord was then inserted into the resulting gap; the egg was sealed with sterile Parafilm and incubated for a further 16 days. (Lower) Thymidine kinase activity of experimental and control pectoral muscles of 18-day-old chicken embryos. N, muscle from unoperated normal embryos; dy, muscle from unoperated dystrophic embryos; N→N, normal muscles innervated by transplanted normal neural tubes; dy→N, normal muscles innervated by transplanted neural tubes from dystrophic embryos. Bars indicate standard errors of means. Note that the normal embryos with transplanted neural tubes from dystrophic embryos (dy→N) develop enzymatic features characteristic of dystrophic muscle (dy). Reproduced from Rathbone, Dimond and Vetrano (1975) courtesy of the authors, and the Editor and publishers of Science, New York)

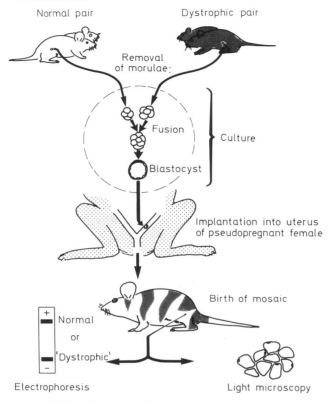

Figure 16.26. The stages in the preparation of a normal-dystrophic mouse chimaera (see text)

received a 'dystrophic' neural tube, whereas this was not found when the transplant had come from another normal animal instead. This experiment, in contrast to the limb-bud transplantations described above, suggests that dystrophy may have a neural aetiology after all (see *Figure 16.25*).

Mouse chimaera study

If dystrophy was indeed a primary myopathy, then a defective gene in the myonuclei must have been expressed; that is, there would be a direct correlation between the *genotype* of the muscle and the presence of dystrophic characteristics (*phenotype*) in that muscle. With the chimaera technique Peterson (1974) was able to test this point in an extremely elegant way. The technique involved fusing together two mouse embryos of which one was dystrophic and the other was normal and of a different strain. The embryos were removed at the 8-cell (morula) stage, prior to their implantation in the uterus, and were then cultured

together for 24 hr; during this time fusion of the embryos took place. The mosaic morula was then transferred to the uterus of a pseudopregnant female and completed its development (*Figure 16.26*). Examination of such a mouse after birth showed that it was indeed a genetic mosaic since its fur had a colour which was intermediate between those of the two strains of mice used in the experiment. The amount of mixing of the genotypes in any tissue could be determined accurately by making use of any differences in isoenzymes between the two strains; in Peterson's experiments malic enzyme was used. It was found that there was no correlation between the genetic origin of the muscles and the presence or absence of dystrophic features. For example, one muscle had an 83 per cent dystrophic genotype and the only detectable abnormality was the occasional central nucleus in the muscle fibres. At the other extreme was a muscle showing the greatest pathological involvement but having no detectable dystrophic genotype. It could be argued that the absence of pathology in a fibre with mainly 'dystrophic' nuclei might be due to a strong beneficial effect of a small number of 'normal' nuclei, but this would hardly account for the degeneration seen in genetically normal muscle. It is obvious that these fascinating results are difficult to explain in terms of a primary myopathic origin for dystrophy, and it would appear that an extramuscular influence, possibly the nervous system, must be responsible for the disease. It is also evident that the chimaera preparation has relevance for understanding the genetic background of muscles in female carriers of the Duchenne dystrophy gene. According to the Lyon hypothesis (page 146) random inactivation of one or other X-chromosome will take place in each

nucleus throughout the body; one would therefore expect that individual muscle fibres would contain mixtures of 'normal' and 'dystrophic' nuclei just as in the mouse chimaeras. In fact, most female carriers show no clinical evidence of dystrophy and special laboratory investigations are required for their detection (page 146). It is interesting that the mouse chimaeras also show no evidence of weakness, even though muscle fibre abnormalities may be demonstrated by microscopy. Therefore in both the female carrier and in the mouse chimaera any effects of the dystrophic genotype seem to be largely suppressed.

CONCLUSIONS

As previously stated, one of the most surprising aspects of these experiments is that, in spite of their direct nature, the results should prove so apparently contradictory. In terms of supporting either a primary muscular or neural origin for dystrophy, the results may be summarized as follows:

Experiment	Indicated origin of dystrophy
Hyperinnervation	Muscle
Parabiosis with X-innervation	Muscle
Tissue culture	Probably muscle
Transplant { Muscle	Muscle or nerve
Limb-bud	Muscle
Neural tube	Nerve
Mouse chimaera	Not muscle

If all the experimental results are to be believed then only one conclusion is possible—dystrophy is indeed initiated by the nervous system but the 'imprinting' occurs very early in development. Once made, the imprint is then permanent, resisting attempts at modification through manipulation of the innervation. The only exceptions were some of the muscle transplantation experiments in which de-differentiation may have restored the susceptibility of the muscle to a neural influence. How is this 'imprinting' achieved? Rathbone, Dimond and Vetrano (1975) suggest that the neural tube induces dystrophy in the muscles and that this

induction is independent of innervation. It is already established that, during development, the neural tube is responsible for inducing differentiation of the mesonephric tubules and the vertebral column; in neither case is innervation involved, the action being mediated instead by inducing-substances released from the neural tube. Rathbone and colleagues point out that in the chick this inductive activity of the neural tube is expressed between 2 and 4 days *in ovo*; this period is after the time at which the neural tube transplants are performed but is before the formation of limb-buds. Hence in the limb-bud transplantation and later experiments dystrophy will behave as a myopathy.

If this interpretation is correct then the truth lies somewhere between the rival myopathic and neural hypotheses of dystrophy. The 'sick motoneurone' hypothesis would be at fault in postulating that dystrophy resulted from an impaired trophic action of the motoneurone on the muscle fibre. In view of the ability of 'dystrophic' nerve to maintain a 'normal' muscle in the parabiotic experiments, this postulate is false, at least in the mouse. If the results are applicable to the human dystrophies, one would have to add that the motoneurone dysfunction (indicated by the motor unit counting and other studies) is the sequel to a genetically-determined abnormality of the neural tube which had induced dystrophy early in fetal development.

Chapter 17

POLYMYOSITIS, MALIGNANT HYPERTHERMIA AND OTHER MYOPATHIES

POLYMYOSITIS

Polymyositis is a non-suppurative inflammatory disorder affecting various muscles of the body; it is thought to arise from dysfunction of the autoimmune system and belongs to the 'collagen vascular' group of diseases. Historically, the first instance of this condition was reported by Wagner in 1863 and the related disorder, dermatomyositis, was described somewhat later, by Unverricht in 1887. Although the disease can arise at any age, the most frequent onset is between 30 and 60; it is twice as common in females as in males. About five new cases per million persons may be anticipated in one year.

Clinical features

The cardinal symptom is a weakness which affects proximal muscles of the limbs more severely than distal ones. Weakness of shoulder muscles causes difficulty in combing the hair or in placing objects on shelves. In the legs the weakness of hip movement is revealed by awkwardness in climbing stairs, rising from a chair and getting out of the bath. Neck muscles are also usually affected and the patient may have difficulty in lifting the head from a flexed position or in raising it up from a pillow. Weakness of bulbar muscles produces difficulty in swallowing (dysphagia) and in phonation (dysphonia), the latter causing the patient to speak with a nasal voice. In a severe case the patient may be doomed to a wheelchair existence or else bedridden; death may supervene from paralysis of respiratory muscles. In other cases the course of the disease varies widely, some patients presenting with an insidious but progressive weakness, others showing spontaneous fluctuations in intensity, and a few exhibiting a brief but rapidly advancing illness (see Pearson and Curvie, 1974).

Associated with the weakness of the muscles may be pain, especially in the arms; the affected muscles may be tender on palpation and feel hardened. Muscle atrophy is usually mild or moderate and appears late. Associated with the muscle abnormalities may be a constitutional disturbance, the patient feeling generally unwell, tiring easily and having a loss of appetite; a fever may also be present. Other tissues may also be affected; of these the skin is the most important, being involved in rather more than half of the cases. In about 40 per cent of patients with polymyositis the skin shows a characteristic dusky-red rash which is distributed across the nose and cheeks ('butterfly' pattern) and may also be found on the forehead, neck, upper chest and arms; in florid cases the subcutaneous tissues are oedematous. Patients with this type of rash are diagnosed as having *dermatomyositis*. Other cutaneous manifestations of this condition include a lilac-coloured suffusion of the upper eyelids (heliotrope rash), hyperaemia

179

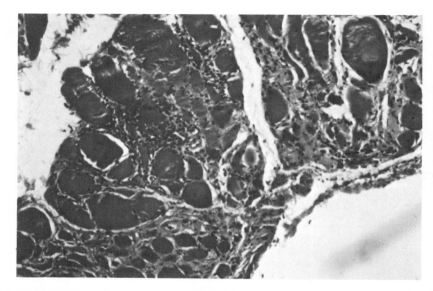

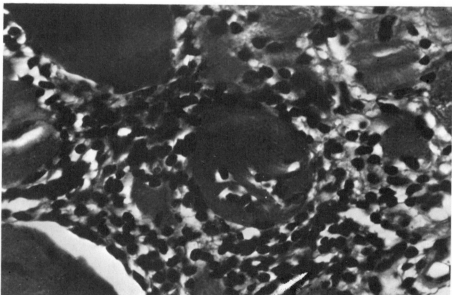

Figure 17.1. Transverse section from a brachial biceps muscle biopsy, obtained from a 64-year-old man with active polymyositis; haematoxylin and eosin staining. At top, with low magnification (×120) can be seen the marked infiltration of the tissue with mononuclear cells; the muscle fibres are of variable size and shape and there is an increase in connective tissue. At bottom, with higher magnification (×480) is shown one of the muscle fibres which has been invaded by mononuclear cells and is probably about to undergo destruction. (Courtesy of Dr J. Groves)

at the bases and sides of the fingernails, and reddened streaks over the backs of the hands and fingers.

Some patients with polymyositis demonstrate other abnormalities; thus, about one-third exhibit *Raynaud's phenomenon*, a transient blanching or cyanosis of the fingers on cooling. A similar proportion of patients have evidence of arthritis, which in some cases appears indistinguishable from *rheumatoid arthritis*. *Scleroderma*, a progressive atrophic condition of the skin and another example of a collagen disorder, may also occur in combination with polymyositis.

Finally, a most important association exists between polymyositis and malignant disease; there is a greater than 50 per cent chance of a neoplasm being present in a male over the age of 40 presenting with dermatomyositis (Arundell, Wilkinson and Haserick, 1960). The tumour is usually a carcinoma originating in the lung, breast, large bowel, prostrate, uterus or ovary.

Special investigations

The erythrocyte sedimentation rate is increased in about half of cases, particularly those in whom the disease is running an acute course accompanied by constitutional upset; it provides a useful indication of the response of the condition to treatment. There may also be rises in the α_2- and γ-globulins and the tests for circulating rheumatoid factor may be positive. The serum creatine phosphokinase (CPK) level is an especially useful test which, like the sedimentation rate, reflects the severity of the disorder; high values are probably related to muscle fibre breakdown and the consequent escape of enzyme into the bloodstream. Muscle biopsy and electrophysiological investigations are considered below.

Treatment and prognosis

Most patients with polymyositis respond to corticosteroids; usually *prednisone* is given, commencing with 60 mg daily in divided doses. When clinical improvement takes place, accompanied by a fall in serum CPK, the dose of prednisone can be reduced gradually. Usually a daily maintenance level of 5–20 mg prednisone will be required for any attempt to reduce the dosage further will result in a relapse; it follows that most patients will need to be treated with prednisone indefinitely. Other immunosuppressive drugs such as cyclosphosphamide and amethopterin have also been tried

but are no more effective than corticosteroids and produce more side-effects.

With treatment about two-thirds of patients recover, the remainder either showing no improvement or else dying; for obvious reasons the prognosis is most serious in the group of patients with an underlying malignancy.

Morphological studies

Light microscopy

Occasionally a specimen of muscle removed at biopsy appears normal on histological examination, despite clinical features and haemotological results strongly suggestive of polymyositis. Such negative findings reflect variations in the incidence and severity of the disease process, not only among different muscles but often between different parts of the same muscle. A myositic region of the muscle may readily be recognized by the presence of *inflammatory cells* which pervade the tissue and tend to form clusters around small blood vessels and degenerating muscle fibres; the cells are mostly lymphocytes. All stages of muscle fibre *degeneration* may be present, ranging from increased eosinophilia, with loss of cross-striations, to complete destruction. Attempts at muscle fibre *regeneration* are usually evident, the new fibres arising either from surviving *myonuclei,* left from the degenerating fibres, or from healthy regions of fibres adjacent to necrotic zones. In specimens of muscle stained with haematoxylin and eosin the regenerating fibres can be recognized by their bluish colour, this being due to the increased amounts of RNA in their cytoplasm (*Figure 17.1*). The simultaneous presence of fibres which are either degenerating, undergoing compensatory hypertrophy or else are in various stages of regeneration, is responsible for the marked variation in fibre diameter which is seen in transverse sections of muscle. In long-standing cases of polymyositis the muscle fibres become separated from each other by increased amounts of connective tissue.

Electronmicroscopy

The high magnification of the electronmicroscope has permitted the above changes to be studied in detail. Within degenerating muscle fibres can be seen autophagic vacuoles and myofibrils undergoing dissolution; the presence of satellite cells signifies that regeneration is already being attempted. The intramuscular capillaries also appear abnormal, both the endothelial cells and the basement-membranes being considerably thickened. One of the most interesting findings is the recent discovery of particles in the sarcoplasm and myonuclei which resemble viruses (Chou, 1967; Chou and Gutmann, 1970).

Electrophysiological studies

Coaxial electrode recordings in an acute case of polymyositis reveal a characteristic combination of discharges as the electrode is introduced into the muscle belly (*insertion activity*) and there may also be short runs of high frequency potentials which start and stop abruptly (*pseudomyotonic discharges*). During volitional contractions the motor unit potentials appear abnormally brief, small and are often complex; on maximum effort they merge into a full interference pattern. These last findings are usually considered to indicate a 'myopathic' type of process, although similar changes can be found at certain stages in a neuropathic disorder

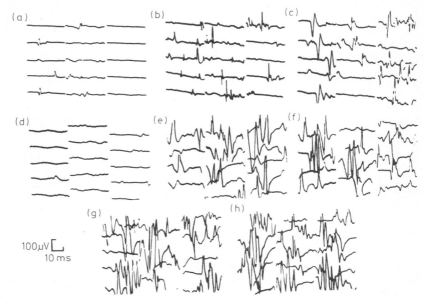

Figure 17.2. Serial EMG recordings from the pectoralis major muscle of a 55-year-old man with polymyositis. Recordings were made with a coaxial electrode during the acute phase (a–c), after 3 years of steroid treatment (d–f), and after a further 2 years (g–h). Note the fibrillations at rest in a, but not in d. During weak effort small brief ('myopathic') potentials are prevalent in b and c while large, prolonged, complex ('neuropathic') potentials predominate in e–h. (Retouched from Mechler (1974) courtesy of the author, and Editor and publishers of Journal of the Neurological Sciences)

spontaneous muscle fibre activity and 'myopathic' motor unit potentials during voluntary contraction. The spontaneous activity consists of *fibrillation potentials and positive sharp waves*, such as are found in denervation (page 75). It is possible that these discharges arise from muscle fibres in which denervation has resulted from destruction of intramuscular motor axons by the inflammatory process. In theory, 'denervation-type' activity could also be generated by segments of a fibre which had become functionally separated from the end-plate region by a necrotic zone; regenerating fibres would also be expected to discharge spontaneously until they had acquired an innervation. In acute polymyositis it is also usual to record an increase in muscle fibre

also (see Fig. 22.5). In relation to this last possibility, the findings of Mechler (1974) in polymyositis are most interesting. This author was able to perform serial EMG examinations on 10 patients, the longest period of observation being 6 years. He observed that in the earliest stages of the disease the EMG findings were as described above, that is, compatible with a 'myopathy'. In time, however, the EMG picture changed to one characteristic of a chronic neuropathic disorder; the density of the interference pattern decreased and individual motor unit potentials became prolonged and complex (*Figure 17.2*). Mechler has given possible reasons for his findings; they include denervation due to involvement of intramuscular motor axons by the inflammatory process, increased extracellular current density caused by an insulating effect of the additional connective tissue around the fibres, and, finally, the transition of motoroneurones from a dysfunctional (sick) state into a non-functional (dead) one (see also page 281).

Motor unit counting studies in polymyositis have not been reported previously but are in keeping with Mechler's results, discussed above. Thus in two patients with acute dermatomyositis there were slight-to-moderate reductions in the populations of functioning motor units in distal muscles of the limbs. Since the evoked potentials of surviving motor units were unusually small, however, the pattern would have been compatible with either a primary myopathy or a dysfunctional neuronal process (see page 112). In patients with long-standing polymyositis the motor unit values are either normal or else show evidence of a chronic neuropathic lesion, that is, there are reduced numbers of units and the survivors generate large potentials.

To summarize the electrophysiological findings, it does seem that a neuropathic process is present in polymyositis; whether this reflects an inflammatory process of the motor axons or whether there is neuronal dysfunction associated with the myopathic disorder remains uncertain.

Aetiology and pathogenesis of polymyositis

The possibility that polymyositis might be an autoimmune disorder is immediately suggested by its association with other diseases considered to have an immunological basis—systemic lupus erythematosus, rheumatoid arthritis, Sjögren's syndrome, and scleroderma. Further pointers in this direction are the infiltrations of lymphocytes which can be seen in specimens of muscle and the fact that polymyositis usually responds to immunosuppressive therapy (see above). Additional evidence suggestive of an immunological disturbance has come from various sources. For example, it is possible to produce a generalized inflammatory myopathy in animals by injecting them repeatedly with muscle prepared from another species, either alone or with Freund's adjuvant (Dawkins, 1965). The pathological features of this myopathy include the presence of scattered muscle fibres showing segmental necrosis and prominent phagocytosis, inflammatory cells in the interstitial spaces and, in chronic cases, moderate atrophy. At about the same time that the myopathic changes appear, that is, 1–2 weeks after the first injection, skin testing shows that the host animal has become sensitized to muscle antigen from the donor. In an extension of

this work, both Kakulas (1966) and Currie (1971) took cells from lymph nodes of affected animals and showed that they attacked 'normal' skeletal muscle fibres in tissue culture. Of greater relevance to the human form of the disease was the related demonstration by Currie and colleagues (1971) that lymphocytes from patients with polymyositis were cytotoxic to cultured muscle fibres. Both *in vivo* and *in vitro*, the lymphoid cells were seen to invade otherwise intact muscle fibres, suggesting that some of the provocative antigens were located internally rather than on the surface of the fibre. As Pearson and Currie (1974) point out 'none of this work has shown whether the lymphoid cells are inherently abnormal, being provoked into action by an external precipitant, or whether such a precipitant has led normal cells to acquire and manifest a potential for cytotoxicity.'

If the disease is indeed autoimmune in origin, what triggers off the initial disturbance? In the case of dermatomyositis, there are reports that some cases have followed treatment with sulphonamides or penicillin (Sheard, 1951) while others have followed an exanthematous illness (Selander, 1950). The possibility that a virus might precipitate polymyositis would not be altogether surprising for it is known that certain ones may induce myositis in lower animals (Rustigian and Pappenheimer, 1949). In man Coxsackie A_2 virus has been isolated from a patient with dermatomyositis and Coxsackie B virus is responsible for the myositic features of Bornholm disease (epidemic myalgia). There is even indirect evidence that the common influenza viruses can produce a myositic illness since a proportion of patients with influenza complain of pain and tenderness in their muscles and exhibit quite marked rises in serum CPK levels (Middleton, Alexander and Szymanski, 1970). The case for a viral aetiology in some patients with polymyositis has been strengthened by the occasional finding of viral-like particles of the myxovirus and picornavirus types in specimens of muscle removed at biopsy and studied with the electronmicroscope (Chou, 1967; Chou and Gutmann, 1970); the picornaviruses include the Coxsackie types. However, the mere demonstration of viral particles does not necessarily indicate an aetiological role for them in polymyositis since Caulfield, Rebeiz and Adams (1968) have observed them in otherwise normal extraocular muscles removed *post mortem*. In considering precipitating factors, it should also be recalled that in some patients polymyositis or dermatomyositis arises as a complication of malignant disease. The presence of tumour appears to render the lymphoid system no longer tolerant of muscle, possibly because a product of the tumour combines with a muscle protein to form an allergen;

alternatively a tumour product may cause cross-sensitization to a component of muscle (Pearson and Currie, 1974).

MALIGNANT HYPERTHERMIA
(Malignant Hyperpyrexia)

Introduction

For the myologist, the condition known as malignant hyperthermia (hyperpyrexia) exerts a fascination which is understandable for several reasons—the disease has only been recognized relatively recently, the clinical features of a pyrexial episode are dramatic and, if not promptly treated, rapidly culminate in death and, finally, the biochemical basis of the disorder is at least partly understood.

It is now agreed that the first description of the syndrome was made by Guedel who, in a monograph on *Inhalational Anaesthesia* published in 1937, reported six affected patients. All of these patients had been anaesthetized with ether and had developed hyperthermia before succumbing. In spite of this clear reference, general awareness of the syndrome was delayed until the contribution of Denborough and Lovell in 1960. These authors, working in Melbourne, Australia, noted a family in which 10 members had died following general anaesthesia; in two of these the temperature had been measured and found to be extremely high (42°C and 43°C respectively). Once attention had been drawn to the condition, it was apparent that similar fatalities had previously been encountered elsewhere and recorded as unexplained anaesthetic deaths. Once such case-history, dating back to 1948, has been recalled by Dr J. F. Riccards of the South Staffordshire Medical Centre and is cited by Isaacs and Barlow (1973).

The anaesthetic was given to a 10-year-old male and the operation was for the suture of a left olecranon process. Premedication was with atropine 0.01 g and Nembutal 0.7 g. Anaesthesia was maintained with gas, oxygen and ether after induction with trilene administered through a semi-closed Boyle circuit. Death occurred one hour and 45 minutes after commencing the anaesthetic and the nature of the symptoms preceding death are recorded as follows:
Induction complicated by slight amount of mucus in respiratory tract. Tensed jaws and pursed lips. Maintenance on 50 per cent gas and oxygen with 5 per cent ether, total flow 6 litres. Esmarch on limb, and face covered with towels. Maintenance difficult owing to mucus in trachea. Anaesthesia had proceeded for about 10 minutes when face was uncovered to display a moderate degree of cyanosis despite hyperpnoea and rich oxygen intake. Cyanosis cleared on full oxygen but returned when gas was added to the mixture. General rigidity was com-

mencing at this stage, with legs and arms in slight flexion and eyeballs deviated upwards and to the right. The operation was hurriedly concluded and 100 per cent oxygen continued. The colour was now flushed and pink but rigidity was increasing. The patient felt hot, the rectal temperature of 108° mounted to over 110° within a few minutes. Over the course of the next hour respiratory function was well maintained but cardiac action became embarrassed with slowing and softening of the pulse. Colour remained pink until 10 minutes before death. Respiratory function failed quickly and suddenly about five minutes before death.

Clinical features

Many of the clinical features of malignant hyperthermia are apparent from the preceding introduction. As already stated, the disease is hereditary, being transmitted by an autosomal dominant gene. The incidence of the condition is difficult to determine, although its increasing recognition suggests that present estimates are too low. Britt and Kalow (1970) have reported five cases of hyperthermia in a total of 71,500 anaesthetics delivered at the Hospital for Sick Children in Toronto over a six-year-period. Since the temperature was monitored routinely on all patients it is unlikely that any instance of hyperthermia was missed; the corresponding crude estimate of incidence would be 1 in 14 000. Since not all patients manifest their hyperthermia trait on their first exposure to a precipitating anaesthetic agent, the true incidence of the condition will be somewhat higher than the value given.

In addition to the tendency to hyperthermia, the patients may show clinical evidence of other muscular anomalies. For example, some patients have unusually bulky muscles or may complain of cramps; in others there may be ptosis, strabismus and various types of hernia. Skeletal abnormalities may also be present including spontaneous dislocations of the hip and patella, a high-arched palate, idiopathic kyphoscoliosis and club foot (Britt and Kalow, 1970).

As already noted, an episode of hyperthermia may be precipitated during anaesthesia; the most common triggering agents are halothane and succinylcholine, the former being an anaesthetic and the latter a depolarizing type of neuromuscular blocking agent (see Fig. 19.4). Other anaesthetics which have been incriminated include diethyl ether, ethyl chloride, methoxyflurane, trichlorethylene, ethylene and cyclopropane. Non-depolarizing muscle relaxants such as *d*-tubocurarine and gallamine may also induce hyperthermia (Relton, 1973). Fatal hyperthermia has also been known to ensue during an attack of influenza.

The most obvious clinical features during an episode of hyperthermia are the muscle rigidity and the rapidly mounting body temperature, the latter usually being accompanied by flushing and sweating of the skin. Initially there is a tachycardia but subsequently the heart rate may slow and become irregular due to the development of arrhythmias; the blood pressure falls and the patient may pass into cardiac failure. The respiratory rate is also increased. In advanced cases the patient is comatose with widely dilated pupils; bilateral Babinski responses may be present. If the hyperthermia is successfully treated the patient will usually notice a smoky red discoloration of his urine during the next 48 hr; this sign indicates the presence of myoglobin, the substance having been released into the circulation from disintegrating muscle fibres. Renal failure may develop in severely-affected patients.

Recently another form of the disease has been recognized in which the mounting body temperature during anaesthesia is unaccompanied by muscular rigidity. Possibly because the diagnosis is delayed the outcome of a hyperthermic episode is equally as hazardous as one in a patient with the rigid type of disease.

Biochemical studies during hyperthermia

Striking biochemical abnormalities can be detected in specimens of blood withdrawn during an attack of hyperthermia. Despite administration of oxygen-rich gas mixtures, the arterial oxygen tension is reduced and that of carbon dioxide elevated. In addition, the destruction of the muscle fibres allows large amounts of potassium to flood the bloodstream; the plasma level of magnesium is also elevated. A metabolic acidosis, with fall in blood pH, is produced by increased concentrations of lactic and pyruvic acids. The damage to the muscle fibre membranes is also signalled by extremely high values of such muscle enzymes as creatine phosphokinase (CPK), aldolase, lactic dehydrogenase and glutamic oxaloacetic transaminase.

Treatment of an acute attack

As in all medicine, the best treatment is prevention and a discussion of the methods available for detecting cases preoperatively is given in the following section (see Britt, 1971, 1974). If an acute episode should develop during anaesthesia a number of actions should be instituted promptly. The inhalational anaesthetics and muscle relaxants must be stopped and major measures undertaken to bring the body temperature down; these include the use of ice-water baths and cold intravenous solutions together with gastric, rectal and wound cooling. Procaineamide and procaine are valuable drugs; one of these should be administered intravenously at a rate of about 0.5–1 mg/kg per minute until the heart rate is controlled. The drug *dantrolene sodium* may prove to be even better; in normal muscle it appears to act on the sarcoplasmic reticulum and prevent calcium activation of the myofilaments from taking place (see page 42). The metabolic acidosis may be controlled with intravenous sodium bicarbonate.

Detection of the malignant hyperthermia trait

In a family known to be at risk for hyperthermia, suspicion that a member carries the trait will be aroused by the presence of any of the musculoskeletal anomalies described above. In addition certain special investigations are of real value, the most definitive being the study of *muscle contracture in vitro*. For this test a specimen of muscle is removed from the patient and, as quickly as possible, a strip some 2 cm long and 3 mm thick is immersed in a physiological bathing solution and connected to a strain gauge. The isometric contractures of the muscle are recorded in response to different doses of caffeine (see page 42) in the presence of halothane. Abnormally large contractures to caffeine alone or to caffeine plus halothane indicate that the suspect carries the trait (Kalow, et al., 1970; Britt et al., 1973; *Figure 17.3*). Unfortunately even such a direct test is not completely reliable for in a minority of patients (about 20 per cent) there is susceptibility to hyperthermia but not to muscular rigidity and the test is therefore negative.

A convenient, though not infallible, test is the *serum creatine phosphokinase* level for in more than half of known cases the value is raised. In order to avoid falsely positive results the test must be conducted in as rigorous a manner as possible.

Another approach is to study the *morphology* of muscle fibres obtained by biopsy. Various abnormalities have been described including wide variations in fibre diameter, the presence of target and targetoid fibres and 'streaming' of the Z-line (Britt *et al.*, 1973). In contrast, and perhaps rather surprisingly in the light of the likely pathogenesis of the disorder (see below), the mitochondria, transverse tubular system and sarcoplasmic reticulum appear normal. In a minority of patients there is evidence of neuropathy for 'fibrotic' intramuscular nerves have been reported (Britt *et al.*, 1973) as have degenerated motor axons and collateral

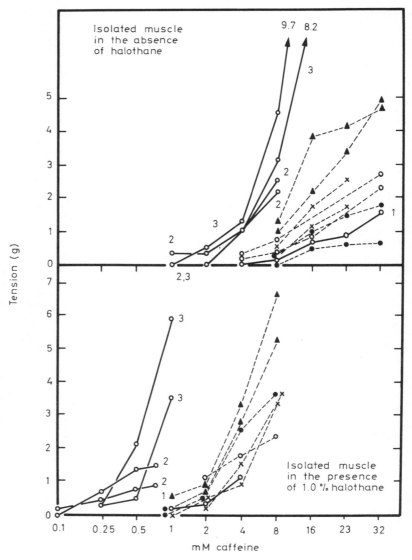

Figure 17.3. Caffeine contractures of various isolated limb muscle specimens taken from volunteers disposed to malignant hyperthermia (full curves) and from controls (interrupted curves). Numbers indicate three different patients of which no. 1 did not display rigidity in association with hyperthermia. From Kalow et al. (1970) courtesy of the authors, and the Editor and publishers of the Lancet)

reinnervation (La Cour, Juul-Jensen and Reske-Nielsen, 1973).

Electromyography has yielded mixed results, some known carriers of the trait proving normal on testing with a coaxial recording electrode (Issacs and Barlow, 1973), others displaying 'myopathic' potentials (Britt *et al.*, 1973) and others having fibrillation activity suggestive of denervation (La Cour, Juul-Jensen and Reske-Nielsen, 1973).

Motor unit counting studies

In unpublished studies carried out in collaboration with Beverly A. Britt and W. Kalow (of the departments of Anaesthesia and Pharmacology respectively, in the University of Toronto) the motor unit counting technique was employed on 22 patients and relatives considered to suffer from the rigid form of the syndrome. In each case the diagnosis had been confirmed by the demonstration of an abnormal sensitivity of biopsied muscle fibres to caffeine and halothane. Motor unit counting was performed on at least three muscles in most patients; the electrophysiological examination was completed by measurements of maximal impulse conduction velocities, sensory nerve recordings and coaxial needle electrode electromyography. In 20 of the 22 patients at least one of the tested muscles exhibited a selective loss of functioning motor units. Of 10 relatives considered not to have the hyperthermia trait, on the basis of normal muscle contracture tests, the motor unit counting results were normal in eight. (One of the two false positives was a policeman with a history of several enforced car crashes and in whom there was other evidence of cervical root or brachial plexus lesions.) These results are of interest in that the neurophysiological testing was carried out without the investigator being aware of the muscle biopsy findings. The success rate for the motor unit counting method in detection was almost 90 per cent and provided a useful validation of the objectivity of the test itself (see Appendix 6.2). It must be acknowledged, however, that both false negative and false positive results can occur; further, the test appears to be of much less value for the detection of patients with the non-rigid form of the disease.

Pathogenesis of the hyperthermic reaction

An understanding of the biochemical disorder underlying the hyperthermic reaction has been greatly facilitated by the fact that a very similar hereditary disease occurs in pigs, affecting animals of the Poland–China and Landrace strains. The existence of this disease is a source of concern in the food industry for attacks can be precipitated by any stressful situation and result in the production of meat unsuitable for human consumption (see Nelson, 1973). From studies on these animals and on susceptible human subjects it has been possible to conceive, at least in outline, the sequence of events which culminates in the production of such excessive amounts of heat. In the first place, it is evident that the triggering agent acts directly on muscle since the fibres undergo contracture even when neuromuscular transmission has been blocked by tubocurarine or succinylcholine. An early key step in the process is the production of high calcium levels in the muscle fibre cytoplasm, probably caused by an anaesthetic-induced inability of the sarcoplasmic reticulum to take up this ion in normal amounts (see page 41). The high calcium concentration now stimulates several catabolic reactions. First, phosphorylase kinase is activated so that increased quantities of lactate and heat are produced by the breakdown of glycogen in the muscle fibre. Secondly, in the rigid form of the disease the free calcium neutralizes the inhibitory action of troponin and enables the myosin cross-bridges to combine with the actin filaments (page 38); in the process ATP is hydrolysed to ADP, the muscle shortens and heat is produced. The muscle fibres will remain shortened as long as calcium and ATP are available. If, however, all the ATP is used up—as happens subsequently—the contracture persists since ATP is normally needed to detach the myosin cross-bridges from the actin filaments (see page 43); this is now the same type of contracture that is seen in *rigor mortis*. A third effect of the high intracellular calcium levels is that some of the ions gain access to the mitochondria, where they uncouple electron transport from oxidative phosphorylation. Electron transport continues, oxygen is consumed, carbon dioxide and heat are produced, but ATP formation is prevented. The lack of ATP will not only contribute to the development of the contracture (see above) but will arrest all the metabolic reactions concerned with the normal maintenance of the integrity of the muscle fibre. The fibre will now start to disintegrate, releasing in the process large quantities of enzymes such as CPK.

GLYCOGEN STORAGE DISEASES

During the past two decades a number of disorders of muscle have been discovered, each of which is characterized by the absence of an enzyme required for the metabolism of glucose or glycogen. These conditions are rare and are inherited, being transmitted by autosomal recessive genes. As described below, the degree of muscle involvement, the presence or absence of associated anomalies, the age of onset and the severity of the clinical features differ among the various syndromes. The classification of these disorders is that devised by Cori (1957).

Type I (Von Gierke's disease; glucose-6-phosphatase deficiency)

Glucose-6-phosphatase is normally found in low amounts in muscles but is an important enzyme in the liver and kidney. It is required for the last step in the breakdown of glycogen to glucose, which is the dephosphorylation of glucose-6-phosphate. The same step is also involved in the conversion of other sugars, such as fructose and galactose, to glucose. As a result the resting blood glucose level is low and does not show the expected rise following the injection of glucagon or adrenaline or the intravenous infusion of fructose or galactose. Instead much of the glucose-6-phosphate is disposed of by anaerobic glycolysis to lactic and pyruvic acid. Clinically, growth is retarded and the liver is grossly enlarged; the muscles are little affected but may be hypotonic. Biochemically, there is a combination of hypoglycaemia, metabolic acidosis, ketonuria and hyperlipaemia; liver biopsy reveals an excess of glycogen and a deficiency of glucose-6-phosphatase.

Type II (Pompe's disease; α-1, 4-glucosidase deficiency; acid maltase deficiency)

The α-1, 4-glucosidase enzyme which has its optimal pH at 4.5–5.0 is also known as acid maltase. It appears to have an important role in lysosomes where it is involved in the hydrolysis of maltose and glycogen to glucose, and in the conversion of maltose to glycogen. Variations in the deficiency of the enzyme can produce infantile, childhood and adult patterns of disease. In its infantile form this disease is the most severe of the glycogen storage diseases, resulting in death within the first 2 years. Within the first few months after birth the child is noticed to be weak and hypotonic. The enlarged tongue may suggest cretinism; the heart is also enlarged and death may result from cardiac failure or from pulmonary infection secondary to poor lung ventilation.

Less severe forms of this disease occur in childhood and in adult life. In both there is a chronic and slowly progressive weakness which mainly affects muscles of the trunk and limb girdle. In these last conditions muscle biopsy reveals degenerating fibres with moderately excessive amounts of glycogen in vacuoles; these vacuoles correspond to lysosomes for it is in these structures that the acid maltase is normally found. In the infantile form the enzyme is absent not only from muscle and liver but also from the heart and the white blood cells, this last deficiency forming the basis of a useful diagnostic test.

Type III (Cori's or Forbes's disease; amylo-1, 6-glucosidase deficiency)

Amylo-1,6-glucosidase deficiency is also known as the 'debrancher enzyme'; together with phosphorylase it is required for the breakdown of glycogen. In its absence only partial glycogenolysis occurs, the residual glycogen having an abnormal structure. The condition usually presents in young children and the clinical features are those of a mild form of type I glycogenolysis.

Type IV (Andersen's disease; amylo-1, 4→1, 6-transglucosidase deficiency)

This is a very rare condition caused by absence of 'brancher enzyme'; it causes an abnormal glycogen to accumulate in many tissues and results in death in early infancy.

Type V (McArdle's disease; myophosphorylase deficiency)

In this disorder, first described by McArdle in 1951, there is lack of an isoenzyme of phosphorylase which appears to be specific to muscle. As a consequence the muscles are unable to break down glycogen to lactic acid during exercise; this abnormality is most readily recognized if a specimen of venous blood is taken from the forearm after a period of ischaemic exercise and with the circulation still arrested. Under more natural circumstances, the patients complain of severe muscle pain during moderate exercise and the muscles may become swollen; the symptoms are relieved by rest but may persist for a day or so. When exercise is carried under ischaemic conditions the muscles rapidly stiffen and maintain their shortened position. In physiological terms this is a *contracture* (page 42), since the shortening is not accompanied by impulse activity in the fibres (McArdle, 1951; Rowland, Araki and Carmel, 1965). After severe exercise myoglobin may appear in the urine.

On examination the patient, usually an adult,

may appear completely normal. Some patients have unusually bulky muscles and in others mild weakness of the proximal muscles may be present. Biopsy specimens of muscle reveal excessive glycogen, mainly in vacuoles beneath the Sarcolemma and in mitochondria; absent phosphorylase activity can be demonstrated histochemically. The condition is associated with a normal life expectancy and patients suffer little incapacity, provided they restrict their exercise; the ingestion of glucose or fructose during exertion may improve tolerance. Motor unit counting studies have been preformed in five patients with this condition; in two of these the results were clearly abnormal (see also Upton, McComas and Bianchi, 1974). Gruener and associates (1968) have shown that a specimen of muscle from a patient with this syndrome resembled a normal preparation in that the fibres underwent contracture in response to calcium ions or caffeine (page 42). The diseased muscle differed, however, in that the contractures were greatly prolonged; the observed abnormality was independent of the surface membrane since the fibres had previously been desheathed, the drugs being applied directly to the sarcoplasm and myofibrils by micropipettes. The persisting contractures could not have resulted from a lack of ATP in the fibres since Rowland, Araki and Carmel (1965) had already demonstrated normal levels in two patients with this disorder at the time of contracture. An alternative possibility considered by Gruener and colleagues (1968) was that there had been a failure to reaccumulate calcium ions by the sacroplasmic reticulum.

Type VI (Hers's disease; hepatophosphorylase deficiency)

Absence of the hepatic isoenzyme of phosphorylase results in a clinical disorder resembling type I glycogenosis but the distinction can be made by the finding of normal serum lactate levels and a normal response to galactose infusion.

Other glycogen storage diseases, including type VII (*phosphofructokinase deficiency*) and type VIII (*hepatic phosphorylase-b-kinase deficiency*) are discussed by McArdle (1974).

MUSCLE DISORDERS WITH MITOCHONDRIAL INVOLVEMENT

A number of rare muscle syndromes have been described in which there is obvious structural or functional evidence of mitochondrial abnormalities. In at least some of these syndromes it is likely that the mitochondrial changes make a major contribution to the disease manifestations. Possibly the most striking of these disorders is the *hypermetabolic myopathy* first described by Ernster, Ikkos and Luft in 1959 (see also Luft *et al.*, 1962). Their patient, a 35-year-old woman, perspired excessively and, in spite of a ravenous appetite, became progressively thinner and developed weakness and wasting of her muscles. Measurements of her basal metabolic rate varied from + 140 to + 210 per cent; she was not thyrotoxic and no other cause could be found for her hypermetabolic state. A muscle biopsy revealed fibres which were packed with mitochondria; biochemical studies showed that the mitochondria possessed very high respiratory rates but were unable to produce the expected amounts of ATP. The excess energy liberated by this 'loosely coupled' respiration appeared as heat. Recently a second case of this syndrome has been described by Affifi *et al* (1972). In passing it should be noted that very high metabolic rates also occur in two other 'primary' muscle disorders—malignant hyperthermia (during the attack), and in the quantal squander myokymia syndrome. In the former condition it is likely that uncoupling may occur (see page 187) but in the latter the situation is unknown.

Other mitochondrial abnormalities may or may not be associated with a frank neuromuscular disorder. These conditions include a *pleoconial myopathy*, first described by Shy, Gonatas and Perez (1966) in an eight-year-old boy who had been 'floppy' during infancy and who displayed the features of a proximal non-progressive myopathy. The possibility that this patient had the normokalaemic form of familial periodic paralysis (page 133) was suggested by occasional exacerbations of weakness, associated with a craving for salt. Although the muscle fibres possessed excessive numbers of mitochondria (hence the term 'pleoconial'), there was no evidence of hypermetabolism as there had been in Luft's patient (see above).

In the same proper Shy, Gonatas and Perez (1966) described an eight-year-old girl with a slowly progressive muscle weakness; there was no hypermetabolism nor had there been any acute episodes of weakness. In muscle fibres of this patient some of the mitochondria were markedly enlarged, measuring up to 5 µm in length, and appeared to be degenerating. The authors referred to this disorder as a *megaconial* myopathy.

These cases are three examples of myopathies with obvious ultrastructural abnormalities suggestive of a metabolic derangement. With each year the number of related or novel diseases increases and in the following section brief accounts of some of these disorders are given; McArdle (1974) or Dubowitz and Brooke (1973) should be consulted for more detailed reviews. All the conditions to be described are examples of congenital myopathies, presumably of hereditary origin.

NEMALINE MYOPATHY

This disorder was described independently by Conen, Murphy and Donohue (1963) and by Shy et al. (1963). The characteristic feature of the disorder is the presence of rod-shaped bodies within the muscle fibres; the rods are considered to be abnormal depositions of Z-disc substance. Similar structures are sometimes encountered as 'nonspecific' findings following polymyositis, denervation, or tenotomy.

CENTRONUCLEAR MYOPATHY
(Myotubular myopathy)

In 1966 Spiro, Shy and Gonatas described a new syndrome in a 12-year-old boy. The child had generalized weakness of muscles (including the external ocular group) and a biopsy revealed that a majority of the fibres possessed central nuclei. The authors suggested that the fibres were in fact myotubes (page 93) and that there had been an arrest in their maturation. It is of interest that an inward migration of myonuclei may also take place after denervation or following work-induced hypertrophy, prior to splitting of the fibre. One may speculate that in each of these situations the internal locations of the nuclei enable messenger-RNA to be supplied more readily to the ribosomes involved with new protein synthesis.

CENTRAL CORE DISEASE

This condition was also first reported by Shy's group (Shy and Magee, 1956); in one family they observed five patients with hypotonia and a mild non-progressive weakness of proximal muscles. Muscle biopsy revealed fibres in which the central regions were largely composed of an amorphous material and were lacking in mitochondria and sarcoplasmic reticulum. The appearance of the cores and their absence of enzyme activity suggests that they were functionally useless. Although the condition may be inherited it is interesting, and possibly of relevance to pathogenesis, that very similar abnormalities may be seen after denervation ('target' or 'targetoid' fibres) and after tenotomy. The interpretation of these findings is difficult, however, for Karpati, Carpenter and Eisen (1972) have shown that the appearance of the cores in tenotomized rat muscle is prevented by prior denervation.

LIPID STORAGE MYOPATHY

In this disorder lipid droplets accumulate within the muscle fibres and it is possible that the underlying metabolic abnormality is one involving carnitine deficiency (Engel and Angelini, 1973).

DISORDERS OF NEUROMUSCULAR JUNCTIONS

The diseases to be described in the next two chapters are those in which a failure of neuromuscular transmission is the principal cause of muscular weakness. The pathophysiology of this type of disorder is now better understood than that of most of the other diseases considered in this book. Of particular value have been the studies of affected neuromuscular junctions with microelectrodes and with the electronmicroscope; before surveying this work it may be found useful to review Chapter 4.

Chapter 18

MYASTHENIA GRAVIS

INTRODUCTION

It is probable that the first clinical description of myasthenia gravis was the following one given by Thomas Willis in 1672:

Nevertheless those labouring with a want of spirits, will use these spirits for local motions as well as they can; in the morning they are able to walk firmly, to fling their arms about hither and thither or to take up any heavy thing; before noon the stock of spirits being spent, which had flowed into the muscles, they are scarcely able to move hand or foot. At this time I have under my charge a prudent and honest woman who for many years has been subject to this sort of spurious palsy, not only in her members, but also in her tongue. She for some time can speak hastily or eagerly, she is not able to speak a word, but becomes suddenly as mute as a fish, nor can she recover the use of her voice for an hour or two.

No further cases were recognized until 1879 when Erb reported a patient with a bulbar form of the disease. The understanding of the disease was next significantly advanced by Jolly (1895) who recorded muscle contractions with a pneumatic capsule and a smoked drum, both during voluntary effort and during nerve stimulation. He was able to show that muscle strength was normal initially but then declined rapidly. Other workers subsequently demonstrated that electrical stimulation of the muscle fibres directly was effective in restoring contractions, although the early investigations must have been susceptible to considerable technical error (see Desmedt, 1973). These studies, together with the resemblance of myasthenia gravis to curare poisoning, the beneficial response to anticholinesterases and the demonstration of normal nerve action potentials (Alajouanine, Scherrer and Bourguignon, 1959), all suggested that the neuromuscular junction was the site of abnormality. Before leaving the history of the disease, mention should be made of Jolly's prediction in 1895 that eserine, an anticholinesterase, would prove useful in the treatment of myasthenia. It was not until 1934 that this prophetic insight was confirmed by Mary Walker.

Clinical features

The disease has a prevalence which is within the range of 1:10 000 to 1:50 000 of the population and is twice as common in females as males. The condition may present at any age, the peak incidence occurring at about 20 years. The initial symptoms may present insidiously or may arise suddenly if precipitated by such factors as emotional disturbance, infection of the upper respiratory tract, pregnancy or anaesthesia. At first the weakness may affect any muscle but certain ones are more likely to be affected than others. For example, weakness of the extraocular muscles may cause the patient to see double when looking in certain directions ('diplopia'). Involvement of the elevators of the upper eyelids (levatores palpebrae superioris) will cause drooping of the lids ('ptosis'; *Figure 18.1*). Other facial muscles may also be affected and there is often weakness of bulbar muscles, causing difficulty in swallowing and in speaking.

Sometimes the disease undergoes spontaneous remission but this is uncommon and it is more usual for the weakness to spread to muscles other than

194

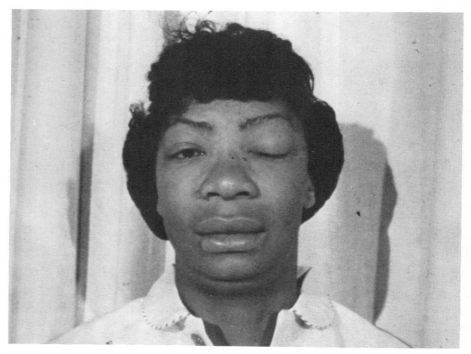

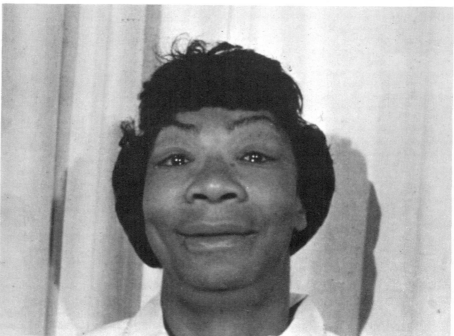

Figure 18.1. Facial appearance of patient with myasthenia gravis before (top) and approximately one minute after (bottom) an injection of Tensilon. Notice how the drooping of eyelids (ptosis) disappears. (Courtesy of Dr H. S. Barrows)

those affected originally. No skeletal muscle is exempt from attack in myasthenia and, in addition to those already described, the extensors of the neck, the shoulder girdle muscles and the hip flexors are most likely to be involved. Weakness of the respiratory muscles is obviously a serious complication and may eventually prove fatal. In a minority of cases some of the muscles become not only permanently weak but also considerably atrophied. A most important and characteristic feature of myasthenia, and one which is of considerable diagnostic value, is the fact that the weakness is aggravated by exertion and improved by rest, being least evident on waking.

Certain other clinical disorders may be associated with myasthenia. Of these, by far the most important is a *thymoma,* which is present in about 10 per cent of cases. One-third of these tumours are malignant and invade other structures in the anterior mediastinum; metastases are uncommon, however. Disorders of the *thyroid gland* are also associated with myasthenia, being found in about 9 per cent of males and in 18 per cent of females (Simpson, 1958; Downes, Greenwood and Wray, 1966). The most common of the thyroid disorders is thyrotoxicosis, but myxoedma, non-toxic goitre and Hashimoto's thyroiditis may also occur. A variety of other diseases have been reported in conjunction with myasthenia and include rheumatoid arthritis, Sjogren's disease, pernicious anaemia, epilepsy and psychotic illness (Simpson, 1974).

Laboratory investigations

The diagnosis of myasthenia gravis may be confirmed by pharmacological, electrophysiological and immunological tests. Undoubtedly the best *pharmacological test* is to observe the effect of administering a quick-acting anticholinesterase drug, edrophonium chloride (Tensilon, Roche Ltd.). Two milligrams of the drug are injected intravenously and, after pausing 30 s to make sure that there is no abnormal sensitivity to the drug, the remaining 8 mg are delivered. Most, but not all, patients with myasthenia will show an improvement in strength within the next minute (*Figure 18.1*). Another test, less commonly employed, is to inject a small dose of tubocurarine intravenously; the myasthenic patient is unusually sensitive to this drug and develops an accentuation of his weakness.

Electrophysiologically, the diagnosis may be confirmed by observing the effects of repetitive stimulation on the evoked compound muscle action potential (*Figure 18.2*). For a patient with generalized myasthenia it is convenient to stimulate the ulnar nerve at the wrist and to record the responses

of the hypothenar muscles with surface electrodes. If the weakness is restricted to facial muscles then it is better to record from these muscles and to stimulate the facial nerve instead.

Whichever muscle is selected for study, the first response is likely to be of normal amplitude but subsequent ones will show a decrement. The degree of decrement will obviously be greater in a severely affected patient and will also depend on the frequency of stimulation. A low stimulus frequency,

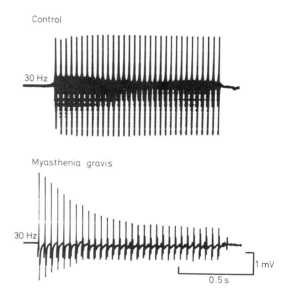

Control

30 Hz

Myasthenia gravis

30 Hz

1 mV

0.5 s

Figure 18.2. (Lower) Decrementing responses in the extensor digitorum brevis muscle of a 35-year-old woman with generalized myasthenia gravis; the peroneal nerve was stimulated at 30 Hz. (Upper) Absence of decrement in the corresponding muscle of a healthy subject

3 Hz for example, has the double advantage of being less painful for the patient and of eliminating possible contamination of the response by movement artefact. At this frequency a decline in response of more than 7 per cent by 1.5 s is abnormal (Slomić, Rosenfalck and Buchthal, 1968).

Sometimes, however, the decrement is only apparent at higher stimulus rates, for example at 50 Hz; at this frequency it is best to regard a fall of 20 per cent or more as significant. If the decline is still not evident, it may be brought out by repeating the stimuli 2 minutes after the cessation of a maximum voluntary contraction (see below). In some patients with undoubted myasthenia the responses to repetitive stimulation may remain normal and falsely negative results may also be obtained with the edrophonium test, described above.

Immunological tests are now being used in several laboratories as aids to the diagnosis of myasthenia gravis; although the techniques are still being refined, the results are already sufficiently promising that this type of test is likely to become the most useful method of diagnosing the condition. In the test of Almon, Andrew and Appel (1974) it is found that the sera of patients with myasthenia gravis will prevent α-bungarotoxin (page 33) from binding to acetylcholine receptors in isolated mammalian muscle; the blocking factor is associated with the globulin component of the plasma proteins. A highly accurate double-antibody test has been devised by Lindstrom and colleagues (1976); in a blind study of sera from patients and controls, the test has proved positive in almost all cases of myasthenia gravis and negative in controls and in patients with other types of neuromuscular disorder.

Treatment

The treatment of myasthenia has several parts. First, a long-acting *anticholinesterase* drug such as pyridostigmine bromide should be given at regular intervals throughout the day, for example at 6-hourly intervals. *Atropine* may be required to suppress muscarinic side-effects. Secondly, *thymectomy* is indicated in cases of medium severity or worse, particularly within the first 5 years of illness; it is also required for any patient with a thymoma. Finally, refractory cases should be given a trial with *cortiscosteroids* and, in some instances, this form of treatment appears life-saving. The most favoured regimen is to give a single large dose of prednisone, for example 100 mg, on alternate days; this dosage may need to be continued indefinitely (see Engel and Warmolts, 1971) but usually some reduction can be achieved.

Prognosis

Despite substantial improvements in drug therapy, in the technique of thymectomy and in intensive care management, patients may still die from myasthenia gravis. The causes of death are usually respiratory arrest or else aspiration pneumonia due to difficulty in swallowing. Patients with a malignant thymoma tend to have an especially poor prognosis due to the severity of the myasthenia, even though the tumour has been excised.

SPECIAL STUDIES IN MYASTHENIA GRAVIS

Although it is generally accepted that a disorder neuromuscular transmission is present in mya thenia gravis there is still no agreement as to tl exact mechanism involved. The defects which a theoretically possible and have been postulated various times, may be classified in the followir way:

I *Presynaptic*
   (*a*) Failure of impulse propagation in axc terminal.
   (*b*) Imparied synthesis of acetylcholine.
   (*c*) Faulty packaging mechanism in vesicles
   (*d*) Impaired release of acetylcholine.
   (*e*) Release of a 'false' transmitter.
II *Intrasynaptic*
   (*f*) Excess diffusion of acetylcholine aw: from the primary synaptic cleft.
   (*g*) Diffusion barrier.
III *Postsynaptic*
   (*h*) Combination of a circulating blockin; agent with acetylcholine receptors.
   (*i*) Depletion of acetylcholine receptors.
   (*j*) Desensitization of acetylcholine recepto
   (*k*) Increased acetylcholinesterase activity.

The evidence which is relevant to this issue h come from many sources and has involved the u of widely differing techniques. It is impossible present all of this data but it is neverthele instructive to review the more important contr butions and then to attempt a synthesis.

Morphological studies

Neuromuscular junctions

Neuromuscular junctions in myasthenia gravis hav been studied with both the light and the electro microscopes. The *light microscope* studies hav mostly been carried out on muscles treated wil methylene blue prior to removal of the biop specimens (Cöers, 1952). This 'vital' staining tecl nique enables the structure of the motor axon including their fine pre-terminal branches and tl endings themselves, to be seen in considerab detail. An alternative technique has been to sta the neuromuscular junctions for cholinesteras Cöers and Woolf (1959; also Woolf and Cöer 1974) in a series of investigations by themselves ar with various collaborators, were able to recogni; two principal abnormalities of the motor nerv endings which they termed 'dystrophic' and 'dy plastic' respectively.

Dystrophic neuromuscular junctions wei

aracterized by branching of a single motor axon as to form multiple end-plates on the same uscle fibre.

Dysplastic junctions were those in which the end-ates were abnormally lengthened on the surface the fibre; some of the terminal expansions appeared shrunken.

In addition some specimens had evidence of coleral reinnervation (page 224).

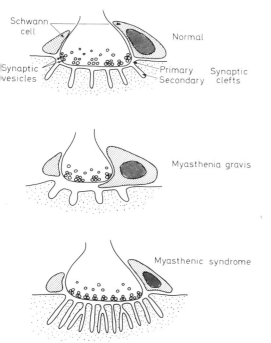

Figure 18.3. Diagrammatic summary of the morphological features of neuromuscular junctions described in myasthenia gravis (middle) and in the myasthenic syndrome (bottom); a normal junction is shown at top for comparison (see text)

Similar findings to those of Cöers and Woolf ave been obtained by MacDermot (1960) and by eske-Nielsen, Dalby and Dalby (1965). A further nportant observation was that both types of neuro-uscular abnormality could be found on muscle pres without any microscopic evidence of de-eneration; this suggested that the neuromuscular sion was a primary event. However, extension of e vital staining technique to other disorders has nown that neither the dystrophic nor the dysplastic aanges are specific for myasthenia since a number : diseases, and dystrophia myotonica in particular, ay show identical abnormalities.

Of the investigations with the *electronmicroscope* at by Santa, Engel and Lambert (1972) is especi-ly thorough, being based on measurements of

synaptic areas and of the sizes and numbers of organelles. The most striking abnormalities noted by these authors were postsynaptic and consisted of a widening of both the primary and secondary synaptic clefts with a reduction in the number of the secondary clefts. Similar findings had been observed previously by Zacks, Bauer and Blumberg (1961). In contrast to these findings the fine structure of the axon terminal appeared well preserved in myasthenia with normal numbers and sizes of synaptic vesicles being noted by Santa and colleagues (1972) and by Johnson and Woolf (1965). The only report to date of a reduction in the number of vesicles appears to be that of Iwayama and Ohta (1962). One presynaptic change which was clearly evident in some of the junctions studied by Zacks and colleagues and by Johnson and Woolf (1965) was a reduction in the size of the terminal axonal expansion; as the axon retracted its place was taken by an extension of Schwann cell cytoplasm. Knowledge of the detailed structure of the myasthenic neuromuscular junction has recently been extended by Fambrough, Drachman and Satyamurti (1973), who used labelled α-bunga-rotoxin to demonstrate the distribution of acetyl-choline receptors on the muscle fibre surface. They found a significant reduction in receptor density at the junction but there was no evidence of receptor spread outside the synaptic area as would have been anticipated in a denervated muscle fibre (page 75). A pictorial summary of the morphological features described by the various workers is given in *figure 18.3*.

Muscle fibre studies

One of the first methodical studies of muscle fibres in myasthenia gravis was that by Dorothy Russell (1953) who examined eight cases at *post mortem* and was able to classify the changes observed in the muscles into three categories:

Type I This was an acute change in which the muscle fibres underwent coagulative necrosis, becoming swollen and then losing their nuclei and myofibrils. There was a pronounced infiltration of inflammatory cells in and around the fibres, in which polymorphonuclear leucocytes and macro-phages predominated.

Type II This change was concerned with the formation of *lymphorrhages*, that is, collections of small lymphocytes around single muscle fibres undergoing atrophy.

Type III This was a simple atrophy affecting single muscle fibres or groups of fibres. The characteristic eosinophilia of the sarcoplasm was retained and the nuclei remained at the periphery of the fibres. There was no loss of cross-striations and no infiltrations of inflammatory cells were seen.

Two of these features deserve special comment. First, the presence of large clusters of lymphocytes (lymphorrhages) around some of the muscle fibres (Type II change) is suggestive of an inflammatory process and would be in keeping with an abnormality of the autoimmune system, as has been postulated for myasthenia gravis (page 207). The second noteworthy feature is the occasional presence of muscle fibre atrophy, sometimes affecting fibres singly and sometimes in groups (Type III change). The presence of scattered atrophic fibres would be anticipated in myasthenia since eventually muscle fibres with severe neuromuscular dysfunction would become denervated and would show the full spectrum of denervation changes, including atrophy. It is of great interest that the atrophy is a late sign of neuromuscular dysfunction in myasthenia for many muscle fibres still appear structurally normal even though their end-plates may show the marked dystrophic and dysplastic changes described above. This discrepancy between the changes at the junction and in the rest of the fibre suggests that there is a period in which the junction is no longer able to excite the muscle fibre but remains capable of supplying it with a trophic influence (see page 72) and that it is only when this trophic influence is lost that the muscle fibre atrophies. But why should some muscles display atrophy of muscle fibres in groups rather than singly? That this is a consistent feature of myasthenia gravis is indicated by the numerous confirmatory reports which have appeared since Russell's (1953) brief allusion to the finding (Steidl, Oswald and Kottke, 1962; Lowenberg-Scharenberg, 1962; Fenichel and Shy, 1963; Brody and Engel, 1964; Garçin, Fardeau and Godet-Guillain, 1965; Lapresle and Fardeau, 1965; Hopf and Ludin, 1968; Brownell, Oppenheimer and Spalding, 1972; Oosterhuis and Bethlem, 1973). For example, Fenichel and Shy (1963) studied 37 biopsies from various limb muscles on myasthenic patients and noted grouped muscle fibre atrophy in 11. The usual interpretation of this abnormality is that it reflects a lesion of the alpha-motoneurone or its axon (page 115) and it is difficult to escape the conclusion that such a lesion must be present in myasthenia gravis; the matter is discussed further on page 207.

(B) Pharmacological studies

The results of these investigations (see Simpson, 1974) may be summarized by stating that, in comparison with the findings in a normal subject neuromuscular transmission in a myasthenic patient is:

(1) Unusually susceptible to *tubocurarine* (which competes with acetylcholine for its receptors).
(2) Resistant to the 'prompt' depressant action of *acetylcholine* injected intra-arterially but more susceptible to the 'late' depressant effect of the drug.
(3) Resistant to *decamethonium* (which combines with acetylcholine receptors and depolarizes with the muscle fibre membrane).
(4) Potentiated by *anticholinesterases* (which prevent the hydrolysis of acetylcholine and hence accentuate its action).

Although germine acetate does not act on the neuromuscular junction, it is convenient to mention the effect of this drug, in view of the interesting study by Flacke et al. (1971). Acting on an earlier suggestion by Jolly (1895) these authors found that the drug produced a significant increase in strength in myasthenic patients. It did so by evoking repetitive impulse activity in those muscle fibres which had responded initially to electrical stimulation of the nerve or to voluntary effort. In turn this repetitive activity depended on a late rise in sodium permeability of the muscle fibre membrane following an impulse (page 24). In effect, Flacke and colleagues were inducing a form of myotonia in order to treat myasthenia—a truly ingenious exercise in neuropharmacology!

Neurophysiological studies

Intracellular investigations

Among the many experimental studies in myasthenia gravis the two microelectrode investigations by Elmqvist and his colleagues in Lund, Sweden have been especially important in shedding light on the nature of the neuromuscular dysfunction (Dahlbäck et al., 1961; Elmqvist, et al., 1964). These authors investigated biopsy specimens of intercostal muscle *in vitro* and examined such factors as the spontaneous electrical activity at the end-plate, the responses of the muscle fibres to stimulation through their nerves, and the sensitivities of the fibres to acetylcholine and other cholinergic drugs. In their first study they found that the miniature end-plate potentials (m.e.p.p.s, page 31) were of normal size but reduced in discharge frequency. With greater experience in the investigation of myasthenic muscle they came to recognize that the real situation was the reverse of that initially reported; most m.e.p.p.s were so small that they would not have been detected in the earlier study and, in fact, their discharge frequency was within the normal range. When the nerve was stimulated the end-plate potentials in some of the muscle fibres were not large enough

the axon-terminal (*presynaptic defect*) Elmqvist and his colleagues considered that it was more likely to involve a faulty mechanism for packaging acetylcholine into the synaptic vesicles than a failure in the synthesis of transmitter. After a nerve

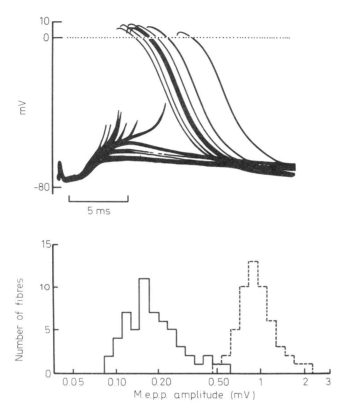

Figure 18.4. (Upper) Intracellular recordings from an intercostal muscle fibre of a patient with generalized myasthenia gravis. When the nerve was stimulated at 5 Hz the evoked response from the fibre often consisted of a subthreshold end-plate potential instead of an action potential. (Lower) amplitudes of miniature end-plate potentials (m.e.p.p.s) in intercostal muscle fibres of myasthenic patients (unbroken line) and control subjects (interrupted line). From Elmqvist et al. (1964) courtesy of the author, and the Editor and publishers of Journal of Physiology)

to cause excitation; other fibres might discharge impulses on some occasions but not on others (*Figure 18.4*). The diminished sizes of the m.e.p.p.s and the end-plate potentials could not have been due to one of the intra- or post-synaptic defects postulated for myasthenia (page 196) since the muscle fibres responded normally to acetylcholine applied from a micropipette and to carbachol and decamethonium administered in the bath solution. Having localized the myasthenic abnormality to

impulse a normal number of vesicles would empty but the acetylcholine released would be insufficient for muscle fibre excitation (*Figure 19.2*). The results of recent studies are at variance with these conclusions. First Ito *et al.* (1976) used gas chromatography and mass spectrometry to demonstrate that myasthenic intercostal muscle actually contained about twice the normal amount of acetylcholine. Secondly, Elmqvist's intracellular findings have been disputed by Albuquerque and his associates

(1976b). While confirming the diminished sizes of the m.e.p.p.s these last workers used a more sensitive iontophoretic technique to demonstrate that the myasthenic end-plates were much less responsive than normal to applied acetylcholine.

Multielectrode studies

Ekstedt and Stålberg (see Ekstedt, 1964) devised a multielectrode containing 13 independent leading-off surfaces; each of these consisted of an insulated platinum wire 25 μm in diameter (*Figure 18.5*). This multilead electrode enabled them to record simultaneously from two (or more) muscle fibres belonging to the same motor unit during a voluntary contraction. The time interval between the impulses of the two fibres during each discharge of the motor unit could then be measured on successive occasions and displayed appropriately (*Figure 18.5*). The authors found that the *fluctuation* in time interval, or '*jitter*', was significantly greater in myasthenic than in normal motor units and they considered that this type of study was useful in the EMG diagnosis of myasthenia (Ekstedt and Stålberg, 1967; Stålberg, Ekstedt and Broman, 1974). The explanation for the increased jitter is to be found in the microelectrode recordings made from single myasthenic muscle fibres by Elmqvist and his colleagues, one of which is displayed in *Figure 18.4*. In this recording it can be seen that the onsets of the action potentials varied by several milliseconds, due to differences in the sizes of the end-plate potentials and hence in the times taken for the depolarizations to reach the firing level of the fibre.

Whole muscle studies

It is standard EMG practice to record, with large surface electrodes, the responses evoked in myasthenic muscles by repetitive supramaximal stimuli delivered to the nerve. In most, but not all patients, a significant decrement can be demonstrated, the extent depending on the frequency and duration of the stimuli and on the severity of involvement of the muscle by the disease process (*Figure 18.2*). The matter has been discussed at length by Desmedt (1966), Slomić, Rosenfalck and Buchthal (1968) and by Özdemir and Young (1971) among others. The decremental responses described are quite in keeping with the excessive fatigability during effort which is such a prominent feature of myasthenia gravis. Further, they can be accounted for in a satisfactory manner by the results of the

microelectrode studies of Elmqvist and colleagues (1964). Of equal interest, however, are the occasions on which muscles display apparently paradoxical responses in the form of *increments* rather than decrements. For example, successive responses may diminish at a low stimulation rate (3 Hz) and increase at a higher rate (20–50 Hz) while at intermediate frequencies the responses may first decline and then enlarge. How can such increments be accounted for? The answer lies in the phenomenon of *post-tetanic facilitation*, which is a feature of normal synapses as well as the abnormal neuromuscular junctions of myasthenia gravis. In essence,

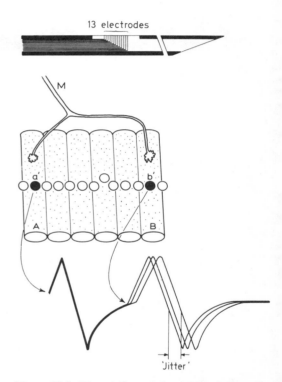

Figure 18.5. (Upper) One of the multilead electrodes devised by Estedt and Stålberg (see text). In this type the cut ends of 13 fine insulated platinum wires are exposed at the side of the stainless steel cannula. (Lower) When the electrode is inserted into a muscle the array of recording leads (circles) is arranged to lie across the muscle fibres. In this diagram muscle fibres A and B are innervated by the same motor axon, M. During a voluntary contraction the action potentials from fibre A are recorded by lead a′ and used to trigger the oscilloscope time base. The discharges from fibre B are recorded by lead b′ and appear after those of fibre A on the oscilloscope sweep. The fluctuation in the intervals separating the discharges from the two fibres is measured and termed the 'jitter' (see text)

it appears that, for a period of 100 ms or so following a nerve impulse, the axon terminal is in a hyperexcitable state such that a second impulse arriving during this period will release an extra amount of transmitter. It has been suggested that the underlying mechanism may involve an increased availability of transmitter following the temporary mobilization of vesicles into strategically favourable positions closer to the axolemma. If the intervals between the nerve stimuli are too great (i.e. more than 100 ms) the mobilization will have worn off and there is instead the effect of less quanta being immediately available for release, due to depletion of vesicles following the first impulse. Because of the small sizes of the m.e.p.p.s in myasthenia gravis, the reduction in available vesicles causes many of the end-plate potentials to become subthreshold for impulse initiation. As fewer muscle fibres become excited so successive evoked action potentials, recorded from the muscle belly, become smaller; the characteristic myasthenic decrement is then observed. If the muscle is allowed to rest additional vesicles are moved into favourable sites for release and the initial response amplitude is regained.

Whole muscle recordings have also shown that in patients with severe mysathenia gravis the terminal motor latency is increased (Preswick, 1965; Slomić, Rosenfalck and Buchthal, 1968); it will be recalled from Chapter 16 that this is the time elapsing between stimulation of the motor nerve close to the muscle and the onset of evoked activity in the latter. In myasthenia the defect is increased by repetitive stimulation; it constitutes further evidence of slowed impulse conduction in the abnormally fine and tortuous motor nerve terminal branches already described (see above).

Motor unit counting studies

Of 10 patients with myasthenia gravis, all below the age of 60, McComas, Sica and Brown (1971) found reduced populations of motor units in half. On the basis of the enlarged motor unit potential amplitudes and of the isometric twitch responses, these authors deduced that the surviving motor units were mostly of the slow-twitch type and had often undertaken collateral reinnervation. It is important to add that the experiments employed very low stimulus repetition rates (usually 0.7 Hz) so that any reduction in motor unit count could not be attributed to 'acute' neuromuscular failure. In this early study only EDB muscles were examined but subsequent work has shown that the motor unit counting technique may also reveal abnormalities in other muscles. Since 1971 a further 10 patients

have been examined and of these motor unit losses have been demonstrated in five (*Figure 18.6*). From this experience it is evident that if the symptoms and signs are confined to the extraocular muscles it is unlikely that motor unit counts in limb muscles will be abnormal. Sometimes, however, a decline from an initially normal motor unit count will be demonstrable if the clinical condition deteriorates, as the following case-report shows.

Patient F. S. was a 41-year-old woman with an 11-year history of myasthenia gravis; the weakness commenced with diplopia but progressed to involve the bulbar musculature, causing her difficulty in swallowing and speaking; there was little involvement of the limb muscles. In addition she suffered from bronchiectasis.

An EMG on 10 January 1974 (Dr M. E. Brandstater) revealed a 15 per cent decrement in the responses of the thenar muscles during repetitive stimulation at 2 Hz. However, the number of functioning motor units in the left thenar muscles (365) was well within normal limits; the M-wave was 10.6 mV. No other EMG abnormality was noted.

Subsequently the patient's clinical condition showed some deterioration; in view of her bronchiectasis she was considered ineligible for treatment with corticosteroids but it was thought worth while performing a thymectomy.

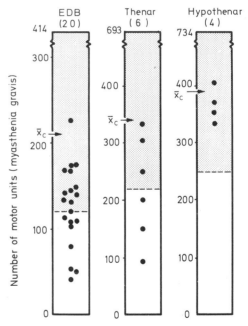

Figure 18.6. Numbers of functioning motor units in the extensor digitorum brevis, thenar and hypothenar muscles of 20 patients with myasthenia gravis. The hatched areas indicate the control ranges for each muscle and the arrows denote the corresponding control mean values

This operation was carried out on 31 March 1974 and an atrophic gland was removed. Although her immediate post-operative course was satisfactory, there was a gradual increase in her muscle weakness during the next 2 months, despite anticholinesterase therapy. On 27 May 1974 she was readmitted to hospital for she required feeding through a naso-gastric tube.

An EMG on 6 June 1974 (Dr A. R. M. Upton) now showed a striking reduction in the left thenar motor unit count (92 units); the M-wave was 6.1 mV, and the potentials of the surviving units were of normal or increased size. There was a slight loss of functioning units in the left extensor digitorum brevis muscle (103 units). As before sensory nerve function and maximal impulse conduction velocities were normal though, interestingly, myotonic activity was noted in the extensor digitorum brevis (EDB). On repetitive stimulation of the thenar, hypothenar and EDB muscles at various frequencies, no significant increment or decrement of the responses was noted.

The following day the patient developed cardiac and respiratory arrests and, despite intensive care, died one week later.

It should be added that, in a study employing a rather different method, Ballantyne and Hansen (1974a) were unable to find reduced EDB motor unit counts in any of their 20 myasthenic patients. This discrepancy between the two studies is discussed later (Appendix 6.1).

The search for a humoral neuromuscular blocking agent

One of the many intriguing features of myasthenia gravis is that the newborn child of a myasthenic mother may have evidence of the disease also. About one in seven of children are affected in this way and recovery, which is both complete and permanent, takes place in 1–12 weeks (Simpson, 1974). These observations strongly suggest that a blocking agent has crossed the placenta from the mother to the child but the fact that only a minority of the neonates at risk are affected could imply that the agent is absent in most adult myasthenics. Further, the neuromuscular junctions of the newborn, because of their immaturity, are likely to react to circulating factors present in concentrations too low to affect junctions in the adult. The studies of Churchill-Davidson and Wise (1963) illustrate this need for caution; in the muscles of *normal* neonates they found evidence of decremental responses to repetitive nerve stimulation together with myasthenic-like resistance to decamethonium.

The observations on neonatal myasthenia and the superficial resemblance between myasthenic weakness and that of curare intoxication have prompted numerous attempts to demonstrate the existence of a humoral blocking agent in myasthenia. Mary Walker, renowned for her introduction of anticholinesterase therapy in myasthenia, reported that ptosis (lid-droop) could occur following release of a tourniquet that had prevented return of venous blood from the exercised limb of a myasthenic patient. An alternative test has been to stimulate motor axons supramaximally and to record the evoked muscle action potentials after the tourniquet has been released in the opposite limb. Using this technique Johns, Grob and Harvey (1956) were unable to find evidence of a circulating blocking agent but a positive result has since been reported by Tsukiyama and colleagues (1959).

In another type of experiment the serum from a myasthenic patient has been applied acutely to the isolated nerve-muscle preparation of an animal. In the first experiment of this kind Wilson and Stoner (1944) employed frog muscle and were able to demonstrate a blocking effect. As with the other tests described above, the results in the hands of different investigators have been extremely variable. For example, Nastuk, Strauss and Osserman (1959), who also used frog muscle, only occasionally found a blocking effect and attributed this to lysis of superficial muscle fibres. In contrast, Parks and McKinna (1966) observed significant reductions in the contractile responses of indirectly stimulated rat diaphragm muscles and were able to reverse the decrement with anticholinesterase drugs. A rather different type of experiment was employed by Toyka and associates (1975), who gave daily injections of immunoglobulin from patients intraperitoneally into mice for periods of 10–14 days. At the end of this time they were able to demonstrate that the treated animals had acquired such myasthenic features as decremental muscle responses to repetitive nerve stimulation, diminished m.e.p.p. amplitudes, and decreased numbers of acetylcholine receptors at end-plates.

A recent and much more sensitive approach to the detection of a circulating blocking agent has been to search for a serum factor which will react specifically with the acetylcholine receptor. In the experiments of Almon, Andrew and Appel (1974), already cited, it was possible to block the combination of labelled α-bungarotoxin with acetylcholine receptors from rat muscle fibres and similar results have since been reported by Bender and colleagues (1975). Using a new immunological technique Lindstrom et al (1976) have also been able to demonstrate circulating antibody to the acetylcholine receptor; their test was nearly always positive in proven cases of myasthenia gravis but was consistently negative in controls and in patients with other types of neuromuscular disease. However, in a more recent study in which *intact* mamalian muscle fibres were examined with intracellular recording and microiontophoretic techniques, it was not possible to demonstrate that myasthenic serum interfered with the combination of acetylcholine and its receptor. To explain this unexpected finding the authors speculated that the immunological factor(s) in myasthenic serum might be exerting a non-specific action on the molecular environment adjacent to the acetylcholine recognition site (Albuquerque et al., 1976a).

ANIMAL MODELS OF MYASTHENIA GRAVIS

The Goldstein model

In an interesting series of experiments Goldstein and his colleagues showed that it was possible to induce an autoimmune inflammatory response in the thymus glands (thymitis) of guinea pigs and rats. They further demonstrated that these animals exhibited a transient block of neuromuscular conduction which had several features in common with myasthenia gravis. The technique employed by these authors was to inject the animals with saline extract of thymus or striated muscle in Freund's complete adjuvant. Two weeks after immunization, collections of small and medium lymphocytes were found in the central medulla of the thymus surrounding the Hassalls's capsules, indicating the presence of 'thymitis'. By this time circulating antibodies to thymus and skeletal muscle could be demonstrated and evidence of impaired neuromuscular function was present. Goldstein was able to show that, not only were there decremental electrical and mechanical responses of the muscles to repetitive stimulation of motor nerves, but that the sizes of the responses were improved by administering anticholinesterases. In later study Goldstein and Hofmann (1968) investigated single muscle fibres of these animals with microelectrodes and noted a further resemblance to myasthenia gravis in that the m.e.p.p.s were diminished in size but had normal discharge frequencies (page 198). Goldstein and Whittingham (1966) proved that the thymus was necessary for the development of the neuromuscular lesion by showing that the latter was absent in animals which had been thymectomized prior to injection of the thymus and adjuvant. In more recent studies Goldstein and Manganaro (1971) have identified two polypeptides from the normal thymus, each having a molecular weight of approximately 7000. One of these, thymin, is considered responsible for inducing neuromuscular block while the other, thymotoxin, is thought to cause the inflammatory responses in the muscles

('myositis') which the experimentally-treated animals commonly show.

Initial reservations concerning the reproducibility of the Goldstein model have been largely dispelled by the confirmatory report of Kalden et al. (1969). In contrast there is still doubt as to the relevance of the model to myasthenia; in particular there is a feeling that the myositic features of the model may be responsible for the neuromuscular block, as sometimes occurs in human polymyositis. The second caution is that, in contrast to myasthenia, the neuromuscular block in the experimental animals is short lived, appearing at about the tenth day and only lasting 7–10 days. In spite of these reservations, the Goldstein model is an intriguing one and there can no longer be any doubt that under certain circumstances a neuromuscular blocking effect can be mediated by the thymus.

The acetylcholine receptor antibody model

The electric organs of fish are profusely innervated and contain very high densities of acetylcholine receptors. From this tissue it is now possible to make highly-purified preparations of the receptors. When such a preparation is injected into rabbits either alone (Heilbronn et al., 1975) or with an adjuvant (Patrick and Lindstrom, 1973), a neuromuscular transmission defect develops. As with the Goldstein model considered above, there is a similarity to myasthenia for the muscle responses to repetitive nerve stimulation show decrements which are eliminated by the administration of anticholinesterase drugs. The value of this new model lies in the fact that the neuromuscular lesion was produced by the acetylcholine receptor itself with contaminating muscle antigens having been eliminated during the purification procedure.

According to Lennon, Lindstrom and Seybold (1975, 1976) the development of the myasthenic illness in rats takes place in two stages, the muscle weakness first appearing at 7–12 days after inoculation and, after full recovery, recurring at about 4 weeks. They noted that this second phase was progressive and that, as in human myasthenia, the weakness could be aggravated by sudden stress. In severely affected rats there was evidence of generalized muscle weakness with difficulty in gripping the cage bars and an inability to reach up for food and water.

Lennon, Lindstrom and Seybold (1976) have analysed the nature of the autoimmune disorder. By skin-testing they showed that thymus-derived lymphocytes (T-cells) became sensitized to acetylcholine receptor at 4–5 days after inoculation of the latter. The sensitized T-cells then reacted with the animal's own acetycholine receptors and released

204

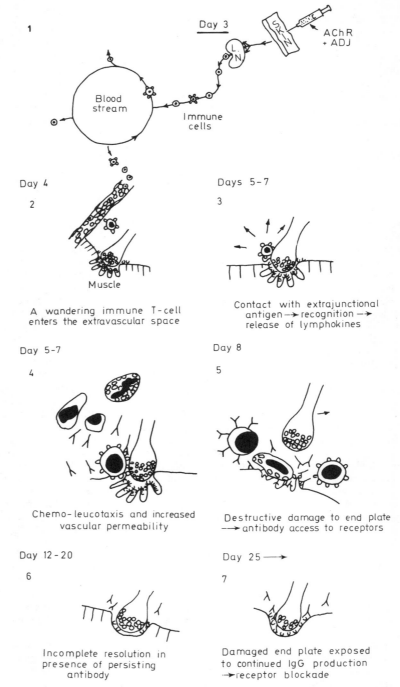

Figure 18.7. *The postulated mode of production of a myasthenia gravis-like illness in animals following the injection of acetylcholine receptor and adjuvant. (From Lennon et al. (1976), courtesy of the authors, and the Editor and publishers of* Annals of the New York Academy of Sciences)

pharmacologically-active *lymphokines;* these in turn increased vascular permeability and caused masses of inflammatory cells to accumulate at the neuromuscular junctions (*Figure 18.7*). Destruction of the synapses then took place and was responsible for the first episode of weakness; during this phase the axon terminals become separated from the postsynaptic membranes. After the acute inflammation response subsided the neuromuscular junctions were partially repaired but now assumed a simpler structure with fewer secondary clefts. Further degeneration of the synapses took place following the appearance of circulating antibody to the acetylcholine receptor; this stage was responsible for the second phase of muscle weakness. Electronmicroscope studies have revealed a strong similarity between the structures of the neuromuscular junctions in this chronic phase of experimental myasthenia and in those of the human disease (Engel *et al.,* 1976). The resemblance is strengthened by the finding of abnormally small miniature end-plate potentials (page 31) in both situations (Lambert, Lindstrom and Lennon, 1975). However, the animal model appears to differ from the human disorder in that the antibody reacts with acetylcholine receptor at some point on the molecule other than its acetylcholine-binding site; in human myasthenia direct competition for the binding site occurs (Almon, Andrew and Appel, 1974).

In spite of this last discrepancy the acetylcholine receptor-induced model of myasthenia appears remarkably similar to the human disease and the outcome of further studies is awaited with interest.

The myasthenic dog

There are now several reports of an illness in dogs characterized by a form of muscle weakness which closely resembles that of myasthenia gravis. This disease, because of its natural occurrence, is probably the best animal model of myasthenia gravis at present. The instances are rare, although the collection of four definite cases and of a further three probable ones in 10 years by the veterinary group in Cambridge, England (Fraser *et al.,*1970) suggests that the diagnosis is usually missed. The disease may affect any breed of dog and the signs develop quite rapidly over the space of a few days; they usually consist of a high-pitched bark, vomiting, and an inability to walk more than a few yards. A barium swallow may reveal gross dilatation of the oesophagus. Electromyograms show the characteristic decremental responses of myasthenia and the animals are invariably and dramatically im-

proved by anticholinesterases. Two of the four dogs studied in detail by Fraser and colleagues (1970) went into spontaneous remissions and required no further medication, as did the animal observed by Zacks, Shields and Steinberg (1966). These last authors carried out an histological and electronmicroscopic study of muscle obtained by biopsy; they found that although no lymphorrhages were present there was the same widening and distortion of the primary and secondary synaptic clefts that has been observed in human myasthenia gravis.

CONCLUSIONS AND SPECULATIONS

There are two questions which have to be answered in myasthenia gravis, as for any neurological disease. First, where is the lesion? Secondly, what is its nature?

Site of the lesion

The possible pre- , intra- and post-synaptic defects which could be responsible for the neuromuscular transmission defect in myasthenia may now be reiterated:

    I *Presynaptic*
       (*a*) Failure of impulse propagation in axon terminal.
       (*b*) Impaired synthesis of acetylcholine.
       (*c*) Faulty packaging mechanism in vesicles.
       (*d*) Impaired release of acetylcholine.
       (*e*) Release of a 'false' transmitter.
    II *Intrasynaptic*
       (*f*) Excess diffusion of acetylcholine away from the primary synaptic clefts.
       (*g*) Diffusion barrier.
    III *Postsynaptic*
       (*h*) Combination of a circulating blocking agent with acetylcholine receptors.
       (*i*) Depletion of acetylcholine receptors.
       (*j*) Desensitization of acetylcholine receptors.
       (*k*) Increased acetylcholinesterase activity.

The attempt to decide between these possibilities is made difficult by the large volume and apparently conflicting nature of the evidence available. Much of this evidence has been presented in the preceding pages and can be summarized in the following way. The microelectrode investigations by Elmqvist's group (page 198), the examination of stained motor end-plates with the light microscope (page 196), the finding of grouped muscle fibre atrophy (page 198) and of a loss of functioning motor units using an electrophysiological technique (page 201) all suggest some kind of presynaptic disorder (possibilities (*a*) to (*e*) above). The beneficial effect of anticholinesterase medication would also seem most readily explicable on the basis of a presynaptic defect in myasthenia. By suppressing the hydrolysis of acetylcholine the drug would tend to compensate for a reduced delivery of the transmitter to its receptors. In addition, a deficiency of released acetylcholine provides a reasonable explanation for the failure of neuromuscular transmission at low impulse discharge frequencies as observed, for example, by Stålberg, Ekstedt and Broman (1974) during weak voluntary muscle contraction. The finding of an increased terminal motor latency in myasthenia (page 201) would also indicate the presence of a presynaptic defect. The effect of such a lesion would undoubtedly be aggravated by an excessive loss of released acetylcholine due to lateral diffusion in the widened primary synaptic clefts (possibility (*f*) above). On the other hand, the ultrastructural studies made with the electron microscope (page 197), the acetylcholine receptor-labelling experiments (page 197) and most of the pharmacological studies favour a postsynaptic defect of type (*i*) (above). Finally, the occurrence of neonatal myasthenia and of transmissible neuromuscular block in some adult patients (page 202) point to the existence of a circulating blocking agent, that is, to possibility (*h*) (above). Stronger evidence for a circulating agent has come from the recent finding of serum antibodies to acetylcholine receptor in myasthenic patients (Almon, Andrew and Appel, 1974; Lindstrom *et al.*, 1976).

In weighing the relative importance of these observations it is legitimate to set aside the results of the pharmacological studies (page 198) since it is now recognized that the actions of drugs at the neuromuscular junction are more complex than had been assumed hitherto, most substances exerting both pre- and post-synaptic effects. One may then turn to the microelectrode studies of Elmqvist and colleagues (1964), for not only are the results detailed and precise but they deal directly with function, rather than with implications of disordered function. These studies reveal several important facts about myasthenia which can probably be accepted without dispute. First, the nerve impulse does reach the axon terminal (excluding possibility (*a*) in the list of possible lesions given above). Second, the transmitter release mechanism appears to be intact (excluding possibility (*d*)). Third, the depolarization produced by each quantum (vesicle) of acetylcholine is too small. It is the reason for this third observation around which the debate is centred, since any of the remaining possibilities

listed above could be responsible. According to Elmqvist and colleagues (1964) and to Dahlbäck and associates (1961) neither an intra- nor a postsynaptic mechanism could be concerned since the muscle fibres responded normally to the iontophoretic application of acetylcholine and to cholinergic drugs administered in the muscle bath solution. They concluded that the packaging of acetylcholine into vesicles was the essential defect in myasthenia gravis. Unfortunately, this explanation is in conflict with the demonstration by Ito *et al.* (1976) of increased acetylcholine in myasthenic muscle and also with Albuquerque *et al.'s* (1976*b*) finding of diminished sensitivity of myasthenic end-plates to applied acetylcholine. Ito *et al.* also found no evidence of a false transmitter excluding possibility (*e*)). Other observations also indicate that there must be a major postsynaptic component to the myasthenic lesions. For example, there is now strong evidence for circulating antibody to acetylcholine receptor in myasthenic patients (Almon, Andrew and Appel, 1974; Lindstrom *et al.*, 1976). In addition, electromicrographs of myasthenic neuromuscular junctions reveal such striking abnormalities of the postsynaptic surface of the muscle fibre that consideration must be given to the possibility that some of the later steps in the transmission process are affected. For example, the widened primary synaptic cleft might allow some acetylcholine to diffuse out of the synapse. Also, the reduced postsynaptic area of membrane caused by the loss and shallowness of the secondary clefts would imply a corresponding reduction in the number of acetylcholine receptors. This last deduction has now been confirmed by Fambrough, Drachman and Satyamurti (1973) using labelled α-bungarotoxin. Admittedly the effect of the loss of receptors would be mitigated to some extent by the proportional depletion of acetylcholinesterase molecules which would also be expected to occur.

In assessing the functional significance of these postsynaptic changes, the safety margin for each step in the transmission process becomes a crucial issue. For a human muscle fibre *in situ* the critical depolarization required to trigger an action potential is usually less than 15 mV (McComas *et al.*, 1968) whereas the full size of the end-plate potential is about 70 mV, suggesting that there are five times as many acetylcholine-receptor interactions as are actually required to excite the fibre. Also relevant to this issue is the work of Barnard, Wieckowski and Chiu (1971) which indicates there are ten times as many acetylcholine receptors as there are molecules of acetylcholine released by a single impulse at a mammalian synapse. However, by measuring the amount of block produced by exposure to α-bungarotoxin, Barnard and colleagues also showed that this surplus of receptors was necessary since the capture of acetylcholine by the receptors was not optimal. Therefore the safety-factor for neuromuscular transmission remains determined by the ratio of the end-plate potential to the critical membrane depolarization, and is approximately five (see Appendix 18.1). Although this is a large safety margin, it would be barely adequate or else insufficient to compensate for the 70–90 per cent loss of acetylcholine receptors demonstrated in myasthenic muscle fibres by Fambrough, Drachman and Satyamurti (1973).

Accepting that there are both pre- and post-synaptic abnormalities and that the latter are mainly, perhaps entirely, responsible for the defect in neuromuscular transmission, which side of the synapse is affected first? A trophic abnormality of the motor axon could affect the muscle fibre and *vice versa*. To answer this point it is necessary to look beyond the neuromuscular junction for other types of evidence. Strong support for a primary post-synaptic defect is the almost invariable finding in myasthenic patients of circulating antibodies to acetylcholine receptor (Lindstrom *et al.*, 1976). Other evidence for a primary post-synaptic lesion would be the presence of atrophic muscle fibres with still normal neuromuscular junctions; this situation must be extremely unusual, however, for more commonly it is the muscle fibres which appear normal even though the end-plates are affected. In contrast, evidence for a primary presynaptic lesion would be the presence of degenerative changes in proximal regions of motor axons or in motoneurones. In myasthenia these structures are considered to be normal although Campbell and Bramwell (1900), in reviewing the early literature, cite occasional cases in which such lesions may have been present. Against this paucity of data must be set the well-documented evidence of grouped muscle fibre atrophy in 10–30 per cent of myasthenic muscles (page 198), a finding which is routinely interpreted as reflecting damage to motoneurones or their axons. There is also the evidence from motor unit counting studies of McComas, Sica and Brown (1971; see also page 201) that about half the patients with myasthenia have a selective loss of functioning motor units in one or more of their muscles.

The explanation of Brownell, Oppenheimer and Spalding (1972), that the evidence of neuropathic changes 'merely indicates an abnormality in the most distal part of the motor nerve fibre, which could well be part and parcel of a disturbance affecting both sides of the neuromuscular synapse' is not convincing. The significance of grouped muscle fibre atrophy, as of the decreased motor

unit populations demonstrated by McComas, Sica and Brown (1971; see below), is that the myasthenic process is not affecting the neuromuscular junctions in a random manner. In some motor units all the junctions have been affected severely so that all the fibres are denervated, whereas other motor units contain relatively normal numbers of innervated fibres. Further, the collateral reinnervation in myasthenia which was found occasionally by Woolf and Cöers (1974; and indicated by the data of McComas, Sica and Brown, 1971, see above) is also relevant for if myasthenia was a *post-junctional* disorder a muscle fibre would be expected to have the same difficulty in forming effective synaptic contacts with a foreign motoneurone as with its original neurone.

In reviewing the above evidence it is apparent that it is still impossible to decide which part of the neuromuscular junction is affected first. If, however, experimental autoimmune (acetylcholine receptor) myasthenia proves a valid model for the human disease, as may well happen, the case for a primary postsynaptic defect will be convincing.

Nature of the lesion

So far only the possible site of the primary lesion in myasthenia gravis has been considered. What is the nature of this lesion? Following the suggestion of Simpson (1960, 1966) and recent experimental work, contemporary opinion seems firmly in favour of an autoimmune mechanism being present. Simpson's hypothesis was based on circumstantial evidence, namely:

(1) Myasthenia resembled systemic lupus erythematosus (SLE), an autoimmune disorder, in being more common in females and in having the highest incidence of onset in the third decade.

(2) Myasthenia may be associated with auto-immune disorders such as rheumatoid arthritis, SLE, Sjögren's syndrome and Raynaud's syndrome.

(3) The infiltrations of lymphocytes within some of the myasthenic muscles were suggestive of an autoimmune disorder.

(4) Simpson incorporated the finding of a high incidence of thymic abnormalities in myasthenia by postulating that this gland had an important role in immune mechanisms. Such a role has since been established (Miller, 1961; see also Yunis, Stutman and Good, 1971, for review) and now constitutes further evidence for an autoimmune disorder in myasthenia.

(5) At about the same time that Simpson put forward his hypothesis, Strauss *et al.* (1960) reported the presence, in a significant proportion of myasthenic patients, of circulating antibody to

the A-band regions of striated muscle fibres. This finding has since been confirmed in many laboratories and also extended by the demonstration that nearly every myasthenic patient with a thymoma carries these antibodies and that they are usually associated with presence of muscle lymphorrhages. More recently it has been shown that nearly all patients with myasthenia gravis carry serum antibodies to acetylcholine receptor (Lindstrom et al., 1976; see also Almon, Andrew and Appel, 1974).

(6) The development of temporary myasthenia gravis in the infants of affected mothers (page 202) must indicate the passage of a humoral factor across the placenta. This humoral factor could well be an antibody, and the unsuccessful attempts to demonstrate a correlation between the presence of antimuscular antibodies in the infant's serum and the development of neonatal myasthenia (Stern, Hall and Robinson, 1964; Oosterhuis, Feltkamp and Van der Geld, 1966) may be irrelevant if only anti-acetylcholine receptor antibody is involved.

(7) Experimental models of myasthenia gravis can be produced by immunizing animals with preparations of muscle, thymus or acetylcholine receptors (page 203).

(8) Immunosuppressive drugs, given in the form of high doses of corticosteroids or of ACTH, are now accepted as beneficial in the treatment of severe cases of myasthenia.

The observations cited above furnish very strong evidence for the presence of an autoimmune disorder in patients with myasthenia gravis and furthermore, one which is probably directed against the acetylcholine receptor. But how is this autoimmune reaction triggered off? It is difficult to believe that abnormal exposure of endogenous receptor is responsible for, even in normal muscle, there are acetylcholine receptors at the ends of fibres which would be exposed to wandering lymphocytes. Nor is there any evidence of myasthenia gravis following conditions in which a massive exposure of receptors would be anticipated, as in crush injuries of limbs, or following denervation of muscles (due to spread of receptors, see page 75). An alternative possibility is that, for some reason, an abnormal acetylcholine receptor is made which then sets off the autoimmune reaction. A third possibility is that an antigen similar to the receptor is presented to the T-cells, possibly by a virus. Certainly the sometimes sudden onset of the disease, the not uncommon history of a preceding respiratory tract infection, and the ability of some patients to improve spontaneously, all raise the possibility of a viral infection as the initiating event. An added possibility is that the virus is a neurotropic one, for in this way one could account for the undoubted neuropathic element in the disease and also perhaps explain why some muscles are involved rather than others. One would also wish to know the role of the presynaptic acetylcholine receptors (page 33) in the pathogenesis of the disease and also whether cholinergic synapses in the central nervous system were affected by the antireceptor antibody. Understanding of the disease would still be incomplete since the high incidence of thyroid disease, particularly thyrotoxicosis, in myasthenia (page 195) would remain to be accounted for. The significance of the relationship between thyrotoxicosis or a similar syndrome and myasthenia is reinforced by Simpson's comment that 'slight exophthalmos and thickening of the upper eyelids is common and many patients complain of excessive sweating even before the use of anticholinesterase drugs' (Simpson, 1974). Excessive sweating is also a feature of quantal squander myokymia and we have observed a patient with this condition who subsequently became myasthenic, complete with thymoma; because of the uniqueness of this event, her case is described separately (Appendix 19.1).

Because of the large number of puzzling observations concerning myasthenia gravis, any attempt to provide a complete account of the disorder must be unusually speculative at present. Even so, there is no denying that the acetylcholine receptor–antibody experiments have provided a very stimulating suggestion as to the nature of the basic pathophysiological abnormality.

Chapter 19

PSEUDOMYASTHENIC SYNDROMES AND OTHER SYNAPTIC DEFECTS

A number of conditions simulate myasthenic gravis in their clinical presentation or else show myasthenic features during electromyography and testing with anticholinesterase drugs. The nomenclature of these conditions is confusing. There appear to be advantages in grouping them together as 'pseudomyasthenic syndromes'.

THE EATON–LAMBERT SYNDROME
(Myasthenic syndrome, Carcinomatous neuropathy, Myopathic–myasthenic syndrome)

In 1953 Anderson, Churchill-Davidson and Richardson reported the case of a 47-year-old man with a recent history of leg weakness which was worse in the evening. The patient was subsequently found to have bronchial carcinoma of the oat cell type. Following bronchoscopy, for which succinylcholine had been administered, the patient remained apnoeic for an hour instead of the usual few minutes. Anderson and his colleagues later demonstrated that the patient was also abnormally sensitive to tubocurarine and that his weakness improved with neostigmine, an anticholinesterase drug. In view of the strong resemblance to myasthenia gravis in these drug responses the authors suggested that the muscle weakness noted previously was of myasthenic origin and they drew attention to the interesting association with bronchial carcinoma. Several similar cases were then reported by others but it was not until 1957

that Eaton and Lambert were able to show that the electromyographic findings differed from those of myasthenia gravis. The condition has since been referred to as the myasthenic or Eaton–Lambert syndrome.

Clinical features

Because of its relationship to bronchial carcinoma, the syndrome is more common in males, with the peak incidence falling within the 50–70 year range. Not all patients have a neoplasm, however, although the neuromuscular syndrome may sometimes precede the appearance of a tumour by several years. Although a bronchial carcinoma is by far the most commonly associated neoplasm, the syndrome has occasionally been seen in conjunction with tumours of the breast, stomach, prostate and rectum.

As with myasthenia gravis, the predominant symptom is weakness; since this affects proximal muscles in the limbs, particularly in the legs, the condition may be misdiagnosed as a myopathy. Although weakness may be accentuated toward the end of the day there is a temporary increase in strength following voluntary effort of a few seconds' duration; tendon reflexes are also enhanced immediately after exercise. In this last respect the syndrome is unlike myasthenia gravis; it also differs in that the extraocular and bulbar muscles are less severely affected than the limb muscles, often being spared altogether.

209

The *treatment* of the myasthenic syndrome is, first, to search thoroughly for a neoplasm, paying particular attention to the chest. Although the prognosis for bronchial carcinoma is poor following surgery, useful remissions of the muscular weakness may sometimes occur following excision of the tumour (see, for example, Anderson, Churchill-Davidson and Richardson, 1953). Medical treatment is of value, the drug of choice being *guanidine;* this substance is given in doses of up to 30 mg/kg daily and acts by increasing the release of acetylcholine from the nerve endings. Anticholinesterases are also worth trying and may add a further improvement.

Special studies

Electrophysiological investigations

Electromyography is invaluable in diagnosis, th crucial aspect being the evoked muscle responses t nerve stimulation. Unlike myasthenia gravis, th first response in the myasthenic syndrome is us usually small; however, there is a similarity in tha successive responses diminish still further, provide the stimuli are given at low repetition rate (1–10 Hz). The most striking difference from myasthenia gravis is seen when the stimuli are give at higher rates (20–50 Hz); the evoked muscl

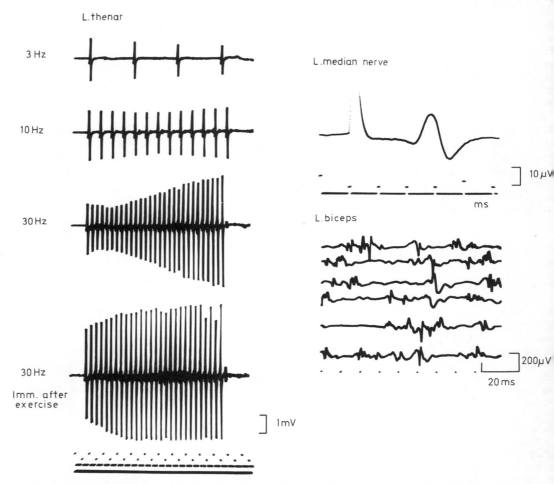

Figure 19.1. Electrophysiological findings in a 61-year-old man with a myasthenic syndrome associated with an occult bronchial carcinoma. At left are the responses of the thenar muscles following repetitive stimulation at a low frequency (3 Hz) and the incrementing responses at a high frequency (30 Hz). The potentiating effect of voluntary effect is seen below. In this patient there was no evidence of an associated sensory neuropathy; note the normal sensory response at the wrist following stimulation of the thumb (top right). Coaxial electrode recording from the biceps brachii revealed mostly small brief volitional potentials (bottom right)

responses grow progressively larger and may be as much as 10 times the size of the initial response (*Figure 19.1*). A similar facilitation can be demonstrated by stimulating the motor nerve as soon as possible after the end of a maximal voluntary contraction. The contrasting EMG findings in myasthenia gravis and the myasthenic syndrome are evident from comparison of *Figures 18.2 and 19.1*. The latter shows oscilloscope recordings obtained from a 61-year-old man with severe weakness of proximal muscles who was subsequently found to have a bronchial carcinoma.

Electromyography may show no other abnormalities but sometimes there is evidence of sensory and motor denervation. In addition, recordings with coaxial electrodes from muscles during voluntary contraction may reveal small, brief potentials of the type customarily interpreted as 'myopathic' (*Figure 19.1, lower right*). In the myasthenic syndrome it is reasonable to attribute these potentials to fragmentation of motor units caused by the presence of inexcitable neuromuscular junctions in a proportion of the muscle fibres.

Microelectrode examinations of intercostal muscle biopsies have been made by Hofmann, Kundin and Farrell (1967) and by Lambert and Elmqvist (1971); the latter study was especially thorough, being conducted on material from 12 patients. Both groups found that the amplitudes and resting discharge frequencies of the miniature end-plate potentials (m.e.p.p.s) were normal but that during nerve stimulation too few quanta (vesicles) of acetylcholine were released from the nerve terminal (*Figure 19.2*). For example, at some neuromuscular junctions the end-plate potential might consist of a single quantum only, whereas in the normal preparation about a hundred quanta are involved in each response to a single nerve impulse. Lambert and Elmqvist also showed that the inability to release acetylcholine was present if the potassium concentration of the bathing solution was raised, for although there was an increase in m.e.p.p. frequency, its magnitude was much smaller than in normal nerve–muscle preparations. In contrast, Lambert and Elmqvist were able to demonstrate that raising the external calcium concentration, or adding guanidine to the bath solution, were both effective in increasing the sizes of the evoked end-plate potentials. These authors also examined the intracellularly recorded muscle fibre responses to repetitive stimulation of motor axons; they found that there was a progressive, and sometimes very striking, enlargement of the end-plate potentials due to the release of

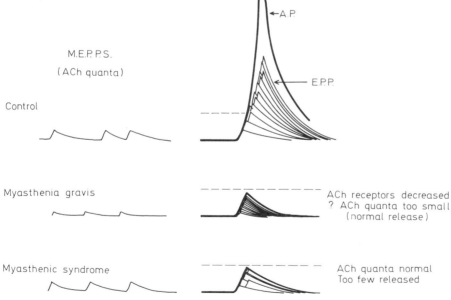

Figure 19.2. *The nature of the neuromuscular transmission defects in myasthenia gravis and the myasthenic syndrome: (left) miniature end-plate potentials (M.E.P.P.S.) in the two disorders; those in the myasthenic syndrome are of normal amplitude but in myasthenia gravis they are diminished; (right) the end-plate potentials (E.P.P.) evoked by single nerve impulses. In neither disorder are these responses large enough to reach the threshold (— — — —) for an action potential (A.P.). In the myasthenic syndrome too few quanta of acetylcholine are released; in myasthenia gravis there are too few receptors and possibly the quanta are small also (see text)*

additional quanta as part of the transmitter mobilization phenomenon (page 29). This last observation provides an explanation for the increase in muscle strength following repetitive nerve stimulation or voluntary contraction which was previously noted as being the distinguishing feature of the myasthenic syndrome.

In summary, then, the neuromuscular transmission defect in the myasthenic syndrome arises from an inability of the impulse in the axon terminal to release sufficient quanta of acetylcholine. The synthesis and packaging of transmitter appear normal, as does the responsiveness of the muscle fibre membrane. These features are contrasted with those of myasthenia gravis in *Figure 19.2*.

Morphological studies

Awad (1968) studied motor nerve endings with the light microscope following vital staining with methylene blue. He observed various changes including axonal swellings, fragmentation of axoplasm, variably sized end-plates, and collateral reinnervation.

Electronmicroscopic investigations have been conducted by Fukuhara *et al.* (1972) as well as by Santa, Engel and Lambert (1972b). The most striking abnormality found by both groups was enlargement of the postsynaptic membrane, caused by increases in the numbers and depths of the secondary synaptic clefts, many of which exhibited branching. The synaptic vesicles within the axon terminal appeared normal. The ultrastructural findings are summarized in *Figure 18.3* and shown in comparison with those of myasthenia gravis. Since, on the basis of microelectrode studies (see above), there is a greater than normal surplus of receptors available for the acetylcholine released, it is difficult to see a functional advantage in the extravagant infolding of the postsynaptic membranes visible with electronmicroscope.

MYOPATHIES AND NEUROPATHIES

The occurrence of increasing fatigability on effort, together with the electro-physiological and sometimes pharmacological features of myasthenia gravis, is not infrequently found in a variety of 'myopathic' or 'neuropathic' disorders once it is looked for. For example, it is recognized in disorders affecting the motoneurone such as amyotrophic lateral sclerosis (Mulder, Lambert and Eaton, 1959) and poliomyelitis (Hodes, 1948).

McComas and colleagues (1973b) showed that the phenomenon was present in the weakened muscle of patients with hemiplegia, presumably because the motoneurones were undergoing trans-synaptic degeneration (Chapter 27). Myasthenic features may also also be found in the course of peripheral neuropathies (Baginsky, 1968; Miglietta, 1971) and are a well-recognized complication of polymyositis. Other myopathies including myotonic and limb-girdle muscular dystrophy (McComas, Campbell and Sica, 1971; Sica and McComas, 1973b) and McArdle's disease (myophosphorylase deficiency; Dyken, Smith and Peak, 1967) may be similarly involved. Brown (1974) has described an interesting abnormality in myotonia congenita, in which a myasthenic-type of decrement can be demonstrated in a rested muscle but not immediately after activity (see also Ricker, Meinck and Stumpf, 1973). Brown and Charlton (1975) have extended their analysis of these pseudomyasthenic syndromes by investigating neuromuscular transmission during regional perfusion of limbs with curare. In the myotonic and lower motoneurone disturbances the curare sensitivity was normal but in Duchenne dystrophy there was a similar hypersensitivity to that found in myasthenia gravis. *Figure 19.3* shows decremental muscle responses to repetitive nerve stimulation in a selection of these myopathic and neuropathic disorders.

One explanation for these phenomena in the neuropathic group of disorders would be that the dysfunctional motoneurones were no longer able to synthesize and transmit an adequate supply of trophic material to maintain the motor nerve endings (see page 15). Support for this concept has come from the recent experiments of Shibuya and associates (1975) in which the sciatic nerves of rats were compressed with ligatures. Six weeks later it was found that repetitive stimulation of the nerve evoked decremental responses in the gastrocenemius muscles and that this abnormality could be reversed with anticholinesterases. In long-standing neuropathies the presence of collateral reinnervation may be an important additional factor since impulse transmission could fail at the points of axonal branching where the safety factor for impulse transmission is lower (Stålberg and Thiele, 1972).

ANTIBIOTICS

It is now recognized that certain antibiotics may also interfere with neuromuscular transmission. The first recorded human case was reported in 1956; the patient was a man who stopped breathing (apnoea) after an intraperitoneal injection of

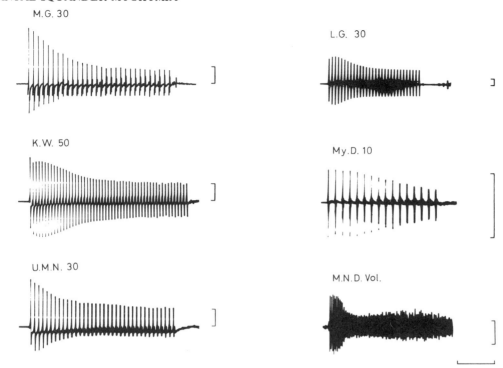

Figure 19.3. Decrementing EDB muscle responses following nerve stimulation in disorders other than myasthenia gravis (MG). Frequency of stimulation (Hz) shown above traces. K.W., Kugelberg-Welander type of spinal muscular atrophy; UMN, upper motoneurone lesion: LG, limb-girdle dystrophy; MyD, myotonic muscular dystrophy; MND, motoneurone disease. In this last record only a single motor unit remained and, instead of employing indirect stimulation, the patient made a maximum voluntary contraction. Vertical calibrations signify 1 mV. Horizontal calibration indicates 1 s for trace lower right only

omycin (Pridgen, 1956). Since that time at least 8 different antibiotics have been judged to have euromuscular blocking properties; apart from omycin they include kanomycin, cholistin, reptomycin, tetracyclines and polymyxin 'ittenger and Adamson, 1972). It may well be that ie various antibiotics interfere with neuromuscular ansmission in different ways but there is no oubt that, for some of these drugs, the most nportant action is the prevention of the release f acetylcholine from the motor nerve terminals. his was clearly demonstrated in the experiments f Elmqvist and Josefsson (1962) in which the 'fects of neomycin on the rat phrenic nerve-aphragm and frog sartorius preparations were vestigated with intracellular recording tech-iques. These authors showed that the miniature id-plate potentials (m.e.p.p.s) did not show the ormal rise in frequency following potassium-iduced depolarization of the motor nerve rminals. Further, following motor nerve stimula-on, the evoked end-plate potentials were frequently of sub-threshold amplitude. As would be expected of an abnormal release mechanism, the blocking effect of neomycin could be overcome by increasing the external calcium concentration. The same authors also demonstrated a relatively mild postsynaptic action of the drug, in that neomycin decreased the sensitivity of the muscle fibre membrane to applied acetylcholine.

QUANTAL SQUANDER MYOKYMIA

(Isaac's syndrome, Continuous muscle fibre activity, Neuromyotonia, Myokymia with impaired muscular relaxation, Pseudomyotonia and myokymia)

Clinical features

The conditions described so far in this chapter have all been characterized by a depression of neuromuscular transmission. In the syndrome termed 'quantal squander' the problem is the reverse, for the axon terminals appear to be spontaneously hyperexcitable. This fascinating but rare disorder was probably described by Schultze (1895) but much of the recent interest in the syndrome stems from the description by Harman and Richardson (1954). The patient reported by these authors was a 58-year-old woman with generalized and continuously-undulating movements of her face, tongue, limbs and trunk. The patient had lost weight and sweated profusely; since she also exhibited a tachycardia and had a raised basal metabolic rate, a diagnosis of thyrotoxicosis was made. With increasing experience of the syndrome, it has become apparent that thyrotoxic symptoms and signs are present in about half of these cases. These clinical features are misleading, for although the basal metabolic rate is raised, specific laboratory investigations of thyrotoxicosis are invariably negative (Gamstorp and Wohlfart, 1959; Isaacs, 1964). Irrespective of the presence or absence of the hypermetabolic features, the best treatment for the excessive muscle activity appears to be diphenylhydantoin (100 mg, three times daily) or carbamazepine (250 mg, four times daily; see Wallis, Poznak and Plum, 1970). A description of a patient with this condition, who subsequently developed myasthenia gravis, is given in Appendix 19.1.

Special studies

Electromyography

Recordings from the affected muscles with coaxial needle electrodes reveal trains of action potentials which, on the basis of small amplitudes and brief durations, are likely to have been generated by single muscle fibres. The discharges characteristically increase and decrease in frequency over a period of several seconds, the maximum rate being about 100 Hz. Sometimes runs of larger and more complex potentials, suggestive of motor unit activity, are seen as well; fasciculation potentials may also be observed. Isaacs (1961) delineated the site of origin of the spontaneous activity by showing that it persisted during general anaesthesia and also following local nerve block; in contrast the activity was abolished by curare and succinylcholine. These results incriminated the motor nerve endings as the site of the lesion but in a patient studied by Wallis, Poznak and Plum (1970) it appeared that some of the spontaneous discharges were arising centrally since a local anaesthetic nerve block reduced, but did not abolish, the muscle activity.

As yet there have been no reports of micro electrode studies in this condition but Isaacs (1964) has nevertheless suggested that the fundamental defect is an excessive spontaneous release of acetylcholine from the nerve endings.

Morphological studies

Muscle biopsy may reveal scattered atrophic fibres (Gamstorp and Wohlfart, 1959) or may be normal (Wallis, Poznak and Plum, 1970). Williamson and Brooke (1972) used the glycogen depletion technique to identify muscle fibres which had participated in the spontaneous activity and the distribution of the fibres suggested that individual motor units had been active.

TOXINS AND THE NEUROMUSCULAR JUNCTION

(A) BACTERIAL NEUROTOXINS

Botulism

Clinical features

The toxins produced by the bacterium, *Clostridium botulinum,* remain the most powerful yet known to man, as little as 0.5 μg of toxin A being fatal. The bacterium is anaerobic and is to be found in soil as well as in animal faeces. Poisoning is fortunately uncommon and usually results from the improper canning or bottling of food; if heat sterilization has been insufficient the spores persist in the food and then germinate in the anaerobic environment. Symptoms of poisoning appear within 48 hours of ingestion of the toxin; initially they consist of double vision (diplopia) and unsteadiness on standing. Subsequently the lower cranial nerves are affected, producing paralysis of speech and swallowing. Unless treatment is available death occurs from respiratory paralysis within a few days. Until the end the patient is fully conscious and is without any disorder of sensation.

Treatment consists of artificial ventilation and is also directed at the cardiac failure which may sometimes develop early in the course of the disease. The most useful drug is undoubtedly guanidine (Cherington and Ryan, 1968) with anticholinesterase and germine monoacetate (Cherington, 1973) also being worthy of trial. Antitoxin should be administered even though there is no convincing evidence that it is effective once paralysis has developed.

Special studies

Electrophysiological investigations

Electromyography reveals small evoked muscle responses following nerve stimulation although the muscle can be shown to respond normally to direct stimulation. Repeating the nerve stimulation at low rates (e.g. 2 Hz) causes further decrement in the muscle responses whereas rapid stimulation (at 50 Hz) produces potentiation; this pattern of behaviour resembles that found in the Eaton–Lambert syndrome (see above and also Cherington, 1973). Measurements of impulse conduction velocity in motor axons are normal. Together, these findings indicate that the paralysis results from a failure of neuromuscular transmission and this is also the conclusion to be drawn from a number of similar studies conducted on animals (see, for example, Guyton and MacDonald, 1947; Burgen, Dickens and Zatmann, 1949).

Microelectrode investigations have been invaluable in elucidating the nature of the transmission defect and, of these studies, that by Harris and Miledi (1971) in the frog appears definitive. The finding of spontaneously occurring m.e.p.p.s indicated to these workers that transmitter was available within the axon terminal and that there was no loss of postsynaptic responsiveness. However, although the nerve impulse still invaded the axon terminal during the phase of paralysis, none of the available transmitter could be released.

Morphological investigations

Harris and Miledi (1971; see above) were able to confirm the earlier observations of Thesleff (1960) that the completely-blocked neuromuscular junction had a normal ultrastructure, as seen with the electronmicroscope. After several days the nerve fibre underwent an important alteration by developing sprouts from the terminal. In the mouse Duchen (1970a) used a combination of cholinesterase staining and silver impregnation to demonstrate that the onset of the sprouting varied among muscles. In the soleus sprouts could be found by the seventh day after local injection of toxin whereas a further 2 weeks elapsed before they were evident in the superficial parts of gastrocnemius. In both muscles some of the terminal sprouts developed into new neuromuscular junctions while the original end-plates could disappear (*Figure 20.2*). Duchen also showed that muscle fibre atrophy developed earlier in the soleus but recovered sooner and was not as profound as that in the gastrocnemius. Interestingly, recovery of muscle function occurred sooner if a nerve was crushed and thereby stimulated to regenerate and form new neuromuscular junctions (Thesleff, Zelená and Hofmann, 1964; Duchen, 1970b).

From electrophysiological and morphological studies it is evident that botulinum toxin blocks the trophic action of nerve on muscle (page 72) in addition to synaptic transmission. Thus, not only are the muscle fibres paralysed but they also display such features as (*a*) a spread of the sensitivity of the membrane to acetylcholine (Josefsson and Thesleff, 1961); (*b*) atrophy with centralization of myonuclei (Duchen, 1970a); and (*c*) an ability to accept a new innervation.

Tetanus

Clinical features

Tetanus is a neurological illness produced by a toxin or toxins formed by the bacterium *Clostridium tetani*. The bacterium is an anaerobe, being found in the soil and in the intestines and faeces of animals. Although unusual mechanisms of infection have been described, in most cases the illness results from contamination of a wound with bacterial spores; these then germinate and the bacilli release their toxins into the bloodstream. Symptoms develop after an incubation period varying from 2 to as many as 100 days. The first symptoms are those of restlessness and of involuntary clenching of the jaw due to intermittent, painless, spasm of the masseter muscles. The spasms then become more frequent and spread to involve other muscles; the limbs stiffen and the back arches (opisthotonos) while retraction of the corners of the mouth produces a grimace (risus sardonicus). The spasms may be precipitated by any disturbance in the environment of the patient such as a sudden noise, a touch or a flash of light; the spasms become increasingly painful and incomplete relaxation occurs between successive episodes. Unless treated, severely infected patients will die from heart failure, asphyxia, bronchopneumonia or simply 'exhaustion'.

The best *treatment* is preventative, by immunizing against the toxin in infancy with an antigenically active but otherwise inert preparation (toxoid). A further dose of toxoid can be given after receipt of any wound likely to be contaminated by the tetanus bacillus. In cases not previously immunized, treatment consists of wound cleansing, the administration of antitoxin (not toxoid) and antibiotics. In addition the patient should be sedated and there are advantages in preventing muscle spasms by the use of muscle relaxants, combined with tracheostomy and positive pressure ventilation.

Special studies

The tetanus toxin has actions on both the peripheral and the central nervous systems; of these the latter action is the more important, being responsible for the spasms. By recording intra-cellularly from motoneurones of cats injected with toxin, Brooks, Curtis and Eccles (1957) were able to show that the postsynaptic inhibition normally mediated by the Renshaw cells had been removed from the motoneurones, so that the latter cells became hyperexcitable.

The action of the toxin on the peripheral nervous system, although not clinically important, is never-theless of interest and it also serves as a model for understanding the mechanisms of the central action of the toxin. The peripheral effect of the toxin is to cause a paralysis and, on the basis of gross recordings with coaxial electrodes from muscles of cats treated with toxin, Harvey (1939) concluded that the neuromuscular junction was the site of action. The nature of the blocking action has been extended by the use of microelectrodes to record intracellularly from muscle fibres in the region of the neuromuscular junctions (for example, Parsons, Hofmann and Feigin, 1966; Kaeser and Saner, 1970; Mellanby and Thompson, 1972). By comparing the sizes of the miniature end-plate

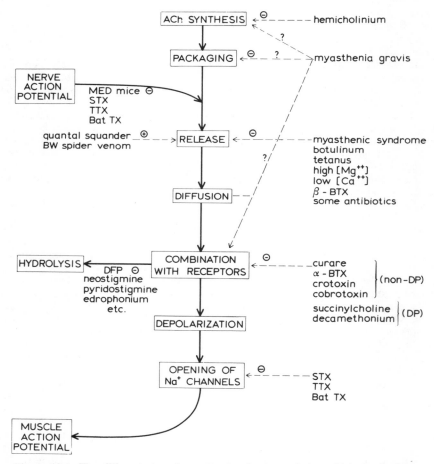

Figure 19.4. The different steps in neuromuscular transmission which can be inter-fered with; details given in text. Bat TX, batrachatoxin; BTX, bungarotoxin; BW, black widow; DFP, difluorophosphate; MED, motor end-plate disease; STX, saxi-tonin; TTX, tetrodotoxin. Depolarizing and non-depolarizing compounds indicated by DP and non-DP respectively. Depression of a step shown by (−), enhancement by (+)

potentials and the responses to nerve stimulation, these authors have agreed that there is a failure on the part of the axon terminals to release the transmitter available. This defect resembles that caused by botulinum toxin (see above) which is, of course, produced by a closely-related bacillus. As in botulism poisoning, there is a loss of neurotrophic action as well as of synaptic transmission; after a few days of paralysis fibrillation potentials and positive sharp waves can be recorded from affected muscles (Prabhu and Oester, 1962). Duchen, Stolkin and Tonge (1972) have shown a further similarity to botulinum intoxication in that the nerve endings of muscles paralysed by tetanus toxin develop sprouts, some of which form new neuromuscular junctions. These authors found that the soleus muscles of mice were much more susceptible to the paralytic action of tetanus toxin than the extensor digitorum longus muscles, an observation presumably related to morphological differences between the neuromuscular junctions in the two muscles (Duchen, 1971). Duchen, Stolkin and Tonge (1972) also noted degenerative changes in the soleus muscle fibres including disruption of the Z-lines, disorganization of myofilaments and the presence of tubular aggregates and abnormal mitochondria.

ANIMAL NEUROTOXINS

In addition to the two bacterial toxins already considered, there are a number of neurotoxins produced by certain animal species. These neurotoxins differ in the mechanisms by which the paralysis is produced, both pre- and post-synaptic actions being employed. In the list given below the sources of the toxin are given in parentheses (*Figure 19.4*).

(I) Presynaptic action
   (*a*) Acetylcholine release blocked
      β-bungarotoxin (the banded krait snake)
   (*b*) Acetylcholine supply exhausted
      Venom of the black widow spider
(II) Postsynaptic action
   Combination with acetylcholine receptors, causing non-depolarizing block
      α-bungarotoxin (branded krait)
      Cobrotoxin (cobra)
      Crotoxin (rattlesnake)
(III) Pre- and post-synaptic actions
   Combination with sodium carriers, causing block of action potentials
   (*a*) No depolarization possible
      Tetrodotoxin (Japanese puffer fish)
      Saxitonin (the flagellate, *Gonyaulax catanella*)
   (*b*) Depolarizing block
      Batrachatoxin (a Columbian species of frog)

Interestingly, the frog *Phyllobates aurotaenia*, which secretes batrachatoxin from its skin, is quite impervious to the toxin whereas the neuromuscular junctions of other species of frog are readily affected (Albuquerque *et al.*, 1973).

DISORDERS OF NERVE FIBRES

The structure of the axon was described in Chapter 2 and an account of the way in which impulses are transmitted along its length was given in Chapter 3. The importance of axoplasmic flow as a bi-directional signalling system operating between the motoneurone soma, axon and muscle fibre, was emphasized in Chapters 2, 8, 9 and 10. With this information in mind, it is now appropriate to study disorders of nerve fibres. These disorders range from transient interference with impulse conduction, which is characteristic of the neurapraxic lesion, to complete destruction of the axon, as after severe mechanical injury. In between these two extremes are the demyelinating disorders (Chapter 21) in which the Schwann cell and its membranes suffer the major pathological injury.

Chapter 20

WALLERIAN DEGENERATION AND FIBRE REGENERATION

If a nerve fibre is cut or crushed, degenerative changes take place in the part of the fibre which has become separated from the cell body of the neurone. In addition the tissue formerly supplied by the nerve undergoes alteration. For example, a denervated region of skin becomes cold, shiny, atrophic and loses hair. In the case of muscle the degenerative events are equally profound and have been discussed elsewhere in relation to the trophic interactions of nerve and muscle (Chapter 8). The purpose of the present chapter is to describe in detail the structural and functional changes which occur in the axon itself after injury. It will be shown that the main trunk of a motor axon differs rather sharply from the axon terminals in the onset and speed of the response to nerve section. Partly for this reason and partly on account of their contrasting functions, the trunk and termination of the axon will be analysed separately in relation to their degeneration processes. A later section of the chapter deals with the remarkable regenerative capacity of the motor axons which, in successful instances, enables them to make new synaptic connections with the muscle fibres.

DEGENERATION OF THE AXON TRUNK (WALLERIAN DEGENERATION)

It is of considerable interest that, at a time when neuromuscular transmission has completely failed (see below), the distal nerve stump still remains capable of initiating and propagating action potentials following electrical stimulation. In the rat usually 24 hr or so elapse after section before electrical activity is impaired and about 80 hr before all the axons become inexcitable. In man and in the baboon impulse conduction in some fibres may persist for as long as 200 hr (Gilliatt and Hjorth, 1972). When the axon commences to break up the process is termed *Wallerian degeneration*, in recognition of Waller (1850) who, many years ago, decribed in detail the changes visible under the light microscope. The observations of Waller have since been confirmed on many occasions and, in addition, the detailed nature of the degenerative changes have been studied with the electronmicroscope; a good recent account is that given by Williams and Hall (1971a, b).

One of the earliest changes is *retraction of myelin* at the *nodes of Ranvier;* this process spreads along the distal stump from the site of the injury and by 1 hr may have involved 20 mm or so of axon. Within the next few hours the nodes show other evidence of increased metabolic activity in the accumulation of mitochondria and lysosomes. At 24 hr the degenerative changes within the *axon cylinder* are well advanced with disruption of the neurotubules, endoplasmic reticulum and neurofilaments being clearly visible. Another early change, already visible within a few minutes of the nerve lesion, is extreme dilatation of the Schmidt–Lanterman incisures (page 12).

The myelin sheath, having already withdrawn slightly at the nodes of Ranvier, now begins to break up with the lamellae peeling off at the

221

nodes. Both at the nodes and at the dilated Schmidt–Lanterman incisures the axons undergo progressive constriction; eventually a series of large 'primary' ellipsoids are formed, each being bounded by the degenerating myelin sheath and cut off from the remainder of the axon. In time the primary ellipsoids become partitioned internally by unfolding of the myelin sheath, while at the ends of the ellipsoids small globules of degenerating myelin become pinched off.

The *Schwann cells* become highly active during the degenerative process, first spreading over the denuded nodes of Ranvier and then undergoing mitotic division so as to form a maximum number of cells at about 15–25 days. The Schwann cells hasten the disintegration of the myelin sheath and engulf some of the lipid droplets. It is probable that a proportion of these cells are transformed into macrophages; however, autoradiographic studies have shown that the majority of macrophages are carried to the degenerating nerve in the bloodstream (Olsson and Sjöstrand, 1969). These haematogenous cells are first seen at about 3 days following the lesion and they are especially active in removing the degenerating myelin. With the passage of time the lipid-laden cells appear to migrate from the endoneurial spaces toward the periphery of the nerve trunk.

If the axon has been crushed rather than cut, the surrounding basement membrane will remain intact and act as a scaffolding for the columns of dividing Schwann cells (bands of Bungner).

DEGENERATION OF THE AXON TERMINAL

It is an interesting observation that, after an axon has been divided, the first severe degenerative changes are seen at the neuromuscular junction rather than in the separated stump of axon. The onset of the changes in the axon terminal depend on two factors; these are the length of the distal stump of axon and the species of animal affected. Miledi and Slater (1970) studied the effect of stump length in the rat by cutting the phrenic nerve either as close as possible to the diaphragm or else in the neck. They found that, when the nerve was divided distally, about 8 hr elapsed before there was any evidence of neuromuscular degeneration in the diaphragm. When the greater length of nerve was left the onset of neuromuscular failure was delayed by approximately 1 hr for each 1.5 cm of axon remaining. This intriguing relationship between the length of the nerve stump and the onset of denervation phenomena is of great significance for an understanding of the nature

of the neurotrophic controlling system (page 85). As already stated, the onset of end-plate failure also depends on the species studied, being much later in man and the baboon than in a smaller mammal such as the rat (Table 20.1). Once the degenerative changes start, however, they proceed rapidly and only 3–5 hr are required for complete disruption of the end-plate. During this time the synaptic vesicles form clumps; the mitochondria swell and their cristae break up into small vesicular pieces; membrane whorls and glycogen bags appear in the axoplasm and lysosomes become evident. At this stage the whole end-plate may become fragmented; meanwhile the Schwann cell sends a cytoplasmic process into the primary synaptic cleft and then completely envelops the degenerating end-plate. It is probable that the Schwann cell assists in the final dissolution of the end-plate. Subsequently the Schwann cell withdraws and, after a month or so, only the sole-plate is left of the original neuromuscular junction.

The electrophysiological behaviour of the end-plate parallels the morphological changes described above. For the first 8 hr or more, depending on the nerve stump length, there is the usual spontaneous discharge of miniature end-plate potentials and electrical stimulation of the axon results in normal neuromuscular transmission. From these observations it would appear that the synaptic vesicles contain normal numbers of acetylcholine molecules and that there is no impediment to the mobilization and release of transmitter from the vesicles. After this latent period is over neuromuscular function fails abruptly; the miniature potentials cease and no postsynaptic response can be detected following nerve stimulation.

NERVE REGENERATION

If an axon is divided and viewed under the microscope axoplasm can be seen to bulge out of the end of the central stump. This extruded material probably reflects the continuing slow flow of axoplasm from the cell body which was originally discovered by Weiss (see Chapter 2). After a few minutes the extrusion ceases, possibly because some of the myelin lamellae have slipped over each other and sealed the exposed end of the cut axon. The end of the fibre now gradually swells; initially this is the result of degenerative changes but the later distension is due to the formation of a growth cone. The changes which subsequently take place in the growth cone have been described with memorable clarity by Cajal (1928) who has also summarized much of the earlier work in this field. In most of Cajal's studies the regenerating fibres had been stained with silver; his drawings are not only elegant but they display his findings in remarkable detail, especially when it is remembered that all the observations were made with an ordinary light microscope. Within 24 hr of nerve section the growing axons were seen to have penetrated into the exudate produced by the wound; sometimes the dilated endings remained single but in other instances they divided into two or more processes. In some of the nerve fibres additional sprouts formed at a distance from the cut end by arising

Sunderland (1947) was able to make observations on the recovery of nerve function in injured military personnel; he noted that the speed of nerve growth depended not only on the time after injury but also on the site of the lesion, being highest after a proximal wound. For example, in the thigh and upper arm the average rate was about 3 mm/day whereas in the hand and foot values of only 0.5 mm/day were observed. Another factor influencing nerve regeneration is a history of previous injury for in such cases recovery is less

TABLE 20.1
Time to Conduction Failure Distal to Nerve Section

Species	Nerve	Time to failure (hr)	Authors
Nerve trunk			
Rabbit	peroneal (lat. popliteal)	71–78	Gutmann and Holubar (1950)
Rat	peroneal (lat. popliteal)	79–81	Gutmann and Holubar (1950)
Guinea pig	peroneal (lat. popliteal)	72–82	Gutmann and Holubar (1950)
Cat	sciatic	72–101	Rosenblueth and Dempsey (1939)
Dog	phrenic	96	Erlanger and Schloepfle (1946)
Baboon	lateral popliteal	120–216	Gilliatt and Hjorth (1972)
Nerve muscle			
Rabbit	peroneal (lat. popliteal)	30–32	Gutmann and Holubar (1952)
Rat	sciatic	24–36	Miledi and Slater (1970)
Guinea pig	sciatic	40–45	Kaeser and Lambert (1962)
Cat	sciatic	69–79	Lissak, Dempsey, and Rosenblueth (1939)
Man	median, ulnar*	85–128	Landau (1953)
Man	facial	120–192	Gilliatt and Taylor (1959)
Baboon	lateral popliteal	96–144	Gilliatt and Hjorth (1972)

* From observation of muscle twitch—no electrical recording. Reproduced from Gilliatt and Hjorth (1972) courtesy of the authors and the Editor and publishers of the *Journal of Neurology, Neurosurgery and Psychiatry*.

from nodes of Ranvier. Recent studies with the electronmicroscope have shown that the growing nerve endings (*growth cones*) are rich in mitochondria, vesicles, dense bodies and lamellar figures. Initially the growth cones are free of surrounding Schwann cell cytoplasm but if they encounter the peripheral nerve stump they will grow preferentially down the tubes formed by the Schwann cells of the stump (*bands of Bungner*). The rate of axon growth was also studied by Cajal, though only approximate values could be given. More recent investigators have agreed that growth is at first slow but subsequently quickens. Gutmann *et al.* (1942) calculated an average velocity of 4.3 mm/day during a period between 13 and 25 days following nerve crush. Jacobsen and Guth (1965) measured the extent of regeneration by stimulating the nerve at the site of crush and attempting to record the compound action potential at different positions in a distal direction. They found that the rate of growth increased until it had reached 3.0 mm/day by the 18th day. In man,

complete; Thomas (1970) has shown that the Schwann cells divide to form large groups associated with multiple axons of varying diameters.

Once the regenerating axons reach the denervated muscle, the endings appear to seek out the sites of the old end-plates in order to establish new neuromuscular junctions. This situation does not arise simply because the axons have been guided back by the peripheral nerve stump; even if the axons are forced to take other pathways they will still run along the denervated muscle fibre until the old end-plate is found (Bennett, McLachlan and Taylor, 1973). Under special circumstances, however, junctions can be made to form outside the original synaptic zone (see below). Once an axon has established successful synaptic connections with the previously denervated muscle, the diameter of the axis cylinder increases (Aitken, Sharman and Young, 1947).

In studies on the regeneration of sciatic nerves in dogs Schröder (1972) found that the myelin

sheath also became thicker, though to a lesser
extent than the axis cylinder. Thus at 12 months
after suture the mean diameter of the axis cylinder
was 79 per cent of normal while that of the myelin
sheath was only 57 per cent. Since the speed of
impulse propagation is directly proportional to
the diameter of the axis cylinder and is also

COLLATERAL REINNERVATION

There is another way in which the nerve supply
a muscle can be restored but this mechanism
only applicable in instances in which the dene
vation has been incomplete. In this type
reinnervation the surviving healthy axons for

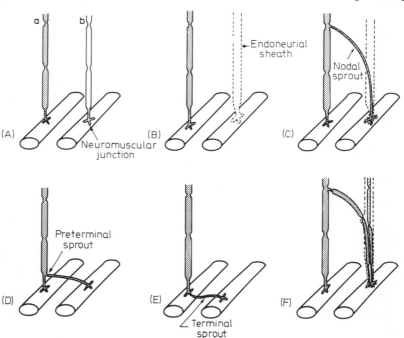

*Figure 20.1. Different types of collateral reinnervation. In (A), axon b is about to
undergo Wallerian degeneration while axon a remains healthy. In (B), the degeneration of b has taken place, leaving the endoneurial sheath intact. In (C) the denervated muscle fibre has been innervated by a nodal sprout from a, which has entered
and followed the endoneurial sheath. In (D) the axon branch has arisen from a prior
to the neuromuscular junction while in (E) the sprout has formed from the terminal
axon expansion. In (F) axon b has regenerated so that the previously denervated
muscle fibre is now supplied by two motoneurones, the respective axons sharing the
same endoneurial sheath*

dependent on the insulating properties of the
myelin sheath (page 239) low values would be
expected in regenerated nerves. In the study by
Hodes, Larrabee and German (1948) values as low
as 50–60 per cent of normal were found in human
nerves 3–4 years after repair by suture. Rather
higher, but still reduced, values were noted in a
recent study by Ballantyne and Campbell (1973)
which included observations on both sensory and
motor fibres. A further change in the appearance
of the new axons is that the nodes of Ranvier are
situated closer together, though in an irregular
manner; this alteration is caused by the proliferation of Schwann cells which takes place during
nerve regeneration (see also page 222).

sprouts which grow across to denervated muscl
fibres in their vicinity and form new neuro
muscular junctions. The sprouts commonly grow
out from the nodes of Ranvier of the health
axon (*nodal sprouts*) but they can also arise
distally, either from the neuromuscular junctio
itself (*terminal sprout*) or from the region o
motor axon immediately in front of it (*pre- o
sub-terminal sprout*). These three branchin
systems are all examples of collateral reinnerva
tion (*Figure 20.1*). The existence of this type o
innervation was first postulated by Exner (1885) i
order to explain the absence of degeneration i
the rabbit cricothyroid muscle following its partia
denervation. Much later, interest in collatera

innervation was revived by the experiments of
eiss and Edds (1945) in the rat in which partial
enervation of leg muscles had been effected by
viding ventral roots entering the lumbosacral
exus. Using a similar preparation, Hoffman
950a) subsequently showed that a nodal sprout
ight sometimes enter the endoneurial tube vacated
 a degenerating axon and follow it down to the
iginal end-plate zone. The importance of
llateral reinnervation lies in the fact that not
ily is it a very powerful compensatory mechanism
it that it is also an extremely common pheno-
enon in neuromuscular diseases. Evidence of its
esence is found in almost every case of partial
enervation, irrespective of aetiology; thus, it is to
 seen in patients with 'central' disorders such as
otoneurone disease and the metabolic and toxic
ying-back' neuropathies (page 274), as well as in
atients with trauma to peripheral nerves. It must
it be imagined that axonal regeneration and
llateral reinnervation are mutually exclusive
covery processes. On the contrary, they occur
multaneously whenever muscle denervation has
en incomplete. Thus, while damaged axons (or
e axons of previously 'sick' motoneurones;
ige 113) are growing back towards the muscle, the
tact axons of healthy motoneurones are already
routing and undertaking collateral reinnervation.

erminal sprouting

erminal sprouting has already been considered as
ie of the mechanisms by which an axon can
idertake collateral reinnervation of a denervated
uscle fibre in its vicinity. The process has a
irther significance, however, in that it enables
motoneurone to either renew or else enlarge exist-
g synaptic connections with its own colony of
uscle fibres. As a result of terminal sprouting
ie new fine axon twigs ramify on the surface of
ie muscle fibre and enlarge the territory of the
id-plate; at the same time the terminal axonic
xpansions are often swollen. From their great
xperience with methylene blue staining Cöers and
Joolf (1959; see also Woolf and Cöers, 1974)
ave provided many examples of the bizarre and
storted innervations which can result. The same
ithors have shown that similar patterns can result
om a variety of nerve and muscle diseases. They
e to be found, for example, in disorders of the
uromuscular junction such as myasthenia gravis,
 myopathies such as dystrophia myotonica and
yotonia congenita, in peripheral neuropathies and
so in less-clearly defined disorders such as ageing
id thyrotoxicosis. In addition particularly clear
:amples of terminal sprouting have been observed

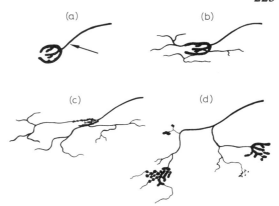

Figure 20.2. Remodelling of muscle fibre innervation
following terminal sprouting, as seen in mouse soleus
muscle fibres after the injection of botulinum toxin
(see text). (From Duchen 1970a, courtesy of the
author, and the Editor and publishers of Journal of
Neurology, Neurosurgery and Psychiatry)

by Duchen and his colleagues (Duchen, 1970a, b;
Duchen, Stolkin and Tonge, 1972) in muscles
poisoned with botulinum or tetanus toxins. The
first evidence of sprouting can be seen as early
as 6 days after the injection of botulinum toxin
into soleus muscles of mice and well before any
degenerative changes are visible in the motor nerve
terminals. *Figure 20.2* and the accompanying
description is reproduced from Duchen's (1970a)
paper. In (*a*) the figure shows a normal nerve ending with a single preterminal axon (arrowed)
innervating the end-plate. Terminal sprouting (*b*)
develops after neuromuscular transmission has
been blocked by the toxin. The nerve sprouts grow
in all direction and branch while the original end-
plate may disappear (*c*). New nerve terminals are
then formed randomly on some of the nerve
sprouts (*d*). It can be seen that the nerve fibres
which were at first terminal sprouts in (*b*) have
now become branched preterminal axons in (*d*).

Having now dealt with the main features of the
neural response to muscle denervation it is
appropriate to consider some of the underlying
phenomena in more detail.

THE STIMULUS FOR NERVE SPROUTING

So far no attention has been given to two of the
most fascinating problems in neurobiology. First,
what is the stimulus which causes an axon to sprout
and, secondly, how do the sprouts find their way
to the denervated muscles fibres? At present it is
not possible to answer either of these questions

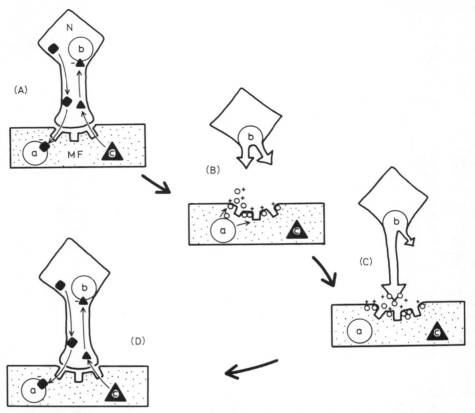

Figure 20.3. Postulated mechanism for axon regeneration and muscle fibre reinnervation following nerve section. In the intact nerve-muscle preparation (A) the sprouting 'apparatus' (b) of the motoneurone (N) is inhibited by centripetal delivery of molecular signals from (c) in the muscle fibre (MF). Similarly (a) in the muscle fibre is prevented from secreting axon-attracting molecules by centrifugal inhibition from the motoneurone. In (B), the axon has been sectioned; (b) is no longer repressed and starts to produce axon sprouts while (a), also unrestrained, secretes attractants which will guide an axon sprout to the site of the original end-plate (C). Once the motor axon has re-established a successful neuromuscular connection, the mutual inhibiting mechanism is reimposed (D)

satisfactorily but it is nevertheless instructive to review some of the experimental observations which must ultimately be incorporated into an acceptable hypothesis.

It is convenient to begin by considering the nature of the stimulus which initiates the sprouting at the central end of a divided nerve fibre. In this situation a signal from the denervated muscle cannot be involved since sprouting will still occur even if the nerve is cut at a distance from the affected muscles. For example, if the sciatic nerve is cut in mid-thigh sprouting will still take place although the central nerve stump is surrounded by the still-innervated hamstring muscles and is at a considerable distance from the denervated muscle fibres below the knee. An alternative suggestion is that

the nerve is stimulated to sprout by some factor(s) released by the degenerating peripheral stump. Yet this is also unlikely for sprouting continues at the cut central end of the nerve after the peripheral stump has been removed. Furthermore Cajal (1928) and others before him had found impossible to induce sprouting in intact axons by placing a length of degenerating nerve in their vicinity.

A third hypothesis seems more attractive than either of the preceding ones. It suggests that the sprouting from the central end of a cut axon takes place because the motoneurone is no longer receiving instructions 'not-to-sprout' from the muscle (*Figure 20.3*). A carrier for such instructions would be the centripetal flow of axoplasm hich is now known to exist. Furthermore (as escribed in Chapter 10) the surge in production of ibosomal RNA in the nucleolus of the moto- eurone occurs sooner if the axon has been ivided close to the cell body. This observation ould be interpreted to mean that the synthesis of rotein, which would be necessary for axonal prouting, is normally repressed by a factor ravelling in the axon toward the motoneurone oma.

What, then, is the role of the peripheral nerve tump in the regeneration process? Although, as lready seen, the degenerating nerve fibres are not ssential for initiating the sprouting reaction, they re valuable nonetheless for the columns of chwann cells provide a favourable pathway for he sprouts to follow. Electronmicrographs reveal hat the growing axons eventually become encircled y extensions of Schwann cell cytoplasm and that myelin sheath is then laid down (see also age 11). Initially there is an over-production of prouts such that these greatly outnumber the ransected axons. As a consequence there may be nore than one sprout in a single Schwann cell ube but with time the situation resolves so that nly one motor axis cylinder usually survives. To Cajal's eyes (Cajal, 1928) the peripheral stump ppeared to be more than a passive guidance system or in his preparations the sprouting fibres took outes which suggested that they were attracted to he stump. He also noted that the attractive property of the stump was lost if it was dried, oiled in water or treated with chloroform or ormalin; it therefore appeared to depend on the itality of the Schwann cells. Whether or not Cajal's deductions are correct, there can be no loubt as to the importance of the peripheral stump n nerve repair. If reunion with the stump is prevented in an experimental animal, or if it fails o take place in a patient because the cut ends of he nerve have become displaced, the axon sprouts ;row in a disorderly manner, often turning back on hemselves. This ramification of the axons and the ttendant proliferation of Schwann cells gives rise o a swelling, or *neuroma*, at the end of the nerve.

This account of nerve sprouting is still incom- plete for it does not explain how collateral einnervation is set in motion or how the sprouts re guided to the original end-plate regions of the lenervated muscle fibres. It will be recalled that n collateral reinnervation axonal sprouts arise rom healthy axons, either at the nodes of Ranvier or else at the motor endings. If the third ypothesis (above) is correct the motoneurone will till be receiving instructions not to sprout from he muscle fibres of its own intact motor unit. These instructions must now be over-ridden by a powerful chemical signal given off from the denervated muscle fibres. This signal must be strongest at the old end-plate regions since this is the part of the fibre to which the sprouts will be attracted (*Figure 20.3*). A satisfactory hypo- thesis must also explain why the sprouting ceases once reinnervation of the muscle fibre has been accomplished. The most likely reason is that the stimulus for sprouting given by the muscle fibre has now been repressed by the successful moto- neurone. From studies of cross-innervated avian muscle by Bennett and Pettigrew (1974b) it seems probable that the strength of this repressive influence will depend on the type of motoneurone involved. These authors suggest that avian moto- neurones supplying 'slow twitch' muscles exert a relatively weak influence which permits the muscle fibre to accept further innervation at about 200 μm intervals down its length. In this way the distributed *en grappe* innervation characteristic of this type of muscle is formed during normal development.

There are only negative observations as to the nature of the factors released by the muscle fibre which stimulates the axon sprouts to form and to grow toward the fibre. Clearly the factor cannot have come from Schwann cells for these may already have withdrawn from the site of the old end-plate before the new axonal sprouts arrive. Nor is junctional cholinesterase likely to be involved for reinnervation still proceeds if the enzyme is inactivated by DFP (Filogamo and Gabella, 1966). Since *d*-tubocurarine and α-bunga- rotoxin are also ineffective in preventing reinnervation, the presence of functioning ACh receptors cannot be a necessary condition for synaptogenesis either (Cohen, 1972; Van Essen and Jansen, 1974). According to Jansen and col- leagues (1973) continuous electrical stimulation of muscle fibres will prevent reinnervation but this is true only for membrane situated at a distance from the original end-plate zone; there is also the dis- ruptive effect of the incessant mechanical activity to take into consideration.

As stated at the onset, none of the answers to the fundamental problems in nerve regeneration and muscle reinnervation is evident at the present time. It must be agreed, however, that the field is a fascinating one and that the eventual solutions are likely to have considerable therapeutic impact.

POLYNEURONAL INNERVATION OR SUPPRESSED SYNAPSES?

In normal mammalian extrafusal muscle each fibre is innervated by only one motoneurone. Consider, however, a partially denervated muscle

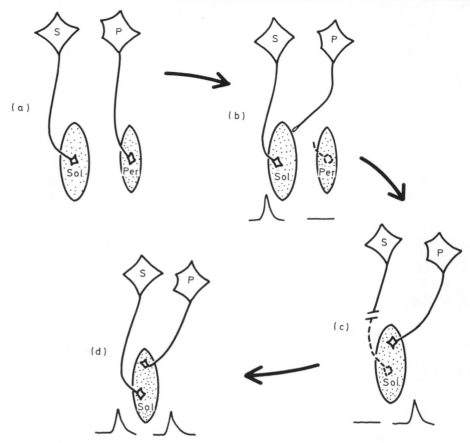

Figure 20.4. Hyperinnervation experiment (a) shows the normal soleus (SOL) and peroneal muscles (PER) with their corresponding motoneurones (S and P respectively). In (b) the peroneal nerve has been cut and the central stump applied to the soleus; no innervation takes place (note absent twitch response below). If the soleus nerve is now divided or crushed, as in (c), the peroneal nerve rapidly forms neuromuscular junctions on the soleus muscle. If the soleus nerve is now allowed to grow back, many muscle fibres will acquire a double innervation (d). (Based on studies of Fex et al. (1966) and others; see text)

in which the twin phenomena of axon regeneration and collateral reinnervation proceed together. What happens if a regenerating axon returns to a muscle fibre which, through collateral reinnervation, has already formed a synapse with a foreign motoneurone? This situation is likely to arise in those disorders in which the peripheral nerve fibre stump is left in continuity even though the axis cylinder has degenerated. It will occur, for example, after a nerve crush or following motoneurone recovery from the 'dying-back' type of neuropathy. In man the observations are few and will be presented later (Chapter 25) but in animals the situation is rather better for several investigations have been directed to this problem. The critical experimental

manœuvres and observations may be summarize in the following way.

First of all, provided the original innervation to muscle is left intact, that muscle is unable to accep further innervation from a foreign nerve (Elsber; 1917). Once the original nerve supply is inte. rupted, either by cutting, crushing or the applica tion of botulinum toxin, the muscle will form ne\ neuromuscular junctions with a foreign nerv presented to it (Fex, Sonnesson and Theslef 1966; Figure 20.4). Curiously, the avidity wit which the foreign nerve is received varies amon muscles, for while the soleus will readily accep innervation from the nerve to extensor digitoru longus (EDL), the latter muscle forms functionin

:uromuscular synapses with the soleus nerve only
ith difficulty (Hoh, 1975). This finding may
flect a general difference between fast-twitch
uscles, like EDL, and slow-twitch muscles, such
 the soleus—upon which most experiments in this
:ld have been conducted.

An extension of this type of experiment has
:en to denervate the rat soleus and to allow it to
ccept a foreign nerve; if the original nerve is now
lowed to grow back to the muscle it is able to
-establish synaptic connections with a large pro-
ortion of fibres, even though these fibres
ready have an ectopic innervation from the
reign nerve. In the study by Frank et al. (1974)
e proportion of doubly innervated fibres in the
uscle was relatively high, being as much as 57 per
nt after a nerve crush. In Tonge's (1974) pre-
ninary report no percentages are given but it is
·ident that some of the newly formed synapses
ith the original nerve remain inactive unless the
reign innervation is interfered with. However,
)th studies clearly show that, under certain cir-
imstances, it is possible to have two functional
napses on the same muscle fibre.

The next question is whether the double innerva-
)n persists, for in embryonic and neonatal muscle
)res of mammals any accessory innervation is
timately rejected (see page 95). There is also
·idence from cross-innervation experiments on
e extraocular muscles of fish that foreign
nervation ceases over a period of two days after
e original nerve supply has been re-established
Iarotte and Mark, 1970); however, the results of
cent single muscle fibre studies on this type of
eparation are at variance with this interpreta-
)n (Scott, 1975). So far as mammalian muscles
e concerned, most of the evidence available is
·mly in favour of the persistence of foreign
napses without any suppression by restoration of
e original nerve supply (Fex et al., 1966; Tonge
)74). The longest period of study to date appears
 be that of Frank and his colleagues (1974, 1975)
ho found that foreign innervation of the rat
leus muscles by the superficial fibular nerve had
·rsisted at least as long as 9 months after its
iplantation. The induction of these doubly-
inervated fibres in adult mammalian muscles
ises interesting questions. For example, do the
o axons belong to motoneurones of the same
pe (see Chapter 6)? If not, does the muscle fibre
:ntain two regions of contrasting biochemical
id contractile properties? If, on the contrary, the
uscle fibre has identical properties throughout its
ngth, which of the two motoneurones is the
)minant one?

Even though the evidence for the maintenance
 doubly-innervated fibres appears so con-

vincing, it is still possible that in some circumstances suppression of synapses occurs in
reinnervated mammalian muscle. The results of
Brown and Butler (1974) on reinnervated intrafusal muscle fibres may prove to be a case in
point. These authors found that in muscle spindles
of the cat the pattern of sensory fibre discharges
following motor fibre stimulation indicated that
the initial reinnervation came exclusively from
alpha-motor axons. Subsequently the spindle

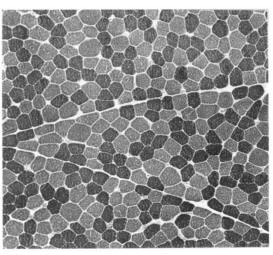

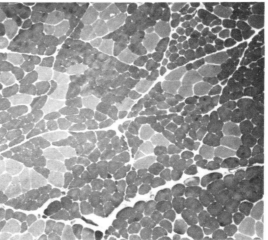

*Figure 20.5. (Upper) Normal mosaic (chequer-board)
pattern of lightly and darkly-staining muscle fibres
(myosin ATPase reaction). (Lower) Following partial
denervation, collateral reinnervation takes place and
groups of muscle fibres acquire similar staining
properties. Specimen obtained from a patient with a
familial chronic peripheral neuropathy. × 60. (Courtesy
of Dr G. Karpati)*

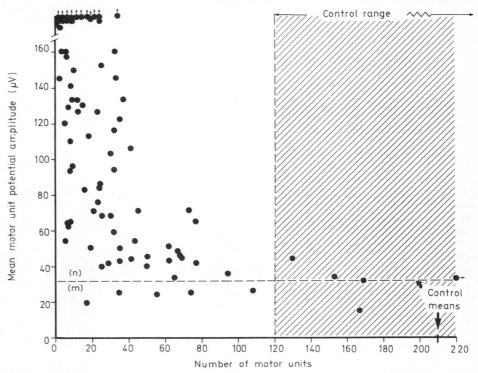

Figure 20.6. Numbers and mean potential amplitudes of functioning motor units in extensor digitorum brevis muscles of patients with motoneurone disease. Values for patients over 70 years were omitted; some muscles were examined more than once (87 observations altogether). The mean number of units in controls (210) is shown by the arrow on the abscissa and the hatched area corresponds to the lower part of the control range. The horizontal interrupted line indicates the mean potential amplitude for controls. It can be seen that the points constitute a hyperbolic relationship between the numbers and sizes of the motor units, that is, the amount of reinnervation undertaken by an EDB motoneurone remains proportional to the number of muscle fibres available for adoption. (It is assumed that the motor unit amplitudes are directly related to the numbers of muscle fibres in each unit)

responses changed to a form which suggested that the slower growing gamma-axons had now reached the spindle and restored the correct innervation of the intrafusal fibres. Although the evidence is indirect, coming from measurements of the numbers and sizes of motor units, the findings in some muscles of patients recovering from toxic or metabolic neuropathies also suggest that synapse suppression may occur (see Chapter 25).

MOTOR UNIT PROPERTIES FOLLOWING REINNERVATION

Before leaving the subject of muscle reinnervation there is one additional aspect which deserves attention; this concerns the properties of the newly-formed motor units. The architectural and functional properties of normal motor units have

already been described; to what extent are those o reinnervated muscle different? It will be recalle that in normal muscle the fibres of the differen motor units overlap. Further, since several types o muscle fibre can be distinguished histochemicall with those of any one motor unit belonging to th same type, the normal appearance of a staine cross-section of muscle is a mosaic or chequer board. Once reinnervation begins in a partiall denervated muscle many neighbouring fibres ma come to be innervated by the same axon. Since th motoneurone controls the biochemical com position of the muscle fibres, all the fibres in th same unit will exhibit similar histochemical staining Thus, instead of the normal mosaic appearance o the muscle, large groups of fibres will be foun with similar staining characteristics. This 'fibre type grouping', when seen in a muscle biopsy, is on

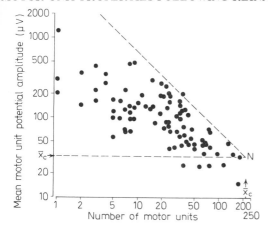

Figure 20.7. Data of Figure 20.6 plotted on logarithmic axes to include potential values for extreme denervation. The point N combines the control mean values for potential amplitudes and numbers of functioning motor units. The slanting interrupted line shows the values of mean potential amplitude which would be obtained if collateral re-innervation was completely successful; if no reinnervation took place the points would be grouped around the horizontal line. As in Figure 20.6 the observed points clearly indicate that considerable collateral reinnervation takes place and that, for an individual EDB motoneurone, the amount of reinnervation remains proportional to the number of denervated muscle fibres available for adoption

of the most useful signs of previous denervation (*Figure 20.5*).

How many fibres can a motoneurone adopt through sprouting? In the study of Kugelberg, Edström and Abbruzzese (1970) the rat tibialis anterior muscle was partially denervated by sectioning one of the ventral roots. Following reinnervation by fibres of the remaining root they found that, on average, the new units were four times larger. Since the enlarged motor unit boundaries corresponded to those of the muscle fibre fascicles, it seemed probable that connective tissue septae within the muscle belly could impede the growth of the axonal sprouts. Even more striking evidence of the power of the collateral reinnervation was obtained by McComas *et al.* (1971b). In patients with motoneurone disease and other chronic denervating disorders they measured the mean sizes of the motor unit potentials and assumed that these would be proportional to the numbers of component muscle fibres (while recognizing that muscle fibre hypertrophy would also influence the results). They found that there was a hyperbolic relationship between the sizes and numbers of surviving motor units; that is, the sizes of the new

units were always proportional to the number of denervated fibres available for adoption. In *Figures 20.6* and *20.7* there is no sign of a limit to the reinnervation capacity; in one patient with motoneurone disease the sole surviving unit generated a potential of 1.2 mV—almost 40 times as large as the mean motor unit potential amplitude of control subjects. When the maximal twitch tensions of the partially denervated muscles were measured it was found that the values remained within the normal range until fewer than 10 per cent of the normal mean population of units were left (*Figure 20.8*). In the most severely denervated muscles the surviving units generated, on average, seven times the normal tension. Since, in such muscles, the twitch tensions remained proportional to the electrical responses it appeared that the motoneurones were able to sustain not only the membranes of the newly-acquired fibres but their myofibrillar contents as well. Whether a partially-denervated muscle is as efficient in continuous work, as opposed to single twitches, is less clear, particularly since Milner-Brown, Stein and Lee (1974a) found no evidence of increased motor unit strength in their experiments. However, some

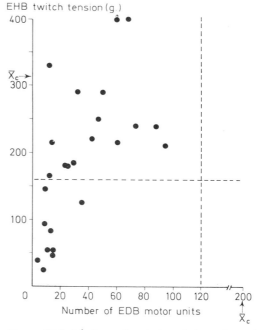

Figure 20.8. Maximum isometric twitch tensions of 25 extensor hallucis brevis muscles with varying degrees of denervation; (— — — —) lower limits of respective normal ranges; X_c, mean control value. (From McComas et al. (1971b), courtesy of the Editor and publishers of Journal of Neurology, Neurosurgery and Psychiatry)

abnormally large single motor unit tensions following reinnervation have been found in the cat soleus muscle by Bagust and Lewis (1974); the same authors noted that there were also newly-formed units which generated unusually small tensions. One factor which may have contributed to Milner-Brown's negative findings is that in some partially denervated muscles there may be impaired neuromuscular function similar to that found in myasthenia gravis. This abnormality may result from the inability of a parent motoneurone to maintain its increased population of neuromuscular junctions satisfactorily; also impulse conduction in the slender new preterminal axons may be unusually hazardous (see also page 212).

One other observation of Milner-Brown's group (1974b) was of special interest and concerned the order of recruitment of motor units during voluntary contraction. In a normal muscle (page 64) progressively larger motor units are called into activity with increasing effort but these workers found that this pattern was completely lost in muscles reinnervated after total nerve section. One interpretation of this result would be that the motoneurones which were most successful in acquiring muscle fibres during early development are not necessarily the most avid adopters in later life. This seems unlikely, however, for the same authors found that in motoneurone disease, in which the muscles undergo progressive denervation and collateral reinnervation takes place, the orderly recruitment pattern was maintained. A more plausible explanation is that, in nerve regeneration following axon division, the occurrence and extent of reinnervation will depend on such simple mechanical factors as the accessibility of the Schwann cells in the peripheral stump to the newly-formed axon sprouts.

CONCLUSIONS

There is perhaps little to add to the excellent descriptions already available of the morphology and electrophysiology of the reinnervation process. In contrast, and in spite of a century of experimental endeavour, there is still ignorance of the cell mechanisms which cause the axon to sprout and then guide the sprouts to their proper destinations. Yet even if these mechanisms remain obscure there is now an increasing awareness of the remarkable effectiveness of the reinnervating process, particularly collateral reinnervation, in restoring muscle strength. The clinical implications of this are clear. Patients may have very substantial muscle denervation without any external evidence being present; only laboratory tests will provide the necessary clues.

Chapter 21

DEMYELINATION AND REMYELINATION

A description of the structure of the myelin sheath and of its formation from the Schwann cell was given in Chapter 2. Now it is appropriate to consider the myelin sheath once more, this time in relation to a group of disorders which have, as their main pathological lesion, a destruction of the sheaths of peripheral and cranial nerve fibres. Interest in these disorders was first established by Gombault (1880) who carried out an investigation which was remarkably comprehensive when considered in relation to the meagre information then available and to the scientific equipment at his disposal. Gombault's experiments were conducted on guinea pigs in which lead poisoning had been induced by administration of the metal in the drinking water. The animals were killed and specimens of peripheral nerve were removed and treated with fixative. Gombault then dissected out single nerve fibres and under the light microscope was able to demonstrate regions in which the myelin was missing. Not only has this type of study remained in vogue, with the electronmicroscope to aid further detail, but Gombault's main conclusions have been amply confirmed by modern investigators. In the last section of his paper Gombault stated that his experimental findings were likely to have clinical relevance since he had observed evidence of demyelination in human nerve fibres which had been damaged and in the ventral roots of a patient with amyotrophic lateral sclerosis. Gombault's predictions were further borne out in the year following his report, when Meyer (1881) published an account of demyelination in the nerve fibres of a patient who had died from diphtheria.

With the accumulation of experimental data, other conditions have been recognized in which a peripheral neuropathy is present and associated with prominent demyelination of the fibres (Gilliatt, 1973; Gamstorp, 1973). Table 21.1 contains a reasonably complete list of these disorders:

It must be stressed, however, that in nearly all of these demyelinating disorders there is some degree of neuronal involvement as well; in specimens of peripheral nerve the neuronal lesions are revealed by losses of axons and the presence of other fibres undergoing Wallerian degeneration (Chapter 20). Again, in any of these conditions, it is common to find that in an individual nerve fibre the myelin sheath may be completely lost between two successive nodes of Ranvier but still present between other nodes; this appearance is termed *segmental demyelination*. The explanation of this patchy involvement lies in the fact that all the myelin between two adjacent nodes will have been formed by the same Schwann cell. If this cell became dysfunctional while its neighbours remain normal, a segmental loss of myelin will result (see also Chapter 2). With reference to Table 21.1, *ageing* has already been dealt with in Chapter 12 where evidence from motor unit counting studies was presented for the existence of progressive motoneurone dysfunction. The effects of *chronic nerve compression* are considered in Chapter 23, in relation to entrapment neuropathies. Apart from ageing, *diabetes mellitus* is now the commonest cause of polyneuropathy in Europe and North America. The numbers of patients with neuropathy from *chronic renal failure* is also increasing, due to the

TABLE 21.1
The Most Frequent Causes of Demyelination in Human
Peripheral Nerves

Ageing
Chronic nerve compression
Diabetes mellitus
Renal failure
Idiopathic polyradiculoneuritis (Guillain–Barré syn-
    drome)
Carcinoma and reticulosis
Diphtheria
Leprosy
Lead poisoning
Vitamin B_{12} deficiency
Familial polyneuropathies:
    Peroneal muscular atrophy
    Friedreich's ataxia
    Déjérine–Sottas
    Leukodystrophies (e.g. metachromatic,
        lipoproteinaemias)

longer survivals achieved by heamodialysis. *Diphtheria,* once a scourge of infancy, has been largely banished by immunization programmes but *leprosy* remains in many parts of the world as the commonest infectious cause of neuropathy. The mode of action of diphtheria toxin on the Schwann cell and myelin sheath has been thoroughly studied and is described on page 237. Of the *hereditary demyelinating polyneuropathies, peroneal muscular atrophy* is encountered most frequently and is considered on page 238. Possibly the most dramatic and interesting of all the demyelinating neuropathies, however, is the 'idiopathic' form, known also as the *Guillain–Barré syndrome;* an account is given in the next section. Finally, this chapter contains an analysis of the effects of demyelination on impulse conduction.

IDIOPATHIC
POLYRADICULONEURITIS

(Acute idiopathic post-infectious polyneuropathy,
Guillain–Barré syndrome, Landry–Guillain–
Barré–Strohl syndrome)

Clinical features

This condition occurs most commonly in an acute form, but it may sometimes become chronic or else exhibit a series of relapses following an initial remission. The four characteristic features of the disease are:

(1) A *paralysis* which frequently commences in the legs and spreads upwards to involve the arms and the muscles of respiration. Sometimes the muscles innervated by the cranial nerves are also affected, causing double vision together with dif-

ficulty in talking and swallowing and also some paralysis of the facial muscles.

(2) A *loss of sensation,* accompanied by a feeling of 'pins and needles', which is most marked in the extremities of the limbs. On examination, numbness to all sensory modalities can be demonstrated in a 'glove-and-stocking' distribution.

(3) A history of *viral infection,* usually involving the upper respiratory tract, approximately 2–4 weeks before the onset of neurological symptoms.

(4) A rise in the protein content of the cerebrospinal fluid with little increase of white cells (*cyto-albuminological dissociation*).

While the presence of all four features makes the diagnosis conclusive, not all are invariably found. Thus, in rather less than half the patients there is no history of a preceding viral infection and in some the paralysis affects the arms and legs simultaneously. In about a quarter of the patients there is a modest rise in CSF leucocytes while in others there may be little or no elevation of the CSF protein. The usual course of the disease is for it to progress for 1–2 weeks and then, after a further few weeks, for recovery to commence. This is usually a slow process and may often be incomplete; some illnesses become chronic or else run relapsing courses. In cases with severe paralysis it may be necessary to perform a tracheostomy and to institute artifical ventilation. Since good evidence exists (see below) that the disease is an immunological disorder, there is a strong case for treating patients with corticosteroids.

Special studies

Pathological

The pathological changes are most marked in the dorsal roots, probably because of their vascularity, but the peripheral nerves are also affected; sometimes the lesions appear to lie in patches with other parts of the nerve remaining functionally normal (see below). With the light microscope individual axons are seen to be demyelinated while others are undergoing Wallerian degeneration (Chapter 20). Inflammatory cells, mainly lymphocytes and somewhat larger mononuclear cells, are found leaving the venules to infiltrate the nerve tissue. With the electronmicroscope the lymphocytes can be observed in the process of attacking the myelin sheaths while rather larger macrophage cells are seen to contain products of the decomposing myelin.

Immunological

Many patients have circulating antibodies to peripheral nerve (Melnick, 1963) and their sera will

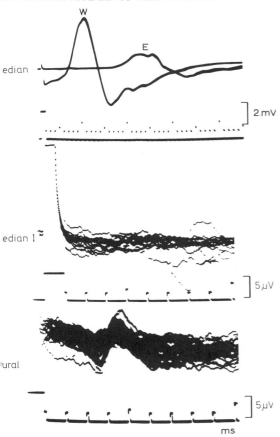

there. The emergent viruses may then contain Schwann cell antigen, presumably myelin basic protein, on their outer surfaces; alternatively the virus and myelin sheath may possess an identical antigenic complex. At any rate, the exposed antigen promotes the production of antibody and lymphocytes by the patient; these then react with the myelin sheath and cause its degeneration. The immunological disorder is discussed further in relation to experimental allergic neuritis (see below), which closely resembles the Guillain–Barré syndrome in man.

Electrophysiological

As expected of a demyelinating neuropathy, the impulse conduction velocities of motor and sensory axons are slowed (page 239) Sometimes the nerve conduction studies reveal that the demyelination is distributed in a patchy manner as in patient N.Q., a 28-year-old woman, who was studied three weeks after the onset of a moderately severe illness. *Figure 21.1* shows that, in this patient, the thenar muscle response was much larger when stimuli were applied to the median nerve at the wrist than at the elbow. This finding, allowing for dispersion of the response, indicated that many axons were inexcitable at some point in the forearm. Even those nerve fibres which were able to propagate impulses to the periphery had electrophysiological evidence of demyelination for their maximum impulse conduction velocity was considerably reduced (21 m/s; lower limit of normal, 45 m/s. Compare *Figures 21.1, upper,* and *3.9*). The focal nature of the demyelinating process in this patient was also shown by the absence of a detectable sensory potential from the thumb in the presence of an almost normal sural nerve potential in the leg (*Figure 21.1*). Serial EMG studies in such patients reveal a gradual increase in the numbers of functioning motor units although full recovery is often not achieved.

Figure 21.1. Electrophysiological findings in patient with Guillain–Barré syndrome: (upper) recordings made from the thenar muscles with surface electrodes following stimulation of the median nerve at the wrist (response W) and at the elbow (response E); (middle) absence of detectable action potential when the thumb was stimulated maximally and the recordings were made from the median nerve at the wrist with surface electrodes; (lower) sural nerve potential of normal amplitude recorded antidromically at the ankle, following stimulation of the nerve over the calf. For significance of findings, see text

cause unfolding and degeneration of the myelin sheaths of axons maintained in tissue culture (Cook et al., 1969; Dubois–Dalecq et al., 1971). Lymphocytes can also be shown to be myelinotoxic (Arnason, Winkler and Hadler, 1969) and will transform on exposure to peripheral nerve antigen (Knowles et al., 1969). These observations, together with the finding of lymphocytes and immunoglobulin deposits in nerve, suggest that the disease is immunologically mediated. The likeliest hypothesis is that during the preceding infection (see above) viruses enter the Schwann cells and replicate

AN ANIMAL MODEL OF THE GUILLAIN-BARRÉ SYNDROME: EXPERIMENTAL ALLERGIC NEURITIS (EAN)

In 1955 Waksman and Adams reported that they had been able to induce an inflammatory disorder of peripheral nerves and nerve roots by an immunological method and they noted its resemblance to the Guillain–Barré syndrome. Their technique had been to make a suspension of rabbit sciatic nerve and to inject small samples, together with Freund's adjuvant (containing heat-killed tubercle bacilli), into the foot-pads of other rabbits (*Figure 21.2*). They observed that after 12 days or more nearly all the injected animals developed the clinical signs of a polyneuropathy. The animals 'tended to lie in a splayed position, with all extremities extended and the head resting on the floor . . . In hopping they were unsteady and erratic . . . Upon landing they would often stagger or lurch to one side . . . the musculature of extremities and trunk was weak and slack.' Most of the affected animals recovered spontaneously after several weeks of illness.

Neuropathological and immunological features

These important results have been confirmed in many laboratories and it is now possible to understand in more detail the immunological mechanisms involved in the pathogenesis. In the first place, it appears that the antigenic component of peripheral nerve is one or both of the two basic proteins contained in myelin. The chemical compositions of these proteins have now been determined. The P1 protein has a molecular weight of 18,100 and contains 168 amino acids; it is identical with one of the

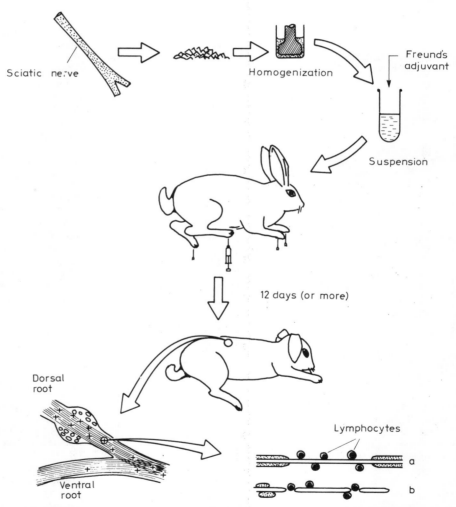

Sciatic nerve

Homogenization

Freund's adjuvant

Suspension

12 days (or more)

Dorsal root

Ventral root

Lymphocytes

a

b

Figure 21.2. Experimental procedure for the induction of experimental allergic neuritis (see text). At bottom left the relative involvement of the dorsal, ventral and mixed roots is indicated (+). At bottom right is shown a fibre with segmental demyelination (a) and a more severely affected fibre undergoing Wallerian degeneration (b)

two basic proteins found in myelin from the central nervous system (Brostoff and Eylar, 1972). The antigenic property of the P1 protein is confined to a small part of the molecule which contains only nine of the amino acids (Westall *et al*, 1971). When injected by itself the P1 protein, or the critical 9 amino acid residue, will induce a demyelinating disorder in both the central and peripheral nervous systems. However, if *intact* peripheral nervous system (PNS) myelin is administered instead only the peripheral nerves and roots are affected and the CNS is spared. Wiśniewski and colleagues (1974) have explained this curious result by suggesting that the antigenic site on the P1 protein is either hidden within the PNS myelin substructure or is conformationally altered so as to be immunologically inert. They further propose that it is the second basic protein of PNS myelin, the P2 protein, which is responsible for experimental allergic neuritis. This protein has a molecular weight of 11 000-12 000 and contains 101 amino acids; when purified and injected with Freund's adjuvant into a variety of animals, it can be shown to produce an inflammatory polyneuropathy (Brostoff *et al.*, 1972).

There is good evidence that, although antibodies to myelin protein can be demonstrated in experimental allergic neuritis (EAN), the degenerative changes are mostly cell mediated. For example, lymphocytes removed from an affected animal will produce demyelination when injected into another animal (Aström and Waksman, 1962) and they are also active when applied to myelinated axons in tissue culture (Lampert, 1969). According to Arnäson, Winkler and Hadler (1969) the lymphocytes cross into the nerve parenchyma through the small veins and, upon exposure to myelin antigen, are transformed into larger cells. These then undergo repeated mitoses before commencing the demyelinating process.

With the electronmicroscope the mononuclear cells can be seen to have penetrated the basement membranes of the Schwann cells with processes which eventually surround the myelin sheaths. The Schwann cells are now isolated from their axons but are not themselves attacked by the mononuclear cells. Instead the mononuclear cells appear to prise apart the tightly-bound spiral of the myelin sheath and cause it to undergo a 'bubbly dissolution' (Lampert, 1969). Eventually the myelin becomes completely stripped from the axis cylinder and is then removed following ingestion by phagocytes (*Figure 21.2, bottom*).

In most animals recovery takes place and is achieved by remyelination of the affected axons. In a small proportion of animals the demyelinating process assumes a chronic course. In such animals the nerve fibres become abnormally thickened so as to form 'onion bulbs'; the thickening is caused by excessive numbers of Schwann cells and their processes (Pollard, King and Thomas, 1975).

DIPHTHERITIC NEUROPATHY

In the Guillain–Barré syndrome and experimental allergic neuritis demyelination is brought about by the direct attack of transformed lymphocytes on the proteins of the myelin sheath. In diphtheritic neuropathy, however, the lesions are caused by the action of the bacterial toxin on the Schwann cells and the pathological consequences are therefore rather different. Experimentally, the effects of diphtheria toxin have been studied in various ways. In early investigations the toxin was injected into animals subcutaneously so that a generalized neuropathy resulted; the study by McDonald (1963a, b) in the cat was particularly thorough, combining the results of clinical, histological and electrophysiological studies. More recently demyelinating focal lesions have been employed instead, the toxin being injected through the connective tissue coat surrounding the nerve fascicles. The results of the pathological investigations will now be considered.

Allt and Cavanagh (1969) injected the sciatic nerves of rats with 'high' or 'low' doses of diphtheria toxin and examined the nerves 3, 7 or 10 days subsequently with both the light and the electron microscopes.

At 3 days after toxin (Figure 21.3, b) the axons appeared normal on light microscopy but the electronmicroscope revealed that some of the terminal myelin loops and inner myelin lamellae were already disorganized and forming debris.

At 7 days after toxin (Figure 21.3, c) there was widening of the node of Ranvier, due to detachment of myelin loops from the axolemma. Also evident at this time was loss of some of the Schwann cell fingers from the node, together with depletion of gap substance. The cytoplasm of the two Schwann cells bordering the node appeared swollen.

At 10 days after toxin (Figure 21.3, d) more extensive widening of the node had occurred, leaving a length of exposed axolemma. In most cases the nodal gaps were greater than 50 μm instead of being the normal 1 μm. Much of the myelin missing from the paranodal region was to be found within the cytoplasm of the Schwann cells. In some instances the whole length of the internode was denuded of myelin, the axon being either bare or else covered with a thin layer of Schwann cell cytoplasm.

Other studies have shown that, in addition to the changes described above, there is an infiltration of macrophages from the blood stream into the vicinity of the degenerating node; these cells appear to assist the Schwann cells in the removal of myelin debris (Webster *et al.*, 1961). If the loss of myelin is not too extensive the missing myelin is replaced by the two Schwann cells bordering the node; attempts at such reparative changes may already be seen by the 10th day. Sometimes, however, the Schwann cell is destroyed by the diphtheria toxin;

ness and wasting of the more distal muscles of the limbs with relatively good preservation of proximal ones. In the legs this differential involvement gives the thigh the appearance of an inverted champagne bottle while the whole leg resembles that of a stork; pes cavus is also commonly found. The weakness of anterior tibial muscles causes the presenting symptom of foot-drop; involvement of the intrinsic

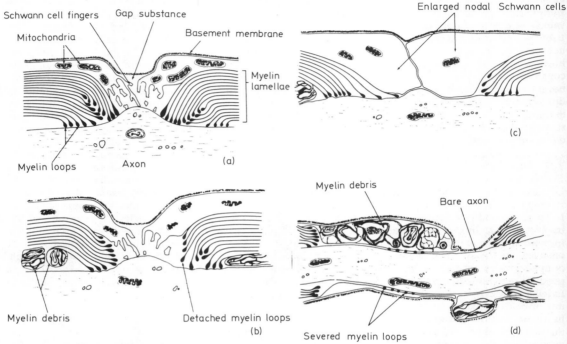

Figure 21.3. Morphological studies of nodes of Ranvier in the sciatic nerves of a normal rat (a) and of animals which had received intraneural injections of diphtheria toxin 3, 7 and 10 days previously (b, c and d respectively). See text for description of changes. (From Allt and Cavanagh (1969) courtesy of the authors, and the Editor and publishers of Brain)

adjacent surviving cells then undergo mitosis and invest the bare axon with cytoplasm and myelin. As a consequence of this cell division a healed nerve fibre may exhibit a surplus of Schwann cells compared with its original population, and some of the internodal distances will be abnormally short. A quantitative example of irregularity in the nodal spacing following remyelination has already been given in *Figure 2.2.* in which the nerve fibre changes due to ageing were displayed.

PERONEAL MUSCULAR ATROPHY

Peroneal muscular atrophy, or Charcot-Marie-Tooth disease, is a group of genetically-determined disorders which eventually result in extreme weak-

muscles of the hand and of the long flexors and extensors of the fingers results in a loss of manual dexterity such that writing and fastening buttons may prove impossible. Following Dyck and Lambert (1968 a, b), peroneal atrophy may be divided into hypertrophic and non-hypertrophic (neuronal) forms. In the hypertrophic form the underlying abnormality is defective myelination of axons, leading to abnormally thin myelin sheaths and segmental demyelination; a striking loss of axons is also present. In an attempt to restore myelin the Schwann cells divide repeatedly and tend to coil round each other so as to produce 'onion bulbs'. The latter structures and the increased connective tissue in the nerve fasciculi are responsible for the enlargement of the nerve trunks which can be detected clinically. Since sensory fibres are also involved, diminished sensation to all somatic modalities is commonly evident in a glove-and stocking distribution. The disease is usually inherited through an autosomal dominant gene but there is also a less frequent and severe autosomal recessive form, the *Déjérine-Sottas* type. In the extremely rare *Refsum* variety, an abnormality of phytanic acid metabolism has been discovered. Because of defective myelination all forms of hypertrophic neuropathy are associated with marked slowing of impulse conduction with values in the 5–25 m/s range. In the *non-hypertrophic* type of peroneal atrophy the lesion is a neuronal one and results in losses of axons with little involvement of myelin sheaths in survivors; consequently impulse conduction velocities are normal or only slightly reduced. In one form of this disorder both motor and sensory axons are affected; in the other form the sensory axons are spared, resulting in a disease which can be regarded as a distal variant of spinal muscular atrophy (page 272).

EFFECT OF DEMYELINATION ON IMPULSE CONDUCTION

In the cats with diphtheritic polyneuropathy studied by McDonald (1963a, b) recordings were made from dorsal root fascicles as well as from single sensory fibres. McDonald found that although some of the axons had ceased conducting in demyelinated regions, the axis cylinders usually remained intact. In less severely-affected fibres he was able to obtain unequivocal evidence of slowed impulse conduction by comparing the velocities with those of fibres of the same receptor type in normal animals. The most extreme instance of slowed conduction in disease has come from experiments on dystrophic mice, in which myelin is absent from most dorsal and ventral root fibres though usually present in the peripheral nerves (Bradley and Jenkison, 1973). It is thought that this abnormality results from a failure of myelination during early development rather than from demyelination (see Chapter 16). Huizar, Kuno and Miyata (1975) stimulated the motor axons of these animals and used intracellar microelectrodes to record antidromically-conducted action potentials in the motoneurone somas. They estimated that the mean impulse conduction velocity was only 2.3 m/s in the amyelinated regions whereas the corresponding value for normal motor roots was about 53 m/s.

Such low velocities in axons which have either lost or failed to acquire myelin sheaths raise the question whether impulse propagation remains saltatory, jumping from one site to another (see page 26), or whether the impulse now flows continuously along the fibre. It turns out that the type of conduction is different in axons which have never been myelinated

(such as the nerve roots of dystrophic mice) from that in axons in which the myelin sheaths have been largely removed (as in diphtheritic neuropathy). To study this problem Rasminsky and Sears (1972) devised a special electrophysiological technique which enabled them to record action potential currents at successive points along the outside of single ventral root fibres (*Figure 21.4, A*). In the normal animal they were able to show that the latency of the recorded current increased in definite steps along the axon, with each step corresponding to the location of a node (*Figure 21.4, B*). These findings were, of course, to be expected if saltatory conduction was occurring. In nerve fibres treated with diphtheria toxin discrete increments of latency were also observed with increasing distance along the axon. In contrast to the findings in the normal animal, in which the conduction time from one node to the next (approximately 1 mm) was about 20 µs, values as large as 600 µs were observed in the demyelinated preparation (*Figure 21.4, C*). These results indicated that, although impulse conduction could be greatly slowed in demyelinated nerve fibres, it remained saltatory to the point of conduction block and did not become continuous.

Why is conduction slowed in these poorly-myelinated axons? The obvious explanation depends on the fact that the affected axon becomes a less efficient cable. The loss of myelin insulation reduces the electrical resistance between the inside and the outside of the axon while the thinner layer of myelin remaining causes the capacitance to increase. Both these factors, decreased resistance and increased capacitance, will allow a large part of the outwardly-flowing action potential current to leak through the internodal region of the axolemma instead of being concentrated at the next node (see page 25). Hence the current must flow for a longer time before the critical depolarization is reached at the node which allows an impulse to be initiated.

A further question is whether the loss of the myelin sheath is the only factor responsible for the reduced impulse conduction velocities in the various neuropathies. For example, in rats made diabetic with streptozotocin, Sharma and Thomas (1975) observed a significant slowing of impulse conduction at a stage when no structural abnormality was visible with the electronmicroscope. Similarly, in the peripheral nerves of dystrophic mice, where the myelin sheaths and nodes of Ranvier appeared perfectly normal, Rasminsky, Bray and Aguayo (1975) found that impulse conduction velocities were approximately one-third lower than in control animals. Such discrepancies suggest that some part of the axon, in addition to the myelin sheath, may be defective in the demyelinating (or amyelinating)

240

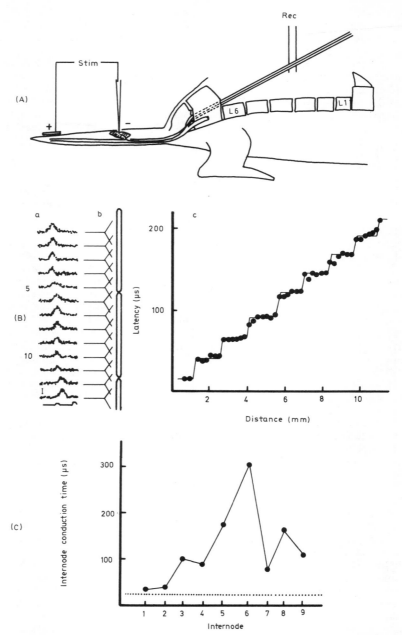

Figure 21.4. Studies of impulse propagation in the normal rat and in an animal treated with diphtheria toxin. In (A) the stimulating electrodes (stim) are shown applied to peripheral nerve fibres in the tail. The recording electrodes consist of two fine wires mounted 400–600 μm apart, which are moved to different positions along the course of a ventral root fibre. In (B, a) are shown the external currents recorded during passage of an impulse; the positions of the recording electrodes in relation to the nodes of Ranvier are shown in b. The increments in the latency of the action current as the electrodes are moved are displayed in c; note their regular nature. Each step corresponds to a node of Ranvier. In (C) are the results for an axon with partial demyelination. Notice the large and irregular values for internode conduction time compared with the average values for a normal axon (..................). (From Rasminsky and Sears (1972), courtesy of the authors, and the Editor and publishers of Journal of Physiology)

ypes of neuropathy. The most obvious possibility s the axolemma; thus, a loss of available sodium arriers in the nodal axolemma could occur if the membrane was itself abnormal or if it was hronically depolarized (for example, by impaired odium pumping secondary to loss of ATP from he damaged Schwann cell fingers).

As described for diphtheritic neuropathy, impulse onduction in demyelinated axons remains saltatory p to the point of block. The situation in axons vhich have never acquired myelin sheaths is diferent, however. First, in the amyelinated ventral oot fibres of dystrophic mice (see above) Raminsky and Kearney (1976) were able to demonstrate that conduction was continuous in the 1–3 m/s ange. Secondly, Bergland (1960) studied impulse onduction in the sciatic nerves of chickens at diferent stages of embryonic development. He found hat the conduction velocities began to undergo a narked increase on the 15th day of development nd that this event coincided with the first apearance of the myelin sheath on electronmicrocopy. Bergland was thus able to show that continuous propagation of the impulse took place in he axons prior to myelination. These findings in myelinated axons are of interest since they demontrate that the entire axolemma is excitable rather han only those regions at which nodes will normally evelop. Even so, it is still theoretically possible hat, were myelination to proceed, membrane xcitability would be suppressed in the internodal egions of the axolemma, perhaps as the result of a rophic influence exerted by the Schwann cell.

EFFECT OF TEMPERATURE ON IMPULSE CONDUCTION IN DEMYELINATED AXONS

The disease multiple sclerosis exercises a particular ascination for the experimental neurologist not only on account of its still undetermined aetiology but also because of the mysterious relapses and emissions that typify its course. It has long been ecognized that the pathological lesion comprises 'plaque' of demyelination in the central nervous ystem, some regions being more susceptible than others. However, it is difficult to conceive of a lemyelinating process which would be sufficiently apid to block impulse conduction within a few hours and to thereby induce the characteristic ymptoms of blindness, weakness, numbness and clumsiness. One possibility is that, in addition to he production of demyelinating lesions, the disease process releases a substance which can bind to the axolemma in the region of the node and exert a ocal anaestetic action. Preliminary evidence for the

existence of such a factor has come from the studies of Bornstein and Crain (1965). These workers took serum from patients undergoing acute exacerbations of multiple sclerosis and added it to preparations of mouse brain and spinal cord in tissue culture. Within 20–50 minutes all the complex trans-synaptic responses to electrical stimulation of the cultures had disappeared. Even faster abolition of electrical activity could be induced by applying serum from rabbits with experimental allergic encephalitis and this block could be made to disappear if normal serum was then substituted. If this intriguing work can be confirmed, the possibility of circulating anaesthetic agents being present in other neurological disorders would seem worthy of exploration.

Multiple sclerosis provides another clue in the study of the demyelinating process in relation to the striking effect of temperature on the clinical features. It has long been recognized that the symptoms and signs of the disease are made more conspicuous if the body temperature is raised (Simons, 1937) and the diagnostic value of this effect has been utilized in the 'hot bath' test. The neurophysiological events underlying this phenomenon have now been investigated in peripheral nerves and the findings are likely to have significance for the full spectrum of neuropathic disorders. In the investigation by Davis and Jacobson (1971) the effect of temperature on impulse conduction was studied on sciatic nerves of frogs and guinea pigs. In some animals the nerves had been crushed between eye forceps; in other guinea pigs experimental allergic neuritis had been induced by injecting the animals beforehand with an emulsion of Freund's adjuvant and sciatic nerve. Irrespective of the nature of the lesion, mechanical or inflammatory, the affected axons were unusually susceptible to raised temperatures. In the guinea pig, for example, impulses in a majority of fibres were blocked at temperatures of 40–41 °C, that is, at values only slightly above the normal body temperature of the animal (38–39 °C).

The analysis of temperature effects on impulse conduction has recently been taken a step further by Rasminsky (1973), who employed the single fibre recording technique devised by Rasminsky and Sears (1972; see above). Like Davis and Jacobson (1971) he found that very modest rises in nerve temperature (for example, 0.5 °C) were sometimes sufficient to block conduction in rat fibres treated with diphtheria toxin and that the block was reversible (*Figure 21.5*). He also noted that, before conduction block took place, the internodal conduction velocity actually increased. This is an interesting observation since, as already seen, demyelinating lesions are associated with reduced impulse conduction velocities and one might have anticipated a further decrease to have occurred before conduction failed altogether. The explanation offered by Rasminsky depends on Tasaki's (1953) concept of a safety factor for the generation of an impulse at a node of Ranvier. The safety factor can be defined as:

$$\frac{\text{current available to stimulate a node}}{\text{current required to excite a node}}$$

molecules will be available for activation in the nodal membrane (see page 241). Once the safety margin is reduced, a temperature effect which would ordinarily be inconsequential may become the critical factor in causing block of impulse conduction. Rasminsky suggests that the effect of the increased temperature is to reduce further the magnitude and duration of the action potential current available to stimulate a node. This reduction

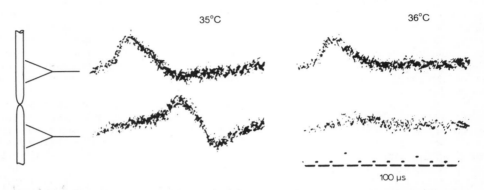

Figure 21.5. The effect of temperature on impulse propagation in an axon treated with diphtheria toxin. At 35 °C there is excitation at the node of Ranvier, shown by the presence of a rather later action current (lower trace) when the recording electrodes are moved beyond the node (downwards in figure). At 36 °C the later action current is abolished, indicating that the node is no longer excited. (From Rasminsky (1973) courtesy of the author, and the Editor and publishers of Archives of Neurology)

The safety factor has not yet been measured for mammalian nerve fibres but for myelinated axons in the toad Tasaki obtained values of between 5 and 7. Indeed, the safety factor is sufficiently large that even if impulse initiation is prevented in two successive nodes of Ranvier, an adequate current can still flow through the axolemma at the next (third) node and induce excitation there. In the case of a demyelinated axon the safety factor will be reduced because, as already seen, a significant fraction of the action potential current will be shunted across the internodal axolemma instead of being concentrated at the node. There is the additional possibility that fewer sodium carrier

comes about because the raised temperature hastens the 'recovery' processes in the axolemma which terminate the action potential; with reference to Chapter 3 these events are the switching-on of the potassium permeability mechanism and the inactivation of the sodium carrier system.

In conclusion, it is clear that the effects of a demyelinating lesion on impulse conduction are much more complex than had hitherto been assumed. Even if the disordered physiology was completely understood, it would still be necessary to explain why the demyelinating factors attack the Schwann cells in preference to the axon cylinder.

Chapter 22

NERVE COMPRESSION

ACUTE LESIONS

Classification

The delicate structure of the nerve fibre makes it very susceptible to mechanical injury. The type and severity of the resulting lesion will depend on many factors, for example, on whether the nerve has been divided, stretched or compressed and, in the last two instances, on the extent and duration of the deformation. The severity of the lesion will also depend on the 'healthiness' of the neurone, for it is a common observation that patients with metabolic or toxic neuropathies are unusually vulnerable to the effects of nerve compression. Two schemes have been put forward for classifying the types of nerve injury, both being based on considerations of nerve structure. Of these schemes Seddon's (1943, 1972) is the simpler since only three grades of disorders are recognized; in order of increasing severity these are:

Neurapraxia—This term refers to a nerve in which there is a temporary loss of function without discontinuity of the axon.

Axonotmesis—This is a total interruption of the axons and their myelin sheaths with preservation of the connective tissue stroma.

Neurotmesis—This term describes a nerve which has either been completely severed or else so seriously disorganized by scar tissue that spontaneous regeneration is impossible.

Sunderland's (1951, 1968) classification is rather more elaborate and a division is made into five degrees of nerve injury.

(1) Interruption of conduction in the axons with preservation of their anatomical continuity.
(2) Loss of continuity of the axons without a breach of the endoneurium.
(3) Complete loss of continuity of nerve fibres but with preservation of the perineurium.
(4) Interruption of nerve funiculi including the perineurial sheath.
(5) Severance of the whole nerve trunk.

Although each type of injury will result in muscle weakness and loss of sensation, the outlook for recovery is strictly related to the type of lesion present. If impulse conduction is blocked but the axon remains in continuity (neurapraxia, or first-degree injury) recovery should follow within a few days or, more usually, weeks. A good prognosis may also be given for second-degree lesions for in these the endoneurial sheath are preserved and can guide the regenerating axons back to the denervated tissue (page 223). The least favourable outlook is clearly for injuries in which the nerve has been completely interrupted. Even though the cut ends of the nerve may be joined together at operation by sutures there is no guarantee that the axon sprouts will find their way to the correct columns of Schwann cells. Since it encompasses a number of fascinating problems in neurobiology, the subject of nerve fibre regeneration has been considered in more detail in Chapter 20. Also of interest, however, is the *neurapraxic lesion* (first-degree nerve injury) for much can be learned from its consequences which are relevant to a discussion of trophic mechanisms.

NEURAPRAXIA

Animal studies

Historically, it is appropriate to begin by acknowledging the contributions of Weir Mitchell, a surgeon in the American Civil War, who described transient palsies following wounds in which bullets has passed close to the nerves. To quote Weir Mitchell, 'This condition of local shock is very curious. A man is shot in the thigh, the ball passes near the sciatic nerve, and instantly the limb is paralysed; within a few minutes, or at the close of a day or a week the volitional control in part returns . . .' (Mitchell, Morehouse and Keen, 1864). A few years later Erb (1876) was able to report the occurrence of similar disorders of nerve function in civilian practice following the accidental compression of peripheral nerves. As one of the pioneers in electromyography Erb also studied the responses of the muscles to electrical stimulation over the motor point (innervation zone) and noted that the reactions of nerve degeneration were absent. Another major advance toward an understanding of the neurapraxic lesion was the experimental study of Denny-Brown and Brenner (1944). These authors devised a mechanical press incorporating a mercury bag; they could insert a segment of cat sciatic nerve into the press while leaving the nerve in continuity. After a desired force had been applied for a certain time the device was removed, the skin incision repaired and the effect on the animal observed during the ensuing days or weeks. At the conclusion of the experiment the sciatic nerve was removed and studied histologically. Later the same workers found that transient constriction of the intact thigh was equally effective in producing a neural lesion. Using the last technique, Denny-Brown and Brenner observed they could produce a nerve block which would persist for 24 hr or more by applying a tourniquet pressure of 700 mm of mercury for 2 hr. Although the muscles might be paralysed for as long as 3 weeks before recovery, the animals gave little evidence of sensory loss. Since muscle contraction could be evoked by electrical stimulation of the nerve below the level of the tourniquet it was evident that the paralysis had resulted from a local block of impulse conduction in the previously compressed region. The experimental lesion was therefore quite comparable to the neurapraxic disorder encountered clinically. When the paralysed nerves were examined with the light microscope, Denny-Brown and Brenner found that the earliest structural abnormality appeared at about 24 hr after the lesion had been made; it consisted of swelling and vacuolation of the axis cylinder throughout the region of compression. After a further 24 hr opposing myelin sheaths had begun to draw apart from each other at the nodes of Ranvier. An interesting observation was that the bared region of axolemma could not be stained with silver. Other abnormalities included the collection of oedema fluid around the nerve fibres and the appearance of macrophage cells. Denny-Brown and Brenner believed that the lesion described had resulted from ischaemia of the sciatic nerve but they were unable to provide a convincing explanation as to why the speed of onset and severity of the induced paralysis should have been increased by the application of progressively larger tourniquet pressures beyond the systolic blood pressure. It is probable that these authors were influenced by the work of Grundfest (1936) who had shown that a pressure of 1000 atmospheres was necessary to block conduction in the frog sciatic nerve. However, Grundfest's experiment had been conducted *in vitro*, the sciatic nerve being kept in a bath of well-oxygenated fluid. In such an experimental situation the compressive force would have been applied even over the nerve. In the *in situ* experiments of Denny-Brown and Brenner the pressure on the nerve would have been uneven, being highest under the cuff and then falling away sharply beyond its edges. One would expect the nerve fibres to have been squashed under the cuff and some of their contents to have been squeezed outwards.

In a more recent experimental study Ochoa *et al.* (1971) have shown that this is exactly what happens. They subjected the hind limbs of baboons to pressures of 1000 mmHg for 1–3 hr, the cuff being applied around the knee. As in Denny-Brown and Brenner's (1944) experiments a paralysis was induced with recovery taking place over several weeks. By a combination of light and electron microscopy the authors found that the damage in the nerve fibres was most severe at the edges of the cuff. In addition they were able to show that, in this region, the nodes of Ranvier had been pushed outwards from the margins of the cuff and had invaginated the adjacent segments of the fibre (*Figure 22.1, c*). Ochoa, Fowler and Gilliatt (1972) suggested that this deformity resulted because the axoplasm which was squeezed along the fibre by the cuff met resistance at the node of Ranvier. Possibly this was because the axis cylinder was narrower at this point; in any event, the effect was for the axoplasm to push the node before it and to thereby invaginate the adjacent internode. Subsequent to the appearance of this lesion demyelination took place. The pressure used by these authors was extremely high (1000 mmHg) but was nevertheless comparable to that used by

Denny-Brown and Brenner. It is therefore curious that the latter authors should not have seen the telescoping lesion in the axons, especially since Ochoa and colleagues were able to recognize it with the light microscope. The findings in these two animal studies are obviously relevant to the neurapraxic lesion which may inadvertently result from the over-long application of a tourniquet during limb surgery. It is less likely that the same pathophysiological derangements are common to 'endogenous' entrapment neuropathies (for example, the carpal tunnel syndrome; see below) for in the latter instances the nerve compression will have involved lower pressures over a longer period of time and will have fluctuated.

The tourniquet experiments enable several important questions to be considered. One of these is the reason for the preservation of sensation at a time when the muscles are severely paralysed following the nerve compression (Denny-Brown and Brenner, 1944). According to Ochoa, Fowler and Gilliatt (1972) the invaginating lesions are largely restricted to fibres with diameters greater than 5 μm, in which case all the α-motor fibres would be vulnerable but a large proportion of cutaneous fibres would be spared. Another question concerns the manner in which the telescoping lesion noted by Ochoa and colleagues (1971, 1972) produces a conduction block. It is doubtful if the burial of the nodal axolemma within the invaginated region of the fibre is sufficient by itself since the safety factor for impulse propagation is high enough for impulses to skip one or two blocked nodes (see page 242). An additional factor may be the high internal resistance of the narrowed core of axoplasm in the region of invagination. Thus the current flowing to the next node during the action potential might then be too small to bring about the critical membrane depolarization (see also page 24). An observation of Denny-Brown and Brenner's which is of great interest in relation to trophic mechanisms, is that the affected muscles did not atrophy nor did they develop fibrillation activity. Thus two signs of denervation were absent, in spite of the fact that

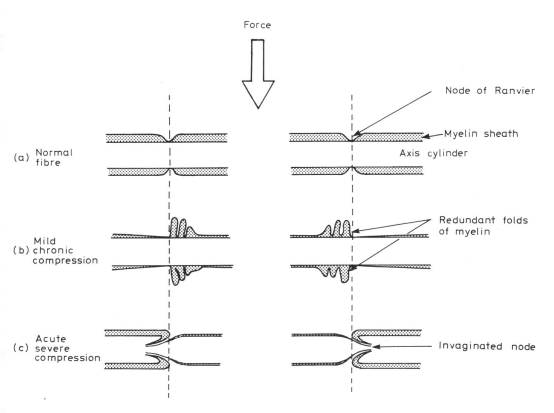

Figure 22.1. The results of compression on axonal structure; note the different effects, depending on the severity of the lesion (see text). (Figure based on findings of Ochoa, Fowler and Gilliatt (1972) and Neary, Ochoa and Gilliatt (1975))

246

NERVE COMPRESSION

the muscles were completely paralysed (see Chapters 8 and 9). Denny-Brown and Brenner drew attention to the significance of this observation with the following statement: 'The lesion, therefore, demonstrates that anatomic continuity of nerve, not receipt of impulses, prevents atrophy

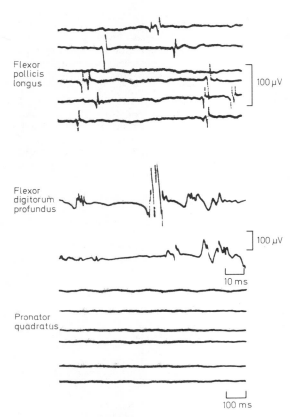

Figure 22.2. EMG findings in the right arm of Case 1. At top is record during attempted contraction of the flexor pollicis longus, showing profuse fibrillation potentials and absence of volitionally-induced activity. Middle section displays the very reduced interference pattern recorded during maximum contraction of the flexor digitorum profundus. Lower section shows absence of volitional or spontaneous activity during attempted use of the pronator quadratus muscle. (From McComas et al. (1974a) courtesy of the Editor and publishers of Canadian Journal of Neurobiological Sciences)

and fibrillation of muscle.' Although the contribution of the neurapraxic lesion toward an understanding of trophic phenomena is already evident, three clinical examples of neurapraxic lesions will now be presented. They serve to emphasize the conclusions from the animal studies but they also

draw attention to certain additional phenomena. More extensive accounts have been published elsewhere (McComas, Jorgensen and Upton, 1974).

Clinical Studies

Case 1 contrasts the electrophysiological findings in three severely-paralysed muscles, the difference depending on whether the underlying nerve lesions are degenerative or neurapraxic.

Mr S. M. was a 23-year-old student who had cut the flexor aspect of the right little finger on the metal lid of a pharmaceutical container. The laceration was deep enough to have severed the tendon of the flexor digitorum profundus; the wound was therefore explored on the day of the accident and the cut ends of the tendon were sutured together. To assist healing of the tendon, a plaster slab was applied over the dorsal aspects of the semiflexed little finger, the hand and the distal two-thirds of the forearm. The slab was firmly bandaged in position and the arm was put into a sling. The patient was aware of some swelling of the hand soon after the operation. One week later he was allowed to discard the sling; the arm felt tight within its bandaging. Four weeks after the injury the plaster was removed and the patient discovered that he was unable to flex the ends of his right thumb and index finger. There was no loss of sensation and his hand was otherwise normal. Eight weeks later (12 weeks after injury) clinical examination revealed some wasting of the flexor muscles in the forearm. There was also weakness of the flexor digitorum profundus (particularly of the part supplying the index finger) and flexor pollicis longus. The clinical diagnosis of an anterior interosseous nerve palsy was confirmed by electromyography, the results of which are set out in *Figure 22.2*: it is probable that the nerve had been compressed by the edge of the bandage around the forearm. From *Figure 22.2 (upper)* it can be seen that the *flexor pollicis longus* (FPL) was completely paralysed for, on attempted contraction, only spontaneously occurring fibrillation activity could be recorded. In the *flexor digitorum profundus* (FDP) the scanty volitional discharges (*Figure 22.2, middle*) confirmed the presence of severe denervation; elsewhere in the muscle fibrillation activity could be recorded. The findings in these two muscles are in contrast to those in the *pronator quadratus. Figure 22.2 (lower)* shows that this muscle was completely paralysed; unlike FDP and FPL, the pronator did not exhibit any fibrillation or sharp wave activity. Again, whereas atrophy of FDP and FPL would have contributed to the muscle wasting visible in the forearm, the belly of the pronator was distinctly *enlarged*. Since all three muscles are supplied by the anterior interosseous nerve it was necessary to presume that the individual muscle branches had been affected differently by the compressive lesion. Thus, in the nerves to FDP and FPL axonal degeneration had probably taken place while the branch to pronator quadratus had sustained a neurapraxic lesion. This last deduction was confirmed by the ability to record an evoked response from the pronator following electrical stimulation of the anterior interosseous nerve distal to the lesion. The spontaneous recovery of muscle function in the patient was studied by Dr Adrian Upton, who had also carried out the initial EMG examination. He observed that, as strength was regained by the pronator quadratus, the striking enlargement of the muscle belly gradually disappeared. The ability of a muscle to respond to a neuropathic lesion by enlargement rather than atrophy is considered elsewhere in relation to the pathogenesis of muscular dystrophy (page 158).

Case 2 demonstrates the value of the motor unit counting technique in enabling the numbers of neurapraxic axons to be determined.

Miss G. L. was an 11-year-old schoolgirl who, 2 months before the EMG examination, had caught her left arm between the rollers of a clothes wringer; the arm had been drawn in to the mid-forearm level. Immediately after the

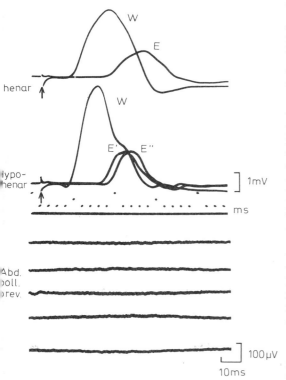

Figure 22.3. Muscle findings in Case 2. (Top) Superimposed traces showing responses evoked in thenar muscles following stimulation of the median nerve at the wrist (response W) and at the elbow (response E). Moment of stimulation indicated by arrow. (Middle) Oscilloscope recordings from hypothenar muscles after stimulation of the ulnar nerve at the wrist (response W) and below and above the elbow (responses E' and E'' respectively). (Lower) Serial sweeps of recordings from abductor pollicis brevis with a coaxial needle electrode; no spontaneous activity visible. From McComas, Jorgensen and Upton (1974) courtesy of the Editor and the publishers of Canadian Journal of Neurological Sciences)

accident she had noticed numbness of the whole hand and muscle weakness; the latter affected all the intrinsic muscles of the left hand together with the extensors of the fingers and wrist. Both sensation and muscle strength had been improving up to the time of study. *Figure 22.3* shows the responses evoked in the thenar and hypothenar muscles following supramaximal stimulation of the median and ulnar nerves. It can be seen that the muscle potentials were much larger when the nerves were excited at the wrist rather than at the elbow. The compact forms and normal configurations of the diminished potentials suggested that the discrepancy had not arisen from dispersion of the muscle responses due to slowed nerve impulse conduction in the arm. Instead the findings must have resulted from neurapraxic lesions in the forearm which had caused local inexcitability of the median and ulnar nerves. Yet in spite of the interruption of the centrifugal flow of impulses, the paralysed muscle fibres showed no other evidence of denervation. On inspection the muscles did not appear wasted, nor could fibrillation potentials and sharp-wave activity be detected during exploration of the muscle with a coaxial electrode (*Figure 22.3, bottom*). Finally, it was unlikely that any collateral reinnervation had occurred (page 224) for the amplitudes of the potentials evoked from the still functioning motor units were not enlarged.

So far the findings are completely in accord with those of Denny-Brown and Brenner in the cat. A problem arises when the motor unit counting results are considered. In the median nerve, for example, it could be shown that only about 29 per cent of the motor axons were in a neurapraxic state and even fewer were able to propagate impulses through the site of the lesion (about 13 per cent). But what of the remaining 58 per cent of axons? The immediate response would be to suggest that these had undergone Wallerian degeneration (page 221) and were therefore no longer excitable below the level of the lesion. This explanation is not convincing, however, for axonal degeneration should have resulted in the muscle fibres developing the full spectrum of denervation changes including fibrillations, atrophy and collateral reinnervation—and yet, as already remarked, these were absent.

Case 3 adds to the interpretative dilemma.

Mrs F. N. was a 48-year-old housewife with a long and complicated history of pain in her neck and lower back. She had undergone five operations without any lasting relief of symptoms. One of these operations was a 'decompression' of the C5, C6 and C7 roots on the left side. On regaining consciousness she found that she was unable to move the fingers and thumb of the left hand and that she had very little strength for movements of the wrist, elbow and shoulder. In addition there was numbness of the thumb, index and middle fingers. These clinical findings had not altered by the time of the first EMG 3 months later. The electrophysiological findings (not shown) included the absence of an evoked potential in the thenar muscles following stimulation of the median nerve at the wrist and elbow. Stimulation of the ulnar nerve yielded a small response in the hypothenar muscles, corresponding to about 25 motor units (*Figure 22.4*).

A second EMG was performed 8 months after the first (11 months postoperatively). On this occasion a substantial response could be evoked in the thenar muscles following stimulation of the median nerve (*Figure 22.5*); the motor unit counting test indicated that about 73 motor units were functional. The hypothenar response was much larger than at the time of the previous EMG and now comprised about 203 motor unit potentials, an almost tenfold increase. In spite of this striking improvement in the electrophysiological findings, hardly any muscle contraction could be detected in the hand; none of the muscles were atrophied, however. As before, the thumb, index and middle fingers were numb and the skin of the hand was shiny and cyanosed.

What can be deduced from these findings? First, at the time of the *second* EMG, it seems that the patient was suffering from a neurapraxic lesion and that this was affecting motor and sensory fibres in the C5, C6, C7, C8 and T1 roots. In this way severe weakness could have been associated with the presence of excitable motor axons in the periphery. Similarly the presence of a neurapraxic lesion could account for the combination of an anaesthetic hand and normal-sized action potentials in digital nerve fibres.

The real problem lies in the interpretation of the results of the *first* EMG, for although the sensory

findings would have been compatible with the existence of a neurapraxic lesion, the motor findings could not be explained on this basis alone. The conventional explanation for the absence of the evoked thenar response on stimulation of the median nerve would be that the motor axons had been more severely-affected than the sensory ones

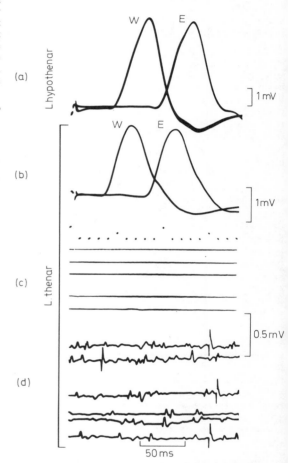

Figure 22.5. Findings in the muscles of the left arm in Case 3 at the second EMG examination. (a) Potentials evoked in the hypothenar muscles by maximal stimulation of the ulnar nerve at the wrist (response W) and at the elbow (response E). (b) Responses evoked in the thenar muscles by maximal stimulation of the median nerve. The smallest intervals on the time scale represent 1 ms. Recordings made with surface electrodes. (c) Absence of spontaneous activity at rest in the left abductor pollicis brevis muscle; recording made with coaxial needle electrode. (d) Incomplete interference pattern in the same muscle during attempted maximal effort (note the falsely 'myopathic' look of many of the potentials). (From McComas, Jorgensen and Upton (1974), courtesy of the Editor and publishers of Canadian Journal of Neurological Sciences)

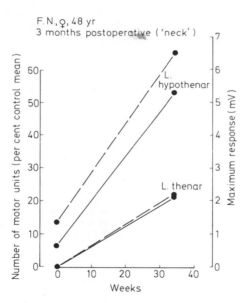

Figure 22.4. Numbers of functioning motor units, expressed as percentages of respective control means, in the thenar and hypothenar muscles of Case 3 at two EMG examinations: (— — — —) maximum evoked muscle responses (M-waves) (see text)

and had degenerated following the root lesion. This interpretation could only have been true for a small proportion of the axons, however, for the thenar muscles were not wasted and very little fibrillation activity could be detected in them. Also, it is doubtful if the motor axons could have grown approximately 800 mm in 320 days since, according to Sunderland (1968), regenerating nerve fibres have difficulty in traversing such great distances; this is possibly the reason why reinnervation of intrinsic muscles of the hand is so uncommon after brachial plexus lesions. A further problem with the degeneration–regeneration explanation is that the compact evoked muscle responses found at the second EMG examination (*Figure 22.5*) suggested that there had not been any slowing of impulse conduction such as would have been expected in regenerated axons. In the light of these considerations two explanations seem possible. In addition to bearing a neurapraxic lesion at the level of the cervical roots, the motor axons must either have become inexcitable in the periphery or else developed non-transmitting neuromuscular junctions. The first explanation is perhaps the less likely of the two since the sensory fibres were certainly excitable in the hand although affected by a neurapraxic lesion in their proximal parts. The remaining possibility, now supported by animal studies (Shibuya *et al.*, 1975), is that a lesion of the motor axon may produce not only a depression of excitability locally but also a loss of synaptic function distally. The synaptic dysfunction could readily be explained by a small reduction in the centrifugal flow of axoplasm as a consequence of the lesion. The importance of axoplasmic flow for the structural and functional integrity of the neuromuscular junction is now well established (see pages 15 and 222. Not only would this explanation suffice for the puzzling results of the second patient (Case 2, above) but it would also provide another explanation for the observation that motor axons appear more susceptible than sensory ones to the effects of ischaemia and nerve compression (see Sunderland, 1968, and Seddon, 1972). Thus not only are the motor axons more vulnerable on account of their relatively large diameters (see page 245) but their axon tips are particularly dependent upon an adequate supply of trophic material. In the third patient one can imagine that, with time, the defect in axoplasmic flow was corrected so that neuromuscular function was restored; at the time of the second EMG only the effect of the proximal neurapraxic lesion remained.

The concept of synaptic failure following an incomplete proximal lesion has been embodied in *Figure 22.6*, which shows the possible effects of increasingly severe compression injuries of nerves

(*at arrow*). In this figure the density of stippling represents the amount of material transported in the axoplasm from the cell body of the motoneurone to the periphery. In the least severe lesion (*b*), slowing of impulse conduction and a slight decrease in axoplasmic flow are the only abnormalities and no peripheral consequences ensue. Section (*c*) depicts the classical neurapraxic lesion in which there is local block of impulse conduction with preservation of axon excitability distally; according to Denny-Brown and Brenner (1974) some demyelination may be expected to occur at the site of the lesion. Section (*d*) illustrates the new concept of neuromuscular junction failure caused by an incomplete proximal lesion of the motor axon; the possibility of inexcitability of the distal axon has not been excluded, however. Even with this lesion there is sufficient flow of axoplasm to sustain the muscle fibre and to prevent the onset of denervation phenomena. In (*e*) a more severe compression interrupts axoplasmic flow; not only will the distal region of the axon degenerate but the muscle fibre will develop the full spectrum of denervation changes. In (*f*) the force of the lesion is sufficient to tear the axon across; the effects are the same as in (*e*).

CHRONIC LESIONS: THE ENTRAPMENT NEUROPATHIES

In this chapter attention has been directed so far to the effects of acute injury on peripheral nerve function; further, in each of the examples cited the lesion resulted from the application of an external force. Consideration must now be given to the consequences of chronic injury and, in particular, to the effects of prolonged compression of nerves by adjacent tissues. That nerves are likely to become damaged at certain points in their courses through 'wear and tear' is now well known; such disorders are referred to as entrapment neuropathies. While it is probable that none of the human peripheral nerves is immune to this type of damage, the commonest lesion by far is that affecting the median nerve at the wrist. This lesion produces the *carpal tunnel syndrome*. The patient, most commonly a middle-aged woman, complains of numbness and tingling in the thumb and adjacent three fingers. The symptoms are aggravated by use of the hand and are also especially severe at night, when they may waken the patient from sleep. Upon examination there is blunting of sensation to light touch and pin-prick over the area of skin felt to be numb. Wasting of muscles may be evident in the lateral part of the thenar eminence. A jolting sensation may be felt in the distribution of the median nerve following sharp percussion over the nerve at the wrist (*Tinel's sign*). Another useful test is that described by Phalen (1966) in which the sensory symptoms are accentuated by maintaining the wrist in a flexed position. The diagnosis may be readily confirmed by electromyography (see *Figure 23.2*). The most effective treatment is to reduce the pressure on the median nerve by dividing the over-

sal interosseous, recognized in the normal subject as the fleshy mound on the back of the hand between the thumb and base of the index finger. Weakness is most easily demonstrated in the adductors and abductors of the fingers. The usual treatment for the type of lesion is to free the ulnar nerve from the cubital groove and to transpose it anteriorly, in

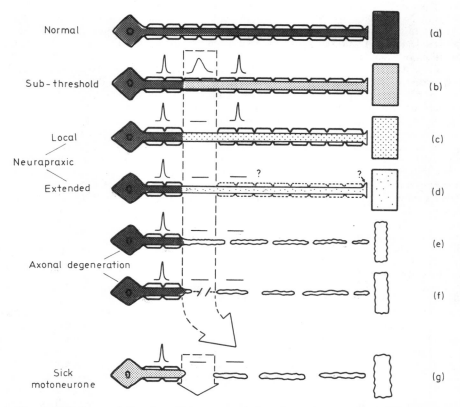

Figure 22.6. Types of disorder which may result from increasingly severe compression of a motor axon; site of compression indicated by tail of arrow. See text for description of changes. (From McComas, Jorgensen and Upton (1974) courtesy of the Editor and the publishers of Canadian Journal of Neurological Sciences*)*

lying transverse carpal ligament (flexor retinaculum); as a temporary measure relief may be obtained by resting the arm, including the use of night splints, or by a local injection of hydrocortisone.

The next most frequently encountered peripheral entrapment neuropathy is the one which involves the *ulnar nerve* as it runs behind the medial epicondyle at the elbow. With this type of lesion numbness and tingling is felt in the little finger and adjacent side of the ring finger. Wasting and weakness may be present in the small muscles of the hand; the best muscle for observing atrophy is the first dor-

front of the medial epicondyle. However, provided further damage to the nerve is prevented, spontaneous remission may often occur (Payan, 1970).

Two other common entrapment neuropathies are those affecting the radial and peroneal nerves. Thus the *radial nerve* may be squashed against the humerus as it passes through spiral groove; this may be caused by a patient falling asleep with his arm hanging over the back of a chair. Numbness is experienced over the dorsolateral aspect of the hand and base of the thumb, while the patient is unable to straighten the fingers and to dorsiflex the wrist.

The *common peroneal nerve* is vulnerable to pressure as it crosses behind the head of the fibula. Sitting for too long with the legs crossed, prolonged squatting, and the wearing of tight knee-high boots are the usual causes of damage. The patient presents with foot drop, being incapable of dorsiflexing the ankle as he lifts the foot from the ground. There is also numbness and tingling on the top of the foot around the cleft separating the big toe from its neighbour.

Some of the *less common entrapment neuropathies* involve:

(1) The median nerve as it passes through the *pronator teres muscle* below the elbow.

(2) The *anterior interosseous* branch of the median nerve.

(3) The deep motor branch of the *ulnar nerve* in the palm.

(4) The *posterior interosseous* branch of the radial nerve.

(5) The *lateral cutaneous nerve of thigh* where it passes under the inguinal ligament.

(6) The *posterior tibial nerve* within the tarsal tunnel.

The characteristic clinical features of these last lesions have been dealt with elsewhere (Koppell and Thompson, 1963; Staal, 1970) and are beyond the scope of this book. Of more interest to the experimental neurologist are considerations of the nature of the traumatic lesion and of the pathological changes which it produces in the nerve.

So far as the first topic is concerned, it is instructive to consider the disorder of the median nerve responsible for the carpal tunnel syndrome. Here the basic assumption is that the lesion results from compression of the nerve and that this is caused by a 'discrepancy between the capacity of the unyielding canal [tunnel] and the volume of its contents' (Entin, 1968). The *capacity of the canal may be reduced* by tightness of the transverse carpal ligament, callus formation or malalignment of bone following fracture of the wrist, and the bony overgrowth associated with acromegaly. The *contents of the canal may be increased* by inflammation of the synovial sheaths surrounding the flexor tendons (as in rheumatoid arthritis), scar tissue following injury, amyloid deposits, tumours and myxoedematous infiltrations. Pregnancy and obesity are also associated with an increased incidence of carpal tunnel syndromes, probably due to excessive amounts of fluid or fatty tissue in the soft tissues of the canal. Apart from these causes of 'static' compression it is probable that other precipitating factors are at play, and one of these is undoubtedly the amount of movement permitted at the wrist. Neary, Ochoa and Gilliatt (1975) report *post-*

mortem evidence of median nerve damage in the carpal tunnel in a 30-year-old man who died after several hours of decorticate rigidity; during this time the wrists had been maintained in a flexed position and the nerve was thought likely to have been compressed under the distal part of the transverse carpal ligament. Another causative factor is that the nerve normally has to slide under the ligament whenever the wrist and fingers are bent or straightened (McLellan and Swash, 1976). Also to be considered is the fact that patients with hereditary neuropathies or with metabolic disorders such as chronic renal failure or diabetes mellitus are very prone to develop median nerve and other entrapment neuropathies. One plausible explanation for this observation is that in each of these conditions the motor (and sensory) neurones are dysfunctional and therefore unable to manufacture and transport normal amounts of trophic messenger substances to the periphery (see Chapter 2). Hence any further reduction of axoplasmic transport due to relatively minor compression of a median nerve in its carpal tunnel would produce degeneration of the motor axons and denervation of the corresponding muscles (see *Figure 22.6, g*).

There is, in fact, some recent evidence that minor compression of the median nerve is very common and that with advancing age it produces pathological changes which may remain subclinical. Neary, Ochoa and Gilliat (1975) carried out *post-mortem* examination of ulnar and median nerves of 12 patients who had died from myocardial infarctions or other conditions not known to predispose to peripheral neuropathies. They found that in both nerves there were often Renaut bodies (whorls of collagen fibres lying beneath the perineurium) at the sites of entrapment and that the perineurial and epineurial tissues were thickened. In about half of the specimens of nerve examined the myelinated fibres also appeared abnormal at the entrapment sites; they exhibited evidence of demyelination or else showed bulbous swellings at the ends of the internodes facing away from the region susceptible to compression. In agreement with these observations is the finding of statistically significant slowing of impulse conduction in median nerve sensory fibres across the carpal tunnels of most normal subjects in middle or later age (Toyonaga and de Faria, unpublished observations). In the next chapter it is suggested that a lesion situated proximally (in the brachial plexus or cervical nerve roots) may accelerate and enhance the effects of minimal compression of the median nerve in the carpal tunnel and a tentative explanation for this is given.

It is of interest that a naturally-occuring pressure neuropathy has been reported in the median and ulnar nerves of guinea pigs; in these animals both nerves run under a cartilaginous bar at the wrist as well as the transverse carpal ligament (Fullerton and Gilliatt, 1967). The myelinated fibres in these animals resemble those described in human *post-mortem* material by Neary, Ochoa and Gilliatt (1975, see above) in that they display swellings at the ends of the internodes furthest from the site of entrapment. With the electronmicroscope Ochoa and Marotte (1973) have shown that the swellings consist of redundant folds of myelin, the latter having apparently been displaced away from the region of compression (*Figure 22.1, b*). In the patient already described by Neary and colleagues with an acute and severe lesion following decorticate rigidity, the teased nerve fibres showed evidence of a more profound abnormality, in that the nodes of Ranvier had been squeezed in an axial direction so as to invaginate the adjacent internodal regions. It will be recalled that this type of lesion could be produced by the application of very high pressures to experimental animals (Ochoa, Fowler and Gilliatt, 1972). It seems

unlikely, however, that deformations of this kind could be an important or consistent feature of the majority of nerve entrapments in which there is a slow but insidious progression of symptoms and the absence of a history of acute injury.

It should also be noted that, whatever the cause of the abnormal force acting upon the nerve (narrowing of the canal, increasing volume of its contents, or excessive sliding and stretching of the nerve), there is the effect on the circulation of the nerve to take into account. Sunderland (1976), in reviewing the pathogenesis of the carpal tunnel syndrome, has agreed that the initial result of compression is obstruction of the venous return from the nerve fascicles, followed by the formation of oedema fluid and then by anoxia due to slowed capillary circulation. Among the evidence supporting a vascular mechanism is the aggravation of symptoms by the application of a venous occlusion cuff, the swelling of the hand during sleep and the almost immediate relief of symptoms after surgical decompression.

Chapter 23

THE DOUBLE CRUSH SYNDROME

Causes of upper limb paraesthesiae (*Figure 23.1*)

The patient with pain and numbness in the arm presents the neurologist with one of his most common problems and, at the same time, provides the electromyographer with the basis of his practice. Lishman and Russell (1961) have given a very full account of the changing trends in clinical diagnosis since the turn of the present century. They describe how attention was directed initially to the brachial plexus, with Gowers (1899) considering the underlying lesion to be an inflammatory process in the nerve sheaths. Gowers thought that the inflammation had reached the nerves from 'fibrositic' areas in the muscle of the neck. Subsequent to this the cervical rib syndrome was recognized and came to account for a proportion of the patients with pain in the arm. Later still it was considered that similar symptoms could occur in the absence of a cervical rib; in such patients the brachial plexus could be compressed either by a fibrous band passing between the transverse process of the seventh cervical vertebra and the first rib, or else by a tonically-contracted scalenus anterior muscle. Walshe (1945) proposed that compression of the lower trunk of the brachial plexus could occur in the absence of a congenital anomaly in those patients with sagging of their shoulder girdles. A further type of plexus lesion was suggested by Wartenberg (1944) and consisted of irritation of the lower part on the first rib during sleep.

Once the occurrence of prolapsed intervertebral discs had been recognized in the lumbar spine, with their attendant clinical features, it was logical to inquire whether a similar type of lesion could affect the neck. Semmes and Murphy (1943) suggested that lateral protrusion of a cervical disc could press on a nerve root and cause symptoms referable to the arm. At operation Frykholm (1951) found that, even when no protrusion could be demonstrated, the sleeve of dura mater investing the nerve root was often thickened and rigid. Both he and Scoville (1946) were sufficiently impressed by their operative results to suggest that lesions of the cervical roots were responsible for most cases of pain in the arm: 'Compression of the nerve roots at the lower cervical vertebral foramens accounts for most of the diagnoses of scalenus anticus syndrome, brachial neuralgia and other obscure neuralgic pains of the shoulder and arm' (Scoville, 1946). In addition to the relatively soft nuclear herniations from cervical discs, the hard bony projections of arthritic cervical spines were also recognized as being likely to impinge on the nerve roots (Liversedge, 1959). A further advance came from Cloward (1960) who investigated the effects of electrical stimulation of the discs and was able to show that some of the pain in the shoulder and arm might have been referred from the innervation of the cervical discs.

At the very time when the cervical roots were being incriminated so strongly as the major cause of brachial neuralgia, attention was abruptly directed elsewhere by the studies of Cannon and Love (1946) and of Brain, Wright and Wilkinson (1947). Both these groups described patients who had suffered from spontaneous compression of the

253

median nerve within its carpal tunnel and who had been treated successfully by section of the transverse carpal ligament. It is of some historical interest that Marie and Foix had encountered this condition in 1913 during the course of an autopsy on a patient with advanced atrophy of the thenar muscles; both median nerves exhibited neuromata immediately proximal to the transverse carpal ligaments (see Chapter 22).

Problems in Diagnosis

While it is possible that so many different types of lesion are capable of producing pain in the arm it is unlikely that all are equally important and one is still faced with the problem of making a diagnosis in the individual patient. It might be thought that these matters could be decided on clinical grounds, either by looking for specific symptoms and signs or else by studying the results of different treatments. A survey of the literature reveals that the

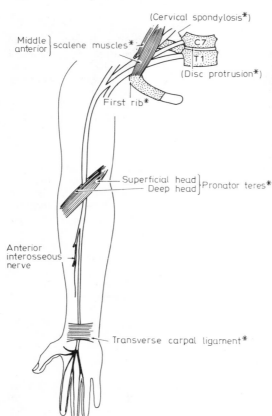

Figure 23.1. Sites of compressive lesions (*) which may produce pain in the territory of the median nerve (see text)

situation is surprisingly complicated and contains a number of apparent contradictions. For example, Scoville (1946) treated 400 patients with brachial neuralgia by operating on the cervical spine and commented that 86 per cent were 'markedly improved'. One interpretation of this result would be that in at least 86 per cent of patients with pain in the shoulder and arm the underlying lesion had involved the cervical roots. However, the surgical treatment involved postoperative rest for the affected limb and, even after this time, it is doubtful whether many patients would have been tempted to use their arms as vigorously as before. One must therefore take into account the possible therapeutic effects of rest and, in this context, the study by Lishman and Russell (1961) is instructive. These authors studied 146 cases of brachial neuralgia and treated the majority with some form of limb immobilization such as bed rest, supporting the arm in a sling, wearing a cervical collar, or applying a plaster cast to the wrist. In most cases the induced rest alone was sufficient to relieve the symptoms and the improvement was often maintained. The excellent consequences of such conservative management require that caution be exercised in the interpretation of surgical studies. An alternative approach would be to look for correlations between the type of conservative treatment which proved successful and the type of lesion suggested by the clinical findings; the presence of such a correlation would suggest that the site of the nerve lesion had been correctly identified. Once again the findings of Lishman and Russell (1961) are relevant: 'Few clear correlations could be found, however, for patients with a carpal tunnel syndrome were often relieved by a sling or light collar, whereas some with pain in the proximal arm were relieved by splinting the wrist. In particular three patients whose symptoms were reproduced by neck movements and two whose symptoms had been aggravated by depression of the shoulders, were eventually cured by treatment at the wrist. Also two patients clearly showing Tinel's sign at the wrist obtained complete relief from neck traction and procaine injections into the scapular muscles respectively.' In patients with such strongly positive physical signs it is unlikely that the initial diagnosis could have been wrong, yet how are these observations to be explained? Further interpretative difficulties arise when the results of careful surgical studies of the carpal tunnel syndrome are considered. Phalen (1966), an authority on this condition, noted that there was no visible evidence of compression in 61 out of 212 exposed median nerves. There is also the fact that some patients with undoubted carpal tunnel syndromes fail to improve after technically satisfactory decompressions of their median nerves (Cseuz *et al.*, 1966). This observation is indeed puzzling, for in laboratory animals with experimental crush injuries nerve regeneration is vigorous and, in any case, only a small population of intact motor axons (e.g. 10–20 per cent) are necessary to provide normal strength in a partially denervated human muscle (McComas *et al.*, 1971b). Another curious feature of distal entrapment neuropathies is that these are commonly multiple.

cases may also have tenderness over the brachial plexus as well.

Electrophysiological studies

The lesson learned from the above studies is that, in order to resolve the pathogenesis of an individual case of brachial neuralgia, it is unwise, and may be

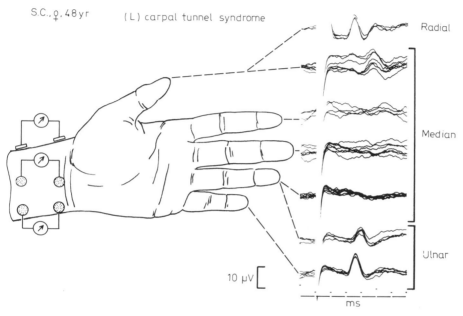

S.C., ♀, 48 yr   (L) carpal tunnel syndrome

Radial

Median

Ulnar

10 μV

ms

Figure 23.2. Sensory nerve studies in patient with a carpal tunnel syndrome on the left side. Notice the slowing of impulses conduction and the small sensory nerve potentials within the distribution of the median nerve. In the ulnar and radial nerves the findings are normal and can serve as useful references for the affected median nerve. Thus, the conduction distances from the stimulating electrodes on the thumb to the recording electrodes over the median and radial nerves are made the same (10 cm), as are the distances from the ring finger to the recording sites over the median and ulnar nerves (13 cm). Inspection of the paired responses from the thumb reveals that impulse conduction in the median nerve is relatively slow while the median nerve response from the ring finger cannot be detected

Thus, not only are ulnar and median entrapment neuropathies often bilateral, but it is now recognized that the two types of lesion exist together in an unexpectedly high proportion of cases (Sedal, McLeod and Walsh, 1973; Buchthal, Rosenfalck and Trojaborg, 1974).

Additional problems arise when patients with atypical brachial neuralgia are considered. Some of these have diffuse pain in the arm without any abnormal physical signs being present while there are others with extensive tenderness over their nerves. For example, pressure upon the median nerve may be as painful when applied at the level of the pronator teres as at the carpal tunnel; such

frankly misleading, to rely solely on clinical information. Fortunately, the problem is no longer as intractable as it might appear for the continued development of electromyography during the past 20 years has made it possible to diagnose peripheral nerve lesions with considerable confidence. The diagnostic tests which the electromyographer has at his disposal are varied but the most important ones for the diagnosis of an entrapment neuropathy are the measurements of impulse conduction velocity in the regions of nerve under suspicion. Such measurements may be performed readily on sensory as well as motor axons and they are usually combined with exploration of appropriate muscles with a coaxial recording electrode. To these standard tests may now be added the estimation of numbers of functioning motor units in the thenar and hypothenar muscles (page 48). In the protocol developed for investigating brachial neuralgia at McMaster University the various tests are combined in the following way. First, the numbers of functioning motor units are estimated in the thenar

impulse conduction also be studied in the opposite ulnar nerve around the elbow. Similarly, abnormalities in both the median and the ulnar nerves raise the possibility of a polyneuropathy being present and so the investigation would be continued with studies of the sural and peroneal nerves and would include a motor unit count in the extensor digitorum brevis.

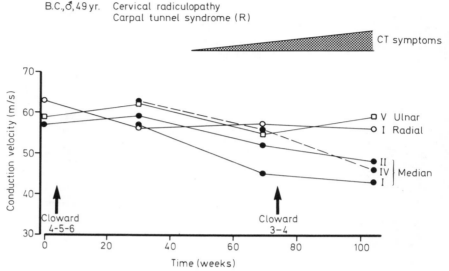

Figure 23.3. Serial EMG findings in a patient who developed a carpal tunnel (CT) syndrome, having presented with proximal symptoms for which Cloward procedures were performed (see text). The values shown are the maximum impulse conduction velocities of sensory fibres in the right median, ulnar and radial nerves. The recordings were made with surface electrodes over the wrist, following stimulation of the appropriate digits (I = thumb). Note the fall in the median nerve conduction velocities and the absence of significant changes in the ulnar and radial nerve values. (Courtesy of Dr A. R. M. Upton)

and hypothenar muscles of the most severely-affected arm. The maximal impulse conduction velocities and terminal latencies are then measured for motor axons of the median and ulnar nerves on this side. The next step is to measure the response amplitudes and impulse conduction velocities for sensory axons of the radial, median and ulnar nerves of both hands, stimulating each digit in turn and recording at the level of the wrist (Figure 23.2). Finally, a coaxial needle electrode is used to record volitional activity and any spontaneous electrical potentials from appropriate muscles on the most severely-affected side. These muscles usually comprise the abductor pollicis brevis, abductor digiti minimi, extensor digitorum, biceps brachii, deltoid, supraspinatus and trapezius; the selection will convey information concerning all the roots between C4 and T1. In some patients the examination is extended further. For example, the discovery of a cubital tunnel lesion on one side requires that

It is obvious that a comprehensive examination of this kind is well suited to detect the presence of single or multiple entrapment neuropathies in a given patient and the additional presence of a cervical root (or brachial plexus) lesion may often be deduced. For example, a patient with a carpal tunnel syndrome would probably also be suffering from a T1 root lesion if the hypothenar motor unit count was reduced without there being any slowing of impulse conduction in the ulnar nerve. In the same patient the existence of an associated C8 lesion would be inferred if it was found that the sensory responses in the digital nerves to the ring and little fingers were significantly diminished.

Using this battery of tests Upton and McComas (1973) investigated 220 unselected patients presenting with pain, numbness or tingling in the hand, sometimes associated with weakness of intrinsic muscles. Then findings are summarized in Table 23.1 from which it can be seen that 85 of the 200 patients had carpal tunnel syndromes, 24 had ulnar neuropathies and six had both types of lesion. The remaining patients were considered to have a radiculopathy or possibly, in some cases, a brachial plexus lesion. Up to this point the findings are as might have been expected for Lishman and Russell (1961), in their study of patients with brachial neuralgia, had also found that irritation of cervical roots and carpal tunnel syndromes were by far the most commonly diagnosed lesions. The feature of the study by Upton and McComas which was remarkable, and was so relevant to the diagnostic problems raised in the introduction, was the following: *81 (70 per cent) of the 115 patients with electrophysiologically-proven entrapment neuropathies also had evidence of cervical root lesions.* In most cases this evidence was electomyographic but in some the presence of a cervical root lesion was inferred from a history of severe neck pain and stiffness and the finding of sensory abnormality corresponding to a dermatomal rather than a peripheral nerve distribution. The radiological findings often supported a diagnosis of cervical root injury but, unless grossly irregular, they were not used as a sufficient criterion in themselves. In connection with radiology, it is both interesting and relevant that one of the six patients with a carpal tunnel syndrome described by Brain, Wright and Wilkinson (1947) was also shown to have bilateral cervical ribs and a Klippel–Feil anomaly.

In some of the patients investigated by Upton and McComas the development of a distal entrapment neuropathy seemed to follow injury to the neck. Inevitably the commonest injury was the so-called 'whiplash' type, which is sustained by the driver or passenger of a car when it is struck from behind and the head is suddenly retroflexed.

The patient described below provided an opportunity to study nerve conduction prior to the onset of his entrapment neuropathy; in this patient there was a history of a cervical root lesion treated surgically.

The patient, a 49-year-old self-employed man, first presented for electromyography with an 18-month history of pain in both shoulders. The pain was more severe on the right side and was especially troublesome at night; it occasionally radiated down the lateral aspect of the forearm. At the first examination (*Figure 23.3*) all the impulse conduction velocities were normal in sensory fibres of the right median, ulnar and radial nerves. The following month a Cloward procedure was performed so as to fuse the 5th, 6th and 7th cervical vertebrae. His symptoms remitted for several months but, shortly before the second EMG, he developed numbness in the fingers and thumbs of both hands. Although the impulse conduction velocities were not significantly changed fibrillation potentials were encountered in the right abductor pollicis brevis and abductor digiti minimi muscles. By the third EMG examination, however, the impulse conduction velocities had fallen in the right median nerve across the wrist; at this time there was clinical evidence, supported by coaxial needle electromyography, of damage to the C4, C5, C6, C8 and T1 roots. A further Cloward procedure was carried out in the 74th week of observation; after a short-lived subjective improvement, the patient noticed that the numbness in both hands had increased, being associated with loss of strength and intermittent cramps of the intrinsic muscles. Phalen's test for carpal tunnel syndrome was positive on both sides and, at the final EMG, further slowing of impulse conduction could be demonstrated in the right median nerve (*Figure 23.3*).

The double crush hypothesis

The findings of Upton and McComas (1973) clearly establish the existence of an association between lesions affecting the cervical roots (or brachial plexus) and those involving the median and ulnar nerves. This association provides an explanation for many of the puzzling features described previously.

TABLE 23.1

Incidence of Cervical and Thoracic Root Lesions among 115 Patients with Carpal Tunnel Syndromes or Ulnar Entrapment Neuropathies*

Peripheral nerve entrapment	Root Lesion		
	Probable	Absent	Possible
Unilateral carpal tunnel	39	13	3
Bilateral carpal tunnel	23	7	0
Unilateral ulnar neuropathy	12	7	1
Bilateral ulnar neuropathy	3	1	0
Carpal tunnel and ulnar neuropathy	4	1	1
Total	81	29	5

* In nine of the patients with probable neck pathology other aetiological factors may also have been involved: diabetes, six cases; arthritis, wrist fracture and alcoholism, one case each

From Upton and McComas (1973), courtesy of the Editor of the *Lancet*

It explains, for example, why patients with carpal or cubital tunnel lesions may suffer from neck or shoulder pain and perhaps have objective evidence of cervical disease. It affords a reason for the persistence of symptoms after the median nerve has been decompressed. In addition, the presence of a second lesion, situated proximally, would account for the normal appearance of some median nerves at exploration as well as for the failure of a median nerve to regenerate adequately following decompression.

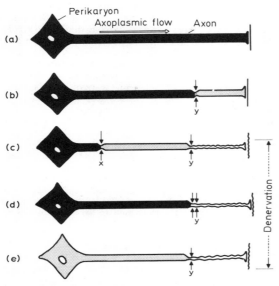

Figure 23.4. The principle of the 'double crush' hypothesis and an explanation for the liability of patients with neuronal disorders to develop entrapment neuropathies. (From Upton and McComas (1973) courtesy of the Editor and publishers of the Lancet)

Since the association between the proximal and distal lesions in the same nerve is too common to be fortuitous, we must assume that in some way one lesion encourages the development of the other. But how? A satisfactory explanation cannot involve the nerve impulse for this is an all-or-nothing event. Provided an impulse can reach the end of a damaged region of axon it will regain its full amplitude before arriving at the second zone of injury: it can tell the axon nothing of the difficulty it had encountered earlier. Lishman and Russell (1961) suggested that injury might release a metabolite at one level and that this might then spread and affect the vulnerability of other regions; they cited the work of Brierley and Field (1949) in which injected radioactive phosphorus was observed to travel rapidly within the connective tissue matrix of rabbit sciatic

nerves. A second possibility is that tethering of a nerve at one point, for example by a prolapsed disc, may cause excessive stretching at vulnerable sites elsewhere (McLellan and Swash, 1976).

A third proposal has been put forward by Upton and McComas (1973). They based their hypothesis on the phenomenon of axoplasmic flow (considered in Chapter 2). The salient features of the hypothesis are given in *Figure 23.4*, which depicts a normal motoneurone (*a*); within the perikaryon (cell body) special 'trophic' messenger substances are known to be synthesized and these are then transported along the axon to the muscle fibres (at *right*). A large body of evidence (reviewed in chapters 8, 9 and 20) indicates that these substances are required for the normal upkeep of the muscle fibres as well as for the motor axon and its terminal. Suppose that in most persons there is a slight compression of axons in the carpal tunnel or in the case of the ulnar nerve, in the cubital tunnel such compression is shown at *y* in (*b*) of Figure 23.4. Provided there is a surplus of trophic material enough will still be delivered beyond the constriction to the muscle fibre and distal axon to prevent their degeneration. The situation will change dramatically if, in the same person, the axon is damaged at another point (at *x*, in *Figure 23.4, c*). Some of the neurotubules and neurofilaments within the axon will now be destroyed at *x* and others will be damaged at *y*; as a consequence the delivery of trophic material beyond *y* will be insufficient to prevent degeneration in the axon and muscle fibre. As noted in Table 23.1, not all entrapment neuropathies arise in this way; in about one-third of patients there is no evidence of a proximal lesion and in these it must be assumed that the distal compression is especially severe (as at *y* in *Figure 23.4, d*).

An extension of the hypothesis provides an explanation for the high incidence of peripheral nerve entrapment syndromes in patients with metabolic disorders such as diabetes mellitus and renal failure, or with hereditary neuropathies (Davies, 1954; Gilliatt and Willison, 1962; Earl *et al.*, 1964). In all these conditions it is reasonable to postulate that the cell body of the motoneurone is affected and is no longer capable of synthesizing a normal amount of trophic material; if so, minor degrees of axon compression will become critical and produce denervation phenomena (*Figure 23.4, e*).

In view of the association between proximal and distal lesions Upton and McComas termed their hypothesis 'the double crush'. They recognized, however, that in some patients the nerve fibres might be affected at more than two levels and that, in some instances, the lesion might not be a compression but rather the damage resulting from sudden stretch (as in a 'whiplash' injury). Further reflection shows that the hypothesis can also account for the presence of multiple peripheral nerve entrapments in the same patient (excluding, of course, those with a polyneuropathy; see above). The explanation lies in the fact that in most patients with cervical disease or injury several roots are affected; if the C6, C7 and C8 roots were seriously involved such a patient would be predisposed to the development of both cubital and carpal tunnel syndromes. In some patients it is the upper cervical roots which are damaged; in these cases a peripheral nerve lesion probably arises because the weakness of trapezius, induced by C3 and C4 lesions, allows the shoulder to droop. The lower part of the brachial plexus is then compressed against the first rib and the proximal lesion is set in train. Finally, although the double crush hypothesis arose from observations on the upper limb, the analogous syndrome has since been recognized in the legs; the patients are those with spontaneous peroneal nerve palsies in association with lumbosacral root lesions.

It might be argued that the cellular mechanism proposed in the hypothesis—the reduction in axoplasmic flow—is speculative. This is not the case, however, since the first evidence for axoplasmic flow came from the experiments of Weiss and Hiscoe (1948) in which a 'damming back' of axoplasm was observed following partial constriction of the axon (page 13). Of still greater relevance to the double crush hypothesis were the further experiments of Weiss and Hiscoe, involving the placement of a second constriction further along the axon. It was then possible to establish that the constriction

of the first site had been incomplete for some of the axoplasm was able to accumulate in front of the distal constriction. In fairness to any opponents of the double crush hypothesis it must be added that the conclusions of Weiss and Hiscoe have since been criticized by Spencer (1972). This author examined electronmicrographs of the region of apparent 'damming'; he noted that although distended nerve fibres were present, the swelling appeared to affect only those axons which were starting to grow back following degeneration at the level of the constriction. In defence of Weiss and Hiscoe's work, it should be pointed out that these authors took pains to induce a very gentle compression and used a sleeve of artery rather than a ligature (as employed by Spencer). A point in favour of Weiss's interpretation is that the existence of 'slow' axoplasmic flow has since been confirmed by numerous isotope studies, although, of course, this does not necessarily mean that a 'bulk' movement of axoplasm is taking place. Finally, in their later work, Weiss and his colleagues had the opportunity to study the detailed structure of the distended regions of axon with the electronmicroscope. They found evidence of stasis of axoplasm in the peripheral rim of the axis cylinder where mitochondria had collected; in contrast it appeared that the core of the axis cylinder was still in motion under the constriction.

In conclusion, it is evident that there is still a need for further experimentation. Nevertheless, sufficient supporting data is available for the 'double crush' hypothesis to seem an attractive possible way of explaining a number of puzzling clinical observations.

DISORDERS OF MOTONEURONES

The final section of this book deals with disorders of motoneurones. In some of these disorders, such as motoneurone disease and spinal muscular atrophy, it is probable that the primary lesion lies within the motoneurone soma; in the toxic and metabolic neuropathies (Chapter 25) there is still uncertainty as to which part of the motor nerve cell is first affected. Thus, even though the first microscopic evidence of abnormality may be restricted to the motor nerve endings, it is quite possible that these changes reflect interference with the synthesis of trophic molecules by the soma, or with their transport down the axon (see Chapter 2). Since the abnormalities are most evident in the periphery, the various disorders are often referred to as the 'dying-back' neuropathies. It will be seen that in the earliest stages of these disorders there may be no effect other than blockage of neuromuscular transmission; the potential reversibility of this type of dysfunction is well illustrated by those patients undergoing treatment for thyrotoxicosis (Chapter 26). More serious involvement of the motoneurone causes the muscle fibre to become fully denervated while the entire motor nerve cell may itself ultimately degenerate.

Chapter 24

MOTONEURONE DEGENERATION

MOTONEURONE DISEASE (AMYOTROPHIC LATERAL SCLEROSIS)

Clinical features

Motoneurone disease is the name given to a disorder in which the anterior horn cells undergo progressive and apparently spontaneous degenerative changes, usually culminating in the death of the patient within a few years. The life expectancy from the time of diagnosis is about 3 years, though considerable variation exists (see below). Approximately one person per 100 0000 of the population dies from the disease each year, the prevalence rate being 2.5–7 per 100 000 (Kurland and Mulder, 1954). Motoneurone disease is about twice as frequent in males as in females, but in both sexes the onset occurs most commonly in the sixth and seventh decades. In the past it has been customary to recognize three clinical variants of the disorder, depending on the presence or absence of pyramidal tract involvement and on the pattern of muscle weakness. These three variants are:

Progressive muscular atrophy

In this form the disease affects the limb motoneurones predominantly and tends to run a slower course. A common presentation is for the patient to notice increasing weakness and wasting of the small muscles of the hands. Eventually proximal muscles in the arms are affected and the legs also

become weak. The patient may notice spontaneous twitchings (fasciculations) in the muscles.

Progressive bulbar palsy

This is the most severe and unpleasant form of the disease, the brunt of the attack falling on the motoneurones within the brainstem. As a consequence the patient suffers from progressive paralysis of the tongue, lips, larynx and palate. There is difficulty in speaking caused partly by the weakness of the tongue, labial and laryngeal muscles and partly by the inability to close off the nasopharynx with the soft palate. A particularly serious consequence of the disorder is the inability to swallow food and liquids properly; this, and the associated difficulty in coughing forcefully, render the patient liable to choking attacks during meals or even from inhalation of his own saliva.

Amyotrophic lateral sclerosis

The most prominent early features of this disorder are the spasticity and weakness which result from degeneration of the corticospinal pathways; the most common clinical presentation is that of difficulty in walking. In time other symptoms and signs of an upper motoneurone lesion are likely to develop and include a spastic weakness of speech and swallowing (pseudobulbar palsy), as well as weakness and clumsiness of the arms. As would be expected in an upper motoneurone type of disorder, the tendon reflexes are extremely brisk and clonus can often be demonstrated; the plantar responses are extensor.

It must be emphasized that many cases are difficult to fit into one of these three categories, since they may show the clinical features of more than one syndrome. For example, patients may have significant weakness and wasting of limb and bulbar

culations are an important diagnostic sign which is likely to be present in all three forms of the disease (Appendix 24.1); the tongue muscles also participte in this activity and may sometimes show it well at a time when it is less evident elsewhere. Muscle *cramps* also commonly occur and may sometimes be the presenting complaint.

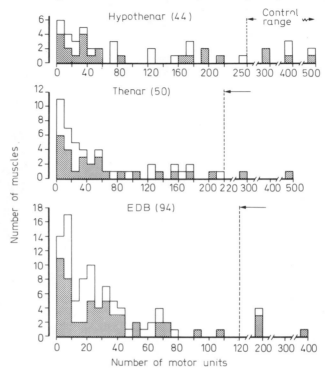

Figure 24.1. Numbers of functioning motor units in patients with motoneurone disease at the time of their initial presentation for electromyography. The lower limits of the control ranges for the hypothenar, thenar and extensor digitorum brevis muscles studied are shown by the interrupted lines and the values for patients below the age of 60 are indicated by the filled columns. Numbers of muscles studied are given in parentheses

muscles as well as florid signs of upper motoneurone disturbance. Even if upper motoneurone signs had been absent in a patient with a clinically pure form of progressive muscular atrophy, an autopsy is likely to show evidence of degeneration in the corticospinal tracts (Friedman and Freedman, 1950). A further point is that, irrespective of the initial presentation, a patient may still develop weakness of bulbar muscles and eventually die from choking or from an aspiration pneumonia. Death may also result from bronchopneumonia secondary to poor ventilation of the lungs; there is an increased incidence of myocardial infarction as well (Liversedge and Campbell, 1974). Again, muscle *fasci-*

There is no *treatment* known to arrest the course of motoneurone disease though to date the search has included vitamins (E and B_{12}), corticosteroids, pancreatic extract, antiviral drugs and guanidine. A trial of anticholinestrase medication is always worth while however, for in some patients myasthenic-like features develop, presumably because the motoneurone cell bodies are unable to sustain full function of the axon terminals (page 212).

A brief clinical description of motoneurone disease having been given, the remainder of the chapter is devoted to certain aspects of the disorder which seem especially interesting at present. Particular mention is made of the results of motor unit counting studies, since they have enabled the severity and progression of the denervation to be measured for the first time. Eighty-seven patients in Newcastle upon Tyne (U.K.) and Hamilton (Canada) were investigated by this method; some of the findings have been briefly reported elsewhere (McComas, Upton and Sica, 1973).

Motor unit counts

the first point to emerge from these studies is the extreme severity of the denervation in some of the muscles at the time when the patient is referred for his or her initial electromyographic examination. In *Figure 24.1* the motor unit populations of the thenar, hypothenar and extensor digitorum brevis muscles have been shown in relation to the lower limits of the normal ranges. Since healthy subjects can be expected to lose function in an increasing number of motor units beyond the age of 60, the values for the 51 patients with motoneurone disease who were aged 60 or less have been shown separately in the figure.

The finding of such severe denervation at the time when the patient first seeks advice has two interesting implications. One of these is that much of the weakness which would otherwise have resulted from the denervation must have been masked. The mechanism responsible for this functional compensation is *collateral reinnervation*, that is, the formation of fresh neuromuscular junctions on denervated muscle fibres by sprouts given off from the axons of surviving motoneurones. A detailed description of this phenomenon has been given elsewhere (page 224) and its functional effectiveness has been stressed (see *Figures 20.6, 20.8*). The second implication from these quantitative studies is that the anterior horn cell degeneration must have been present well in advance of the development of symptoms.

To obtain more information about the rate of denervation it is necessary to make serial estimates of motor unit numbers in individual patients. It is found that the results differ markedly from case to case or even between muscles of the same patient, as was shown in one 59-year-old lady with a 3-year history of weakness of bulbar muscles.

At the first examination there was evidence of severe denervation of distal muscles in the limbs which was strikingly asymmetrical. Thus the left extensor digitorum brevis muscle (EDB) was estimated to have 130 motor units (within the normal range) whereas the right EDB had only 15 units; similarly in the hands the right hypothenar muscles had a full complement of units (about 549) whereas the corresponding muscles on the left were

already well depleted (about 179 units). Within the next seven months there were dramatic reductions in the numbers of motor units in the better two muscles, while the ones already partially denervated showed proportionately less change. At the time of the next examination, 4 months later, there were signs that the rate of the degenerative process had slackened in the motoneurone pools supplying the muscles which had just undergone such rapid denervation (left EDB and right hypothenar).

The same phenomenon of a rapid loss of motor units followed by a levelling-off was noted in the EDB muscle of patient T.H., a 51-year-old man

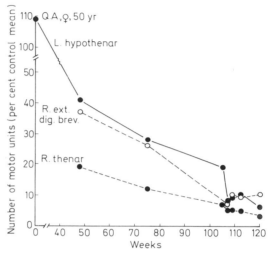

Figure 24.2. Serial estimates of numbers of functioning motor units in a 50-year-old woman with motoneurone disease. Note the progressive and widespread loss of units (see text)

with a 1-year history of muscle weakness. Within the space of only 10 weeks the motor unit count in the muscle had fallen from about 167 to 37 but in the ensuing 10 months no further loss took place. Although these results demonstrate that some motoneurones are able to withstand the degenerative process better than others, all cells may succumb eventually for we have also encountered 19 muscles in which fewer than six motor units remained, as well as four in which there had been total denervation.

The results shown in *Figure 24.2* were chosen for illustration, partly because they demonstrated progressive reductions in the motor unit populations of all three muscles tested, but also because the first EMG examination was made before the onset of weakness.

The patient, a 50-year-old woman, had presented with numbness and tingling in the ring and little fingers of her left hand. Electrophysiological examination revealed a normal hypothenar motor unit population and no evidence of ulnar nerve or cervical root lesions; the sensory symptoms eventually resolved spontaneously. Approximately 9 months later she began to notice increasing weakness of her arms and legs. The weakness was confirmed on physical examination and found to be associated with slight atrophy, fasciculations and bilateral upper motoneurone signs. An EMG examination now revealed significant reductions in the motor unit populations of the hypothenar, thenar and extensor digitorum brevis muscles with enlargement of surviving units. The steady downhill course is evident from *Figure 24.2* and was unaffected by a course of prednisone in high dosage; the patient developed progressive bulbar palsy and died one year after the last examination.

Sometimes a patient with undoubted motoneurone disease defies a pessimistic prognosis by manifesting a remarkably slow deterioration, sometimes with temporary remissions; several examples have been reported by Engel and colleagues (1969). In the series of 87 patients studied in Newcastle and Hamilton there is a similar patient, in whom the motor units counting studies substantiated the clinical findings.

moderate muscle atrophy. Upper motoneurone involvement was indicated by abnormally brisk tendon reflexes and the presence of Babinski responses bilaterally. In spite of the 5-year history of weakness, she was still able to walk without assistance, to work as a bank clerk and to perform normal household duties. During her illness E. Q. had been treated at various times with anti-cholinesterase drugs, pancreatic extract and vitamin E; she had also received medication for an associated depression and anxiety state.

At the first EMG examination (5 years after the onset of symptoms) evidence of severe chronic denervation was found in small muscles of the hand and foot by means of the motor unit counting technique. Signs of denervation in proximal muscles of the limbs were obtained during examination with a coaxial needle electrode. In contrast to the marked muscle abnormalities, there was no electrophysiological evidence of sensory neurone involvement in the upper or lower limbs. At the end of the first year of observation no significant change had occurred in the populations of motor units in the hypothenar and EDB muscles, though there appeared to be some increase in the thenar population (*Figure 24.3*). At the 69th week of observation the patient felt considerably weaker and asked for further EMG examination;

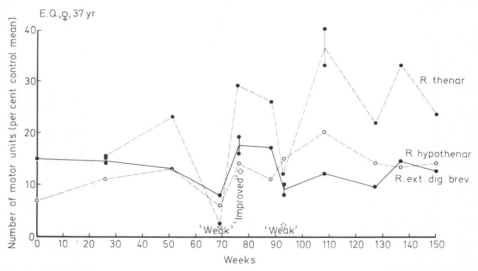

Figure 24.3. Serial estimates of numbers of functioning motor units in a 37-year-old woman with a slow and fluctuating form of hereditary motoneurone disease (see text)

Patient E. Q., a woman, was 37 years of age at the time of her initial EMG examination. She had not been exposed to any neurotoxic chemicals, nor had she suffered from poliomyelitis earlier. However, her mother had died at the age of 52 following a 5-year history of progressive muscle weakness and had been diagnosed as having motoneurone disease. Since the age of 32 the propositus had noticed an increasing loss of strength which was generalized, affecting muscles of the trunk and neck as well as proximal and distal muscles of the limbs; speech and swallowing were unaffected. In addition to the signs of widespread muscle weakness, there was evidence of

this disclosed definite deteriorations in the numbers of functioning motor units in all three muscles tested. After consideration, the patient gave informed consent for an empirical trial with corticosteroids and was admitted to hospital for observation at the 75th week. At admission, however, she volunteered that her strength had improved and an EMG (at 76 weeks) revealed considerable improvement in the functioning motor unit populations, particularly in the thenar group (*Figure 24.3*). The clinical and electrophysiological amelioration persisted up to the time of the next EMG (at 88 weeks). On the next occasion of study two of the motor unit counts were again depressed, the patient complaining of further loss of strength. The patient was next investigated at 108 weeks and it was found that all three motor unit populations were larger, the thenar complement being greater than on any of the previous six occasions. Although the patient was unaware of any increase in strength it is likely that her self-assessment had been influenced adversely by a profound depression. Further examinations, at 127, 137 and 150 weeks, disclosed continuing variations in the thenar count but comparative stability in the values for the EDB and hypothenar muscles (*Figure 24.3*).

In summary, the motor unit counting studies in this patient revealed that no additional persisting muscle denervation had occurred during the 3-year period of observation. Equally remarkable were the fluctuations in the numbers of functioning motor units; it should be stressed that these variations were too great to have been accounted for on the basis of experimental error. The only explanation remaining for these changes is that they reflected the repeated transition of motoneurones between healthy and dysfunctional ('sick') phases.

Aetiology of motoneurone disease

Perhaps the most fascinating aspect of moto-neurone disease is its aetiology. The interest in this subject and the enigmatic nature of the problem is reflected in the long and varied list of possibilities which has been adduced to date. This list includes the following:

Lead poisoning
Manganese poisoning
Poliomyelitis
'Slow' virus infection
Carcinoma
Malabsorption
Trauma
Electric shock
Disordered carbohydrate metabolism
Genetic

Some of these possibilities will be discussed further.

Lead poisoning

It is well known that chronic lead poisoning may give rise to a neurological syndrome with a close resemblance to motoneurone disease. Indeed, in the first description of motoneurone disease by Aran (1850) three of the 11 patients had been exposed to lead and two of these had previously suffered from lead poisoning. During the last century potential sources of lead poisoning were common for the substance was used in paints, hair dyes, cosmetics, glazing and water pipes. Although these sources have since diminished or else disappeared altogether others have arisen to take their place; perhaps the most important and widespread of these is the lead contained in the exhaust fumes from petrol engines. A modern investigation of the possible role of lead in motoneurone disease was undertaken by Campbell, Williams and Barltrop (1970). In a study of 74 patients these authors obtained a history of severe exposure to lead in 11, compared with four in a control group matched for age and sex (p = <0.05). At the time of study, however, there was no evidence from bone biopsies of an increased body burden of lead. In spite of this negative result the authors still consider it possible that the nervous system may have previously had increased exposure to lead following release of the mineral from the skeleton, for example, as a result of osteoporosis or limb-fracture.

Poliomyelitis

Zilkha (1962) first drew attention to a group of 11 patients in whom the occurrence of moto-neurone disease had followed between 17 and 43 years after an attack of poliomyelitis; he pointed out that the incidence of this association was far higher than would have been expected by chance. Some of these patients had signs of an upper motoneurone lesion and all showed muscle fasciculations; the muscle atrophy was slowly pro-gressive. Confirmatory evidence of an association between the two diseases was found by Poskanzer, Cantor and Kaplan (1969) and the relatively benign nature of the late motoneurone disorder has been stressed by Mulder, Rosenbaum and Layton (1972).

Slow virus

A type of tick-borne encephalitis occurs in the Soviet Union and leaves muscle wasting and fasci-culations as its sequelae. This observation raised the possibility that motoneurone disease might be a viral infection and prompted Zil'ber and his associates (1963) to inoculate monkeys with extracts of spinal cord and medulla from patients who had died from motoneurone disease. Four of the seven monkeys which had received intracerebral inoculations developed signs of muscle weakness and wasting after an interval of 6 months to 3 years; the disorder could be transmitted to other animals. Unfortunately this work could not be duplicated in the United States, even when tissue for inoculation was provided by Zil'ber (Gibbs and Gajdusek, 1969; see also Johnson, 1969).

Carcinoma

Patients with carcinoma, particularly of the bronchial type, are prone to suffer neuronal degeneration which may affect virtually any part of the nervous system (Brain and Norris, 1965). Since the degeneration can take place without any evidence of metastic tumour in the affected region, it is termed a 'remote' effect of the neoplasm. One example has already been considered in Chapter 18; this is the pseudomyasthenic syndrome of Eaton and Lambert. Another of the carcinomatous syndromes consists of progressive muscle wasting and weakness; the resemblance to motoneurone disease is strengthened by the frequent finding of fasciculations on clinical examination (Brain, Croft and Wilkinson, 1969) and at electromyography (Campbell and Paty, 1974). In addition some patients display pyramidal tract signs (Norris and Engel, 1964; Brain, Croft and Wilkinson, 1969) but in most cases the stretch reflexes are depressed rather than increased (see Norris, McMenemy and Barnard, 1969). The study by Campbell and Paty (1974) is of particular interest in that these authors included in their investigation a group of 30 unselected patients with bronchial carcinoma. Included among the battery of electrophysiological tests was the estimation of functioning motor unit numbers in the EDB muscle. In 10 of 26 patients tested the EDB count was found to be reduced and only five patients appeared completely normal on further electrophysiological testing.

Disordered carbohydrate metabolism

One of the first intimations that a disorder of carbohydrate metabolism might be present in motoneurone disease came from the work of Cumings (1962) who noted an abnormality of pyruvate metabolism in 15 of 36 patients. It was then found that a high proportion of patients exhibited a diabetic type of response to loading with glucose and that the reaction to intravenous tolbutaminde was also abnormal; in contrast the blood glucose fell normally after the injection of insulin (Steinke and Tyler, 1964; Ionasescu and Luca, 1964). The implication from these studies was that there was a failure in insulin secretion by the pancreatic islet cells; this defect has now been confirmed by measurements of plasma insulin levels, following the administration of a 50 g glucose load (Gotoh et al., 1972). A relationship between motoneurone disease and diabetes mellitus is also suggested by the observation that in both conditions impulse

conduction in sensory nerve axons is unusually resistant to ischaemia (Shahani and Russell, 1969; Shahani, Davies-Jones and Russell, 1971). It is of further interest that diabetes is associated with Friedreich's ataxia (Hewer, 1968), in which motoneurone degeneration also occurs.

The possibility that the exocrine function of the pancreas might also be abnormal in motoneurone disease was raised by Quick and Greer (1967) but two subsequent studies have not shown any derangements (Brown and Kater, 1969; Utterback et al., 1970). Similarly the treatment of patients with pancreatic extracts now appears to be of little value.

On the basis of the studies reported above, the presence of a pancreatic endocrine deficiency in a significant proportion of patients with motoneurone disease must be regarded as proven. One obvious interpretation of this curious association would be to postulate that any impairment of carbohydrate metabolism in the cell bodies of the motoneurones would lead to their eventual destruction. Indirect support for such an hypothesis comes from the susceptibility of patients with diabetes mellitus to develop polyneuropathies. Yet the situation must be more complex than this, for in diabetes mellitus the rate of neural degeneration is much slower, affecting sensory as well as motor neurones, in spite of the fact that the disorder of carbohydrate metabolism may be far more severe than in motoneurone disease. To cloud the issue further, marked degeneration of motoneurones may occur in patients with abnormally high serum insulin levels resulting from pancreatic islet-cell tumours.

Genetic influence

Fewer than 10 per cent of patients with motoneurone disease give a history of a similar condition affecting another member of the family. In such families the disease appears to be transmitted by an autosomal dominant gene. In the series of 87 patients in Newcastle and Hamilton there were two with positive family histories, compared with five in a population of 58 patients studied by Kurland and Mulder (1954). The clinical features of these cases may be indistinguishable from those of others with motoneurone disease but in some mild sensory loss is also present (Wechsler, Brock and Weil, 1929) and degenerative changes may be evident in the posterior columns of the spinal cord (Hirano, Kurland and Sayre, 1967). One patient with a remarkably slow progression of a familial form of the disease has already been described (see above).

Motoneurone disease in Guam
(see Mulder and Espinosa, 1969)

In the aftermath of World War II, with its heavy involvement of U.S. forces in the Pacific, it was noticed that there was an unusually high incidence of motoneurone disease in Guam, one of the islands in the Mariana group (Koerner, 1952). Death records on the island reveal that the disease had already been recognized at the turn of the century; because of their isolation, the islanders were unaware that they were succumbing to a disease which was uncommon elsewhere in the world. Not all the inhabitants of Guam display this susceptibility to motoneurone disease for while it is prevalent in the Chamorros it is infrequent in the Filipinos and the other racial groups. Of equal relevance is the observation that Chamorros who have emigrated from Guam to California remain prone to the disease (Torres, Iriarte and Kurland, 1957). Although other aetiological factors have been explored, a hereditary influence still appears to be the most likely explanation for the high incidence in the Chamorros. Recently another 'pocket' of motoneurone disease has been discovered in the Kii peninsula of Japan (Kusui, 1962) and here a hereditary factor may also be at play.

Other aetiological factors

Even now, the list of possible aetiological influences in motoneurone disease is far from complete. For example, Ask-Upmark (1950) described the onset of the disease in five patients following *gastric resection* (see also Ask-Upmark and Meurling, 1955). The importance of these observations is diminished by the inability of Stiel (1967) to find a similar case in a series of 125 patients with motoneurone disease studied by him. The occurrence of a neurological syndrome indistinguishable from motoneurone disease has been reported in *primary hyperparathyroidism* (Patten *et al.*, 1974) and undergoes remission once the parathyroid adenoma has been removed. An association between motoneurone disease and *physical trauma* has been proposed (Alpers and Farmer, 1949) while *electrical shocks* have also been incriminated (Panse, 1930). Finally, there is a suspicion that the disease may be more common in former *athletes* (Critchley, 1962).

THE AGEING HYPOTHESIS OF MOTONEURONE DISEASE

In the preceding section a multitude of possible aetiological factors have been discussed in connection with motoneurone disease. In each instance the observed facts are either gently persuasive or else apparently irrefutable. For example, in a small proportion of cases the disease *is* clearly inherited, in another group of patients there *is* a significant association with a previous episode of poliomyelitis, and so on. A sensible solution to the dilemma would be to acknowledge that there are many ways of killing motoneurones and that the same end-result will be common to all, namely weakness and wasting of muscles and perhaps fasciculations as well. In a similar way the presence of upper motoneurone signs in many patients can be explained by postulating that the same causative agent produces neural degeneration elsewhere in the central nervous system. A multifactorial hypothesis of this kind is not fully satisfactory, however, for it leaves unanswered two major problems. The first of these is that, for the majority of patients with motoneurone disease, it is impossible to incriminate any of the causative factors discussed above. For example, in the Newcastle-Hamilton series of 87 patients there were only two with family histories of motoneurone disease, two had suffered from poliomyelitis in childhood, one had been treated for carbon tetrachloride poisoning 40 years earlier, three volunteered that they had suffered severe electric shocks in the course of their occupations, and none had evidence of carcinoma. Deletion of these eight cases from the series leaves 79 patients (91 per cent) unaccounted for in terms of aetiology. The second major problem is that a simple multifactorial hypothesis leaves unexplained one of the most striking features of motoneurone disease, this being the age incidence of the disease. In all the studies reported to date the most common age of onset is between 50 and 65 years, two of the mean values being 64 (Kurland, Choi and Sayre, 1969) and 52 (Friedman and Freedman, 1950; see also Mulder, 1957). Examination of the mortality statistics for the whole United States between 1959 and 1961 yields a mean age at *death* of 64.4 years (see Kurland, Choi and Sayre, 1969) and about 3 years would require to be subtracted from this value in order to give the corresponding mean age of onset. For the 87 patients in Newcastle and Hamilton series the mean age of onset was 54.5 ± 11.9 years, the youngest case being a 17-year-old girl and the eldest an 80-year-old man; the pooled values for each decade are shown in *Figure 24.4* (*upper*).

The existence of such a marked tendency for the disease to occur in later life immediately raises the possibility that an ageing factor is involved. For this possibility to be pursued, it would be desirable to know the effect of ageing on motoneurones within the normal population. Much of this ground has already been covered in Chapter 12, from which it was clear that there is little reliable anatomical information available regarding numbers of motoneurones, ventral root fibres, and peripheral motor axons in man. In mice and rats the situation is rather better for evidence

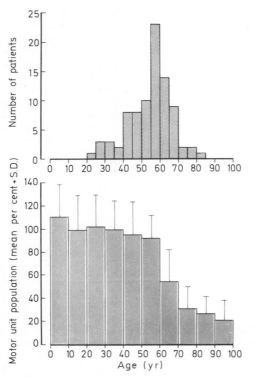

Figure 24.4. (Upper) Ages of 87 patients with motoneurone disease when symptoms first appeared; (lower) numbers of functioning motor units in 503 muscles of 250 healthy subjects, expressed as percentages of respective control means, and plotted as means for each decade (see text)

was presented for a relatively modest loss of moto-neurones, particularly towards the end of the animal's life span. Even so, the mere existence of a motoneurone soma in the ventral horn does not necessarily signify that the cell was behaving normally prior to death.

By using the electrophysiological technique for estimating numbers of functioning motor units (McComas et al., 1971a; see page 48) it is possible to overcome many of the problems inherent in this type of study and furthermore the results are applicable to man during life. Figure 24.4 (lower) shows the numbers of functioning motor units in a total of 503 muscles

(EDB, thenar, hypothenar and soleus) belonging to 250 subjects aged 7 months to 97 years, all of whom were regarded as being in good health for their ages. The result for each muscle has been expressed as a percentage of the mean number of motor units for that particular muscle in normal subjects below the age of 60. The pooled percentage values have then been averaged for each decade and their standard deviations calculated. Apart from a slight fall during the first decade, the motor unit population remains remarkable stable until about 60. Beyond the age of 60, however, there is a very definite loss of functioning motor units. This fall was found in all the muscle preparations examined, being rather greater for the thenar and extensor digitorum brevis muscles than for the hypothenar group. Figure 24.4 also shows that in the ninth and tenth decades there seems to be a reduction in the intensity of the ageing process. As pointed out on page 105 this is probably an artefact, for at this age the population will consist of survivors who, owing to chance or to some physical endowment (conceivably the persistence of unusually large numbers of motor units) have lived beyond the average life expectancy. In an un-selected elderly population, a better estimate of the rapidity of the ageing process might be obtained by extrapolating the difference between the sixth and seventh decades. If this manoeuvre is permissible, the normal ageing process would account for approximately 3.9 per cent of the original motor unit population per annum after the age of 60.

It must be stressed that the data obtained is con-cerned with numbers of functioning motor units rather than numbers of α-motoneurones. It is quite possible that some of the motor unit loss is due to such factors as ischaemia or demyelination of nerves, either of which could cause the motor axons to become inexcitable in the periphery. In their study of the EDB muscle Campbell, McComas and Petito (1973) paid particular attention to the vasculature of the legs in an attempt to exclude patients with ischaemic neuropathies. The same authors also looked for indirect evidence of demye-lination from the measurements of maximal and minimal impulse conduction velocity in motor axons. Although the presence of peripheral factors could not be excluded, the authors thought it more likely that the observed reduction in numbers of motor units resulted from increasing motoneurone dysfunction during ageing.

The interest in these results comes from their comparison with the age incidence for the onset of motoneurone disease, shown at the top of Figure 24.4 for the 87 patients in the Newcastle-Hamilton series. It can be seen that the peak incidence for the start of the disease occurs at the same time that motoneurones are beginning to fail as part of the normal ageing process. This quite striking coincidence presents a new aetiological factor for consideration in the genesis of moto-neurone disease, namely that the disease simply represents the 'fast' end of the normal moto-neuronal ageing process. Thus at any given age beyond 60 some 'normal' subjects will have fewer motor units than others (reflected in the standard deviations of *Figure 24.4, lower*), indicating that the ageing process is running a faster course or has begun sooner. If a large control population were to be examined, there would be a strong likelihood of encountering some subjects who were losing motoneurone function very rapidly. If questioned, they would probably admit to feeling more easily fatigued than usual and their relatives might volunteer a remark to the effect that the subject was 'not the man he was' or 'never quite the same after his last cold' and so on. On electrophysio-logical examination the diminished motor unit values, with relative sparing of sensory nerve function, would be quite compatible with a diagnosis of the progressive muscular atrophy variant of motoneurone disease. In the initial control survey of EDB muscles conducted in New-castle upon Tyne one subject, a 65-year-old man, was discovered in this category. This subject also showed fibrillations in other muscles; unfor-tunately he was lost for follow-up and no informa-tion is available as to his progress.

The problem with the ageing hypothesis of moto-neurone disease is that it is difficult, if not impossible, to test directly. The evidence presented above is purely circumstantial and, for this reason, the hypothesis remains tenable only so long as other aetiological factors can be excluded. As demanded of a satisfactory hypothesis, it can account for certain other observations in motoneurone disease. One of these is the frequent finding of neuro-fibrillary degeneration in cerebral neurones of patients with motoneurone disease from Guam (Hirano *et al.,* 1969) and from the Kii peninsula (Shiraki, 1969). The significance of the neuro-fibrillary tangles is that they are a recognized feature of ageing brains as well as of the Alzheimer type of pre-senile dementia. There is no evidence, however, that neurofibrillary degeneration is unusually prominent in the nervous systems of patients with idiopathic motoneurone disease.

The ageing hypothesis also provides an alter-native explanation for the association of pancreatic islet-cell dysfunction with motoneurone disease, considered previously. Since diabetes mellitus also has its peak incidence in later life it is conceivable that both diseases are manifestations of an accelerated ageing process. In this context it is

interesting, and possibly relevant, that the beta cells of the pancreatic islets are now thought to resemble the nervous system in being derived from neural crest ectoderm (Pearse, 1969; but see Pictet *et al.,* 1976). The ageing hypothesis can also accom-modate many of the aetiological observations cited earlier. Thus any factor which interferes adversely with the metabolism of motoneurones would be

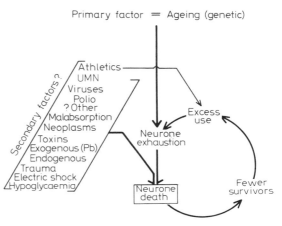

Figure 24.5. Summary of the factors which have been held responsible for motoneurone disease (see text). Of these the most important (primary) factor is considered to be ageing, itself genetically determined. Notice how the onset of denervation may lead to further loss of moto-neurones by 'exhaustion' of the survivors; UMN, upper motoneurone lesion. (From McComas, Upton and Sica (1973) courtesy of the Editor and publishers of the Lancet)

likely to hasten the ageing process in those cells subsequently. The source of this interference could obviously vary; for example, it might consist of a chemical such as lead or manganese, or it might be a physical stimulus such as a severe electric shock. Alternatively the interference might consist of excessive metabolic activity of the motoneurone and consideration of the trophic role of the neurone suggests how this might occur. From Chapter 2 it will be recalled that the neurone soma is normally required to synthesize a variety of messenger sub-stances which are then conveyed via the axon to the muscle fibres. These 'trophic' substances are necessary for the maintenance of the normal structure and function of the muscle fibre (Chapters 8 and 9). If the muscle fibres are forced to undergo hypertrophy through excessive work the motoneurone will probably be required to make extra amounts of neurotrophic material to support them. In this way the neurones might become prematurely exhausted in former athletes, account-ing for the suspicion that motoneurone disease is commoner in such individuals (Critchley, 1962).

The motoneurones would also be expected to supply extra trophic material if their motor unit territory was enlarged through collateral reinnervation (page 224). Premature neuronal exhaustion should then take place in any condition involving chronic partial denervation and this could account for the occurrence of motoneurone disease some years after poliomyelitis (see above). The same consideration can be applied to the denervation which occurs during the ageing process itself. As more and more muscle fibres become denervated, so the sizes of the surviving motor units will become larger and the corresponding motoneurones will suffer premature exhaustion. Finally, in those patients with motoneurone disease showing marked pyramidal tract involvement, there will be the added factor of trans-synaptic degeneration to take into account (Chapter 27). In *Figure 24.5* an attempt has been made to show the way in which the primary factor (ageing) can be integrated with the various secondary factors to cause motoneurone degeneration and how, once started, the latter process becomes self-perpetuating.

So far no consideration has been given to the nature of the ageing effect on motoneurones. Several lines of indirect evidence suggest that the most important factor influencing motoneurone ageing is a genetic one:

(1) From motor-unit counting studies in rats and mice it seems that in each species there is a loss of functioning motoneurones with advancing age. Thus the number of motoneurones is appropriate for the genetically determined lifespan of the species.

(2) In man it is accepted that longevity is hereditary and it seems inconceivable that active life in old age could be accomplished without substantial motor unit populations.

(3) There are several hereditary disorders in which motoneurones die prematurely. These include a familial form of 'adult' motoneurone disease, the spinal muscular atrophies, peroneal muscular atrophy, wobbler disease of mice, and Guam motoneurone disease (possibly hereditary).

It cannot be argued from the above observations that the genetic influence on the motoneurone is a direct one without the involvement of some other system (e.g. immunological). Convincing proof would require additional experiments such as the determination of lifespans of neural cultures taken from various species and at different times from the same species. This omission does not detract from the hypothesis, however, for the latter requires only the existence of a genetic influence without the need to specify its mechanism.

SPINAL MUSCULAR ATROPHY

Toward the end of the last century Werdnig (1891) and Hoffmann (1893) described infants exhibiting a severe and progressive form of generalized muscle weakness with fatal outcome. Autopsy studies subsequently showed that the muscle changes were secondary to degeneration of motoneurones in the spinal cord and brainstem. Since that time it has become evident that less severe forms of spinal muscular atrophy exist with their clinical onsets during childhood, adolescence or adult life. Although the age of onset and severity of the disease varies so extensively there is an increasing tendency to separate the spinal muscular atrophies into two categories—the severe infantile type, or *Werdnig–Hoffmann disease,* and the later onset type with slower progression, or *Kugelberg–Welander* type. Both conditions are thought to be genetic in origin and to arise from autosomal recessive genes; however, the possibility cannot be excluded that in some patients a different aetiology is involved.

Infantile spinal muscular atrophy (Werdnig–Hoffmann)

In most cases of infantile spinal muscular atrophy the presence of muscle weakness is obvious immediately after birth or within the first few weeks of life. If a healthy sibling is already present in the family, the mother may have noticed that the movements of the abnormal fetus were comparatively feeble. At birth the baby appears limp and floppy; the arms and legs are motionless and the face is without expression. Feeding is difficult and the weakness of the intercostal muscles is revealed by the drawing-in of the lower intercostal spaces in inspiration. During development most children remain unable to raise their heads and few can sit without support. Unlike adult patients with motoneurone disease, the tendon reflexes are absent and there are no signs of upper motoneurone involvement. The weakness is progressive and death usually occurs before 18 months, most commonly from bronchopneumonia. In a minority of cases the disease, although presenting in infancy, runs a slower course and may occasionally appear to become arrested. Although severely crippled, the patients may survive into their teens or even longer. *Muscle biopsy* reveals masses of small rounded muscle fibres and it is possible that some of these have never received a nerve supply during embryonic development. Mingled with these small fibres are larger innervated ones, some of which appear to have undergone compensatory hyperrophy (*Figure 24.6*). *Electromyography* is fraught with interpretative problems, especially since it is sometimes difficult to goad normal babies into producing full interference patterns; in addition there is usually a paucity of the large prolonged complex potentials typical of chronic denervation in the adult. Fibrillations may be encountered, however, and Buchthal and Olsen (1970) have described a characteristic type of spontaneous motor unit activity in which regular discharges at 5–15 Hz are maintained during sleep or under sedation.

Late-onset spinal muscular atrophy (Kugelberg–Welander)

This category of spinal muscular atrophy embraces remarkably varied clinical features. As already stated, inheritance is usually through an autosomal recessive gene but sometimes autosomal dominant or X-linked recessive modes of transmission are involved. The onset of the disease may be in childhood, adolescence or in adult life. The pattern of muscle involvement also varies; most frequently the proximal muscles of the limbs are affected, together with the muscles of the hips, shoulder girdle and trunk. Since some patients also demonstrate pseudohypertrophy of their calf and other muscles, it may be impossible to distinguish them from cases of limb-girdle muscular dystrophy. Further, since in many patients the muscle biopsy and electromyogram may show a mixture of 'myopathic' and 'neuropathic' features, there seems little point in continuing to regard the two conditions as separate entities. This view is not generally accepted, however, but is defended on pages 160–165, in relation to the pathogenesis of the muscular dystrophies.

In a minority of patients with spinal muscular atrophy the pattern of weakness is different; it may either be generalized or else it may be restricted to the distal muscles of the limbs. In about half of all cases fasciculations can be observed in the proximal muscles and very occasionally the presence of extensor plantar responses indicates that the corticospinal tracts are involved; the tendon reflexes are usually depressed, however. The progression of the disease is also variable. Many cases remain able to walk and enjoy a normal life expectancy; at the other extreme is the young adult or adolescent with severe spinal deformity who is doomed to a wheelchair existence and runs the risk of premature death from bronchopneumonia.

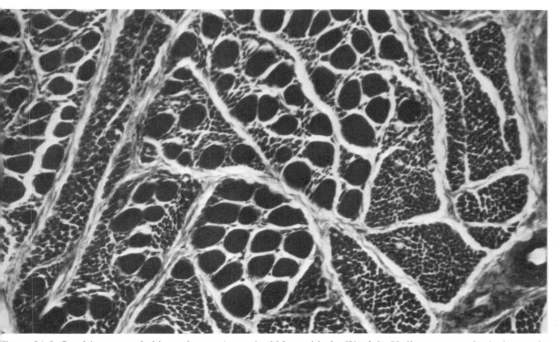

Figure 24.6. Quadriceps muscle biopsy from a 4-month-old boy with the Werdnig–Hoffmann type of spinal muscular atrophy, stained with haemotoxylin and eosin. Notice the relatively large rounded fibres in the centre of the figure and the masses of much smaller fibres to either side. It is probable that the smaller fibres had never received an innervation during development. 120 ×.

Chapter 25

TOXIC AND METABOLIC NEUROPATHIES

There are many chemicals which are known to damage neurones and it is convenient to classify them according to their type as in Table 25.1. Although the list is far from complete, it does contain the most important neurotoxic agents and it also draws attention to their variety. Apart from the heavy metals, the substances listed are the products of an advancing industrial and pharmaceutical technology and undoubtedly many new causes of toxic neuropathy may be anticipated in the future. Previously it was thought that neurotoxic agents produced their effects by causing demyelination of the axons. In 1954, however, Cavanagh published the results of a study of triorthocresylphosphate poisoning in the hen and reported that demyelination was only found in nerve fibres undergoing degeneration of their axis cylinders. This association led him to postulate that the primary lesion involved the neurone and that the demyelination was a secondary event—just as the myelin sheath disintegrates following proximal section of the nerve fibre. Cavanagh also noted that the axon degeneration was more marked in distal regions of nerve fibres and that long axons were more severely affected than short ones. To explain this distribution of the pathological changes he suggested that a 'dying-back' process was taking place; the toxin interfered with the metabolism of the neuronal cell-body such that it was no longer able to sustain the full length of its axon, the farthest part then degenerating. Although an exogenous toxin had been employed in these experiments, Cavanagh drew attention to the similarity of the neural lesion to that occurring in the course of

diseases such as peroneal muscular atrophy and motoneurone disease (Chapter 24) and suggested that common mechanisms might be involved.

Since this important paper investigations have been made of the 'dying-back' phenomenon following the deliberate application of a number of neurotoxic substances. The agent which has been most thoroughly studied in experimental animals is *acrylamide* and the following account of its action illustrates many structural and functional features shared by the other toxic neuropathies.

AN EXPERIMENTAL MODEL FOR STUDYING NEUROTOXICITY: ACRYLAMIDE

Chemistry

The acrylamide molecule (monomer) consists of two parts; and amide group and a vinyl group conjugated with it:

$$
(\beta)\ \underset{\underset{\displaystyle H\ (\alpha)}{|}}{\overset{\overset{\displaystyle H}{|}}{C}} = \underset{\underset{\displaystyle H}{|}}{\overset{\overset{\displaystyle H}{|}}{C}} - \underset{}{\overset{\overset{\displaystyle O}{\parallel}}{C}} - \underset{\underset{\displaystyle H}{|}}{\overset{\overset{\displaystyle H}{|}}{N}}
$$

$$
\underbrace{}_{\text{vinyl}} \quad \underbrace{}_{\text{amide}}
$$

The compound readily undergoes additive reactions at the β-position, especially with thiols and amino groups.

Jses

Acrylamide readily undergoes polymerization to form polyacrylamide and it is this property which makes it so useful in industry. The high molecular weight polymers are employed to strengthen paper and chipboard, to treat industrial and municipal effluents, and to increase oilwell production by fracturing the strata and forcing oil to the surface. Other uses include the manufacture of grouting agents, adhesives, electrophoretic gels and coatings for metals; it also has applications in photography. In North America alone, three firms produce over 50 million pounds of the acrylamide monomer each year (see Spencer and Schaumberg, 1974).

Metabolism

It is the acrylamide monomer which possess neurotoxic qualities; the various polymers appear inert. It is therefore important to reduce contamination of the polymers by the monomer; the Food and Drug Administration of the United States does not allow more than 0.05 per cent monomer in the polymers used for the manufacture of paper containers for food. The substance can be absorbed through the skin in addition to passage through the respiratory and alimentary tracts. Once absorbed acrylamide is widely distributed in the body, with the highest levels being found in the blood, with progressively less being present in the kidney, liver, brain, spinal cord and sciatic nerve (Hashimoto and Aldridge, 1970). Following homogenization of the brain the substance can be demonstrated in all subcellular fractions and it appears that it reacts strongly with proteins, especially those containing sulfhydryl groups. Experiments with labelled acrylamide have shown that 60–85 per cent is

excreted by 3–4 days (Ziegler, 1969), two-thirds of this material appearing in the urine in an unchanged form.

Human toxicity

The first cases of acrylamide poisoning in man were identified in 1954, the affected individuals being engaged in the manufacture of acrylamide from acrylonitrile. Since that time further cases of poisoning have been reported from many parts of the world and the various clinical features of the syndrome have been clearly described (see Spencer and Schaumberg, 1974). Thus, in those patients with cutaneous exposure to the chemical, the first signs are erythema and peeling of the palms and these are followed by somnolence, easy fatigability and weight loss. More definite evidence of central and peripheral nervous system involvement is delayed for several weeks. The most striking features are those of a sensory and motor polyneuropathy, giving rise to numbness and tingling in the hands and feet, unsteadiness of gait, and clumsiness of movements requiring manual dexterity. Muscle strength is reduced and atrophy may be visible, particularly of the intrinsic muscles of the hands; the tendon reflexes are depressed or absent. Involvement of the central nervous system is suggested by the presence of tremor, ataxia, vertigo and past-pointing; excessive sleepiness, mental dysfunction and EEG abnormalities provide further evidence.

Once further exposure to acrylamide is prevented the symptoms and signs of peripheral neuropathy gradually diminish; in mildly affected cases a complete clinical recovery may ensue within 2–12 months (Garland and Patterson, 1967) whereas a neurological deficit may persist in patients with severe poisoning.

Morphological studies

One of the most complete sets of light microscopic observations on acrylamide neuropathy is that of Hopkins (1970) who induced the disorder in baboons by including the substance in their food. Hopkins found that the main pathological changes in the nerve fibres were those of Wallerian degeneration (Chapter 20). The axons were fragmented and displayed clumping of the neurofilaments together with the formation of digestion chambers (autophagic vacuoles). Both sensory and motor fibres were involved and the larger diameter axons were affected more than the smaller ones. By studying the same nerves at different levels it was possible to demonstrate that the degenerative

TABLE 25.1

Chemical Agents Known to Cause
Neuronal Degeneration

Heavy Metals: Arsenic, gold, lead, mercury
Industrial organic substances:
   Solvents: Carbon tetrachloride, hexane, trichlorethylene
   Insecticides and herbicides: DDT, dieldrin, aldrin
   Others: Triorthocresylphosphate, acrylamide
Drugs:
   Antimitotic: Vincristine, vinblastine, nitrogen mustards
   Chemotherapeutic: Isoniazid, furan group, sulphonamides, chloroquin
   Sedatives: thalidomide, glutethimide
   Others: Disulfiram, hydrallazine, imipramine, oxidase inhibitors, ergotamine, diphenylhydantoin.

changes were most prominent in the distal parts of the axons, this being the abnormality characteristic of a 'dying-back' process (see above). Although it has not been possible to study specimens of human nerve during the stage of florid neuropathy, Fullerton (1969) was able to show that the largest diameter fibres had been affected in the sural nerves of three patients undergoing recovery from acrylamide toxicity.

Further details of the degenerative process have been established by electromicroscopic investigations in cats with neuropathy (Prineas, 1969a, b; Schaumberg, Wiśniewski and Spencer, 1974). At high magnifications it can be seen that there is a hyperplasia of the neurofilaments which causes the axon to become distended in the paranodal regions. The swellings also contain dense bodies, granules, vesicles and mitochondria. Some of the organelles within the axon are enclosed by a membrane; Spencer (1971) has suggested that the membrane has been formed by Schwann cells in an attempt to sequester and remove the abnormal organelles from the axon. More distally the axon can be seen to break up into the ovoids characteristic of Wallerian degeneration.

Even while some axons are degenerating others may have already started to regenerate, the sprouts growing along the bands of Bungner towards the periphery (see Chapter 20). Proximal to the region of frank degeneration the myelin sheath may appear abnormal with retraction occurring at the nodes of Ranvier. Although it is possible that this change is a primary effect of acrylamide on the Schwann cell, it is perhaps more likely to reflect secondary involvement of the Schwann cell by a 'failing' axon. If the amount of myelin retraction is small the defect is made good during the recovery period by the preparation of fresh myelin by the two Schwann cells on either side of the node. More extensive denudation of the axolemma is repaired by the formation of an extra Schwann cell by mitosis and by subsequent myelination so as to form an intercalated segment (Hopkins, 1970).

The study of Schaumberg, Wiśniewski and Spencer (1974), already referred to, is of interest for another reason, inasmuch as these authors compared the dying-back process in different types of nerve ending. In cats treated with acrylamide they observed that the Pacinian corpuscles in the fore- and hind-feet were the first terminals to exhibit axonal changes. Degeneration of sensory terminals in the muscle spindles followed, occurring first in the annulospiral endings and then in the various secondary ones.

The changes in the neuromuscular junctions of rats with acrylamide neuropathy were investigated by Tsujihata, Engel and Lambert (1974). After 20 days of exposure the terminal motor axons wer swollen with neurofilaments and largely deplete of synaptic vesicles and mitochondria. At a mor advanced stage of toxicity one or more of the axo terminals had disappeared from individual enc plates leaving much of the postsynaptic surface c the muscle fibre membrane exposed or else covere by an extension of the Schwann cell; complet denervation was not seen, however, for at least on axon terminal remained at each end-plate. I microelectrode studies Swift and Lambert (1974 found that the frequency of miniature end-plat potentials fell and that the store of acetylcholin quanta dropped to half or less of the original value both changes would be anticipated from the loss c synaptic vesicles observed on electromicroscopy Thirty days after the acrylamide had been stoppe the postsynaptic areas denuded of axon could n longer be found, indicating that axon regeneratio had taken place. Even after 60 days of recovery however, the axon terminals had not regained thei full complement of mitochondria and synapti vesicles.

Nerve conduction studies

In baboons treated with acrylamide Hopkins an Gilliatt (1971) followed the changes in impuls conduction in both motor and sensory nerves. Thei investigation is noteworthy not only for clarity c the electrophysiological recordings but also for th number of times that some of the experimenta animals were studied; in one animal recording were made on 15 occasions over a period of 2 months (see their Figure 4). In this last animal it wa found that the number of functioning sensory an motor fibres continued to decline after acrylamid had been stopped and no sign of recovery could b detected until more than 200 days had elapsed These authors attributed the moderate loss i impulse conduction velocity to the preferentia involvement of larger diameter fibres.

EXAMPLES OF TOXIC AND METABOLIC NEUROPATHIES IN MAN

Vincristine neuropathy

With the motor unit counting technique o McComas and colleagues (1971a) it has bee possible to study many patients with toxic neuro pathies. In 15 of these patients the neurotoxi agent was the drug *vincristine;* this substance is on of the Vinca alkaloids derived from the periwinkl

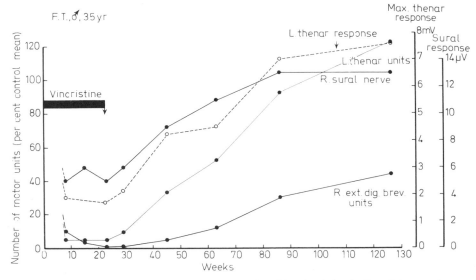

Figure 25.1. Recovery from a neuropathy induced by vincristine in Case 1 (see text)

lant and, because of its ability to stop mitotic ctivity, has been used extensively in the treatment f malignant disease. Thirteen of the patients in this eries suffered from acute leukaemia and the nanging motor unit values in one of these has een reported previously (McComas *et al.*, 1974b).

ne of the remaining two patients was a 34-year-old umber (Case 2 of McComas, Upton and Jorgensen, 975) who underwent surgery for an embryonal carci- oma of the testis; the tumour was removed and a ock dissection of the pelvic lymph nodes was carried ut. In addition he was treated with a course of intra- enous vincristine, methotrexate, cyclophosphamide and -fluorouracil which was repeated at 3-weekly intervals. 'hen seen 8 weeks after commencing this therapy the atient displayed marked weakness and wasting of limb uscles, particularly in the extremities; he was also suffer- g from severe numbness and tingling in the hands and et. An electrophysiological examination at this time owed that there had been a substantial loss of function- g motor units in the thenar and extensor digitorum revis (EDB) muscles on both sides (*Figure 25.1*); in ontrast the left hypothenar value was normal (290 units) nd the right moderately reduced (93 units). Profuse brillation activity was detected in the right EDB muscle ith a coaxial electrode. *Figure 25.1* also shows that the mplitude of the compound action potential of the right ural nerve was at the lower limit of the normal range μV); diminished values were noted in digital branches f the radial, median and ulnar nerves. Following this itial EMG examination the 5-day course of chemo- erapy was repeated at 3-weekly intervals until April 973 (24 weeks, *Figure 25.1*); by this time the patient's eakness had increased and only three functioning motor nits could be demonstrated in the right EDB muscle. In ew of the deteriorating neurological condition vincristine

was withdrawn but treatment with the other drugs main- tained at 3-weekly intervals. At examination 5 weeks later (29 weeks; *Figure 25.1*) it was evident that recovery had already started in thenar muscles, both the maximum evoked response and the number of functioning motor units being larger. At 45 weeks the right EDB count was rising and the sensory responses, including that of the right sural nerve, were larger. At this stage the 5-day courses of chemotherapy (5-fluorouracil, methotrexate and cyclophosphamide) were given at 6-weekly, rather than at 3-weekly, intervals. By the time that the patient was next seen (86 weeks, *Figure 25.1*) the population of excitable motor units in the left thenar muscles had grown still further, now lying well within the control range; the functional muscle fibre bulk, indicated by the maximum response, had increased to a similar extent. The right EDB motor unit population had also grown while the right sural nerve response had attained the mean amplitude determined for control subjects in this laboratory (13 μV). At the final examination (126 weeks, *Figure 25.1*) the thenar muscle values had increased still further (within the control range) and the recovery in sural nerve function appeared to have been completed. Of all the electrophysiological parameters examined, only the number of motor units in the right EDB muscle remained abnormal; even in this instance there had been an improvement to 44 per cent of the control mean from a minimum value of 1 per cent (only three units were detected at the 24th and 29th weeks).

The findings in this patient have been presented because they illustrate certain features found to be common to patients with toxic and metabolic neuro- pathies.

(1) There is a constant difference between muscles in their susceptibility to functional denerva- tion. The extensor digitorum brevis is always

affected most severely, the thenar group less so, and the hypothenar muscles exhibit considerable resistance. It will be recalled that there is the same differential susceptibility in ageing; it is also found in the neuropathies of thyrotoxicosis and renal failure (see below), as well as in the Duchenne and myotonic types of muscular dystrophy (see Chapter 16).

(2) Although a muscle may be severely denervated, the affected motoneurones display remarkable powers of recovery, provided sufficient time elapses after the withdrawal of the toxic agent. The same neuronal resilience is also apparent from the work of Hopkins and Gilliatt (1971) on acrylamide neuropathy in the baboon, referred to earlier.

(3) The loss of functioning motor units in the extensor digitorum brevis muscle, expressed proportionally, is always greater than the diminution in the size of the evoked sural nerve response. Similarly, in the hands, the relative loss of thenar motor units exceeds the reduction in the amplitudes of the median sensory nerve potentials. It could be argued that the method conventionally employed for examining nerve conduction in sensory axons involves electrical stimulation and does not test the part of the axon most likely to be affected in a toxic

or metabolic neuropathy, the receptor terminal (see Spencer and Schaumburg, 1974; also above). This is a valid point but even when the receptors are tested with a mechanical vibrator, sensory function still appears to be better preserved than motor function (unpublished studies with Dr C. de Faria and Dr K Toyonaga). This disparity is rather surprising for the electronmicroscopic investigations of Spencer and Schaumburg (1974) showed that the structure of the motor axon terminal was maintained for a longer period than that of the various sensory receptors, at least in the dying-back neuropathy induced by acrylamide. In this patient the finding of fibrillation potentials in the right EDB muscle indicated that denervation of the discharging muscle fibres had been complete. It is therefore probable that the motor axon terminals which had previously supplied these fibres had undergone Wallerian degeneration and that the subsequent recovery in the number of motor units had been effected by axonal regeneration.

Renal neuropathy

The next protocol to be presented shows that a more subtle derangement of neuromuscular

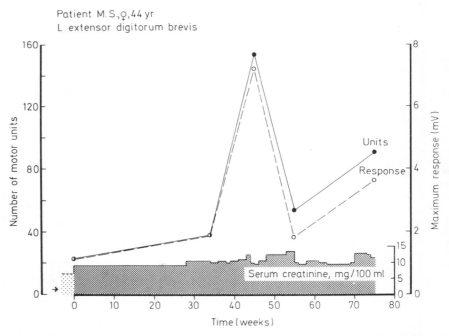

Figure 25.2. Fluctuating neuropathy in Case 2, a patient with chronic renal failure (see text). (From McComas, Upton and Jorgensen (1975a) courtesy of the Editor and publishers of Canadian Journal of Neurological Sciences)

function can occur under certain circumstances. Although the motor axon terminals appeared incapable of transmitting excitation, there was indirect evidence that they were still present in a non-degenerate form.

The patient concerned, M.S. (Case 4 of McComas, Upton and Jorgensen, 1975a), was one of 50 patients with chronic renal failure in whom repeated electrophysiological testing was performed. She presented in July 1972 as a 44-year-old woman with symptoms of nausea, vomiting, shortness of breath, angina of effort, swelling of her ankles and haematuria. Her kidneys were enlarged on abdominal palpation and were shown radiologically to be polycystic. Her blood pressure, measured while erect, was 150/100 Hg; her fundi appeared normal and no abnormalities were noted on examination of her nervous system. Laboratory examination revealed the following serum electrolyte values (mEq/l): sodium, 137; potassium 5.0; chloride, 107; bicarbonate, 17. Other biochemical values (in mg per cent) were: calcium, 8.5; phosphorus, 6.2; blood urea nitrogen, 85; creatinine, 6.5. She had a normochromic anaemia (haemoglobin, 8.8 g per cent). At this stage her only medication was Aldomet 250 mg, three times daily. Upon electrophysiological examination a severe loss of functioning motor units was noted in the left EDB muscle (*Figure 25.2*) such that only about 23 were left. The motor unit potentials of the surviving functional units were of normal size (mean ± 46 μV) and no spontaneous activity could be detected during exploration of the muscle with a coaxial electrode. In contrast to EDB the hypothenar motor unit population was normal (417 units). Sensory nerve responses were diminished in the sural nerves but normal elsewhere. At the second EMG examiniation (34 weeks) the left EDB still showed severe functional denervation while the hypothenar muscles remained normal; a thenar study showed moderate denervation (166 units). The third electrophysiological study was undertaken at 45 weeks; on this occasion the muscle responses were strikingly improved. The EDB motor unit count (153 units) was now well within the normal range (above 120 units) and *Figure 25.2* shows that there had been a proportional increase in the maximum evoked muscle response. In keeping with the EDB results, the thenar muscles also showed a significant improvement with a motor unit count of 286 (normal, above 220) and an enlarged maximum muscle response. *Figure 25.2* shows that this recovery of muscle function was not associated with any measurable improvement in renal function for the serum creatinine had risen to 9.9 mg per cent while the other biochemical values were not significantly different from those obtained initially. Her clinical condition was slightly better for she no longer suffered from ankle swelling or chest pain while the nausea and breathlessness were less marked. By the time of the next electrophysiological examination, 10 weeks later, a clear deterioration in muscle function had taken place, the motor unit counts and maximum muscle responses having fallen in EDB (*Figure 25.2*) and in the thenar muscles. The patient now felt more breathless on exertion and the serum creatinine had risen to 13.4 mg per cent and the blood urea nitrogen to 100 mg per cent; the serum electrolytes

were not significantly different. At the next examination (75 weeks) there had been some improvement in EDB function but a further decline in that of thenar muscles while, for the first time, the hypothenar muscles showed evidence of involvement. Once again the serum electrolytes were unchanged while the creatinine had fallen to 11.4 mg per cent and the blood urea nitrogen to 60 mg per cent. Following this visit blood dialysis was started; within 6 months there had been a return to thenar and hypothenar muscle function to normal but the left EDB could no longer be tested because of the proximity of the peroneal nerve to the arteriovenous fistula.

The interest of this case lies in two observations. First, at a time when only a small number of motor units continued to function in the EDB muscle, the inexcitable muscle fibres displayed no other evidence of denervation. Thus, the muscle belly was not atrophied, no fibrillations or sharp-wave potentials could be recorded with a coaxial electrode, and the normal sizes of the evoked motor unit potentials suggested that collateral reinnervation had not taken place. From studies of neurapraxic lesions of axons (Chapter 22) it is known that these parameters of denervation are not caused by a loss of nerve fibre impulses and must therefore depend on the absence of a chemical neurotrophic influence instead (see also Chapters 2 and 9). If these considerations are applied to patient M.S. it seems likely that, at a time when there was a severe loss of functioning motor units, the motor axon terminals were still present and conveying a chemical neurotrophic influence to the muscle fibres even though the neuromuscular junctions were inexcitable. This suggestion is supported by the second observation of interest in this patient—the striking, albeit transient, recovery of motor unit function at the third occasion of study. The compact form of the evoked muscle responses recorded at this time indicated that the recovery had not been associated with remyelination or regeneration of the motor axons. A more plausible explanation is that the 'silent' synapses had started to transmit once more; the matter is discussed again on page 281.

Disulfiram neuropathy

The case history of a third patient will now be given because it illustrates another type of neuronal recovery mechanism.

Unlike the first two patients, in whom recovery could be attributed to axon regeneration and to the 'switching-on' of non-transmitting synapses respectively, in the third patient collateral reinnervation (page 224) appeared to be the main mechanism. In this last patient it is probable that the neuropathy had resulted from the use of disulfiram. This patient, K.S., was a 37-year-old woman with a 20-year history of chronic alcoholism involving the consumption of beer and spirits. In June 1972 treatment was started with disulfiram (Antabuse), 0.5 g orally each day. Twelve weeks later the patient sought advice for tingling and numbness in the left hand and forearm, blurred vision, and unsteadiness while walking. On examination no sensory abnormalities were noted except for Rombergism; her ankle jerks were present but diminished. In view of a long and complicated psychiatric history involving numerous transitory symptoms a decision was made to continue the disulfiram under strict

population (141 units; lower limit of normal range, 220 units). In contrast the left hypothenar value was borderline (249 units; lower limit of normal, 250 units). It is of interest that the maximum evoked response in the right EDB was only 25 μV, which suggested that even in the three remaining motor units there had been a loss of muscle fibres. In terms of the neurogenic hypothesis of McComas and colleagues (1971, see Chapter 13), this observation indicated that the three corresponding motoneurones had entered a dysfunctional ('sick') phase. The

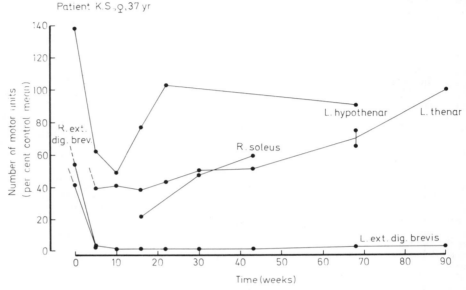

Figure 25.3. Case 3: development of, and recovery from, a neuropathy which had probably been induced by disulfiram (see text)

clinical surveillance. By November 1972, 19 weeks after starting treatment, the sensory symptoms had become more pronounced; a burning sensation and a feeling of numbness were present in both feet. On examination, sensation to light touch and pin-prick was diminished up to the mid-calf with loss of vibratory sensibility at the ankles; joint-position and temperature sensations appeared to be present. The ankle jerks could no longer be obtained but other tendon reflexes were normal. There was a suggestion of wasting of the calf muscles but dorsi- and plantar-flexion of the ankles were of normal strength. No abnormality was noted in the arms. A clinical diagnosis of progressive polyneuropathy was made and the disulfiram was stopped. In fact this diagnosis had already been suggested 3 weeks earlier on the basis of a slightly reduced number of functioning motor units in the left EDB muscle (112 units; lower limit of normal, 120) and a sural nerve response which was at the lower end of the normal range for amplitude (5 μV).

At the second EMG examination, 5 weeks after the first, it was evident that the functional muscle denervation had progressed (*Figure 25.3*). There were now only three motor units remaining in the right EDB and there was a moderate depletion of the left thenar

left EDB muscle was explored with a coaxial electrode; no volitional activity could be detected even though the maximum evoked response was composed of seven small increments. These findings could be explained by a failure of impulse propagation in regions of the axons proximal to the ankle or by an inability of the descending facilitatory pathways to excite the surviving motoneurones. The presence of fibrillations and sharp wave activity indicated that many axons had degenerated, rather than merely exhibiting a block of impulse conduction (see McComas, Jorgensen and Upton, 1974). In spite of the severe deterioration in muscle function the sural nerve responses had not changed significantly, being 6 μV on both sides.

At the third examination (10 weeks; *Figure 25.3*) the left hypothenar and EDB motor unit counts had fallen still further, even though the patient was no longer receiving disulfiram. During the remainder of the period of observation (from 19 to 90 weeks) functional improvement took place in all the muscles studied but the rates and extents varied. *Figure 25.3* shows that although both the hypothenar and thenar muscles recovered completely, the process was much swifter in the former. In distinction to the hand muscles, the EDB muscle showed very little improvement in the number of functioning motor units, since these had only risen to five from a minimum of two in the space of 80 weeks. *Figure 25.4 (upper)* shows that the EDB was a more effective muscle nonetheless for the maximum evoked response had increased to 1.52 mV from a value of 75 μV, a 20-fold increase. This disproportionately large increase in muscle response relative to the increase in number of motor units provided the evidence that collateral reinnervation had been the main recovery mechanism for the EDB muscle in this patient. The phenomenon of collateral reinnervation has been considered in more detail in Chapter 20 and has also been represented in *Figure 25.5 (a, lower right)*.

Inspection of *Figure 25.4 (lower)* raises a problem; for what type of neuronal recovery process could have been responsible for the findings in the thenar muscles? In these it can be seen that the number of functioning motor units more than doubled while the maximum evoked muscle response showed no significant alteration. In order to explain these curious results it is necessary to consider the findings at the first EMG study. On this occasion the number of functioning thenar units was greatly decreased but the sizes of the surviving units, as reflected by the amplitudes of their evoked potentials, were increased; it is therefore probable

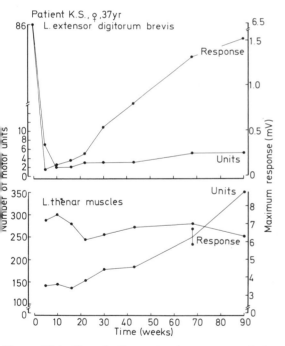

Figure 25.4. Case 3: the contrasting recovery of the numbers of functioning motor units and of functional muscle fibre mass ('response') in the extensor digitorum brevis (upper section) and in the thenar muscle group (lower section) (see text). (From McComas, Upton and Jorgensen (1975a), courtesy of the Editor and publishers of Canadian Journal of Neurological Sciences)

that substantial collateral reinnervation had already taken place. Since the maximum muscle response did not enlarge subsequently, the recovering motoneurones must have resumed synaptic connections with muscle fibres which had already been adopted by 'foreign' motoneurones. This situation would obviously result in hyperinnervation of fibres, similar to that produced experimentally following the crushing or sectioning of nerves in the presence of a secondary innervation (page 228). In these last experiments it was shown that the double innervation could persist, possibly indefinitely. If this were also the case in patient K.S., the *estimated* number of motor units would still be too low, for the increments, upon which the estimate is based, would include unusually large potentials (due to persisting collateral reinnervation) as well as rather smaller potentials (due to neuronal recovery). The fact that a normal complement of motor units *was* estimated suggests that an additional process must have occurred, namely the reclamation of muscle fibres from 'foreign' motoneurones by the newly-recovered 'original' neurones. So far this phenomenon has not been demonstrated in animal experiments, other than in those of Brown and Butler (1974) on spindle reinnervation (page 229), and caution should therefore be exercised before the suggested interpretation is accepted. It should be added, however, that none of the experimental models were of the type considered here since all involved axonal degeneration of the original innervation.

It is now convenient to summarize in diagram form the concepts of neuronal dysfunction and recovery which have emerged from these studies on neuropathic patients. At the top of *Figure 25.5 (I)* is shown a healthy motoneurone with just two of the muscle fibres comprising its motor unit. At each of the neuromuscular junctions excitation of the muscle fibre can take place following the arrival of an impulse from the neurone soma. The neuromuscular junctions are also the site of transfer of trophic substances from axon to muscle fibre and *vice versa*. The earliest stage of neuronal dysfunction is that of *partial synaptic failure*, in which a neuromuscular junction becomes incapable of synaptic transmission while still remaining able to convey a neurotrophic influence. This is the type of junction which has been termed a 'silent' synapse by McComas, Upton and Jorgensen (1975b) and a 'non-transmitting' one by Dennis and Miledi (1974); it will be recalled that the latter authors had encountered this phenomenon as a transient phase during axon regeneration (page 77). At first restricted to a proportion of the neuromuscular junctions within a motor unit (*Figure 25.5, II*), the partial dysfunction eventually involves all the synapses (*Figure 25.5, III*). Since the chemically-mediated neurotrophic influence remains, the non-excitable muscle fibres do not show certain of the other features of denervation; thus the fibres do not atrophy, they do not discharge fibrillations or positive sharp waves, and they do not attract a new innervation from other motoneurones. These non-excitable fibres can be regarded as '*functionally*' denervated. '*Full*' denervation takes place only when the neuromuscular junction loses its ability to transmit the neurotrophic influence; the synapse is in a stage of total *synaptic failure* (*Figure 25.5, IV*) and may

now show microscopic evidence of degeneration. If the neurotoxic insult is severe the degenerative process will spread proximally towards the neurone soma, giving rise to the characteristic 'dying-back' appearance of the axons. In man it is not yet possible to trace the extent of the dying-back process in motor axons with electrophysiological techniques since an unknown proportion of the impulse activity evoked in a muscle nerve will have emanated from large diameter sensory fibres. As a consequence neuropathological studies are needed to determine the amount of dying back in motor axons; from these studies it is clear that all degrees

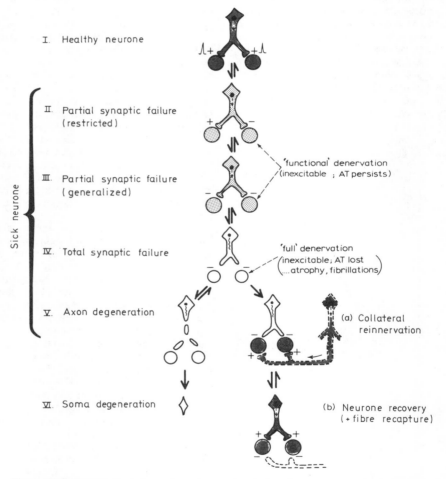

Figure 25.5. Hypothetical stages in motoneurone dysfunction (see text). The postive and negative signs indicate excitable and non-excitable neuromuscular junctions respectively. The density of the stippling is related to the amount of axoplasmic transport (AT), also shown by arrows directed away from motoneurone soma. (From McComas, Upton and Jorgensen (1975a) courtesy of the Editor and publishers of Canadian Journal of Neurological Sciences*)*

are possible, the most severe culminating in the degeneration of the neurone soma (*Figure 25.5, VI*). In contrast the dying-back process can be studied quite easily in sensory axons using electro-physiological techniques, for recordings can readily be made from a purely cutaneous nerve such as the sural or saphenous; digital nerves are also accessible for study and contain joint afferents in addition to skin receptor fibres. It is interesting that, in cats poisoned with acrylamide, it is possible to detect a stage of sensory neurone dysfunction in which the muscle spindle endings are unable to respond to a mechanical stimulus but can be excited electrically (Sumner, 1975). Although the structure and function of a sensory receptor obviously differ from those of a motor axon terminal, this finding by Sumner could be regarded as a sensory counter-part to the silent synapse phenomenon at the neuromuscular junction.

Returning now to the muscle, any fibres which have been fully denervated will become available for collateral reinnervation; in some way the fibres appear to stimulate the formation of sprouts from the neighbouring axons of healthy surviving moto-neurones (see page 227 and *Figure 25.5, a*). This stage is recognized electromyographically by the presence of unusually large or prolonged motor unit potentials.

The last feature of neuronal recovery to be considered is that of *muscle fibre recapture* (*Figure 25.5, b*). In this the original motoneurone appears able to reactivate (or regenerate) its neuro-muscular junction and then to suppress the foreign innervation. If the reality of this stage can be confirmed it would indicate that the original moto-neurone is somehow able to exercise a proprietorial right over the muscle fibres of its motor unit; how this domination over foreign motoneurones might be achieved is unknown.

Apart from its relevance to toxic and metabolic neuropathies, the scheme outlined in *Figure 25.5* is crucial to an understanding of the sick motoneurone hypothesis for the various elements within it can be combined in such a way as to duplicate many of the features observed in some of the myopathies. The subject is discussed more fully in Chapters 13 and 28. There is, however, one cautionary note. Although a dying-back process can be readily observed in a variety of toxic, metabolic, and other neuropathies, there is no convincing evidence so far that the primary lesion is within the neurone soma as postulated by Cavanagh (1954). On the one hand Cavanagh and Chen (1971) were able to demonstrate an inhibition of protein synthesis prior to the clinical development of a toxic neuropathy and a similar finding has been made by Asbury, Cox and Kanada (1973). Against this is the finding

of *increased* uptake of lysine and methionine by the spinal cords of animals with acrylamide neuro-pathy, as found by Hashimoto and Ando (1973). If protein synthesis were impaired, a reduced amount would be available to the axon for its continued upkeep; the consumption of proteins by the proximal region of axon would leave insufficient to flow to the distal region and to prevent degenera-tion from taking place there. Further, the hypothesis does provide an explanation as to why the largest and longest axons would be the first to show dying-back changes, since these would normally require a relatively greater amount of axoplasmic material for their sustenance.

An alternative explanation for the dying-back phenomenon is that axoplasmic flow, rather than protein synthesis, is interfered with. In the case of colchicine and vincristine, there is good experi-mental evidence that local application of these sub-stances to nerve will block axoplasmic transport (Albuquerque *et al.,* 1972; Hofmann and Thesleff, 1972) but this does not mean that substances chemically unrelated will act in the same manner. So far as acrylamide neuropathy is concerned the evidence is conflicting, for while Pleasure, Mischler and Engel (1969) found slow axoplasmic flow to be reduced, Bradley and Williams (1973) were unable to confirm this observation. The latter authors did find a decrease in the velocity of the fast crest but they felt that this was unlikely to have been responsible for the dying-back features observed. In renal failure interesting observations have been made by Brimijoin and Dyck (1974) who used the enzyme dopamine-β-hydroxylase as a marker for fast axoplasmic transport in excised specimens of sural nerve. In one patient, who had clinical evidence of a sensory and motor neuro-pathy, there was a significant reduction in the rate of transport while in a second patient, without signs of a neuropathy, transport was normal.

A third possibility is that the neurotoxic agent in a dying-back neuropathy acts directly on the distal region of the axon and affects it more severely than the soma. This situation might arise if the axon was particularly vulnerable to the toxic substance or alternatively if the latter was distributed pre-ferentially in the nerve endings. In keeping with this last possibility is the observation of Ando and Hashimoto (1972) that more [^{14}C]-acrylamide accumulates in the distal half of the mouse sciatic nerve than in the proximal half. In an extension of this work Ando (1973) was able to show that the accumulation of acrylamide distally had not resulted from transport of this substance from the soma; thus, the effect was still present if the nerve had been ligated.

From what has been said it is clear that the mode

of action of the neurotoxic agents remains largely unknown and that further studies of protein synthesis are required, together with more detailed investigations of axoplasmic flow. Even when definitive answers have been obtained on these various points, the results will still only have provided indirect evidence as to the likely mechanism of action of the toxic agent. A quite different approach may be needed to give a conclusive answer to the basic question as to whether the agent is acting on the soma or the distal axon.

Chapter 26

REVERSIBLE MOTONEURONE
DYSFUNCTION IN THYROTOXICOSIS

In the preceding chapter a patient was described in whom a neuropathic process had arisen as a complication of *chronic renal failure*. This disorder, and *diabetes mellitus,* constitute the two most frequent causes of 'metabolic' neuropathies. Other conditions which can be included with this category are *hypoglycaemia, porphyria* and *hepatic failure.* In certain other disorders, all of them rare, a degenerative neuropathy occurs in association with a well-defined metabolic abnormality which may, or may not, be the cause of the neural lesion. Included in this last group of disorders are *Bassen–Kornweig's disease* (absent beta-lipoproteins), *Tangier disease* (absent alpha-lipoproteins), *Fabry's disease* (ceramide trihexosidase deficiency) and *metachromatic leucodystrophy* (aryl sulphatase A deficiency). In some of these conditions there appears to be a generalized abnormality of cell membranes resulting in the formation of defective myelin sheaths; axonal degeneration may also occur.

The recently described metabolic neuropathy of *primary hyperparathyroidism* is of particular interest in that it may simulate motoneurone disease and will disappear if the parathyroid adenoma is removed (Patten *et al.,* 1974; see also page 269). One of the best examples of a potentially reversible metabolic neuropathy is that occurring in *thyrotoxicosis;* it appears that the neuronal dysfunction is relatively subtle, resulting in impaired synaptic transmission while leaving trophic function largely undisturbed. In terms of the scheme outlined in *Figure 25.5* the dysfunction corresponds to stages II and III (partial synaptic failure). Since the presence of a neuropathic disorder in thyrotoxicosis is not generally recognized and since neuromuscular function has been studied in some detail by the motor unit counting technique of McComas *et al.,* (1971a) an account of the findings may now be given (see also McComas *et al.,* 1973a, 1974a).

Clinical features

The close relationship between the thyroid gland and the neuromuscular system is indicated by the fact that overactivity of the gland may be associated with four different neurological syndromes—myasthenia gravis, periodic paralysis, and thyrotoxic 'myopathy' and ophthalmopathy. The first two syndromes have been discussed in chapters 18 and 15 respectively; it is the thyrotoxic 'myopathy' which is of present concern. The precise incidence of this last condition is difficult to determine. Clinically, most patients with hyperthyroidism tire easily and part of their loss of weight may be due to muscle atrophy. Frank weakness of muscles, particularly proximal ones of the limbs, occurs in rather more than half the patients (Ramsay, 1969; Whitfield and Hudson, 1961). Much less common are spontaneous twitchings and cramps of affected muscles.

In contrast to the high incidence of 'myopathic' features in thyrotoxicosis, only scant mention has been made of a possible neuropathic complication. Birket-Smith and Olivarius (1957) described one patient with 'polyradiculitis' while Bronsky,

Kaganiec and Waldstein (1964) reported four cases of the Guillain–Barré syndrome associated with thyrotoxicosis. The last authors thought that, in some way, thyrotoxicosis predisposed to the development of the neuropathy. In a third study, by Ludin, Spiess and Koenig (1969), a prospective approach was adopted; these authors investigated extensor digitorum brevis muscles with coaxial recording electrodes and found evidence of denervation in eight of 13 patients with thyrotoxicosis. Despite these reports the consensus of opinion is that neuropathic changes in thyrotoxicosis are infrequent and, if present, signify an additional aetiological factor (Engel, 1972).

Morphological studies of muscle and nerve

In spite of the presence of clinical and EMG features indicative of muscle disease, biopsy specimens of muscle often appear normal on microscopical examination (Havard et al., 1963; Engel, 1966). In other cases mild atrophy of muscle fibres appears as the only abnormality, but in a small proportion of cases there are obvious degenerative changes in the fibres accompanied by infiltrations of macrophages and lymphocytes ('lymphorrhages'). Electronmicroscopy has shed little further light for, although the mitochondria may appear abnormal, the changes are slight and are non-specific (Engel, 1966). Abnormal deposits of polysaccharide material in extraocular muscles were reported by Asboe-Hansen, Iversen and Wichmann (1962); similar accumulations, shown by electronmicroscopy to consist of glycogen, have since been demonstrated under the sarcolemmae of limb muscle fibres (Engel, 1966; Gruener et al., 1975).

Although the motor innervation has not been studied as much as the muscle fibres, the findings are nevertheless of interest for Havard and colleagues (1963) were able to demonstrate swellings in the terminal motor axons and also clubbing of the end-plates. Woolf and Cöers (1974) in a review article on the anatomy of intramuscular nerve endings, include a photograph (their Figure 8.5) showing prominent axonal sprouting in a patient with thyrotoxic myopathy; the frequency of this type of abnormality is not stated.

Electrophysiological studies

There have been several accounts of conventional EMG studies in thyrotoxicosis, all of which have shown the features characteristic of a 'myopathic' disorder, that is, the presence small, brief and sometimes complex motor unit potentials which merge into a full interference pattern on maximal effort. Using such criteria Ramsay (1966) found evidence of myopathy in 92.6 per cent of thyrotoxic patients while Havard and colleagues (1963) reported an incidence of 80 per cent. The investigation by Sanderson and Adey (1952) is of additional interest in that these workers were able to show that the brief 'myopathic' potentials regained their normal durations following successful treatment of the endocrine disorder. It is not surprising that the

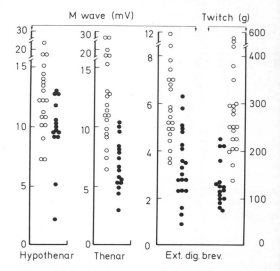

Figure 26.1. Maximum evoked muscle responses (M-waves) and isometric twitch tensions in 20 patients with thyrotoxicosis (●), and in a matched population of control subjects (○). (From McComas et al. (1974a), courtesy of the Editor and publishers of Journal of Neurology, Neurosurgery and Psychiatry)

contractile properties of muscle have also been studied in thyrotoxicosis, in view of the usual clinical finding of abnormally brisk tendon reflexes. These apparently rapid contractions contrast with the sluggish responses in hypothyroidism. Many recording systems have been devised for recording the ankle jerk in thyrotoxicosis, most of them depending on the movement of the unrestrained ankle following percussion of the Achilles tendon. This is a very inferior way to study muscle contraction and relaxation; it is much better to record the isometric twitch tension following maximal stimulation of the appropriate motor nerve. Among studies of the latter type, that by Lambert and associates (1951) is exemplary; these authors were able to show that the twitch became abnormally slow in hypothyroidism while in thyrotoxicosis the values for duration lay at the fast end of the normal range. More recently Takamori, Gutmann and Shane (1971) have analysed the twitch kinetics and suggested that the

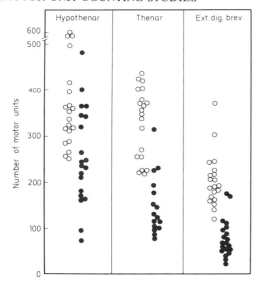

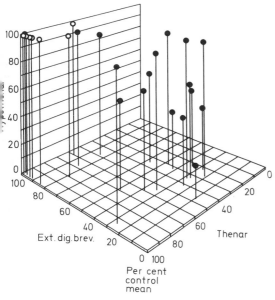

Figure 26.2. (Upper) Numbers of functioning motor units in the hypothenar, thenar and extensor digitorum brevis muscles of 20 patients with thyrotoxicosis (●) and in a matched population of control subjects (o). Notice that the hypothenar muscles are less severely involved than the others. (Lower) Simulated 3-dimensional display of the above results in those patients (●) and control subjects (o) in whom all three muscle groups had been investigated. Control values greater than means shown as 100 per cent. Notice again the clear separation between the results for patients and controls and the relative sparing of the hypothenar muscles in the former. (From McComas et al. 1974a), courtesy of the Editor and publishers of Journal of Neurology, Neurosurgery and Psychiatry)

fast twitch in hyperthyroidism results from shortening of the 'active state' duration (page 41). Possibly this effect is mediated through the potentiation, by thyroid hormone(s), of β-adrenergic receptor activity within the muscle fibres (see also Marsden and Meadows, 1970).

Microelectrode recordings from muscle fibres have been undertaken in rats made thyrotoxic by triiodothyronine (Hofmann and Denys, 1972) and also in patients, using the intercostal muscle biopsy technique (Gruener et al., 1975). In both studies it was found that the resting membrane potentials of many diseased fibres were reduced and that a proportion of the fibres could not be activated, even on direct stimulation. By hyperpolarizing the fibres and repeating the stimulation Gruener and colleagues were able to show that the diseased fibre membranes were less excitable than normal ones.

Motor unit counting studies

McComas and colleagues (1974a) investigated 20 patients with thyrotoxicosis; they were all below the age of 60 but were otherwise unselected. The patients, 19 of whom were female, had not been treated for more than one week with radio-iodine; control subjects, matched both for age and sex, were also studied.

In this study it was first of all shown that there was a reduction in functional muscle mass in thyrotoxicosis; this was indicated by reductions in the amplitudes of the maximum evoked muscle action potentials (M waves) and in the isometric muscle twitch tensions (*Figure 26.1*). The numbers of functioning motor units were then estimated in the thenar, hypothenar and extensor digitorum brevis (EDB) muscles. It was observed that in each patient at least one of the motor unit estimates was reduced. *Figure 26.2* demonstrates another interesting result—the loss of functioning motor units tended to be greater in the EDB muscle and thenar muscles, while the hypothenar muscles were less severely affected. A similar difference in motor unit vulnerability has been commented upon previously, for it was shown to occur in ageing, myotonic and Duchenne dystrophy, renal failure and toxic neuropathies.

As has been discussed earlier, the finding of a loss of functioning motor units is not sufficient evidence in itself of a neuropathic disorder for the same situation might arise in the course of a myopathy. To distinguish between these two possibilities requires knowledge of the sizes of the surviving motor units, normal or increased sizes suggesting a neuropathy and smaller ones indicating either a neuropathy or a myopathy (page 119). In

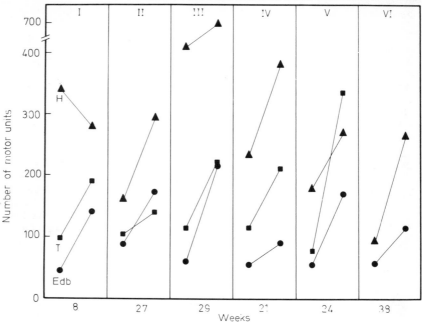

thyrotoxicosis the surviving motor units, as judged by the amplitudes of their evoked potentials, are significantly enlarged—at least in EDB. It therefore seems probable that a neuropathic disorder is present in thyrotoxicosis; whether a myopathic condition exists independently is uncertain, especially since some or all of the myopathic features might be secondary. It would be interesting to know the efficacy of axoplasmic transport in thyrotoxicosis; the finding of swellings in terminal motor axons by Havard and colleagues (1963) could indicate that axoplasmic flow had been interfered with.

One of the attractions of the metabolic neuromyopathies for the investigator is that they are potentially reversible and this is certainly true of hyperthyroidism, as *Figure 26.3* (*upper*) indicates. In this figure the numbers of functioning motor units have been shown in six patients, each of whom was studied following their return to a euthyroid state. It can be seen that each of the previously depleted populations of motor units showed an increase. Two additional patients were studied on a number of occasions before and after treatment; in these cases the speed of recovery of motor unit function is impressive (*Figure 26.3, lower*).

Although only thyrotoxicosis has been considered in detail in this short chapter, the unexpected but nevertheless striking electrophysiological findings raise the possibility that muscle weakness in other metabolic disorders may also have a latent neural component.

Figure 26.3 (Upper) Recovery of motor unit function in six patients treated for thyrotoxicosis. Periods of observation (weeks) shown at bottom of columns. ▲ ■*, and* ● *indicate values for hypothenar, thenar and extensor digitorum brevis muscles respectively. (From McComas et al. (1974a), courtesy of the Editor and publishers of Journal of Neurology, Neurosurgery and Psychiatry). (Lower) Serial studies on a further two patients with thyrotoxicosis, showing recovery. (Courtesy of Dr K. Toyonaga)*

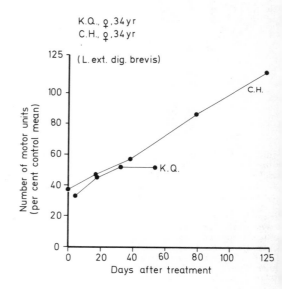

Chapter 27

TRANS-SYNAPTIC MOTONEURONE DEGENERATION

INTRODUCTION

It was shown in Chapter 8 that the removal of the trophic influence of the motoneurones, as following severance of their axons, resulted in the development of certain degenerative changes in the muscle fibres. The nature of the electrical and biochemical influences responsible for the normal trophic action of the motoneurone was considered in Chapter 9. In other chapters the possibility has been raised that some of the features of diseased muscle fibres, seen in conditions hitherto regarded as primary myopathies, may instead have resulted from withdrawal or modification of neurotrophic activity. Thus, a large part of this book has dealt, directly or indirectly, with the trophic effects of the motoneurone on its colony of muscle fibres.

The question might now be asked as to whether trophic interactions are peculiar to the motoneurone and its muscle fibres or whether they are property of all neurones making synaptic connections with each other or with other types of target tissue. In the case of skin and its innervation the answer is known, for denervated skin develops obvious changes which have been labelled 'trophic'; they include atrophy and a loss of hair. Muscle and skin are special examples of innervation, however, for in both tissues the nerve supply is distributed in a relatively simple manner; this is most obvious in skeletal muscle, where each fibre receives its total innervation from a single motoneurone. The situation is very different in the central nervous system where individual neurones may receive synaptic inputs from tens, if not hundreds, of other nerve cells. If a trophic action exists, is it mediated at each of the synapses or are some neural pathways much more important than others in this respect?

In considering these points, the basic question 'are there trophic interactions in the mammalian central nervous system?' can be answered convincingly in the affirmative. The best evidence has come from experiments on the visual system, in which it has been shown that section of the optic nerve is followed by degeneration in the lateral geniculate body and, later, in the visual cortex itself (Glees and Le Gros Clark, 1941; Cook, Walker and Barr, 1951; Goldby, 1957; Hess, 1957; Matthews, Cowan and Powell, 1960).

Further, in the intact visual system injected [³H]-proline can be demonstrated to pass from the eye to the cortex (Grafstein, 1971) and putative neurotrophic substances might follow a similar route. It is difficult to extrapolate from these findings to motoneurones for the latter cells receive many neural inputs, either descending from the brain or coming from such segmental sources as muscle spindles, Golgi-tendon organs, cutaneous receptors and Renshaw cells.

It seems to be widely assumed that the descending pathways, at least, are relatively ineffectual sources of trophic activity. This philosophy finds expression in a type of experiment devised by Sarah Tower to investigate the effects on muscle of disuse, as opposed to denervation. In this experiment the alpha motoneurones are rendered electrically inactive, but are assumed to remain otherwise intact, by transecting the spinal cord rostrally and caudally and by dividing the dorsal roots (Tower, 1937). Even though some workers (for example, Barron, 1933; Young, 1966) have described degeneration of motoneurones after rostral section of the cord in animals, others have attributed this finding to interference with the local blood supply at operation

by Reske-Nielsen, Harmsen and Ovesen (1971) will be considered later in the chapter.

MOTOR UNIT COUNTING STUDIES

In an attempt to resolve the question of possible trans-synaptic degeneration of human motoneurones, McComas (1973c) investigated 40 patients who had been rendered hemiplegic or

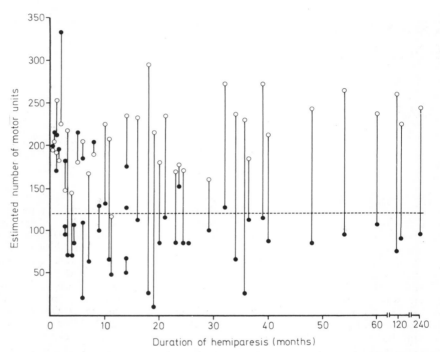

Figure 27.1. Numbers of functioning motor units in the extensor digitorum brevis muscles of patients with hemipareses following cerebrovascular lesions. Values for normal and hemiparetic sides shown by o and ● respectively; (------------------) indicates the lower limit of the control range. (From McComas et al. (1973b) courtesy of the Editor and publishers of Journal of Neurology, Neurosurgery and Psychiatry)

(Klinkerfuss and Haugh, 1970). In man, opinion is also divided for although Charcot (1893) reported the presence of motoneurone degeneration at autopsy following upper motoneurone lesions, his contemporary Déjérine (1889) was unable to recognize similar changes. Nevertheless Déjérine did note marked degeneration in a proportion of the peripheral nerve fibres; this is of great interest, for the finding of a neurone with an intact cell body and a degenerating axon would now arouse suspicion that a 'dying-back' process was taking place (see page 274). Because of its pertinence to recent electrophysiological data, the morphological study

hemiparetic after cerebrovascular lesions (see also McComas et al., 1971c). In each patient they estimated the numbers of functioning motor units in the extensor digitorum brevis (EDB) muscle on the two sides, using the electrophysiological method described in Chapter 6. They reasoned that any degeneration of motoneurones would produce a corresponding reduction in the number of functioning units. Their findings are displayed in Figure 27.1. It can be seen that, for the first 2 months after the stroke, there was no significant difference in the numbers of motor units between the two legs. After this critical period, however, a striking reduction in motor units took place on the side of the hemiparesis, such that only about half of the original population remained functional. In 27 patients with hemiparesis for longer than 2 months, the mean number of EDB units on the weakened side was 93.7 ± 8.4, compared with a value of 216.7 ± 7.9 units for the normal side (p = <0.001). Inspection of *Figure 27.1* gives no hint of a continuing loss of units once the critical 2-month period was over, nor is there statistical evidence of a correlation between the length of illness (beyond 2 months) and the number of surviving units (r = −0.02). In a recent study utilizing the same electrophysiological method Serratrice and associates (1975) have also been able to demonstrate a loss of functioning motor units on the side of the hemiplegia.

McComas and colleagues attempted to define some of the properties of the remaining motor units by measuring their evoked potential amplitudes. They found that the motor unit potentials were significantly larger in the affected EDB muscles compared with the contralateral controls (means 49.7 ± 3.2 μV and 31.2 ± 1.4 μV respectively; p = <0.001). Closer examination of the results revealed a further point of interest in that the enhancement of the motor unit potentials was not apparent until 20 months or more had elapsed following the cerebrovascular episode (*Figure 27.2*). Insofar as the size of a motor unit potential is an indication of the number of muscle fibres in that unit, these results suggested that collateral reinnervation of denervated muscle fibres by surviving motoneurones was deferred for a considerable period of time. The EDB isometric twitch studies were also of value for they showed that the surviving motor units tended to have relatively slow twitches, the contraction times for the normal and affected sides being 72.0 ± 2.2 and 81.7 ± 2.9 ms respectively (p = <0.01). No difference could be detected in the maximal impulse conduction velocities of peroneal nerve motor axons between the normal and affected legs, though the time elapsing between stimulation of the nerve at the ankle and the onset of the EDB muscle response ('terminal latency') was greater on the affected side. This last observation, and the finding of decremental muscle responses during repetitive nerve stimulation in approximately one-third of cases (*Figure 19.3*), indicated that function in the distal parts of the motor axons was compromised. In terms of the 'sick motoneurone hypothesis' (Chapter 13) it suggested that a proportion of the motoneurones were surviving in a 'sick' or 'dysfunctional' state.

The results of the various electrophysiological investigations in this study having been summarized, *Figure 27.3* gives a diagrammatic representation of the changes which are thought to have taken place

in the spinal cord and muscle following the acute hemiplegic lesion. At top (*a*) is shown, in simplified form, the normal situation in which an alpha-motoneurone (*mn*) innervates part of a muscle (*m*) and itself receives synaptic inputs from higher centres (*cortex*) as well as from such segmental sources (*seg*) as the muscle spindle. In (*b*) a cerebrovascular lesion destroys neurones in the motor cortex or segments

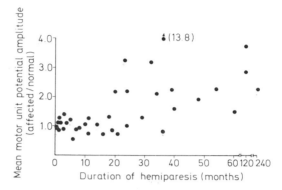

Figure 27.2. Increasing amplitudes of motor unit potentials in extensor digitorum brevis muscles following hemiparesis. Results expressed as fractions of the mean amplitudes on the normal sides. (From McComas et al. (1973b) courtesy of the Editor and publishers of Journal of Neurology, Neurosurgery and Psychiatry)

of the axons issuing from them; Wallerian degeneration takes place in the remainders of the axons beyond the lesion. Deprived of their trophic input from the cortex, the motoneurones enter a dysfunctional state (*stippling*) during which their synaptic connections with some of the muscle fibres become ineffective. All these changes appear to take place in the first 2 months after the stroke; at the end of this time a motoneurone may lose all functional connections with its colony of muscle fibres. This change coincides with the reduction in the functioning motor unit population to approximately half its original size. The most likely explanation for this major event is that the motoneurones have indeed undergone trans-synaptic degeneration (*Figure 27.3, c*). The only other possibility would be that the peripheral nerves had been inadvertently damaged as, for example, by compression of the peroneal nerve behind the head of the fibula. The nerve conduction studies gave no evidence of this complication and, furthermore, care was taken to reject from the study any patients with below-knee calipers. It would also be expected that nerve injury would occur, not at 2 months, but in the first few days or

292

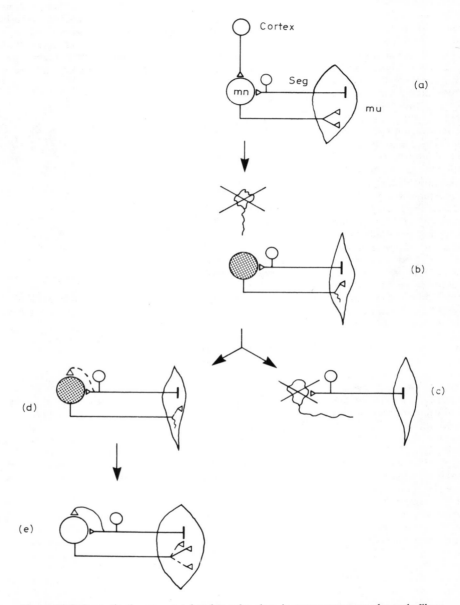

Figure 27.3. Synaptic changes postulated to take place in motoneurones and muscle fibres on the side of a hemiparesis. For description see text. (From McComas et al. (1973b) courtesy of the Editor and publishers of Journal of Neurology, Neurosurgery and Psychiatry)

eeks immediately following the stroke, at a time hen the weakness was greatest and the patient had et to learn the trick of manoeuvring himself about. lso, the loss of motor units following a hemi- egia is not peculiar to EDB, for similar changes ave since been noted in the thenar and hypothenar uscles. It would therefore be necessary to postulate e presence of multiple nerve entrapments in order account for all the denervation noted.

Even though the observed changes must reflect ans-synaptic degeneration of the motoneurones, e motor unit counting studies give no clue as to e pathological state of the neurones and their xons. However, the finding of fibrillation and arp wave potentials by Goldkamp (1967) and otermans (1968) in muscles on the side of the emiplegia indicates that the neuromuscular junc- ons are not simply 'silent' (non-transmitting); generation of the axon terminals, and possibly of e axon trunks too, must have taken place age 282). The best information on this point has me from autopsy studies of spinal cords in patients ying at various times after fractures of the neck. four such cases Reske-Nielsen, Harmsen and vesen (1971) observed a striking loss of moto- urones, even well below the level of the lesion. rviving neurones were often ballooned and the issl substance was pushed to the periphery of the ell body. The findings of these authors are related those of McComas and colleagues (1971c, 1973b) another way, for Reske-Nielsen and associates 971), using histological techniques, also observed evidence of muscle denervation in the first 2 onths after injury. The reality of this critical riod following an upper motoneurone lesion ust therefore be regarded as established.

The story does not finish here, however, for many f the motoneurones which survive appear able to gain their normal vigour, the best manifestation of is being their readiness to adopt denervated uscle fibres by the process of collateral reinnerva- on (page 224). In the electrophysiological studies f McComas and colleagues (1971c, 1973b) the esence of this phenomenon had to be inferred om the enlarged sizes of the evoked motor unit otentials (see above). With the intravital staining chnique (page 196) Reske-Nielsen, Harmsen and vesen were able to see direct evidence of axonal routing in biopsied specimens of the tibialis nterior and peroneus brevis muscles. In this last udy sprouting was recognized as early as 41 and 3 days after the lesion, even though other features f denervation could not be detected in the muscle this time. From Table IV of Reske-Nielsen, armsen and Ovesen (1971) most collateral rein- ervation appears to have taken place by 14 onths post-injury. This is rather shorter than the

20-month period found by McComas and colleagues (1973b) but, upon this issue, the histological find- ings are obviously more reliable.

Which factors are responsible for restoring the vigour of the surviving motoneurones? There is no definite answer to this question but McComas and associates (1973b), on the basis of observations from other laboratories, were able to make a sug- gestion. They noted that in experiments on the cat, sprouting of incoming dorsal root fibres appeared to take place after the cord had been sectioned rostrally (McCouch, Austin, Liu and Liu, 1958). The implication is that these new fibres would grow towards the alpha-motoneurones and take over the synaptic sites occupied by the terminals of the corticospinal tract fibres before their degeneration (Appendix 27.1). The McComas group (1973) suggested that the new synapses established on a motoneurone by the sprouts from incoming dorsal root axons would restore some of the missing trophic input to the motoneurone and thereby enable it to regain its normal function (*Figure 27.3, d and e*). Other questions deserve consideration also. For example, why should only half the motoneurone pool show the features of the trans-synaptic de- generation? Why, in five of the 46 patients studied by McComas and colleagues (1973b), should the motor unit values have been normal even though the hemiplegia was as severe as in the other patients displaying losses of motor units? Further, do the striking abnormalities encountered in the above study indicate that the corticospinal pathway is more important than other fibre systems in mediat- ing a trophic influence on the motoneurones? The answer here is uncertain, for there is no information as to the extent of motoneurone degeneration fol- lowing section of other pathways, such as the dorsal roots.

McComas *et al* did not attempt to define the neuronal origin of the descending fibre pathways responsible for maintaining the trophic influence on the motoneurones. It is likely that in most of their patients the cerebrovascular lesion consisted of a haemorrhage into the internal capsule. If so, the 'neurotrophic' cells would lie within the cerebral cortex rather than the brainstem. In other studies the occurrence of muscle atrophy has provided a clue as to the origin of the trophic influence on the motoneurones; thus the fact that a tumour of the hemisphere or meninges can produce contralateral muscle atrophy would also implicate the cerebral cortex as the trophic source (Silverstein, 1955). This is still only a partial answer to the question for the massive spinal projection from each cerebral hemi- sphere has a wide field of origin, involving the parietal lobe as well as the frontal one (Levin and Bradford, 1938). This point has been demonstrated electrophysiologically in man by Penfield and Boldrey (1937) who were able to produce movements in conscious patients by electrical stimulation of the exposed postcentral gyrus on the opposite side. Some workers, indeed, have insisted that the parietal lobe is the sole source of the trophic influence (Silverstein, 1931; Botez, 1971) but others have pointed out the difficulty in reconciling this view with the presence of contralateral muscle wasting in some hemiplegic patients not showing any evidence of the parietal lobe type of sensory loss (Fenichel, Daroff and Glaser, 1964). Partly for this last reason, and partly on account of other experimental observations, it seems more likely that it is the motor cortex which normally supplies the trophic influence to the motoneurones. The most obvious evidence in favour of the motor cortex is the association between muscle wasting (or loss of functioning motor units) and a cerebral lesion on the opposite side which must have included the motor cortex in order to account for the combination of weakness, increased tendon reflexes and a Babinski response. A more specific observation is that extirpation of the motor strip will produce contralateral muscle wasting in chimpanzees whereas lesions of the postcentral gyrus appear to be ineffective (Fulton, 1936, 1949). One interesting suggestion which has been put forward is that, irrespective of whether frontal or parietal lobe mechanisms are involved, there is a relationship between hemispheric dominance and muscle wasting. Thus Botez (1971), in an extensive study of patients with cerebral tumours, noted that muscle wasting was commonly associated with lesions of the minor hemisphere but was infrequently encountered if the dominant hemisphere was involved instead. This relationship was not observed in the study by McComas and colleagues (1973b); for example, six patients had bilateral spastic weakness and in four of these the EDB motor unit populations were reduced on both sides.

It is debatable whether trans-synaptic degeneration of motoneurones can account for all the muscle wasting observed. In Chapter 20 it was shown that in other disorders muscles may suffer very severe denervation and yet be compensated fully by collateral reinnervation from remaining motoneurones. Since in hemiplegia about half the motoneurones are left, one must surmise that these survivors are incapable of initiating sufficient axonal sprouting to prevent some denervation atrophy from taking place. An alternative suggestion is that some of the wasting is due to disuse; while this might account for atrophy in a large proximal muscle such as the quadriceps femoris, experiments using plaster casts to produce immobilization have shown that disuse causes little wasting in relatively small distal muscles such as the thenar group (Sale, unpublished observations). A third possibility, which has found favour in the past, is that the muscle wasting is secondary to a vasomotor disturbance initiated by the cortical lesion (Feudell and Fischer, 1956). It is certainly true that the skin on the side of the hemiplegia is usually colder and is often pale or cyanosed; however, measurements of muscle blood flow and temperature have shown normal vasomotor responses following warming and cooling of the body (Uprus et al., 1935; Sturup et al., 1935). At present then, the most likely explanation for muscle wasting, at least in distal muscles, is inadequate collateral sprouting following denervation of muscle fibres.

CONCLUSIONS

In conclusion, there now seems good evidence that trans-synaptic degeneration of motoneurones does occur following lesions of the contralateral motor cortex or emergent fibres and that it affects, in an irreversible manner, approximately half the motoneurone pool. The critical time at which the degenerating motoneurones become no longer able to excite the muscle fibres is about 2 months after the upper motoneurone lesion. Although axonal sprouting is undertaken by surviving motoneurones it may occur too late or be insufficiently vigorous to prevent some denervation atrophy of the muscle fibres from taking place.

It might be added that although this chapter has been concerned mainly with motoneurones the results, and those of experiments on the visual system cited earlier, have relevance to other regions of the central nervous system. Thus, whenever a population of neurones or axons has been destroyed, many of the cells to which they had projected will also undergo degeneration, and the process may then be repeated at the next station in the neural pathway. A lesion may be well localized at the onset, but with time its effects may be observed, functionally if not structurally, in an increasingly large part of the nervous system.

Chapter 28

CONCLUSIONS

In the first part of this book an attempt has been made to provide a reasonably detailed description of the normal physiology of the motoneurone and muscle fibre. The information concerning structure, although smaller in amount, is nevertheless sufficient to enable the physiological considerations to become intelligible. In terms of existing knowledge, the correlation between structure and function is perhaps most complete in the examples of neuromuscular transmission and of muscle contraction. In other areas there are serious gaps in our knowledge, particularly at the macromolecular level just beyond the resolving power of the electronmicroscope. For example, despite various hypothetical models and recent studies of antibiotics with ionophore properties, little is known of the specialized molecules which regulate the permeability of the nerve and muscle fibre membranes. There is also ignorance concerning the mechanism whereby calcium ions are transported from the lateral sacs of the sacroplasmic reticulum to the reactive sites on the actin filaments. Perhaps the most fascinating of the still unresolved problems, however, are the identities of the special trophic messenger molecules which pass between the motoneurone, muscle fibre and Schwann cell. As has been shown, the structural and functional integrity of the three different types of cell depend on this molecular traffic. If a motor axon is severed the part which is now isolated from the motoneurone soma degenerates, as do the associated Schwann cells; the muscle fibre is also affected, becoming very much smaller and showing evidence

of altered biochemistry and of abnormal membrane function. But the reverse is also true for, when permanently deprived of its connection to muscle fibres, a motoneurone may undergo irreversible degeneration. When the biochemistry of this trophic activity has been elucidated, the knowledge is likely to have profound implications for the treatment of neuromuscular disease. Furthermore, the information gained from the study of nerve and muscle may well prove crucial for an understanding of the trophic phenomena which are known to exist in the central nervous system. In Chapter 27, for example, it was shown that motoneurones underwent trans-synaptic degeneration when their inputs from certain descending pathways were removed. It is probable that less florid instances of neuronal disuse, or for that matter, of overuse, can result in potentially reversible structural and functional changes at individual synapses elsewhere in the brain and spinal cord. Such changes are likely to be responsible for conferring on the nervous system its important property of behavioural plasticity; for example, by strengthening certain synaptic connections at the expense of others, fresh skills can be learned, information memorized, and new reflex behaviour acquired.

In examining the trophic relationship between the motoneurone and the muscle fibre it is clear that the metabolic demands made on the motoneurone are the greater. Through the synthesis and transport of messenger molecules each neurone must support a large number of muscle fibres, in

295

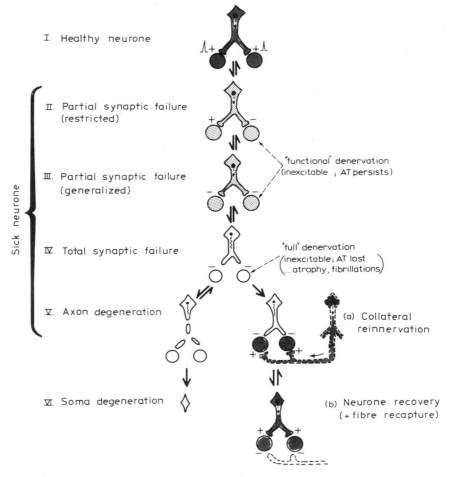

I. Healthy neurone

Sick neurone

II. Partial synaptic failure (restricted)

III. Partial synaptic failure (generalized)

'functional' denervation (inexcitable ; AT persists)

IV. Total synaptic failure

'full' denervation (inexcitable; AT lost ...atrophy, fibrillations)

V. Axon degeneration

(a) Collateral reinnervation

VI. Soma degeneration

(b) Neurone recovery (+fibre recapture)

Figure 28.1. Hypothetical stages in motoneurone dysfunction (see page 281). The positive and negative signs indicate excitable and non-excitable neuromuscular junctions respectively. The density of the stippling is related to the amount of axoplasmic transport (AT), also shown by arrows directed away from motoneurone soma (see text). (From McComas Upton and Jorgensen (1975a), courtesy of the Editor and publishers of the Canadian journal of Neurological Sciences)

some cases more than a thousand. Even sustenance of its own axon is a major undertaking since, as first shown by Weiss (see Chapter 2), the soma is continually synthesizing and renewing the cytoplasm of the axis cylinder. The high metabolic activity of the motoneurones has an unfortunate consequence in that it makes the cells particularly vulnerable to adverse systemic factors. We see evidence of this susceptibility in the neuropathies associated with chronic renal failure and diabetes mellitus and in those due to the action of such drugs as vincristine (page 276). It would be surprising if the neuronal metabolism responsible for

trophic function was not upset in other circumstances as, for example, during any period of profound debilitation. In this context it is intriguing that one of the patients described in Chapter 25, who had made a satisfactory recovery from a vincristine-induced neuropathy (page 277), volunteered that his paraesthesiæ returned during bouts of influenza.

Adding to the problem of maintaining adequate axoplasmic transport is the tendency of axons to undergo compression at certain vulnerable sites. Thus the median nerve is subjected to pressure at the wrist, while the ulnar nerve may be damaged at the elbow and the peroneal nerve at the head of the fibula. It is possible that the propensity of the peroneal nerve for trauma is responsible for the extreme subsceptibility of the extensor digitorum brevis muscle to generalized denervating disorders; if so, denervation would result because the reduced flow of axoplasm from 'sick motoneurones' was diminished still further by axonal compression at the head of the fibula. One of the puzzling features of the extensor digitorum brevis muscle is the histological evidence of denervation in apparently healthy adults below the age of 60, in the absence of a progressive fall in motor unit population. This discrepancy may be explained by drawing upon some of the ideas already put forward. We can suggest that during life the motoneurones are repeatedly affected by adverse systemic factors or perhaps the axons are repeatedly traumatized; after the muscle fibres become denervated many are annexed by collateral sprouts from surviving axons. This collateral reinnervation gives rise to groups of muscle fibres with similar staining reactions and to large, prolonged and complex EMG potentials. Unless the motoneurones have been irreversibly damaged, their axons will regenerate and will then re-establish synaptic connections with some of the muscle fibres; in some cases the original moto-neurones may win back some of their lost territory. If these suppositions are correct certain muscles would be expected to have normal numbers of motor units but display histological and EMG features associated with chronic denervation. This

concept of lability of motoneurone function has received some support from studies of patients in chronic renal failure and in the recovery phase of thyrotoxicosis, for in both circumstances the fluctuations in motor unit counts far exceed the experimental error. Even in apparently healthy subjects, random EMG studies may occasionally disclose such 'abnormal' features as widespread muscle fasciculations, unexpectedly low motor unit counts and incremental muscle responses during repetitive nerve stimulation.

It is implicit from this concept of fluctuating neuronal behaviour that there must be several gradations of altered neuromuscular function between normality on the one hand, and frank denervation on the other. These stages have been described in Chapter 25 and are displayed again in *Figure 28.1*: the recognition of these stages is relatively easy and depends on the comparison of motor unit counts, maximum evoked muscle responses and the presence or absence of spon-taneous electrical activity on coaxial needle examination (*Figure 28.2*).

Even if motoneurones have avoided irreparable harm from metabolic, toxic or traumatic mishaps in earlier life, the cells must ultimately fall victim to the degenerative processes which accompany ageing. Unlike some of the other studies of the effects of old age on the neuromuscular system, the recent investigation by Campbell, McComas and Petito (1973) suggests that much of the muscle weakness and wasting is secondary to the inability

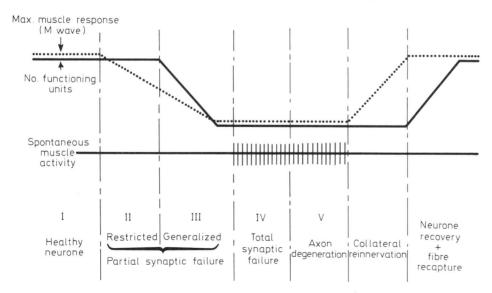

Figure 28.2. Electrophysiological features of muscles, as revealed by EMG, during the various stages of motoneurone dysfunction. (From McComas, Upton and Jorgensen (1975a), courtesy of the Editor and publishers of the Canadian Journal of Neurological Sciences)

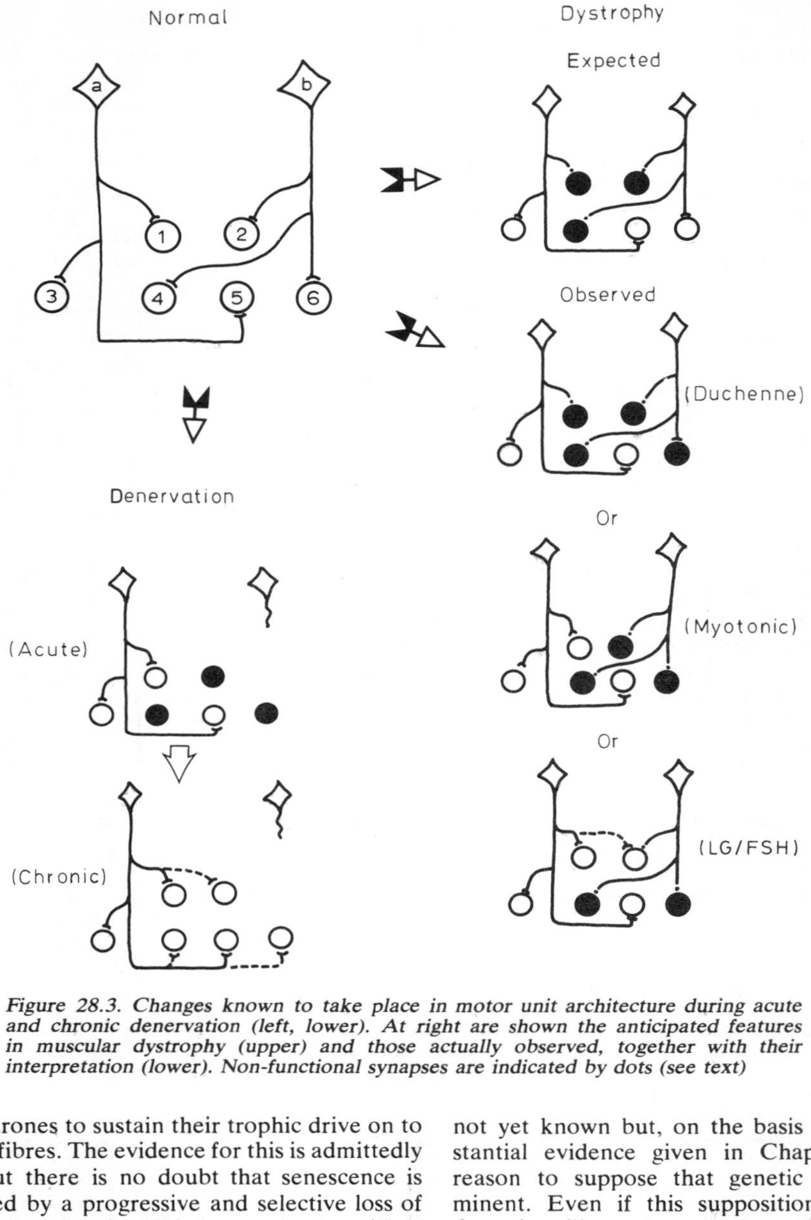

Figure 28.3. Changes known to take place in motor unit architecture during acute and chronic denervation (left, lower). At right are shown the anticipated features in muscular dystrophy (upper) and those actually observed, together with their interpretation (lower). Non-functional synapses are indicated by dots (see text)

of motoneurones to sustain their trophic drive on to the muscle fibres. The evidence for this is admittedly indirect, but there is no doubt that senescence is accompanied by a progressive and selective loss of functioning motor units. This last study also differs from most others in identifying a critical age for the onset of the ageing defects in the nervous system. In a large population of healthy subjects this critical age is around 60 but, as in all physiological parameters, there is a significant variation about the mean such that much older subjects may be encountered in whom the populations of motor units are still within the normal range. The factors responsible for this loss of neuronal function are not yet known but, on the basis of rather circumstantial evidence given in Chapter 12, there is reason to suppose that genetic factors are prominent. Even if this supposition proves correct, there is still much more that one would wish to know. The most important question is whether the genetic influence is one which affects the motoneurones directly or whether the neuronal changes are secondary to an age-induced failure of some other tissue. Answers to such fundamental questions would not seem to be beyond the present bounds of experimental neurobiology. One would also wish to know whether the tempo of the ageing process is hastened in motoneurones which have been used excessively, for example, in athletes or in workers engaged in heavy manual work. Beyond the hint that motoneurone disease may be commoner in former athletes (Critchley, 1962) there is no literature available on this topic.

Undeniably, much of the present debate in the neurology of the peripheral nervous system concerns the possibility that many conditions formerly thought to involve only muscle fibres (i.e. the 'primary myopathies') may instead be associated with significant abnormalities of the nervous system. If this is indeed the case, the further possibility arises that the pathological changes in the muscles may have been caused by the abnormal innervation, rather than occurring as primary events. The fact that, in the normal animal, the contractile and biochemical properties of the muscle fibre can be shown to be governed by the motoneurone is an inducement to consider this last possibility seriously. Similarly, the observation that dystrophic-like features can be produced in muscles by chronic denervation is interesting and relevant circumstantial evidence, but its value is somewhat limited since various unrelated procedures may achieve the same result (for example, muscle ischaemia or the administration of drugs which inhibit monoamine oxidase activity). Rather better evidence is the finding of denervation phenomena in the muscles of patients considered to have myopathies. Within this category of evidence the motor unit counting results appear crucial and, possibly for this reason, have been subjected to much critical debate. The counting technique itself has been described in Chapter 6 and the theoretical significance of the experimental results has been analysed in Chapter 13 and can be conveniently reviewed with the aid of *Figure 28.3*. Two motor neurones *a* and *b* are shown (*top left*), *a* innervating muscle fibres 1, 3 and 5 and *b* supplying fibres 2, 4 and 6. The diagram shows the normal overlap of the motor unit territories. In a truly neuropathic disorder (at *left*) motoneurone *b* degenerates with fibres 2, 4 and 6 showing the consequent denervation phenomena (*shaded fibres*). Provided sufficient time elapses neurone *a* undertakes axonal sprouting (*interrupted lines*) and will incorporate the denervated fibres into its motor unit territory. Since the motoneurone determines the biochemical features of the muscle fibres, histochemical studies will show groups of muscle fibres with similar staining properties rather than the mosaic pattern of normal muscle (see *Figure 20.5*). With the motor unit counting technique one would expect to find reduced numbers of functioning motor units with the surviving units generating enlarged potentials; in practice, this is indeed observed (see *Figure 28.4, upper*). In dystrophy (*Figure 28.3, right*) one

would anticipate that a primary muscle disorder would affect the muscle fibres within the various units in a random manner, for example, such that fibres 1, 2 and 4 would degenerate and fibres 3, 5 and 6 would be spared. Investigation of such a muscle with the motor unit counting technique

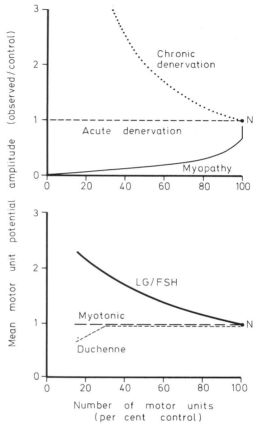

Figure 28.4. (Upper) The relationship between the sizes and numbers of motor units which is observed in denervating disorders and that anticipated to occur in myopathic conditions. (Lower) The relationship actually observed in the various types of dystrophy (see text) N, normal values

would reveal a normal number of motor units but with the sizes of the units being diminished (see also *Figure 28.4, upper*). However, as has been shown in Chapter 16, these theoretical predictions are not borne out experimentally. In each type of dystrophy many patients exhibit a loss of functioning motor units with the surviving units tending to be slightly diminished in Duchenne dystrophy, of normal size in myotonic dystrophy, and somewhat enlarged in the limb-girdle and facioscapulohumeral forms. These findings are displayed in *Figure 28.4* (*lower*), and their interpretation, in terms of motor unit populations, is set out in *Figure 28.3* (*right*) which shows the largely selective involvement of the motor units in the three types of dystrophy, with the presence of some collateral reinnervation in the limb-girdle and facioscapulohumeral forms. Since in the Duchenne and mytonic dystrophies the motoneurones of the still functional motor units appeared unable to undertake collateral reinnervation, McComas and colleagues (1971f) postulated that these neurones were to some extent dysfunctional or 'sick'. Given certain assumptions, they further showed that it was possible to estimate the proportions of 'healthy', 'sick' and functionally 'dead' motoneurones in a patient with dystrophy and also the average duration of the phase of neuronal dysfunction and the annual rate of cell loss. Further experience has shown that some of these concepts require modification. For example, serial examination of 'young' patients (8–9 years) with Duchenne dystrophy has shown that any loss of functioning motor units present initially is not increased over a 3-year period. However, the sizes of the motor units become smaller suggesting that muscle fibres continue to become inexcitable and to degenerate. These new observations are in keeping with the earlier finding of McComas, Sica and Currie (1971) that in Duchenne dystrophy there is no correlation between the age of the patient and the number of functioning motor units. The presence of such a correlation would, of course, have suggested that there was a progressive loss of functioning units. These more recent studies have also shown that, in contrast to the earlier report, a modest enlargement of motor units may *occasionally* occur at an *early* stage of Duchenne dystrophy. In terms of the sick motoneurone

hypothesis, this observation would suggest that a small proportion of motoneurones were still healthy and able to form collateral axonal sprouts. Limited axonal branching may also be inferred from the multielectrode studies of Stålberg (1977) and Stålberg, Trontelj and Janko (1972) which have revealed an increased density of muscle fibres within some of the motor unit territories. The prolonged and complex muscle action potentials noted by Desmedt and Borenstein (1973) may also be explained in terms of collateral sprouting.

The motor unit counting technique has also shown that there is a neural component in certain other disorders, usually regarded as being of primary myopathic origin. These conditions are listed in Table 28.1 and have been ranked in order of the severity and incidence of the functional denervation. For example, whereas a loss of motor units may be encountered in almost any patient with myotonic dystrophy or severe thyrotoxicosis, it has only been demonstrated in about half of patients with myasthenia gravis, McArdle's syndrome and myotonia congenita.

In this part of the chapter care has been taken to talk about the presence or absence of a neural component in the 'primary myopathies' and, indeed, this is all that may safely be deduced from the results of the motor unit counting technique. In theory, however, the involvement of the nervous system in the primary myopathies is open to four interpretations which, in the case of the hereditary disorders, are as follows:

(1) The motoneurones, muscle fibres and possibly other cells may be fundamentally abnormal due to the action of a single defective gene ('pleiotropic' gene action). The degeneration in each type of tissue would proceed independently.

TABLE 28.1

'Muscle Disorders' Found to Have a Loss of Functioning Motor Units, together with the Incidence of this Abnormality

Condition	Incidence
Ageing	All subjects
Upper motoneurone disorders	
Thyrotoxicosis	
Malignant hyperthermia	
Polymyositis and dermatomyositis	
Muscular dystrophy:	Most (60–90%)
Myotonic	
Limb-girdle	
Facioscapulohumeral	
Duchenne	
Myasthenia gravis	
McArdle's disease	
Myotonia congenita	About half
Scleroderma	

(2) Irrespective of possible lesions elsewhere, the muscle degeneration is primary and any motoneurone changes are secondary, being caused by a loss of trophic influence from the periphery (see Chapter 10). This is the traditional concept of these disorders.

(3) Irrespective of possible lesions elsewhere, the motoneurone changes are the primary event with the muscle fibre degeneration resulting from a loss of the peripherally-directed trophic influence; this is the sick motoneurone hypothesis described in Chapter 13.

(4) The primary action of the abnormal gene is upon a third tissue, other than nerve and muscle, with the neuromuscular system being involved secondarily. The vascular hypothesis of muscular dystrophy (Appendix 16.2) falls within this category as would any hypothesis involving a deficiency factor or a circulating toxic agent.

In the case of myotonic muscular dystrophy it has long been known that tissues other than nerve and muscle are defective as revealed by the occurrence of cataracts, gonadal atrophy, frontal baldness and thickening of the skull. The recent description of biochemical and morphological abnormalities in the red cells in this type of dystrophy and in the Duchenne, limb-girdle and facioscapulohumeral forms would provide further evidence of a pleiotrophic gene defect. This does not resolve the question, however, as to whether the muscle and neural degenerations are both primary events and largely independent of each other (hypotheses 1 and 2). The fact that, in the various myopathies, the losses of muscle fibres follow a motor unit pattern and that in some muscles grouped muscle fibre atrophy may be evident, strongly suggests that at least some of the changes in the muscles are of neural origin. Similarly the presence of enlarged motor units in the limb-girdle and facioscapulohumeral dystrophies, for example, indicates that muscle fibres may fare much better if they can lose their original innervation and be adopted by 'better' motoneurones. This observation also suggests that some of the muscle changes are neurally induced.

To argue beyond this point in man is unrewarding since, both for ethical or practical reasons, the type of evidence which is necessary for a conclusive answer is unobtainable. This impasse may be circumvented by turning to animal models of muscle disease. While keeping in mind the possibility that these models may not mimic the human disease in their pathogenesis, there is a danger in becoming overcautious to the point of inaction. For example, were it to be shown that in each type of animal dystrophy the pathogenesis was the same, it would be unlikely that the origins of the human forms would be any different. Apart from allowing the mechanism of the disease to be analysed completely the animal models also deserve study in that they provide a testing ground for experimental treatments.

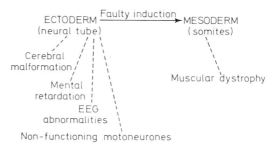

Figure 28.5. Revised concept of the pathogenesis of muscular dystrophy (see text)

At the present time the animal models have convincingly reinforced the concept of abnormal motoneurones in dystrophy. In the mouse it has been shown that there is defective myelination, abnormal axoplasmic flow, slowed impulse conduction, and ultrastructural changes in the nerve terminal (see Chapter 16). The presence of these striking abnormalities raises obvious doubts as to whether the motoneurones would be able to supply an adequate trophic influence to the muscle fibres. Surprisingly, however, it appears that they are able to do so, as shown by the parabiotic cross innervation experiments described on page 173. These clear-cut results, now reported by three different teams of investigators, certainly appear to disprove the sick motoneurone hypothesis in its original form, in so far as it applied to the animal dystrophies. Yet how can the findings be reconciled with some of the muscle transplant results, as well as with the spinal cord transplant experiment of Rathbone and his colleagues and the mouse chimera study of Peterson (see pages 174–178)? At present the only visible solution to this problem is to invoke the concept of an abnormal inductive influence of the neural tube on the muscle-forming mesoderm at an early stage in the development of the embryo. Because of an inherent ectodermal defect the development of the neural tube might also proceed abnormally, giving rise to such phenomena as cerebral malformation, mental retardation and EEG dysrhythmias, together with malfunctioning motoneurones (*Figure 28.5*). Although these abnormalities may be seen in Duchenne dystrophy, the most florid examples of central nervous system involvement occur in a congenital form of muscular dystrophy recently reported from Japan (Segawa *et al*, 1970; Kamoshita *et al*, 1976).

So far as the muscle is concerned, once the dystrophic imprint has been made by faulty induction, it appears resistant to later modification by any alteration of its innervation. Conversely, it is difficult to make normal muscle dystrophic by manipulating the nerve supply unless (perhaps) the muscle can be made to 'regress' by preliminary mincing. The final answer to the vexed problem of the pathogenesis of dystrophy may thus come to lie somewhere between the myopathic and neural hypotheses. This concern with pathogenesis is, of course, not a reason for neglecting to study the course of the disease within the muscle fibre and it will still be necessary to establish whether the muscle fibres degenerate because of leaky membranes, ruptured myofilaments or for some other reason (see page 148). As regards a cure, it may still be possible to bypass the nervous system and to treat the muscle fibres directly.

In conclusion it may seem that, in the light of the present controversy surrounding the motor unit counting technique, it is unwise to hang so much speculative material on its results. Yet in assessing the balance between fact and speculation, it can be seen that several of the conclusions drawn from the motor unit counting results have since been verified by other approaches. For example the significance of 60 as the age at which loss of functioning motor units commences in man is now supported by the multielectrode studies of Stålberg. In healthy subjects this author has found electrophysiological evidence of collateral reinnervation in the seventh decade but not before (Stålberg, 1974). Regarding the possibility of transsynaptic degeneration of motoneurones, not only has this phenomenon been demonstrated at autopsy by Reske-Nielsen, Harmsen and Ovesen (1971) but these authors, like ourselves, have identified a 2-month period following the upper motoneurone lesion before the denervation changes are apparent in the muscle. In the myotonic form of muscular dystrophy the losses of motor units have been confirmed by other electrophysiological studies (see Chapter 16). A recent autopsy study has shown a loss of motoneurones in a patient diagnosed during life as having limb-girdle dystrophy (Tomlinson, Walton and Irving, 1974). Denervation, sufficient to cause grouped muscle fibre atrophy and therefore presumably of central origin, is now recognized as occurring in a proportion of patients with myasthenia gravis (page 198) and with malignant hyperpyrexia (LaCour, Juul-Jensen and Reske-Nielsen, 1973). In relation to thyrotoxicosis, patients occasionally develop a severe neuropathy with evidence of denervation being found by muscle histology and conventional electromyography (Feibel and Campa, 1976). Clearly the possibility exists that a milder neuropathy may occur more commonly, being detected only by a sensitive technique such as motor unit counting. It is in Duchenne dystrophy that the findings of losses of motor units are most seriously at variance with other published results. Even here, however, recent findings compatible with neural involvement have come from single fibre electromyography. Thus Stålberg (1977) has observed some motor units with abnormal clustering of fibres, as might have occurred after collateral reinnervation, while a small fraction of motor axons have impaired impulse transmission.

Irrespective of its final status, the neural hypothesis has played some part in bringing new life to the long-established area of neuromuscular diseases. Some of the experimental methods used to test the hypothesis have been of extreme elegance (pages 173–178) and will doubtless find other uses. There is now an awareness that tissues other than muscle may be abnormal in the so-called primary myopathies. Finally, and rather ironically, the examination of the nervous system in murine dystrophy has led to the discovery of the most satisfactory model presently available for studying the effect of defective myelination on impulse conduction. If, in addition to these contributions, the hypothesis has helped to bring a rational therapy for any of the presently untreatable neuromuscular disorders a little nearer, so much the better.

APPENDICES

APPENDIX 3.1—INTRACELLULAR RECORDING IN MAN

As stated in Chapter 3, it is possible to measure the potentials across the membrane of a muscle fibre directly by using the intracellular recording technique. This technique involves the insertion of a very fine electrode (*microelectrode*) through the cell membrane; a larger electrode is placed in the fluid bathing the muscle, or in some other extracellular location, and is used as a reference. The microelectrode is made from a length of glass capillary tubing which is heated in its central region and then rapidly drawn out so as to form two electrodes with tapering ends. With automatic electrode-pulling machines it is possible to manufacture electrodes with reasonably consistent dimensions; for muscle fibre studies the tips of the microelectrodes should have external diameters of 1 μm or less. After the glass tubing has been drawn it is filled with a concentrated salt solution so as to enable it to conduct electricity; the solution of choice for recording is 3 M potassium chloride; because potassium and chloride have similar ionic mobilities there is less tendency for anomalous potentials to form at the electrode tips due to unequal diffusion of ions. The most suitable electrodes for recording from human muscle fibres have d.c. resistances in the 8–15 MΩ range; the anomalous 'tip' potentials should not be more than 5 μV. For intracellular stimulation, rather larger electrodes may be required since otherwise the electrode will change during the passage of current; potassium citrate is commonly used as the filling solution.

Types of preparation

Three different methods have been employed for intracellular recording from human muscle fibres.

In vitro method (*Figure A3.1, a*)

In this method a piece of muscle is removed, mounted in a bath and covered with a physiological solution. In practice, the only fibres which are readily accessible and sufficiently small to be excised intact are those of the external intercostal muscles (Dillon *et al.*, 1955). This limitation would be a serious drawback in the study of any patient in whom the neuromuscular disorder was not generalized; in practice, it has given results of great interest and theoretical value in myotonia (page 127), myasthenia gravis (page 198) and the Eaton-Lambert syndrome (page 211). The advantages of the method are considerable. It offers great mechanical stability of the preparation and recording electrode so that prolonged investigation of single fibres is practicable. The floor of the muscle chamber can be transilluminated allowing the outlines of the fibres to be distinguished and also the small intramuscular nerve bundles. In addition the bathing solution can be rapidly changed, thereby enabling the effects of altered ionic composition to be observed on the membrane parameters.

In situ cannula method (*Figure A3.1, b*)

This technique was devised independently by Beránek (1964) and by Riecker *et al.* (1964). A stainless steel hypodermic cannula is inserted through the skin and into the muscle belly. The tip of a microelectrode is then driven gently out of the cannula so as to penetrate the neighbouring muscle fibres. The disadvantage of the method is that the cannula inevitably damages the fibres at, and just beyond, its end; these fibres will therefore have falsely low resting potentials. Although deeper

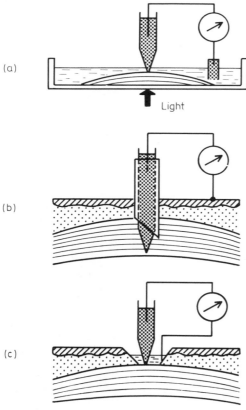

(a)
Light

(b)

(c)

Figure A3.1. The three methods used for penetrating human muscle fibres with micro-electrodes: (a) in vitro; (b) in situ cannula; (c) in situ open. (See text)

fibres can be sampled, the 'tip' potential (see above) then becomes larger and causes artefactual problems. If major changes in membrane potential are a feature of the disease process under study, the method is useful; also, by stimulating through a Wheatstone bridge circuit the same microelectrode can be used to check whether or not the fibres are directly excitable. One of the best applications of this technique has been to follow the changes in membrane potential and excitability during an attack of familial periodic paralysis (see Brooks, 1969; also page 136).

In situ open method (*Figure A3.1, c*)

If muscle is to be removed for histological or other examination, it is justifiable to make microelectrode recordings beforehand. Once the surface of the muscle belly has been exposed, the edges of the skin incision are retracted so as to form retaining walls for the physiological bathing solution. The superficial fibres can then be sampled with a microelectrode but must, of course, be rejected for morphological studies. The problems with this method are its inconvenience and the mechanical instability introduced by vascular, respiratory and other movements of the tissue. If it is important to study limb muscle in its normal milieu, however, measurements may be made more reliably with this method than with the cannula technique.

Measuring techniques (*Figure A3.2*)

The intra- and extra-cellular recording electrodes are connected to the terminals of a d.c. amplifier; because of the high resistance of the electrodes it may be necessary to insert an impedance matching device (input coupler) earlier in the circuit. The measuring device may be an oscilloscope, voltmeter or a pen recorder. The latter has the advantage of economy and it provides a permanent record of resting potentials; conversely the rapid response of the oscilloscope allows potential transients to be recorded more accurately. The advantage of a digital voltmeter is that the observer bias on visual measurements is eliminated. Returning to the input circuit, *Figure 3A.2* shows how junction potentials can be largely avoided by using non-polarizable electrodes of silver chloride mounted in an agar gel containing mammalian bathing fluid.

APPENDIX 3.2

Kao (1966) has given a fascinating and full account of tetrodotoxin (TTX) poisoning. It appears that one of the earliest references appeared in the first Chinese pharmacopea, *Pen-T'so Chin* (The Book of Herbs), which was written during his life of the Emperor Shun Nung (2838–2698 B.C.). The Chinese still refer to the tetrodon fish as Ho-Tun (piglet of the river) but, in view of the ability of the fish to inflate itself, it is more popularly known as the 'puffer' or 'blow' fish. The first Europeans to visit China and Japan were warned of the dangers of eating the fish. This did not deter the famous eighteenth-century navigator and explorer, Captain Cook, who believed that he had eaten the same species of fish previously without ill effect.

After the second occasion Cook was able to give the following account of his experience (Cook, 1777):

Having no suspicion of its being of a poisonous nature [referring to the fish] we ordered it to be dressed for supper; but very luckily, the operation of drawing and describing took up so much time that it was too late, so that only the liver and roe were dressed, of which the two Mr Forsters and myself did but taste. About three o'clock in the morning, we found ourselves seized with an extraordinary weakness and numbness all over our limbs. I had almost lost the sense of feeling, nor could I distinguish between light and heavy bodies of such as I had the strength to move, a quart pot, full of water, and a feather being the same in my hand.

APPENDIX 3.3—THE MEASUREMENT OF IMPULSE VELOCITY IN THE SLOWEST CONDUCTING MOTOR AXONS

Two methods are available for estimating the impulse conduction velocities in the slowest-conducting α-motor axons.

(1) In the method of *Thomas, Sears and Gilliatt 1959*) a stimulus, S_1, is delivered to the nerve at a site close to the muscle while a second stimulus, S_2, is applied more distantly; the corresponding responses evoked in the muscle are R_1 and R_2 respectively (see a and b in *Figure A3.3*). If both stimuli are made supramaximal and S_1 is given a few milliseconds before S_2, the response R_2 disappears. The explanation for this is that the impulses initiated in motor axons by S_1 will travel along the nerve in opposite directions. The impulses proceeding antidromically (towards the elbow in *Figure A3.3*) will collide with those passing towards the muscle from the stimulus S_2; the two volleys of impulses then undergo mutual extinction. If the intensity of S_1 is now diminished so as to become slightly submaximal, a small R_2 can be detected. This response will have been mediated by the axons with the highest thresholds to electrical stimulation at S_2 and, by analogy with the results of animal experiments, are presumed to be the slowest conducting. If S_1 is now reduced further R_2 grows progressively larger (c in *Figure A.3.3*) since there are fewer impulses travelling antidromically to cause collisions. The *difference* in the latencies of the maximum and minimum R_2 responses (t') is measured, using high amplification (*Figure A3.3, d*). This value can then be expressed as a percentage of the latency (t) of the maximal R_2 response, the latter reflecting activity mediated by the fastest-conducting fibres. The disadvantages of the method are that: (a) it does not measure the absolute conduction velocity of the slowest-conducting fibres but only their impulse conduction time relative to that of the fastest-conducting fibres; (b) the thresholds of the fibres are governed by their positions within the nerve trunk as well as by the biophysical properties of the fibres themselves; (c) an undamaged region of fibre may have a low threshold at the point of stimulation but, because of localized demyelination distally, the fibre may have a slow impulse conduction velocity. Such fibres would be missed by the technique.

(2) The method of *Hopf (1962, 1963)* also employs two stimuli but depends on the minimum time required to prevent impulse collision. As

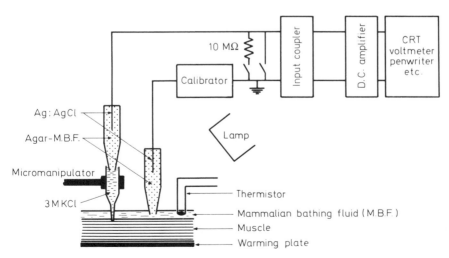

Figure A3.2. The complete system for measuring membrane potentials (shown with in vitro method). (See text)

306

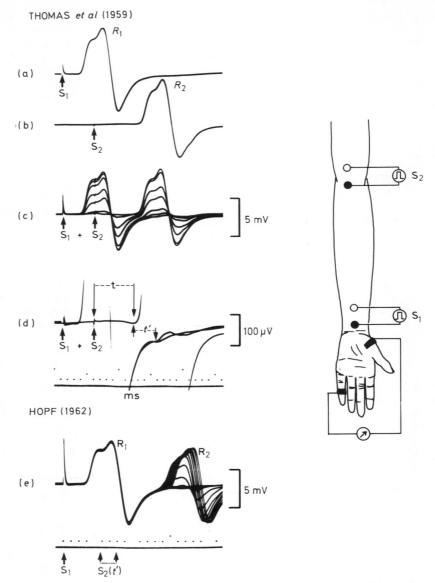

THOMAS *et al* (1959)

R_1

(a)

S_1

(b)

S_2

R_2

(c)

S_1 + S_2

5 mV

(d)

S_1 + S_2

100 µV

ms

HOPF (1962)

R_1

R_2

(e)

5 mV

S_1 $S_2(t')$

S_2

S_1

Figure A3.3. Two techniques for estimating impulse conduction velocities in the slowest-conducting motor axons of the median nerve. The positions of the stimulating and recording electrodes are shown at right, the cathodal stimulating electrodes being black. (a) shows the thenar muscle response R_1 following maximal stimulating of the nerve at the wrist (S_1). (b) shows the response R_2 maximal stimulation at the elbow (S_2). In (c), the intensity of S_2 is kept maximal and that of S_1 is gradually increased. Due to impulse collision the response R_2 becomes progressively smaller and finally disappears, as shown on the superimposed traces. (d) shows two superimposed traces; first, when S_1 is zero and the full R_2 response is recorded; second, when S_1 is almost maximal and only a small R_2 is left; t' is the time elapsing between onsets (arrowed) of the two R_2 responses while t is the time between S_2 and the maximal R_2, S_1 being omitted. In (e) is shown method of Hopf (1962, 1963) in which S_1 and S_2 are kept supramaximal and the interval between them is gradually increased. The smallest R_2 response occurs when the antidromic impulses in the fastest conducting fibres have passed the stimulating electrodes at the elbow and the fibres have recovered from their absolutely refractory periods. When R_2 is maximal, all the motor axons, including the slowest conducting ones, will have recovered following the passage of the impulses past the elbow. t' is the additional time between S_1 and S_2 which is required for the R_2 response to grow from its minimal to its maximal size: it is shown on the superimposed traces. See text for the calculation of velocities in the 'slow' fibres

before stimuli (S_1 and S_2) are applied at two points with S_1 preceding S_2; both stimuli are made supra-maximal. At first S_2 elicits no response from the muscle because of impulse collision with the volley initiated by S_1. S_2 is then progressively delayed in relation to S_1 until a small muscle response is seen (R_2). This response will have been elicited by the fastest-conducting motor axons; they will have had time to recover from the passage of the antidromic action potential from S_1 and can be excited by S_2. Next S_2 is delayed further until R_2 becomes maximal. The extra period of stimulus delay for R_2 to grow from its smallest to its largest values is then measured (t', in *Figure A3.3, e*). If t is the latency of the maximal R_2 muscle response (reflecting activity mediated by the fastest-conducting fibres) then the ratio of the conduction velocity of the fastest conducting fibres V_f) to that of the slowest conducting fibres (V_s) will be

$$t + t' : t$$

V_f can be measured in the conventional way (see page 26 and *Figure 3.9*) and hence

$$V_s = V_f \times \frac{t}{t + t'}$$

The disadvantage of the method is that it is often difficult to determine whether R_2 has become maximal as t' is increased. Also, a small error will be introduced into the measurement of V_s on account of the slowest-conducting fibres having rather longer refractory periods than the fastest-conducting fibres.

APPENDIX 6.1—THE MOTOR UNIT COUNTING TECHNIQUE: ATTACK AND DEFENCE

After the electrophysiological technique for counting motor units was first reported it attracted many criticisms, most of which had been anticipated in the initial paper (McComas *et al.,* 1971a). Since the results obtained with this method provided the basis of the neural hypothesis (McComas, Sica and Campbell, 1971) and, in an updated form, have now been given in this book, it is appropriate that the criticisms should be examined once again.

Unreliability of the extensor digitorum brevis (EDB) muscle

Although the EDB muscle had previously been much used in clinical electromyography, the largely unexpected motor unit results obtained by the McComas method led to a histological examination of this muscle. Jennekens, Tomlinson and Walton (1972) found evidence of grouped muscle fibre atrophy, even in young adults who had suffered accidental death. In an EMG study with coaxial electrodes Rosselle and Stevens (1973) reported that 87 per cent of healthy young subjects had evidence of denervation and that 29 per cent had abnormal spontaneous activity (fibrillations and/or positive sharp waves). If, in normal subjects, the EDB muscle was so susceptible to denervation, presumably through accidental trauma to the peroneal nerve, one might reasonably expect that this tendency would be increased in patients disabled by neuromuscular disease.

Rebuttal

(1) The EMG findings of Rosselle and Stevens (1973) are contrary to the experience of other electromyographers (see Ballantyne and Hansen, 1974a). Campbell, McComas and Petito (1973) studied EDB muscles of normal subjects and did not find fibrillations in any, though it is certainly true that the volitional interference pattern is not as full in this muscle as in other intrinsic muscles of the hand and foot.

(2) In their 1971b paper McComas and colleagues acknowledged that some denervation might occur in the normal EDB but pointed out that it was not sufficient to cause a detectable decline in motor unit population before the age of 60. A similar conclusion has been reached by Ballantyne and Hansen (1974a).

(3) McComas, Sica and Currie (1971) found that a loss of functioning motor units could be demonstrated in some patients with an early stage of muscular dystrophy, even though these patients were not disabled and therefore particularly prone to inadvertent nerve trauma.

(4) McComas, Sica and Upton (1974) were able to show that losses of functioning motor units could be demonstrated in muscles other than EDB, such as the thenar and hypothenar groups and soleus.

(5) In relation to these last results, the same authors were unable to demonstrate any evidence of localized nerve trauma since sensory nerve function was normal.

Motor axon branching

Bradley (1974) has suggested that axon-branching may be present at the sites of stimulation and that, in effect, parts of motor units, rather than total motor units, may be responsible for the response increments.

Rebuttal

(1) On the basis of the study by Eccles and Sherrington (1930) it is unlikely that more than a small fraction of motor axons divide 6–8 cm from the points of entry of the nerves into the respective muscle bellies, this being the approximate distance from the stimulating cathode to the EDB muscle.

(2) Even if branching was present, the whole motor unit would probably fire, since the impulse travelling antidromically in one branch should activate the other branch(es) at the point of bifurcation. Further, as the stimulus intensity was raised and other branches were excited directly, the late components in the response should disappear, but in practice this is not observed.

(3) There is no *a priori* reason why motor axons in patients with 'primary myopathies' would show more extramuscular branching than in controls. However, a branching effect may be responsible for the misleadingly high motor unit counts found by Peyronnard (1975) *following partial denervation* in the EDB muscles of monkeys. In discussion Peyronnard has suggested that intermittent failure of impulse conduction occurs at newly-formed branching points in nerve fibres undertaking collateral reinnervation. The impulse blocking would cause the evoked muscle responses to fluctuate, the variations being indistinguishable from those caused by alterations in the numbers of functioning (whole) motor units. If the results are applicable to man, the blocking effect could mean that partial denervation might be missed at an early stage of a disease process or at a certain time after nerve injury, but it would not detract from the significance of the results in those patients who *did have* low estimates of functioning units. It should also be stated that the branching anomaly did not appear in a number of patients studied by the McComas group in whom the time course of the denervating process was carefully documented. Thus it was possible to observe a severe loss of functioning units with little change for many weeks afterwards, even though the increasingly large evoked muscle response indicated that collateral reinnervation was taking place (see *Figure 25.4, upper,* for example).

Unrepresentative sampling

Small motor units not detected

Panayiotopoulos, Scarpalezos and Papapetropoulos (1974) have claimed that very small motor units

would not have been detected by the method of McComas *et al.* (1971a) and that this could account for the apparent loss of motor units in Duchenne dystrophy.

Rebuttal (1) If many very small units were present in dystrophy, it would still be necessary to explain why the surviving, detectable, units have normal sizes, since the non-random involvement of the motor units would not be in keeping with a myopathy (see page 113).

(2) The claim of Panayiotopoulos and Scarpalezos to have observed very small unit potentials using a new technique is unacceptable. They claim that by comparing single oscilloscope traces taken at two different stimulus intensities, they can recognize potentials smaller than 3 μV (Scarpalezos and Panayiotoupolos, 1973) or 4 μV (Panayiotopoulos, Scarpalezos and Papapetropoulos, 1974). However, inspection of their records (Figure 1 of Panayiotopoulos and colleagues, 1974) reveals a 'noise' level as high as 8 μV in some traces and it is therefore a logical impossibility for these authors to be able to detect evoked responses smaller than this without recourse to a signal enhancement procedure. *Figure A6.1* illustrates the problems in interpretation which arise if only single traces are viewed and the improved resolution which is obtainable by a superimposition technique.

(3) Panayiotoupolos, Scarpalezos and Papapetropoulos (1974) have obtained a mean number of motor units in EDB muscles of controls which is almost double that of Ballantyne and Hansen (1974a); these last workers also claim to have devised an improved counting method (see below). Obviously both groups cannot be correct in their methodology.

Large motor units not detected

Feasby and Brown (1974) state that the motor units which participate in the F-wave response generate larger potentials than those units sampled by the incremental stimulation technique and that the samples are therefore unrepresentative.

Rebuttal (1) Assuming that the F-wave responses of Brown and Feasby are indeed those of single motor units, it is quite possible that the corresponding motoneurones are activated because of some special biophysical feature of the axon-soma complex. Since the incremental stimulating technique of McComas *et al.* (1971a) excites axons which have low thresholds mainly because of their positions in the nerve trunk, the resulting samples are probably not seriously biased in favour of unduly large (or small) motor units. As might be expected from animal studies of motor unit populations, the samples do occasionally include motor units with large potentials as the histogram in *Figure 6.5* illustrates. Such occurrences have been responsible for some of the lower values in the normal distribution of motor unit numbers; nevertheless, the finding of even smaller values in patients would still be indicative of abnormality.

'Dangers' of amplitude measurements

Ballantyne and Hansen (1974a) have pointed out that if the motor unit potentials in each sample are unusually brief and are discharged earlier or later than the potentials of the remainder of the motor unit population, the estimate of their number will be misleadingly high. If, however, the potentials are compared on the basis of area (i.e. voltage × time) rather than amplitude (i.e. voltage), a more accurate estimate will be obtained. They then describe a computer-based method for area comparisons; the area of each new increment is determined by subtracting the preceding (averaged) evoked response from the new one.

Rebuttal (1) In an extensive experience with motor unit counting, McComas and colleagues have always found it possible to obtain samples of motor unit potentials which, in their summated form, closely resemble the maximum evoked responses in terms of duration and configuration. This similarity has been as true for complex potentials, such as those of soleus (*Figure A6.1*), as for the simple diphasic ones of EDB and the thenar group (*Figure 16.7*). Certainly nothing has been seen approaching the hypothetical responses of Ballantyne and Hansen (see their *Figure 6, lower section*).

(2) If area measurements are performed on some of our dystrophic material, reduced estimates are still found. For example, in patient X.N. (*Figure 16.7*) the estimates for the soleus muscle, when based on comparisons of amplitude and area, were 120 and 152 units respectively; both values are well below the lower limit of the normal range (542 units).

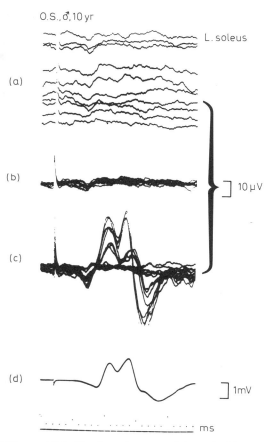

O.S., ♂, 10 yr

L. soleus

(a)

(b)] 10 μV

(c)

(d)] 1mV

ms

Figure A6.1. Muscle action potentials evoked in the soleus muscle of a 10-year-old boy with Duchenne dystrophy. In (a) the individual traces suggest the presence of a response to weak stimulation of the posterior tibial nerve but there are random deflections of similar amplitude elsewhere in the record (i.e. 'noise'). If the traces are superimposed, however, a 4 μV evoked response can be clearly differentiated from the background noise (b). In (c) slightly stronger shocks are used and a total of seven increments are seen in the 80 μV response. In (d) maximum stimulation yields a response of 2.7 mV for an estimated 236 units. An estimate based on 11 increments gave a value of 220 units (lower limit of normal, 542 units). (From McComas (1975) courtesy of Dr W. G. Bradley and Excerpta Medica)

Conflict with conventional electromyography

Engel and Warmolts (1973) have remarked that in the so-called myopathies the interference pattern recorded with a coaxial needle electrode during maximal effort appears full and that it is therefore difficult to reconcile this with the loss of functioning units found by the incremental counting technique of McComas et al. (1971a).

Rebuttal The density of the interference pattern is an insensitive technique for detecting denervation. In patients with truly neuropathic lesions McComas *et al.* (1971a) found that a muscle may be 70 per cent denervated, as estimated by the incremental technique, and yet appear to have a full interference pattern (see also *Figure 6.1, e*).

Validation of the motor unit counting method

In man

It is difficult to compare the electrophysiologically-derived estimates of motor unit numbers with the results of axon counts in man since in the latter type of study there are several uncertainties in deciding how large a fraction of the axons are alpha-motor. Nevertheless in two specimens of peroneal nerve McComas *et al.* (1971a) found that the values from anatomical studies were within the upper part of the electrophysiologically-determined range. Another test of the technique in man has been to apply it to the detection of patients with the 'rigid' malignant hyperthermia trait. The advantage of studying this disorder is that, in most cases, it is impossible to judge whether or not a subject is likely to be affected on the basis of physical appearance. In a 'blind' study of 32 suspects, with B. A. Britt and W. Kalow, the motor unit results were compared with those of *in vitro* tests for muscle contracture thresholds (see page 185). Assuming that the latter test was completely reliable, the motor unit counting technique was correct on 28 occasions. This correlation was unlikely to have arisen by chance (p = 0.001).

In animals

(1) In the rat soleus muscle Eisen *et al.* (1974) found that there was good agreement between electrophysiological and anatomical estimates of motor unit populations in (*a*) normal animals, (*b*) animals with an induced ischaemic myopathy, and (*c*) animals with chronic denervation. In (*a*) and (*b*) the motor unit counts were normal but in (*c*) it was reduced.

(2) In *normal* monkeys subjected to dorsal rhizotomy Peyronnard (1975) has found good agreement between anatomical and electrophysiological estimates of the EDB motor unit populations, the latter estimate being about 10 per cent lower than the former.

Mitigating factors

In considering possible causes of the discrepancies between the findings of the McComas team and of the other groups, certain additional factors should be taken into account.

(1) McComas and colleagues never stated that a loss of functioning motor units was an invariable finding in muscular dystrophy or myasthenia gravis. Some patients *do* have normal values and in their 1974b paper the McComas group argued that in most of these instances it was probable that the muscles were not significantly affected by the disease process. Their evidence was that the maximum evoked electrical and mechanical responses were within the normal ranges.

(2) In *myasthenia gravis* the McComas group have now studied 20 patients and found losses of motor units in half (see page 201). However, their patients were more severely affected than those studied by Ballantyne and Hansen (1974a, b) for the latter patients were all ambulant and none were severely disabled. In contrast two of the patients investigated by the McComas group died from their myasthenia within 6 months of examination and a third required a permanent tracheostomy.

(3) The demonstration of chronic muscle denervation is essential for a diagnosis of spinal muscular atrophy to be made and in this context the motor unit counting technique has proved itself a sensitive diagnostic technique. The problem arises as to whether, *on the basis of other criteria*, these patients might be judged to have *limb-girdle or facioscapulohumeral dystrophy* instead. The distinction between these types of dystrophy, on the one hand, and spinal muscular atrophy, on the other, may be impossible on the basis of clinical features, serum CPK level and muscle biopsy. So far as electromyography is concerned, Ballantyne and Hansen (1974a) imply that such a distinction can readily be made but the experience of the McComas group is that, with exhaustive sampling of muscles, it is difficult to do so with any confidence in most patients (see page 161 and *Figure 16.14*). It therefore seems probable that the discrepancy between the reported findings in limb-girdle and facioscapulohumeral dystrophies may well reflect differences in diagnosis rather than in methodology. One must nevertheless accept that among the patients who satisfy all diagnostic criteria for these dystrophies, there is a group who have normal motor unit counts (McComas *et al.*, 1974b).

(4) *For Duchenne dystrophy* no mitigating factors appear to exist. Against the negative findings of Panayiotopoulos and colleagues (1974) and of Ballantyne and Hansen (1974c) must be set the positive findings, not only of McComas, Sica and Currie (1971) but of their subsequent co-workers (Drs Brandstater, Law, Petito and Upton; data pooled in *Figure 16.6*).

Which technique is best?

The method of Panayiotopoulos *et al.* (1974) is unacceptable because of the impossibility of recognizing, on single oscilloscope sweeps, evoked responses smaller than the noise level of the recording system. The Ballantyne and Hansen (1974a) method is theoretically superior to the original technique of McComas *et al.* (1971a) but in practice its advantages are largely illusory. As stated above, temporal factors in sampling are not a problem and the new method does not solve the two greatest practical difficulties with the counting techniques. One of these is in deciding whether or not a change in evoked response has occurred and the other is in separating the thresholds of the motor axons to electrical stimulation. In relation to the first matter, both methods depend on visual inspection of the oscilloscope trace for any reproducible changes in the amplitude or configuration of the evoked responses. In relation to the second point, the similar thresholds of axons give rise to the phenomenon of 'alternation' such that, at a certain constant stimulus intensity, the response fluctuates because different combinations of units have been excited (McComas *et al.*, 1971a). Since each fluctuation may be misinterpreted as recruitment of a further motor unit rather than as a different combination of previously excited units, the estimated number of units may be falsely large. McComas and associates attempt to compensate for the effect of alternation by limiting the number of stimuli. Thus, when response fluctuation begins to appear the stimulus intensity is increased slightly as soon as a new increment has been 'confirmed' *once* by superimposition. Their experience of alternation is such that, unlike Ballantyne and Hansen, they would not have found it possible to average more than the first few increments evoked by repeated stimulation at given intensities.

Because of the vagaries of alternation and increment detection, the McComas group believe that any theoretical advantages in measuring response areas, rather than amplitudes, are of minor consequence. The great practical advantage of amplitude measurements is that they can be made quickly from the storage oscilloscope screen without the need to employ a computer.

Notwithstanding the present arguments over methodology, it is hoped that other workers will not be discouraged from trying out a new technique which, in the hands of several groups of investigators, has now been shown to have considerable value in the diagnosis of recognized denervating disorders.

APPENDIX 14.1—THE DISCOVERY OF THE MYOTONIC GOAT

The introduction of the myotonic goat into medical science is too interesting a story for it not to be included in a book on neuromuscular disorders. The following account of these fascinating animals was given by Clark, Luton and Cutler (1939).

In middle Tennessee and portions of adjacent states there occurs a variety of goat which has the same general appearance as the ordinary type of goat, but which is endowed with a peculiarity of behavior that causes it to be called 'nervous'. When one of these animals is suddenly frightened, excited, or faced with some emergency which requires action, instead of being able to run or jump, it becomes rigid in a part or all of the voluntary musculature and for a short time cannot move. If one of them attempts to run and becomes rigid, it falls over and lies with legs outstretched and stiff.

During such a spasm the goat has the general appearance of an animal in decerebrate rigidity, with legs rigid in extension, and with the tonic contraction of the muscles of the neck and trunk holding the animal in the position of opisthotonos. The eyes are open widely, and the eye-balls are fixed in position with the gaze directed forward and slightly downward. As a rule the legs are not only extended but also are in slight abduction, though one goat was observed whose legs during the rigidity were in such a degree of adduction that its feet were crossed. All the muscles seem equally firm on palpation, so the position of the legs appears to be determined by the resultant of the forces of contraction of the various muscle groups. There are no fibrillary twitchings or choreiform movements.

Such attacks last from a few seconds to more than a minute, during which time the goat may be pushed over or handled as if it were a wooden image. The muscles gradually relax and voluntary movement returns, though the residual stiffness causes difficulty in walking for a few steps. After such an attack, the animal may be perfectly normal for a while, and cannot be thrown into another spasm until after a period of rest or relative inactivity.

There has been much speculation concerning the origin of these animals. One of the most knowledgeable authorities on this score is Dr Virgil LeQuire, Professor of Pathology at Vanderbilt University, Nashville, Tennessee. Dr LeQuire was once kind enough to show the author the flock of myotonic goats which he keeps on his beautiful farm. He has also given permission for the following letter to be reproduced; It was sent to a Mr R. J. Goode of Glastonburg, Alabama by Dr H. H. Mayberry of Marshall County, Tennessee.

Dr. Mr Goode:
    I do not recall the exact date, but early in the 1880s, a stranger appeared one day at the home of my neighbour, Mr J. M. Porter. Besides the clothes on his back, the man's only possession was a sacred cow, three nanny goats and one billy. Mr Porter invited them all to stay and they all did.

During the months the man was there, the Porters never succeeded in finding out from whence the stranger had come. It was believed by some, however, that he had arrived, rather circuitously, from Nova Scotia. Many things about the man mystified the Porters but they were most impressed I think by the fact that his goats were subject to strange fits or fainting spells, the like of which had never been seen before in these parts.

The goats were indeed interesting, and one day after I had seen one of these incredible attacks for myself, I offered the man $36·00 for his goats. At that time, he refused to even consider selling them, but he did promise to let me know if he ever decided to part with them.

About a month later, accompanied as usual by his cow and his goats, he appeared at my home and said he would sell the goats. I paid him for them; and both he and their former owner settled down at my place, the stranger putting in his time working on the farm. Not once while he was there did the stranger ever eat at my table. He took all his meals in the barn where the sacred cow was kept.

At the end of about three weeks, the stranger and his sacred cow left, going over to Lick Creek, a little town in Maury County, Tennessee. There he promptly married an old lady by the name of Barnhill. On her farm that summer the stranger raised an excellent corn crop. But one night after the crop was in, without any warning to his wife, he left with the sacred cow and was never heard of again.

From the goats which I bought from this man I raised a number of other goats and sold them in different parts of Kentucky and Tennessee. These goats were, I am sure, the progenitors of all such goats in this section of the country, and from which you say it is quite possible that the entire breed originated from this source.

Sincerely yours,
Dr H. H. Mayberry

There are many interesting anecdotes concerning the goats. One of the most humorous belongs to Mr Goode, the recipient of Dr Mayberry's letter and himself a breeder of the animals; it is fitting that he should have the last word on the subject.

I've heard a story about a new hired man who, a few days before a barbecue, was given a scatter gun and told to go into the back pasture and kill one of the goats. He was advised that the goats were very shy and that he should be very careful not to apprise them of his presence until ready to shoot. After crawling up cautiously, he picked out a nice fat kid, took careful aim, and fired. Goats dropped in every direction, some thirty animals collapsing simultaneously. Aghast, and without waiting for the resurrection, he ran back to the house, 'I don't know how it happened,' he panted. 'I only fired once but I killed every damn one of them goats.'

APPENDIX 16.1—POLIOMYELITIS AND MUSCULAR DYSTROPHY

The conventional explanation for the association of poliomyelitis and muscular dystrophy in a patient would be coincidence but, rather surprisingly, there is at least a hint that the two disorders may be related. Dr Hira Branch, a specialist in physical medicine in Flint, Michigan, has drawn the author's attention to a series of nine children, eight of them boys, whom he had personally observed between 1948 and 1957. In each child there had been a typical poliomyelitis-like illness and, after recovery from the acute pyrexial episode, the weakness had slowly progressed over the next few years. In six children striking enlargement of the calf and thigh muscles had developed and all the children came to walk with a lordotic gait; in none was there a positive family history of Duchenne dystrophy. These nine cases of 'dystrophy' had been noted in a population of 893 cases of poliomyelitis observed during the same 10-year period. These values give an incidence of 1008 dystrophy patients per 100,000 poliomyelitis cases, which is at least 50 times greater than the incidence of Duchenne dystrophy in the general population.

Dr Branch speculated that in some patients without family histories of neuromuscular disorders an illness indistinguishable from Duchenne dystrophy had been caused by the poliomyelitis virus. However, it is difficult to explain the higher incidence of such illnesses in males unless the dystrophy-inducing effect of the poliovirus was somehow augmented by the presence of the Y-chromosome within the motoneurone soma. Since poliomyelitis has now disappeared as a major source of illness the answers to these speculations may never be forthcoming.

APPENDIX 16.2—THE VASCULAR HYPOTHESIS OF DUCHENNE DYSTROPHY

One of the many puzzling features of Duchenne muscular dystrophy is the distinctive pathology of the muscle lesions. In this type of dystrophy, more than any other, regions of muscle fibres can be seen undergoing frank necrosis; immediately adjacent fibres commonly exhibit similar changes. Rather than incriminate denervation as a cause for these lesions of muscle fibre groups, W. K. Engel and his associates suggested that a vascular mechanism was involved. Their evidence was based largely on the fact that lesions of similar appearance could be produced in animals by interfering with the blood supply in various ways. For example, aortic ligation followed by the injection of 20–80 μm dextran particles to produce embolization was effective, as was aortic ligation and treatment with vasoactive amines (Hathaway, Engel and Zellweger, 1970;

Mendell, Engel and Derrer, 1971). Although there was no evidence of increased serum levels of 5-hydroxytryptamine (5-HT) or noradrenaline in patients with Duchenne dystrophy, the same group of workers have found that there was a diminished uptake of 5-HT by the platelets (Murphy, Mendell and Engel, 1973). If uptake of 5-HT was blocked experimentally in rats by the administration of imipramine, the treated animals developed a myopathy which further resembled Duchenne dystrophy by involving proximal muscles most severely (Parker and Mendell, 1974). Parker and Mendell (1974) have now modified the vascular hypothesis by suggesting that the degeneration of the muscle fibres in Duchenne dystrophy is caused, not by occlusion of muscle arterioles and capillaries as previously supposed, but by the accumulation of monoamines in the fibres. The authors cite the finding of intrafibrillar fluorescence of the monoamine type by Wright, O'Neill and Olson (1973) as further evidence. The elimination of vascular occlusion as a necessary part of the hypothesis enables the modified version to be reconciled with the findings of normal muscle blood flow in dystrophy (Paulson, Engel and Gomez, 1974), and of a largely-normal microvasculature on electronmicroscopy (Jerusalem, Engel and Gomez, 1974a).

APPENDIX 16.3—THE MEMBRANE HYPOTHESIS OF MUSCULAR DYSTROPHY

The notion that dystrophy might result from a defect of the muscle fibre membrane is an appealing one. To begin with, there is good electrophysiological evidence of membrane abnormality from the finding of low resting membrane potentials in both human and animal types of dystrophy (see Chapter 16), while the phenomenon of 'peripheral' myotonia in dystrophy is clearly of membranous origin (Chapter 14). The 'leakiness' of dystrophic mouse fibres for the enzyme aldolase (Zierler, 1961) and the high levels of serum enzymes in some patients with dystrophy, particularly of the Duchenne type, also point to the existence of abnormal membranes. Recently, the hypothesis has gained further ground from the demonstration, in preparations of membranes, of altered phosphorylation of endogenous proteins by protein kinases. This abnormality was shown to be present not only in the muscle fibre membranes of patients with myotonic muscular dystrophy (Roses and Appel, 1974) but in their red cell membranes also (Roses and Appel,

1973). Other work from the same laboratory, using measurements of electron spin resonance, has shown that the erythrocyte membranes of patients with myotonic dystrophy appear less polar and more fluid (Butterfield et al., 1974). However, the most striking demonstration that something is indeed wrong with red cell membranes has come from photographs of these cells with the scanning electronmicroscope. After a washing in normal saline, the cells from patients with Duchenne, limb-girdle or facioscapulohumeral dystrophy differ from those of controls in that there is a large population with surface projections (echinocytes). An abnormally high incidence of deformed cells is also observed in carriers of Duchenne dystrophy (Matheson and Howland, 1974). It should be noted that, dramatic though these changes are, they are not unique to dystrophy for they are commonly associated with liver disease, splenectomy, uraemia and the haemoglobinopathies. Furthermore, extreme care must be taken in preparing the blood samples for study since the red cells of normal subjects will become deformed if fixation is delayed. (Miller et al., 1976). Danger also exists in extrapolating from red cell membranes to sarcolemma since an abnormality of lipid composition is demonstrable in the former (Kunze et al., 1973) but not in the latter (Peter et al., 1975). In spite of this cautionary note the possibility that generalized membrane abnormalities exist in dystrophy is an exciting one and it could conceivably explain the progressive ultrastructural changes in Duchenne dystrophy described by Cullen and Fulthorpe (1975). It will be recalled (page 148) that these workers found that segments of myofibrils became overcontracted, so that a tearing of the fibril took place elsewhere. Cullen and Fulthorpe have postulated that the overcontraction (actually a 'contracture', page 42) might occur if calcium ions are not pumped back efficiently by the sarcoplasmic reticulum. In keeping with this suggesion are the results of biochemical investigations of fragmented sarcoplasmic reticulum (Sugita et al., 1967; Peter and Worsford, 1969; Samaha and Gergely, 1969) and the finding of slowed isometric muscle twitches in Duchenne dystrophy (see, for example, McComas and Thomas, 1968b). It should be added that the localized contracture phenomenon may well be a feature of other types of dystrophy in addition to the Duchenne type. The possibility of a calcium disorder being present is strengthened by Cosmos's (1964) earlier finding of an abnormal distribution of this ion within dystrophic chick muscle fibres. Mokri and Engel (1975) suggest that calcium might also accumulate by passing from extracellular fluid into regions of fibres where the sarcolemma is no longer intact.

APPENDIX 16.4—'ANTICIPATION' IN MYOTONIC DYSTROPHY

When members of a family with myotonic dystrophy are examined it often appears that the manifestations of the disease are more severe in successive generations. In the first generation there may be no more than early cataracts; in the second, muscle weakness may present in middle age, while in the third there may be the triad of muscle weakness, stiffness and mental deficiency in childhood. This apparent progression has been termed 'anticipation'. A memorable but tragic example of the social degradation which affected families suffer has been given by Caughey and Myrianthopoulos (1963); it involves a European monarchy and reflects interesting detective work on the part of the authors.

A dissenting note on the reality of anticipation was sounded by Penrose (1948), who attributed the findings to epidemiological artefacts. He pointed out that only a mildly-affected case of myotonic dystrophy would be able to marry and have children whereas a severe case might occur randomly in the next generation, giving the appearance of anticipation. Also, in a family survery only the more severely involved children would be detected since any mildly-affected ones would develop the disease in later life. Although Penrose's points are valid, they do not altogether dispose of the anticipation phenomenon. The most striking evidence that some undetermined factor(s) can modify the expression of the myotonic dystrophy gene has come from Harper and Dyken (1972). These authors studied the family histories of 35 cases of severe infantile myotonic dystrophy and found that in all but one instance the mother was the affected parent. They postulated that a humoral agent from the mother had accelerated the course of the disease in the fetus. An alternative explanation could depend on the fact that, at fertilization, the ovum donates considerably more cytoplasm, including mitochondrial DNA, than does the sperm.

The author has seen two cases of myotonic dystrophy presenting at birth with generalized muscular hypotonia associated with respiratory and feeding difficulties. In both instances the mother had been the affected parent. While accepting the invariability of the transmission pattern in such cases, can this phenomenon, together with Penrose's arguments, completely account for the clinical impression of anticipation? One of Penrose's arguments was that only mildly-affected cases would be likely to marry whereas more severe cases would be expected to occur randomly in his or her progeny. However, it is equally true that there should also be mild cases among the children and, by using coaxial needle electromyography, it is probable that any such cases could be detected during electrophysiological examination. In unpublished studies with A. R. M. Upton and F. Petito, this reasoning has been put to test. In 14 families with myotonic dystrophy the members of two generations have been subjected to motor unit counting in one or more muscles, together with measurements of maximal isometric twitch tensions. The advantage of this approach is obvious; instead of relying on subjective impressions of muscle strength, the performance of the individual muscles can be accurately assessed. In the second generations of these 14 families there were 20 affected individuals and 11 normal siblings, yielding a disease incidence of 66 per cent. Since, for a disorder transmitted by an autosomal dominant gene, one would expect half the offspring to be affected, it is unlikely that any mild cases had been overlooked. When the electrophysiological data was compared, it was found that 15 of the children already had more advanced stages of the disease than their parents, in spite of the difference in ages. Included in this survey were six children born to four affected fathers; in these families too, the disease was more severe in the second generation. The conclusion from this study is that anticipation is a real phenomenon and is not a statistical artefact; although the most severe form of the disease, that responsible for neonatal weakness, is transmitted through the mother, anticipation is also evident when the father is dystrophic.

APPENDIX 16.5

It is interesting that if the data of Montgomery (1975) is recalculated from that author's Table 7 and the text a significant neural influence emerges in the parabiotic experiments involving tibialis anterior, though not in those on the extensor digitorum longus. Thus the tetanic tension generated by 1 mg of wet 'normal' tibialis anterior muscle fell from 3.97 g to 3.0 g if it was reinnervated by a 'dystrophic' rather than a normal sciatic nerve. Conversely, the tension produced by 1 mg of wet 'dystrophic' muscle rose from 1.85 g to 2.8 g if reinnervation was undertaken by a 'normal' rather than a 'dystrophic' nerve.

APPENDIX 18.1

In the experiments of Barnard, Wieckowski and Chiu (1971) the safety factor, determined experimentally, was only about 2. However, the experiments were conducted *in vitro* and under these circumstances the muscle fibre resting potential falls and the membrane excitability is somewhat diminished.

APPENDIX 19.1—MYASTHENIA GRAVIS PRECEDED BY QUANTAL SQUANDER MYOKYMIA

The following brief report describes a patient with an apparently unique combination of neurological illnesses, all of which fell within a 3-year period. Of particular interest is the fact that two of these disorders involved the neuromuscular junction and affected transmission in quite different ways.

At the start of her illness in June 1971 O.V. was a 46-year-old white woman; she was married with two healthy children aged 17 and 20 and she worked as a nurse. Both parents had died from myocardial infarction and there was no history of neuromuscular disease in the family. Apart from two episodes of pulmonary embolism in 1967, for which no source was discovered, O.V. had always been healthy and she indulged actively in a number of sports.

'Encephalitic' illness

In June 1971 she began to feel vaguely unwell. During the next month, while on holiday in Europe, she started to tire easily, lost her appetite and developed blurring of vision in all directions together with photophobia. She also suffered from frequent severe headaches and had numerous bouts of excessive perspiration.

In August 1971 was admitted to hospital in a stuporose condition and shortly afterwards was observed to have a grand mal seizure; no residual neurological deficit was found 1 hr later. She then underwent a number of laboratory investigations including repeated serum electrolytes (with calcium), CSF analysis on two occasions, and haematological examination. The results of all these tests were within normal limits; her sedimentation rate was 14 mm/hr and no L.E. cells could be detected. However, three successive serum *CPK estimations were abnormal,* values of 465, 159 and 158 mu/ml being found (upper limit of normal 50 mu/ml for laboratory).

A radiological examination of the cerebral circulation was conducted using four-vessel angiography and no abnormalities were noted; a pneumo-encephalogram was also normal (Dr Z. Strassberg). A radiological examination of the chest indicated the presence of an *irregular lobulated mass in the anterior mediastinum.*

An EEG (Dr D. Levy) revealed poorly-organized rhythms but no definite evidence of focal abnormality.

During her 2-week stay in hospital the headaches and photophobia disappeared and no further seizures were noted. It was thought likely that she had recovered from an attack of *encephalitis,* the cause of which was unknown, and she was discharged.

Quantal squander myokymia

After being at home for 3 weeks the patient was readmitted on account of general ill health together with a number of new symptoms. She now complained that she was perspiring profusely throughout the day and night and that she was unusually thirsty. As before she tired easily and she felt weak; she had lost 15 lb during the previous month. Of particular concern to her were very painful muscle spasms which would last for 10–20 s; they were most severe in her calf muscles but could occur elsewhere. On examination she had a pulse rate of 70/min, was sweating profusely and exhibited a coarse generalized tremor. Her muscles were observed to be repeatedly developing cramps, during which they became hard; in addition there were generalized fasciculations, though not involving the tongue. Her tendon reflexes were symmetrically brisk and her plantar responses were flexor.

A number of laboratory investigations were undertaken. As before haematological and serum electrolyte studies were normal, as were tests of thyroid function (1^{131} uptake, T4, T3 suppression, and serum cholesterol) and estimations of 24-hour urinary catecholamines and vanilmandelic acid. A muscle biopsy taken from the left gastrocnemius revealed that the majority of fibres were normal but a few scattered angulated small fibres were present, suggestive of early denervation. Histochemical staining for DPNH reductase showed a normal mosaic pattern of fibres. An EMG (Dr M. Brandstater) disclosed that sensory nerve responses and impulse conduction velocities were normal but that, upon coaxial needle examination of the limb muscles, generalized brief runs of single muscle fibre potentials were frequent; these were described as myokymic; fasciculation potentials were also present. An intravenous Tensilon (edrophonium chloride, Roche Ltd) test had been performed during the previous stay in hospital and was negative.

In spite of the information available the diagnosis of quantal squander myokymia was not made until the following year. She was treated with Dilantin, 300 mg/day, and made a good recovery in that both the spontaneous muscle cramps and the excessive perspiration gradually ceased during the next 2 years.

Figure A19.1 (upper) shows some of the residual spontaneous muscle activity in the right lateral gastrocnemius muscle. The brief trains of muscle fibre potentials (myokymia) are no longer present but there are still single discharges of fibres while the larger and more complex potentials suggest that some of the other activity was arising in the motor nerve. The *middle* section shows superimposed traces of the hypothenar muscle responses to stimulation of the ulnar nerve at the wrist. Repetitive firing of a proportion of the muscle fibres is suggested by the consistent irregularities of the base-line following the main evoked response (M-wave).

The *lower* section of the figure displays the reduction in the numbers of functioning motor units and in the amplitude of the M-wave in the right extensor digitorum brevis muscle during a 3-year period of observation.

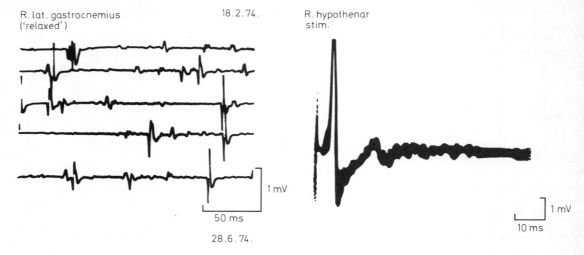

R. lat. gastrocnemius ('relaxed')

18.2.74.

R. hypothenar stim.

1 mV

50 ms

1 mV

10 ms

28.6.74.

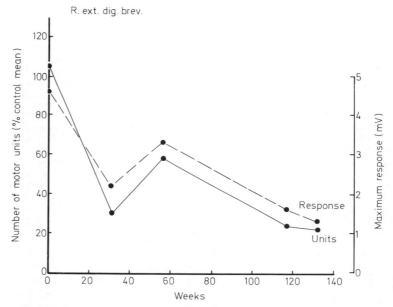

R. ext. dig. brev.

Response

Units

Figure A19.1. Electrophysiological recordings from a patient with quantal squander myokymia who subsequently developed myasthenia gravis (see text). (Top left) shows spontaneous electrical activity in the right lateral gastrocnemius muscle, recorded with a coaxial electrode. At this stage of her illness the brief runs of muscle fibre potentials (myokymia) had disappeared and only single discharges were evident. The amplitude and form of some discharges suggested that they had resulted from motor axon activity (see text). (Top right) Super-imposed traces of hypothenar muscle responses following stimulation of the ulnar nerve at the wrist. Repetitive firing was a consistent feature of the responses (shown as baseline ripple). (Lower) Successive motor unit counts and maximum evoked responses in the extensor digitorum brevis muscle of the same patient

Malignant thymoma

The presence of a mass in the anterior mediastinum was noted on radiological examination at the time of her first admission to hospital in August 1971. An operation was performed in the following month (Dr A. Parisi) and a thymoma was found: the tumour was lobulated and hard: it had infiltrated the anterior mediastinum and was adherent to the upper lobes of both lungs, the pericardium and the innominate vein. The tumour was dissected away and an apparently complete removal achieved: there has been no radiological evidence of recurrence in the ensuing four years. Histological examination of the excised tumour revealed a highly cellular tissue comprising lymphocytes and sheets of epitheloid cells.

Herpes zoster

In June 1972 she developed the typical vesicular eruption of herpes zoster the cutaneous distribution of the seventh and eighth thoracic roots on the left side. For a period of several months afterwards she experienced distressing post-herpetic neuralgia.

Myasthenia gravis

In May 1974 she complained of increasing muscle weakness. Her symptons, supported by examination, included double vision on looking to the right, three episodes of left-sided facial weakness, and difficulty in swallowing and in raising her head. A Tensilon test was now positive and repetitive stimulation of the right ulnar nerve at 30 Hz evoked the decremental muscle responses characteristic of myasthenia gravis (see *Figure 18.2*).

She was treated with anticholinesterase medication (pyridostigmine bromide: Mestinon, Roche Ltd.) and atropine but her initial improvement was followed by deterioration. In June 1974, while in hospital, she suffered a respiratory arrest but was promptly intubated and ventilated artificially. After 8 days without improvement a tracheostomy was performed. For several weeks she was sustained by intravenous feeding but eventually a gastrostomy was performed.

Her anticholinesterase therapy was discontinued on the day of her respiratory arrest and instead methyl prednisolone 100 mg was given by intramuscular injection on alternate days. After 2 weeks a slow improvement started, the artificial respiration being discontinued after a further 3 weeks and the gastrostomy feeding being stopped rather later. At present (August 1975) she leads an almost normal life, being able to perform housework and to travel abroad. She has no diplopia or ptosis and only slight weakness of bulbar and limb musculature: she is currently maintained on prednisone, 45 mg on alternate days, and Mestinon 90 mg 4-hourly during the day.

APPENDIX 24.1—FASCICULATIONS AND CRAMPS

The importance of muscle fasciculations as a physical sign in the diagnosis of motoneurone disease has already been mentioned. They are recognized as irregular, slowly-repeating, contractions of part of a muscle which cause visible movements of the overlying skin. They correspond to the discharges of single motor units and in partially-denervated muscle are associated with relatively large, prolonged and often complex potentials in the electromyogram. Fasciculations must not be confused with *fibrillations*, which have been considered elsewhere (page 75): the latter type of activity results from the spontaneous excitation of single muscle fibres following denervation. In contrast to fasciculations, fibrillations cannot be detected in a muscle through the thickness of the skin: the fibrillation potentials are discharged regularly (1 or more impulses per second) and are usually brief diphasic potentials of small amplitude.

In the diagnosis of motoneurone disease care must be taken to distinguish the condition from other causes of muscle fasciculations. One such cause is severe *thyrotoxicosis*, for in this disorder too there may be muscle weakness and wasting in association with prominent fasciculations. Fasciculations, usually restricted to one part of the body, may also be seen in conditions in which there is degeneration or irritation of motoneurones, ventral roots or peripheral motor axons: they may be seen, for example, in patients with spinal cord tumour, syringomyelia and prolapsed intervertebral disc. The most difficult distinction, however, is between motoneurone disease and the syndrome of *benign fasciculations*. In the latter disorder the patient usually becomes aware of the spontaneous flickering movements of his muscles and seeks medical advice on their account. The fasciculations may be confined to a group of muscles (usually the calf muscles) or else they may be widespread: at times painful muscle cramps may develop. Motor unit counting reveals normal values or else denervation limited to a few muscles only: in these muscles the rate of cell loss is too low to have produced significant alterations in the motor unit counts one year later. In spite of the good prognosis which may be offered to affected individuals it is possible that the condition may nevertheless represent a restricted variant ('forme fruste') of motoneurone disease.

Equally fascinating and mysterious are the transient fasciculations which may affect muscles of otherwise healthy subjects after bouts of severe exercise. It is difficult to envisage a lesion of the motoneurones which could be responsible for this phenomenon and it is more likely that the spontaneous action potentials arise in the intramuscular portions of the motor axons. One possibility would be that they result from mechanical stresses imposed on the axons during exercise; alternatively the axons could be excited by metabolites released from damaged segments of muscle fibres. Even in motoneurone disease, where the site of the lesion is known to be the cell soma, the majority of the fasciculations appear to arise in the periphery since the activity persists after spinal anaesthesia, nerve block or nerve section (Forster and Alpers, 1944; Forster, Borkowski, and Alpers, 1946). In this disorder it is probable that the distal regions of the axons become excessively excitable, either as part of the dying-back process (page 274) or as a consequence of the extra branching following collateral reinnervation.

There is some suggestion that, in the period where the motor unit is fasciculating, the motoneurone itself may be inexcitable. Trojaborg and Buchthal (1965) found that only 2 out of 177 fasciculating units could be recruited during weak or moderate voluntary contraction.

Life fasciculations, *muscle cramps* can occur in health and disease. In the latter situation they can complicate motoneurone disease and any other disorders affecting the neurone soma, including those of toxic or metabolic origin. They are, for example, a frequent complaint of patients who are either developing, or are recovering from, vincristine-induced neuropathies. In normal subjects cramps tend to occur at night or upon wakening in the morning; they are most common in the muscles of the calf and sole and are usually precipitated by voluntary movement. EMG studies show that the cramps are associated with high-frequency discharges of motor unit potentials; the activity can be stopped by passive stretch of the muscle. Lambert and his colleagues have studied healthy subjects predisposed to cramps and have shown that attacks can be induced by stimulating motor nerves distal to anaesthetic blocks. The authors conclude that the naturally-occurring cramps, like fasciculations, can originate in the periphery and that the intramuscular regions of the axons, very likely the terminals, are probably the generator-sites (Lambert, Elmqvist and Goldstein, 1969).

APPENDIX 27.1

Direct proof of this type of synaptic plasticity has been obtained in the septal nuclei of the rat by Raisman and Field (1973).

REFERENCES

A supplementary list of recent articles cited in the text is appended at the end of this reference list.

ABERFIELD, D. C., HINTERBUCHNER, L. P. and SCHNEIDER, M. (1965). 'Myotonia, dwarfism, diffuse bone disease and unusual ocular and facial abnormalities (a new syndrome).' *Brain* **88**, 313–322

ADAMS, R. D., DENNY-BROWN, D. and PEARSON, C. (1962). *Diseases in muscle. A study in pathology.* 2nd edn. New York: Harper and Row

ADRIAN, E. D. and BRONK, D. W. (1929). 'The discharge of impulses in motor nerve fibres. Part II. The frequency of discharge in reflex and voluntary contractions.' *Journal of Physiology,* **67**, 119–151

ADRIAN, E. D. and GELFAN, S. (1933). 'Rhythmic activity in skeletal muscle fibres.' *Journal of Physiology,* **78**, 271–287

ADRIAN, R. H. and BRYANT, S. H. (1974). 'On the repetitive discharge in myotonic muscle fibres.' *Journal of Physiology,* **240**, 505–515

ADRIAN, R. H., COSTANTIN, L. L. and PEACHEY, L. D. (1969). 'Radial spread of contraction in frog muscle fibres.' *Journal of Physiology,* **204**, 231–257

AFFIFI, A. K., IBRAHIM, M. Z. M., BERGMAN, R. A., ABU HAYDAR, N., MIRE, J., BAHUTH, N. and KAYLANI, F. (1972). 'Morphological features of hypermetabolic mitochondrial disease. A light microscopic, histochemical, and electron microscopic study.' *Journal of Neurological Sciences,* **15**, 271–290

AITKEN, J. T., SHARMAN, M. and YOUNG, J. Z. (1947). 'Maturation of regenerating nerve fibres with various peripheral connexions.' *Journal of Anatomy,* **81**, 1–22

AITKEN, R. S., ALLOTT, E. N., CASTLEDEN, L. I. M. and WALKER, MARY (1937). 'Observations on a case of familial periodic paralysis.' *Clinical Science,* **3**, 47–57

ALAJOUANINE, T., SCHERRER, J. and BOURGUIGNON, A. (1959). 'Enregistrement simultané de la réponse électrique du nerf et du muscle dans la myathénie.' *Revue Neurologique,* **100**, 238–241

AL-AMOOD, W. S., BULLER, A. J. and POPE, R. (1973). 'Long-term stimulation of cat fast-twitch skeletal muscle.' *Nature (London),* **244**, 225–227

ALBUQUERQUE, E. X., BARNARD, E. A., CHIU, T. H., LAPA, A. J., DOLLY, J. O., JANSSON, S., DALY, J. and WITKOP, B. (1973a). 'Acetylcholine receptor and ion conductance modulator sites at the murine neuromuscular junction:

evidence for specific toxin reactions.' *Proceedings of the National Academy of Sciences (U.S.),* **70**, 949–953

ALBUQUERQUE, E. X., LEBEDA, F. J., APPEL, S. H., ALMON, R., KAUFFMAN, F. C., MAYER, R. F., NARAHASHI, T. and YEH, J. Z. (1976a). 'Effects of normal and myasthenic serum factors on innervated and chronically denervated mammalian muscles.' *Annals of the New York Academy of Sciences.* **274**, 475–492

ALBUQUERQUE, E. X., RASH, J. E., MAYER, R. F. and SATTERFIELD, J. R. (1976). 'An electrophysiological and morphological study of the neuromuscular junction in patients with myasthenia gravis.' *Experimental Neurology.* In press

ALBUQUERQUE, E. X., SCHUH, F. T. and KAUFFMAN, F. C. (1971). 'Early membrane depolarization of the fast mammalian muscle after denervation.' *Pfluegers Archiv; European Journal of Physiology,* **328**, 36–50

ALBUQUERQUE, E. X., WARNICK, J. E., SANSONE, F. M. and DALY, J. (1973b). 'The pharmacology of batrachotoxin. V. A comparative study of membrane properties and the effect of batrachotoxin on sartorius muscles of the frogs, *Phyllobates aurotaenia* and *Rana pipiens.*' *Journal of Pharmacology and Experimental Therapeutics,* **184**, 315–329

ALBUQUERQUE, E. X., WARNICK, J. E., TASSE, J. R. and SANSONE, F. M. (1972). 'Effects of vinblastine and cholchicine on neural regulation of the fast and slow skeletal muscles of the rat.' *Experimental Neurology,* **37**, 607–634

ALLEN, J. E. and RODGIN, D. W. (1960). 'Mental retardation in association with progressive muscular dystrophy.' *American Journal of Diseases of Children,* **100**, 208–211

ALLT, G. and CAVANAGH, J. B. (1969). 'Ultrastructural changes in the regions of the node of Ranvier in the rat caused by diphtheria toxin.' *Brain,* **92**, 459–468

ALMON, R. R., ANDREW, C. G. and APPEL, S. H. (1974). 'Serum globulin in myasthenia gravis: inhibition of α-bungarotoxin binding to acetylcholine receptors. *Science,* **186**, 55–57

ALNAES, E. and RAHAMIMOFF, R. (1975). 'On the role of mitochondria in transmitter release from motor nerve terminals.' *Journal of Physiology,* **248**, 285–306

ALPERS, B. J. and FARMER, R. A. (1949). 'Role of repeated trauma by pneumatic drill in production of amyotrophic lateral sclerosis.' *Archives of Neurology and Psychiatry (Chicago)*, **62**, 178–182

ANDERSON, H. J., CHURCHILL-DAVIDSON, H. C. and RICHARDSON, A. T. (1953). 'Bronchial neoplasm with myasthenia; prolonged apnoea after administration of succinylcholine.' *Lancet*, **ii**, 1291–1293

ANDO, K. (1973). 'Study on the transport of acrylamide to the peripheral part of the rat sciatic nerve.' *Proceedings of the Osaka Prefectural Institute of Public Health*, **11**, 45–48. Cited by Spencer, P. S. and Schaumburg, H. H. *Canadian Journal of Neurological Sciences*, **1**, 152–169, 1974

ANDO, K. and HASHIMOTO, K. (1972). 'Accumulation of (^{14}C)-acrylamide in mouse nerve tissue.' *Proceedings of the Osaka Prefectural Institute of Public Health*, **10**, 7–12

ARAN, F. A. (1850). 'Réchèrches sur une maladie non encore décrite du système musculaire (atrophie musculaire progressive).' *Archives générales de médecine*, **24**, 4–35, 172–214

ARNASON, B. G. W., WINKLER, G. F. and HADLER, N. M. (1969). 'Cell-mediated demyelination of peripheral nerve in tissue culture.' *Laboratory Investigation*, **21**, 1–10

ARNOLD, N. and HARRIMAN, D. G. F. (1970). 'The incidence of abnormality in control human peripheral nerves studied by single axon dissection.' *Journal of Neurology, Neurosurgery and Psychiatry*, **33**, 55–61

ARUNDELL, F. D., WILKINSON, R. D. and HASERICK, J. R. (1960). 'Dermatomyositis and malignant neoplasms in adults.' *Archives of Dermatology and Syphilology*, **82**, 772–775

ASBOE-HANSEN, G., IVERSEN, K. and WICHMANN, R. (1962). 'Progressive exophthalmos: muscular changes and thyrotropin content in serum.' *Acta Endocrinologica*, **11**, 376–399

ASBURY, A. K., COX, S. C. and KANADA, D. (1973). '^{3}H leucine incorporation in acrylamide neuropathy in the mouse.' *Neurology (Minneapolis)*, **23**, 406

ASHLEY, C. C. and RIDGWAY, E. B. (1968). 'Simultaneous recording of membrane potential, calcium transient and tension in single muscle fibres.' *Nature (London)*, **219**, 1168–1169

ASHLEY, C. C. and RIDGWAY, E. B. (1970). 'On the relationships between membrane potential, calcium transient and tension in single barnacle muscle fibres.' *Journal of Physiology*, **209**, 105–130

ASK-UPMARK, E. (1950). 'Amyotrophic lateral sclerosis observed in 5 persons after gastric resection.' *Gastroenterology*, **15**, 257–259

ASK-UPMARK, E. and MEURLING, S. (1955). 'On the presence of a deficiency factor in the pathogenesis of amyotrophic lateral sclerosis.' *Acta Medica Scandinavica*, **152**, 217–222

ASTRÖM, K. E. and WAKSMAN, B. H. (1962). 'The passive transfer of experimental allergic encephalomyelitis and neuritis with living lymphoid cells.' *Journal of Pathology and Bacteriology*, **83**, 89–106

AU, K.-S. and YEUNG, ROSE T. T. (1972). 'Thyrotoxic periodic paralysis.' *Archives of Neurology*, **26**, 543–546

AWAD, E. A. (1968). 'Motor-point biopsies in carcinomatous neuropathy.' *Archives of Physical Medicine* **49**, 643–649

AXELSSON, J. and THESLEFF, S. (1959). 'A study of supersensitivity in denervated mammalian skeletal muscle.' *Journal of Physiology*, **147**, 178–193

BAGINSKY, R. G. (1968). 'A case of peripheral neuropathy displaying myasthenic EMG patterns.' *Electroencephalography and Clinical Neurophysiology* **25**, 397

BAGUST, J. (1974). 'Relationships between motor nerve conduction velocities and motor unit contraction characteristics in a slow-twitch muscle of the cat.' *Journal of Physiology*, **238**, 269–278

BAGUST, J. and LEWIS, D. M. (1974). 'Isometric contractions of motor units in self-reinnervated fast and slow twitch muscles of the cat.' *Journal of Physiology* **237**, 91–102

BAGUST, J., LEWIS, D. M. and WESTERMAN, R. A. (1973) 'Polyneuronal innervation of kitten skeletal muscle.' *Journal of Physiology*, **229**, 241–255

BAKER, P. F., HODGKIN, A. L. and SHAW, T. I. (1962a). 'Replacement of the axoplasm of giant nerve fibres with artificial solutions.' *Journal of Physiology*, **164**, 330–354

BAKER, P. F., HODGKIN, A. L. and SHAW, T. I. (1962b). 'The effects of changes in internal ionic concentrations on the electrical properties of perfused giant axons.' *Journal of Physiology*, **164**, 355–374

BALLANTYNE, J. P. and CAMPBELL, M. J. (1973). 'Electrophysiological study after surgical repair of sectioned human peripheral nerves.' *Journal of Neurology, Neurosurgery and Psychiatry*, **36**, 797–805

BALLANTYNE, J. P. and HANSEN, S. (1974a). 'A new method for the estimation of the number of motor units in a muscle. 1. Control subjects and patients with myasthenia gravis.' *Journal of Neurology, Neurosurgery and Psychiatry*, **37**, 907–915

BALLANTYNE, J. P. and HANSEN, S. (1974b). 'Computer method for the analysis of evoked motor unit potentials. 1. Control subjects and patients with myasthenia gravis.' *Journal of Neurology, Neurosurgery and Psychiatry*, **37**, 1187–1194

BALLANTYNE, J. P. and HANSEN, S. (1974c). 'New method for the estimation of the number of motor units in a muscle. 2. Duchenne, limb-girdle and facioscapulohumeral, and myotonic muscular dystrophies.' *Journal of Neurology, Neurosurgery and Psychiatry*, **37**, 1195–1201

BARANY, M. (1967). 'ATPase activity of myosin correlated with speed of muscle shortening.' *Journal of General Physiology*, **50** (Suppl., part 2), 197–218

BARANY, M. and CLOSE, R. I. (1971). 'The transformation of myosin in cross-innervated rat muscles.' *Journal of Physiology*, **213**, 455–474

BARCROFT, H. and MILLEN, J. L. E. (1939). 'The blood flow through muscle during sustained contraction.' *Journal of Physiology*, **97**, 17–31

BARI and ANDREW (1964). Cited by Andrew, W. (1971). In *The Anatomy of Ageing in Man and Animal*, p. 231. New York: Grune and Stratton

BARNARD, E. A., DOLLY, J. O., PORTER, C. W. and ALBUQUERQUE, E. X. (1975). 'The acetylcholine receptor and the ionic conductance modulation system of skeletal muscle.' *Experimental Neurology*, **48**, 1–28

ARNARD, E. A., WIECKOWSKI, J. and CHIU, T. H. (1971). 'Cholinergic receptor molecules and cholinesterase molecules at mouse skeletal muscle junctions.' *Nature (London)*, **234**, 207–209

ARNARD, R. J., EDGERTON, V. R. and PETER, J. B. (1970a). 'Effects of exercise on skeletal muscle. I. Biochemical and histochemical properties.' *Journal of Applied Physiology*, **28**, 762–766

ARNARD, R. J., EDGERTON, V. R. and PETER, J. B. (1970b). 'Effects of exercise on skeletal muscle. II. Contractile properties.' *Journal of Applied Physiology*, **28**, 767–770

ARRON, D. H. (1933). 'Structural changes in anterior horn cells following central lesions.' *Proceedings of the Society of Experimental Biology and Medicine*, **30**, 1327–1329

ARWICK, D. D., OSSELTON, J. W. and WALTON, J. N. (1965). 'Electro-encephalographic studies in hereditary myopathy.' *Journal of Neurology, Neurosurgery and Psychiatry*, **28**, 109–114

ASMAJIAN, J. V. (1963). 'Control and training of individual motor units.' *Science, N.Y.*, **141**, 440–441

ASTIAN, J. and NAKAJIMA, S. (1974). 'Action potential in the transverse tubules and its role in the activation of skeletal muscle.' *Journal of General Physiology*, **63**, 257–278

LMAR, J. and EYZAGUIRRE, C. (1966). 'Pacemaker site of fibrillation potentials in denervated mammalian muscle.' *Journal of Neurophysiology*, **29**, 425–441

NDER, A. N., RINGEL, S. P., ENGEL, W. K., DANIELS, M. P. and VOGEL, Z. (1975). 'Myasthenia gravis: a serum factor blocking acetylcholine receptors of the human neuromuscular junction.' *Lancet*, **i**, 607–609

NNETT, M. R., FLORIN, T. and WOOG, R. (1974). 'The formation of synapses in regenerating mammalian striated muscle.' *Journal of Physiology*, **238**, 79–92

NNETT, M. R., MCLACHLAN, Elspeth and TAYLOR, R. S. (1973). 'The formation of synapses in reinnervated mammalian striated muscle.' *Journal of Physiology*, **233**, 481–500

NNETT, M. R. and PETTIGREW, A. G. (1974a). 'The formation of synapses in striated muscle during development.' *Journal of Physiology*, **241**, 515–545

NNETT, M. R. and PETTIGREW, A. G. (1974b). 'The formation of synapses in reinnervated and cross-reinnervated striated muscle during development.' *Journal of Physiology*, **241**, 547–573

NNETT, M. R., PETTIGREW, A. G. and TAYLOR, R. S. (1973). 'The formation of synapses in reinnervated and cross-reinnervated adult avian muscle.' *Journal of Physiology*, **230**, 331–357

RÁNEK, R. (1964). 'Intracellular stimulation myography in man.' *Electroencephalography and Clinical Neurophysiology*, **16**, 301–304

RG, D. K. and HALL, Z. W. (1975). 'Increased extrajunctional acetylcholine sensitivity produced by chronic post-synaptic neuromuscular blockade.' *Journal of Physiology*, **244**, 659–676

RGLAND, R. M. (1960). 'Newer concepts of myelin formation correlated to functional changes.' *Archives of Neurology*, **2**, 260–265

BERGMANS, J. (1970). '*The Physiology of Single Human Nerve Fibres*. Louvain: Vander

BERGSTRÖM, J. (1962). 'Muscle electrolytes in man.' *Scandinavian Journal of Clinical Laboratory Investigation*, Suppl. **68**

BERL, S. and PUSZKIN, S. (1970). 'Mg^{2+}-Ca^{2+} activated adenosine triphosphatase system isolated from mammalian brain.' *Biochemistry*, **9**, 2058–2067

BIEMOND, A. and DANIELS, A. P. (1934). 'Familial periodic paralysis and its transition into spinal muscular atrophy.' *Brain*, **57**, 91–108

BIGLAND, BRENDA V. and LIPPOLD, O. C. J. (1954). 'Motor unit activity in the voluntary contraction of human muscle.' *Journal of Physiology*, **125**, 322–325

BIRKET-SMITH, E. and OLIVARIUS, B. de F. (1957). 'Polyradiculomyopathia in transient thyrotoxicosis.' *Danish Medical Bulletin*, **4**, 217–219

BIRKS, R. I. and DAVEY, D. F. (1969). 'Osmotic responses demonstrating the extracellular character of the sacroplasmic reticulum.' *Journal of Physiology*, **202**, 171–188

BISBY, M. A. (1975). 'Inhibition of axonal transport in nerves chronically treated with local anaesthetics.' *Experimental Neurology*, **47**, 481–489

BISCHOFF, R. and HOLTZER, H. (1969). 'Mitosis and the process of differentiation of myogenic cells *in vitro*.' *Journal of Cell Biology*, **41**, 188–200

BISCHOFF, R. and LOWE, M. (1974). 'Cell surface components and the interaction of myogenic cells.' In *Exploratory Concepts in Muscular Dystrophy II*, Ed. by A. T. Milhorat, pp. 17–29. Amsterdam: Excerpta Medica

BLACK, J. T., BHATT, E. P., DEJESUS, P. V., SCHOTLAND, D. L. and ROWLAND, L. P. (1974). 'Diagnostic accuracy of clinical data, quantitative electromyography and histochemistry in neuromuscular disease. A study of 105 cases.' *Journal of the Neurological Sciences*, **21**, 59–70

BLUMCKE, S. and NIEDORF, H. R. (1965). 'Elektronenoptische untersuchungen an Wachstumsendkolben regenerierender peripherer nervenfasern.' *Virchow's Archiv fur pathologische Anatomie und Physiologie*, **340**, 93–104

BODIAN, D. (1964). 'An electronmicroscopic study of the monkey spinal cord. I. Fine structure of normal motor column. II. Effects of retrograde chromatolysis. III. Cytologic effects of mild and virulent poliovirus infection.' *Bulletin of Johns Hopkins Hospital*, **114**, 13–119

BOEGMAN, R. J., WOOD, P. L. and PINAUD, L. (1975). 'Increased axoplasmic flow associated with pargyline under conditions which induce a myopathy.' *Nature (London)*, **253**, 51–52

BORNSTEIN, M. B. and CRAIN, S. M. (1965). 'Functional studies of cultured brain tissues as related to "demyelinative disorders".' *Science, N.Y.*, **148**, 1242–1244

BORNSTEIN, M. B., IWANAMI, H., LEHRER, G. M. and BREITBART, L. (1968). 'Observations on the appearance of neuromuscular relationships in cultured mouse tissues.' *Zeitschrift für Zellforschung*, **92**, 197–206

BOTEZ, M. I. (1971). 'Some clinical findings concerning muscular atrophy of central origin.' *European Neurology*, **5**, 25–33

BOWDEN, R. E. M. and GUTMANN, E. (1944). 'Denervation and re-innervation of human voluntary muscle.' *Brain*, **67**, 273–313

BOYD, I. A. and DAVEY, Mary R. (1968). *Composition of Peripheral Nerves*. Edinburgh: Livingstone

BRADLEY, W. G. (1974). *Disorders of Peripheral Nerves*. Oxford: Blackwell

BRADLEY, W. G. and JAROS, E. (1973). 'Axoplasmic flow in axonal neuropathies. II. Axoplasmic flow in mice with motoneurone disease and muscular dystrophy.' *Brain*, **96**, 247–258

BRADLEY, W. G. and JENKISON, Margaret (1973). 'Abnormalities of peripheral nerves in murine muscular dystrophy.' *Journal of Neurological Sciences*, **18**, 227–247

BRADLEY, W. G. and WILLIAMS, M. H. (1973). 'Axoplasmic flow in axonal neuropathies. I. Axoplasmic flow in cats with toxic neuropathies.' *Brain*, **96**, 235–246

BRAIN, Lord, CROFT, P. and WILKINSON, Marcia (1969). 'The course and outcome of motor neuron disease.' In *Motor Neuron Diseases*. Ed. by F. H. Norris, Jr and L. T. Kurland, pp. 20–27. New York and London: Grune and Stratton

BRAIN, Lord and NORRIS, F. H. JR (Eds.) (1965). *The Remote Effects of Cancer on the Nervous System*. New York and London: Grune and Stratton

BRAIN, W. R., WRIGHT, A. D. and WILKINSON, MARCIA (1947). 'Spontaneous compression of both median nerves in the carpal tunnel. Six cases treated surgically.' *Lancet*, **i**, 277–282

BRANDSTATER, M. E. and LAMBERT, E. H. (1969). 'A histochemical study of the spatial arrangement of muscle fibres in single motor units within rat tibialis anterior muscle.' *Bulletin of the American Association of Electromyography and Electrodiagnosis*, **82**, 15–16

BRANDSTATER, M. E. and LAMBERT, E. H. (1973). 'Motor unit anatomy. Type and spatial arrangement of muscle fibres.' In *New Developments in Electromyography and Clinical Neurophysiology*. Ed. by J. E. Desmedt, Vol. 1, pp 14–22. Basel: Karger

BRAY, J. J. and HARRIS, A. J. (1975). 'Dissociation between nerve-muscle transmission and nerve trophic effects on rat diaphragm using type D botulinum toxin.' *Journal of Physiology*, **253**, 53–77

BRIERLEY, J. B. and FIELD, E. J. (1949). 'The fate of an intraneural injection as demonstrated by the use of radio-active phosphorus.' *Journal of Neurology, Neurosurgery and Psychiatry*, **12**, 86–99

BRIMIJOIN, S. (1975). 'Stop-flow: a new technique for measuring axonal transport, and its application to the transport of dopamine-β-hydroxylase.' *Journal of Neurobiology*, **6**, 379–394

BRIMIJOIN, S. and DYCK, P. J. (1974). 'Axonal transport of dopamine-β-hydroxylase by abnormal sural nerves.' In *Dynamics of Degeneration and Growth in Neurons*. Ed. by K. Fuxe, L. Olson and Y. Zotterman. Oxford: Pergamon

BRITT, Beverley A. (1971). 'Comment during discussion on "Malignant hyperthermia with subsequent uneventful general anaesthesia".' *Anaesthesia and Analgesia*, **50**, 1107–1111

BRITT, Beverley A. (1974). 'Malignant hyperthermia a pharmacogenetic disease of skeletal and cardia muscle.' *New England Journal of Medicine*, **29(** 1140–1142

BRITT, Beverley A. and KALOW, W. (1970). 'Malignan hyperthermia: a statistical review.' *Canadian Anae thetists' Society Journal*, **17**, 293–315

BRITT, Beverley A., KALOW, W., GORDON, A., HUMPHREY J. G. and REWCASTLE, N. B. (1973). 'Malignant hyper thermia: an investigation of five patients.' *Canadia Anaesthetists' Society Journal*, **20**, 431–467

BRODY, I. A. and ENGEL, W. K. (1964). 'Denervation c muscle in myasthenia gravis.' *Archives of Neurolog* **11**, 350–354

BRONSKY, D., KAGANIEC, G. I. and WALDSTEIN, S. S. (1964 'An association between the Guillain-Barré syndrom and hyperthyroidism.' *American Journal of Medic Sciences*, **247**, 196–200

BROOKE, M. H. and ENGEL, W. K. (1969). 'The histc graphic analysis of human muscle biopsies with regar to fibre types 1. Adult male and female.' *Neurolog (Minneapolis)*, **19**, 221–233

BROOKE, M. H. and KAISER, K. K. (1970). 'Muscle fibr types: How many and what kind?' *Archives of Neurc logy*, **23**, 369–379

BROOKE, M. H. and KAISER, K. K. (1974). 'The use an abuse of muscle histochemistry.' In *Trophic Functior of the Neuron (Symposium)*. Ed. by D. B. Drachmar *Annals of the New York Academy of Sciences*, **228** 121–144

BROOKS, J. E. (1969). 'Hyperkalaemic periodic paralysi Intracellular EMG studies.' *Archives of Neurolog* **20**, 13–18

BROOKS, V. B., CURTIS, D. R. and ECCLES, J. C. (1957). 'Th action of tetanus toxin on the inhibition of motc neurones.' *Journal of Physiology*, **135**, 655–672

BROOKS, V. B. and THIES, R. E. (1962). 'Reduction c quantum content during neuromuscular transmission. *Journal of Physiology*, **162**, 298–310

BROSTOFF, S., BURNETT, P., LAMBERT, P. and EYLAR, E. H (1972). 'Isolation and characterization of a protein fron sciatic nerve myelin responsible for experimenta allergic neuritis.' *Nature New Biology*, **235**, 210–212

BROSTOFF, S. W. and EYLAR, E. H. (1972). 'The proposec amino acid sequence of the P1 protein of rabbit sciati nerve myelin.' *Archives of Biochemistry and Bio physics*, **153**, 590–598

BROWN, G. L. and HARVEY, A. M. (1939). 'Congenita myotonia in the goat.' *Brain*, **62**, 341–363

BROWN, J. C. (1974). 'Repetitive stimulation and neurc muscular transmission studies.' In *Disorders o Voluntary Muscle*, 3rd edn. Ed. by J. N. Walton pp. 958–972. Edinburgh: Churchill Livingstone

BROWN, J. C. and CHARLTON, J. E. (1975). 'Study o sensitivity to curare in certain neurological disorder using a regional technique.' *Journal of Neurolog Neurosurgery and Psychiatry*, **38**, 34–45

BROWN, J. C. and KATER, R. M. H. (1969). 'Pancreati function in patients with amyotrophic lateral sclerosis *Neurology (Minneapolis)*, **19**, 185–189

BROWN, M. C. and BUTLER, R. G. (1974). 'Evidence fo innervation of muscle spindle intrafusal fibres by branches of α-motoneurones following nerve injury.' *Journal of Physiology*, **238**, 41–43P

BROWN, W. F. (1972). 'A method for estimating the number of motor units in thenar muscles and the changes in motor unit counting with ageing.' *Journal of Neurology, Neurosurgery and Psychiatry*, **35**, 845–852

BROWN, W. F. (1973). 'Functional compensation of human motor units in health and disease.' *Journal of the Neurological Sciences*, **20**, 199–209

BROWNELL, Betty, OPPENHEIMER, D. R. and SPALDING, J. M. K. (1972). 'Neurogenic muscle atrophy in myasthenia gravis.' *Journal of Neurology, Neurosurgery and Psychiatry*, **35**, 311–322

BRUMLIK, J. and CUETTER, A. C. (1969). 'Denervation myotonia: a subclinical electromyographic finding.' *Electromyography*, **9**, 297–310

BRYANT, S. H. (1962). 'Muscle membrane of normal and myotonic goats in normal and low external chloride.' *Federation Proceedings*, **21**, 312

BRYANT, S. H. (1969). 'Cable properties of external intercostal muscle fibres from myotonic and nonmyotonic goats.' *Journal of Physiology*, **204**, 539–550

BRYANT, S. H. and MORALES-AGUILERA, A. (1971). 'Chloride conductance in normal and myotonic muscle fibres and the action of monocarboxylic aromatic acids.' *Journal of Physiology*, **219**, 367–383

BUCHTHAL, F., GULD, C. and ROSENFALCK, P. (1955). 'Propagation velocity in electrically activated muscle fibres in man.' *Acta physiologica Scandinavica*, **34**, 75–89

BUCHTHAL, F., GULD, C. and ROSENFALCK, P. (1957). 'Multielectrode study of the territory of a motor unit.' *Acta Physiologica Scandinavica*, **39**, 83–104

BUCHTHAL, F. and OLSEN, P. Z. (1970). 'Electromyography and muscle biopsy in infantile spinal muscular atrophy.' *Brain*, **93**, 15–30

BUCHTHAL, F. and ROSENFALCK, Annelise (1966). 'Evoked action potentials and conduction velocity in human sensory nerve.' *Brain Research*, **3**, 1–222 (Special issue)

BUCHTHAL, F. and ROSENFALCK, P. (1958). 'Rate of impulse conduction in denervated human muscle.' *Electroencephalography and Clinical Neurophysiology*, **10**, 521–526

BUCHTHAL, F. and ROSENFALCK, P. (1966). 'Spontaneous electrical activity of human muscle.' *Electroencephalography and Clinical Neurophysiology*, **20**, 321–336

BUCHTHAL, F., ROSENFALCK, P. and ERMINIO, F. (1960). 'Motor unit territory and fibre density in myopathies.' *Neurology (Minneapolis)*, **10**, 398–408

BUCHTHAL, F., ROSENFALCK, Annelise and TROJABORG, W. (1974). 'Electrophysiological findings in entrapment of the median nerve at wrist and elbow.' *Journal of Neurology, Neurosurgery and Psychiatry*, **37**, 340–360

BUCHTHAL, F. and SCHMALBRUCH, H. (1970). 'Contraction times and fibre types in intact human muscle.' *Acta Physiologica Scandinavica*, **79**, 435–452

BUCHTHAL, F., SCHMALBRUCH, H. and KAMIENIECKA, ZOFIA (1971a). 'Contraction times and fibre types in neurogenic paresis.' *Neurology (Minneapolis)*, **21**, 58–67

BUCHTHAL, F., SCHMALBRUCH, H. and KAMIENIECKA, ZOFIA (1971b). 'Contraction times and fibre types in patients with progressive muscular dystrophy.' *Neurology (Minneapolis)*, **21**, 131–139

BULLER, A. J., DORNHORST, A. C., EDWARDS, R., KERR, D. and WHELAN, R. F. (1959). 'Fast and slow muscles in mammals.' *Nature (London)*, **183**, 1516–1517

BULLER, A. J., ECCLES, J. C. and ECCLES, Rosamond M. (1960a). 'Differentiation of fast and slow muscles in the cat hind limb.' *Journal of Physiology*, **150**, 399–416

BULLER, A. J., ECCLES, J. C. and ECCLES, Rosamond M. (1960b). 'Interactions between motoneurones and muscles in respect of the characteristic speeds of their responses.' *Journal of Physiology*, **150**, 417–439

BULLER, A. J. and LEWIS, D. M. (1965). 'Further observations on the differentiation of skeletal muscles in the kitten hindlimb.' *Journal of Physiology*, **176**, 355–370

BULLER, A. J., MOMMAERTS, W. F. H. M. and SERAYDARIAN, K. (1969). 'Enzymic properties of myosin in fast and slow twitch muscles of the cat following cross-innervation.' *Journal of Physiology*, **205**, 581–597

BURGEN, A. S. V., DICKENS, J. and ZATMAN, L. J. (1949). 'The action of botulinum toxin on the neuromuscular junction.' *Journal of Physiology*, **109**, 10–24

BURKE, D., SKUSE, N. F. and LETHLEAN, A. K. (1974). 'Isometric contraction of the abductor digiti minimi muscle in man.' *Journal of Neurology, Neurosurgery and Psychiatry*, **37**, 825–834

BURKE, R. E. (1967). 'Motor unit types of cat triceps surae muscle.' *Journal of Physiology*, **193**, 141–160

BURKE, R. E., KANDA, K. and MAYER, R. F. (1975). 'The effect of chronic immobilization on defined types of motor units in the cat medial gastrocnemius.' *Society for Neuroscience, 5th Annual Meeting, New York.* Abstract no. 1174

BURKE, R. E., LEVINE, D. N., SALCMAN, M. and TSAIRIS, P. (1974). 'Motor units in cat soleus muscle: physiological, histochemical and morphological characteristics.' *Journal of Physiology*, **238**, 503–514

BURKE, R. E., LEVINE, D. N., TSAIRIS, P. and ZAJAC, F. E. III (1973). 'Physiological types and histochemical profiles in motor units of the cat gastrocnemius.' *Journal of Physiology*, **234**, 723–748

BURKE, R. E., LEVINE, D. N., ZAJAC, F. E. III, TSAIRIS, P. and ENGEL, W. K. (1971). 'Mammalian motor units: physiological-histochemical correlation in three types in cat gastrocnemius.' *Science, N.Y.*, **174**, 709–712

BURKE, R. E. and TSAIRIS, P. (1973). 'Anatomy and innervation ratios in motor units of cat gastrocnemius.' *Journal of Physiology*, **234**, 749–765

BURKE, W. E., TUTTLE, W. W., THOMPSON, C. W., JANNEY, C. D. and WEBER, R. J. (1953). 'The relation of grip strength and grip strength endurance to age.' *Journal of Applied Physiology*, **5**, 628–630

BUTTERFIELD, D. A., CHESNUT, D., ROSES, A. D. and APPEL, S. H. (1974). 'Electron spin resonance studies of erythrocytes from patients with myotonic muscular dystrophy.' *Proceedings of the National Academy of Sciences of the United States of America*, **71**, 909–913

BYERS, Margaret R., FINK, B. R., KENNEDY, R. D., MIDDAUGH, M. E. and HENDRICKSON, Anita E. (1973). 'Effects of lidocaine on axonal morphology, microtubules, and rapid transport in rabbit vagus nerve *in vitro*.' *Journal of Neurobiology*, **4**, 125–143

CACCIA, M. R., BOIARDI, A., ANDREUSSI, L. and CORNELIO, F. (1975). 'Nerve supply and experimental myotonia in rats.' *Journal of the Neurological Sciences*, **24**, 145–150

CACCIA, M. R., NEGRI, S. and PRETO PARVIS, V. (1972). 'Myotonic dystrophy with neural involvement.' *Journal of the Neurological Sciences*, **16**, 253–269

CAJAL, S. R. (1928). *Degeneration and Regeneration of the Nervous System*. Vol. 1. Trans. and ed. by R. M. May. London: Oxford University Press

CAMPA, J. F. and SANDERS, D. B. (1974). 'Familial hypokalemic periodic paralysis. Local recovery after nerve stimulation.' *Archives of Neurology*, **31**, 110–115

CAMPBELL, A. M. G., WILLIAMS, E. R. and BARLTROP, D. (1970). 'Motor neurone disease and exposure to lead.' *Journal of Neurology, Neurosurgery and Psychiatry*, **33**, 877–885

CAMPBELL, H. and BRAMWELL, E. (1900). 'Myasthenia gravis.' *Brain*, **23**, 277–336

CAMPBELL, M. J. and McCOMAS, A. J. (1970). 'The effects of ageing on muscle function.' In *5th Symposium on Current Research on Muscular Dystrophy and Related Disease, London*. Abstract No. 6. London: Muscular Dystrophy Group of Great Britain

CAMPBELL, M. J., McCOMAS, A. J. and PETITO, F. (1973). 'Physiological changes in ageing muscles.' *Journal of Neurology, Neurosurgery and Psychiatry*, **36**, 174–182

CAMPBELL, M. J., McCOMAS, A. J. and SICA, R. (1970). 'An electrophysiological study of dystrophia myotonica.' *Journal of Physiology*, **209**, 28–29P

CAMPBELL, M. J. and PATY, D. W. (1974). 'Carcinomatous neuromyopathy: 1. Electrophysiological studies. An electrophysiological and immunological study of patients with carcinoma of the lung.' *Journal of Neurology, Neurosurgery and Psychiatry*. **37**, 131–141

CANGIANO, A. (1973). 'Acetylcholine supersensitivity: the role of neurotrophic factors.' *Brain Research*, **58**, 255–259

CANNON, B. W. and LOVE, J. G. (1946). 'Tardy median palsy: median neuritis: median thenar neuritis amenable to surgery.' *Surgery*, **20**, 210–216

CAPALDI, R. A. (1974). 'A dynamic model of cell membranes.' *Scientific American*, **230**, 26–33

CARLSON, B. M. (1970). 'Regeneration of the rat gastrocnemius muscle from sibling and non-sibling muscle fragments.' *American Journal of Anatomy*, **128**, 21–31

CARLSON, B. M. and GUTMANN, E. (1972). 'Development of contractile properties of minced muscle regenerates in the rat.' *Experimental Neurology*, **36**, 239–249

CARSON, M. J. and PEARSON, C. M. (1964). 'Familial hyperkalaemic periodic paralysis with myotonic features.' *Journal of Paediatrics*, **64**, 853–865

CASPARY, E. A., CURRIE, S. and FIELD, E. J. (1971). 'Sensitized lymphocytes in muscular dystrophy: evidence for a neural factor in pathogenesis.' *Journal of Neurology, Neurosurgery and Psychiatry*, **34**, 353–356

CAUGHEY, J. E. and MYRIANTHOPOULOS, N. C. (1963). *Dystrophia Myotonica and Related Disorders*. Springfield, Ill.: Thomas

CAULFIELD, J. B., REBEIZ, J. J. and ADAMS, R. D. (1968).

'Viral involvement of human muscle.' *Journal Pathology and Bacteriology*, **96**, 232–234

CAUSEY, E. and HOFFMAN, H. (1955). 'Axon sprouting partially deneurotized nerves.' *Brain*, **78**, 661–688

CAVANAGH, J. B. (1954). 'The toxic effects of tri-ortho cresyl phosphate on the nervous system. An exper mental study in hens.' *Journal of Neurology, Neur surgery and Psychiatry*, **17**, 163–172

CAVANAGH, J. B. (1964). 'Peripheral nerve changes ortho-cresyl phosphate poisoning in the cat.' *Journ of Pathology and Bacteriology*, **87**, 365–383

CAVANAGH, J. B. and CHEN, F. C. K. (1971). 'Amino ac incorporation in protein during the "silent phase before organo-mercury and p-bromophenylacetylure neuropathy in the rat.' *Acta neuropathologica (Berlin* **19**, 216–224

CECCARELLI, B. and HURLBUT, W. P. (1975). 'The effec of prolonged repetitive stimulation in hemicholiniu on the frog neuromuscular junction.' *Journal Physiology*, **247**, 163–188

CHACO, J. and TAUSTEIN, I. (1969). 'Myotonia dystr phica and Friedreich's ataxia in one patient.' *Europea Neurology*, **2**, 123–126

CHARCOT, J. M. (1887). 'Dégénerations secondaires c cause cérébrale (fin): Amyotrophies consécutives.' I *Oeuvres Completes de J. M. Charcot*, **4**, 235–24 Paris: Bureaux du Progres Medical

CHERINGTON, M. (1973). 'Botulism: electrophysiologic and therapeutic observations.' In *New Developmen in Electromyography and Clinical Neurophysiolog* Ed. by J. E. Desmedt. Vol. 1, pp. 375–379. Bas Karger

CHERINGTON, M. and RYAN, D. W. (1968). 'Botulism ar guanidine.' *New England Journal of Medicine*, **27** 931–933

CHOU, S. M. (1967). 'Myxovirus-like structures in a ca of human chronic polymyositis.' *Science, N.Y.*, **15** 1453–1455

CHOU, S. M. and GUTMANN, L. (1970). 'Picornavirus-lik crystals in subacute polymyositis.' *Neurology (Minnea polis)*, **20**, 205–213

CHU, L. W. (1954). 'A cytological study of anterior hor cells isolated from human spinal cord.' *Journal c Comparative Neurology*, **100**, 381–413

CHUNG, C. S., MORTON, N. E. and PETERS, H. A. (1960 'Serum enzymes and genetic carriers in muscula dystrophy.' *American Journal of Human Genetic* **12**, 52–66

CHURCHILL-DAVIDSON, H. C. and WISE, R. P. (1963 'Neuromuscular transmission in the newborn infant *Anaesthesiology*, **24**, 271–278

CLAMANN, H. P. (1970). 'Activity of single motor uni during isometric tension.' *Neurology (Minneapolis* **20**, 254–260

CLARK, A. W., MAURO, A., LONGNECKER, H. E. and HURL BUT, W. P. (1970). 'Effects of black widow spider venor on the frog neuromuscular junction. Effects on the fir structure of the frog neuromuscular junction.' *Natur (London)*, **225**, 703–705

CLARK, S. L., LUTON, F. H. and CUTLER, J. T. (1939). ' form of congenital myotonia in goats.' *Journal c Nervous and Mental Disease*, **90**, 297–309

CLOSE, R. I. (1972). 'Dynamic properties of mammalian skeletal muscles.' *Physiological Reviews*, **52**, 129–197

CLOWARD, R. B. (1960). 'The clinical significance of the sinu-vertebral nerve of the cervical spine in relation to the cervical disk syndrome.' *Journal of Neurology, Neurosurgery and Psychiatry*, **23**, 321–326

COËRS, C. (1952). 'The vital staining of muscle biopsies with methylene blue.' *Journal of Neurology, Neurosurgery and Psychiatry*, **15**, 211–215

COËRS, C., TELERMAN-TOPPET, NICOLE and GERARD, J-M. (1973). 'Terminal innervation ratio in neuromuscular disease.' *Archives of Neurology*, **29**, 210–222

COËRS, C. and WOOLF, A. L. (1959). *The Innervation of Muscle: A Biopsy Study*. Oxford: Blackwell Scientific Publications

COHEN, CAROLYN (1975). 'The protein switch of muscle contraction.' *Scientific American*, **233**, 36–45.

COHEN, L. and MORGAN, Juliet (1976). 'Diethylstilbestrol effects on serum enzymes and isoenzymes in muscular dystrophy.' *Archives of Neurology*, **33**, 480–484

COHEN, M. W. (1972). 'The development of neuromuscular connexions in the presence of D-tubocurarine.' *Brain Research*, **41**, 457–463

COLQUHOUN, D., RANG, H. P. and RITCHIE, J. M. (1974). 'The binding of tetrodotoxin and α-bungarotoxin to normal and denervated mammalian muscle.' *Journal of Physiology*, **240**, 199–226

CONEN, P. E., MURPHY, E. G. and DONOHUE, W. L. (1963). 'Light and electron microscope studies of ''myogranules'' in a child with hypotonia and muscle weakness.' *Canadian Medical Association Journal*, **89**, 983–986

CONN, J. W., FAJANS, S. S., LOUIS, L. H., STREETEN, D. H. P. and JOHNSON, R. D. (1957). 'Intermittent aldosteronism in periodic paralysis.' *Lancet*, **1**, 802–805

CONRAD, J. T. and GLASER, G. H. (1964). 'Spontaneous activity at myoneural junction in dystrophic muscle.' *Archives of Neurology*, **11**, 310–316

COOK, J. A. (1777). *A Voyage Towards the South Pole and Around the World*. Vol. ii, pp. 112–113. London: Straham and Cadell

COOK, S. D., MURRAY, M. N., WHITAKER, J. N. and DOWLING, P. (1969). 'Myelinotoxic antibody in the Guillain-Barré syndrome.' *Neurology (Minneapolis)*, **19**, 284

COOK, W. H., WALKER, J. H. and BARR, M. L. (1951). 'A cytological study of transneuronal atrophy in the cat and the rabbit.' *Journal of Comparative Neurology*, **94**, 267–291

CORBIN, K. B. and GARDINER, E. D. (1937). 'Decrease in number of myelinated fibres in human spinal roots with age.' *Anatomical Record*, **68**, 63–74

CORI, G. T. (1957). 'Biochemical aspects of glycogen deposition disease.' *Modern Problems in Padiatrics*, **3**, 344–358

COSMOS, Ethel (1964). 'Intracellular distribution of calcium in developing breast muscle of normal and dystrophic chickens.' *Journal of Cell Biology*, **23**, 241–252

COSMOS, Ethel (1973). 'Muscle-nerve transplants. Experimental models to study influences on differentiation.' *Physiologist*, **16**, 167–177

COSMOS, Ethel and BUTLER, Jane (1972). 'Differentiation of muscle transplanted between normal and dystrophic chickens.' In *Research in Muscle Development and the Muscle Spindle*. Ed. by B. Q. Banker, R. J. Przyblski, J. P. Van Der Meulen and M. Victor, pp. 149–162. Amsterdam: Excerpta Medica

COSTANTIN, L. L. (1970). 'The role of sodium currents in the radial spread of contraction in frog muscle fibres.' *Journal of General Physiology*, **55**, 703–715

COSTANTIN, L. L. and PODOLSKY, R. J. (1967). 'Depolarization of the internal membrane system in the activation of frog skeletal muscle.' *Journal of General Physiology*, **50**, 1101–1124

COTTER, Mary, HUDLICKÁ, Olga, PETTE, D., STAUDTE, H. and VRBOVÁ, Gerta (1972). 'Changes of capillary density and enzyme pattern in fast rabbit muscles during long term stimulation.' *Journal of Physiology*, **230**, 34–35P

CREESE, R. (1968). 'Sodium fluxes in diaphragm muscle and the effects of insulin and serum proteins.' With an appendix by D. J. Jenden. *Journal of Physiology*, **197**, 255–278

CREESE, R. and NORTHOVER, Jean (1961). 'Maintenance of isolated diaphragm with normal content.' *Journal of Physiology*, **155**, 343–357

CREESE, R., SCHOLES, N. W. and WHALEN, W. J. (1958). 'Resting potentials of diaphragm muscle after prolonged anoxia.' *Journal of Physiology*, **140**, 301–317

CREUTZFELDT, O. D., ABBOTT, B. C., FOWLER, W. M. and PEARSON, C. M. (1963). 'Muscle membrane potentials in episodic adynamia.' *Electroencephalography and Clinical Neurophysiology*, **15**, 508–519

CRITCHLEY, M. (1962). In 'Discussion on motor neurone disease.' *Proceedings of the Royal Society of Medicine*, **55**, 1032–1033

CSEUZ, K. A., THOMAS, J. E., LAMBERT, E. H., LOVE, J. G. and LIPSCOMB, P. R. (1966). 'Long-term results of operation for carpal tunnel syndrome.' *Mayo Clinic Proceedings*, **41**, 232–241

CULLEN, M. J. and FULTHORPE, J. J. (1975). 'Stages in fibre breakdown in Duchenne muscular dystrophy. An electron-microscopic study.' *Journal of Neurological Sciences*, **24**, 179–200

CUMINGS, J. N. (1962). 'Biochemical aspects of motoneurone disease.' *Proceedings of the Royal Society of Medicine*, **55**, 1023–1024

CURRIE, S. (1971). 'Experimental myositis. The *in-vivo* and *in vitro* activity of lymph-node cells.' *Journal of Pathology*, **105**, 169–185

CURRIE, S., SAUNDERS, M., KNOWLES, M. and BROWN, A. D. (1971). 'Immunological aspects of polymyositis.' *Quarterly Journal of Medicine*, **40**, 63–84

DAHLBÄCK, O., ELMQVIST, D., JOHNS, T. R., RADNER, S. and THESLEFF, S. (1961). 'An electrophysiological study of the neuromuscular junction in myasthenia gravis.' *Journal of Physiology*, **156**, 336–343

DASGUPTA, A. and SIMPSON, J. A. (1962). 'Relation between firing frequency of motor units and muscle tension in the human.' *Electromyography*, **2**, 117–218

DASTUR, D. K. and RAZZAK, Z. A. (1973). 'Possible neurogenic factor in muscular dystrophy: its similarity to denervation atrophy.' *Journal of Neurology, Neurosurgery and Psychiatry*, **36**, 399–410

DAVIES, D. M. (1954). 'Recurrent peripheral-nerve palsies in a family.' *Lancet*, **ii**, 266–268

DAVIES, D. V. (Ed.) (1967). *Gray's Anatomy*, 34th ed., p. 1234. London: Longmans

DAVIS, C. J. F. (1970). 'Prolonged Nembutal narcosis of the cat and its effects upon the isometric contraction characteristics of fast twitch and slow twitch skeletal muscle.' Ph.D. Thesis, University of Bristol, Bristol, England. Cited by D. M. Lewis, C. J. C. Kean and J. D. McGarrick (1974). In *Annals of the New York Academy of Sciences*, **228**, 105–120

DAVIS, F. A. and JACOBSON, S. (1971). 'Altered thermal sensitivity in injured and demyelinated nerve. A possible model of temperature effects in multiple sclerosis.' *Journal of Neurology, Neurosurgery and Psychiatry*, **34**, 551–561

DAVIS, R. and KOELLE, G. E. (1967). 'Electron microscopic localization of acetylcholinesterase and non-specific cholinesterase at the neuromuscular junction by the gold thiocholine and gold-thiolacetic acid methods.' *Journal of Cell Biology*, **34**, 157–171

DAWKINS, R. L. (1965). 'Experimental myositis associated with hypersensitivity to muscle.' *Journal of Pathology and Bacteriology*, **90**, 619–625

DEFARIA, C. (1976). 'Motor unit estimates in the human abductor pollicis longus muscle.' In preparation

DÉJÉRINE, J. (1889). 'De la névrite périphérique dans l'atrophie musculaire des hemiplegiques.' *Comptes Redus Hebdomadaires des Séances et Mémoires de la Société de Biologie*. **41**, 523–530

DeLORME, T. L. (1945). 'Restoration of muscle power by heavy resistance exercises.' *Journal of Bone and Joint Surgery*, **27**, 645–667

DENBOROUGH, M. A. and LOVELL, R. R. H. (1960). 'Anaesthetic deaths in a family.' *Lancet*, **ii**, 45

DENNIS, M. J. and MILEDI, R. (1974). 'Non-transmitting neuromuscular junctions during an early stage of end-plate reinnervation.' *Journal of Physiology*, **239**, 553–570

DENNY-BROWN, D. E. (1929). 'The histological features of striped muscle in relation to its functional activity.' *Proceedings of the Royal Society, Series B*, **104**, 371–411

DENNY-BROWN, D. and BRENNER, C. (1944). 'Paralysis of nerve induced by direct pressure and by tourniquet.' *Archives of Neurology and Psychiatry (Chicago)*, **51**, 1–26

DENNY-BROWN, D. and NEVIN, S. (1941). 'The phenomenon of myotonia.' *Brain*, **64**, 1–18

DESMEDT, J. (1959). 'The physio-pathology of neuromuscular transmission and the trophic influence of motor innervation.' *American Journal of Physical Medicine*, **38**, 248–261

DESMEDT, J.. E. (1966). 'Presynaptic mechanisms in myasthenia gravis.' In *Myasthenia Gravis*. Ed. by K. E. Osserman. *Annals of the New York Academy of Sciences*, **135**, 209–246

DESMEDT, J. E. (1973). 'The neuromuscular disorder in myasthenia gravis.' In *New Developments in Electromyography and Clinical Neurophysiology*. Ed. by J. E. Desmedt. Vol. i, pp. 241–304. Basel: Karger

DESMEDT, J. E. and BORENSTEIN, S. (1973). 'Collateral reinnervation of muscle fibres by motor axons of dystrophic motor units.' *Nature (London)*, **246**, 500–501

DESMEDT, J. E., EMERYK, BARBARA, RENOIRTE, P. and HAINAUT, K. (1968). 'Disorder of muscle contraction processes in sex-linked (Duchenne) muscular dystrophy with correlative electromyographic study of myopathic involvement in small hand muscles.' *American Journal of Medicine*, **45**, 853–872

DEVREOTES, P. N. (1975). 'Acetylcholine receptor turn over in membranes of developing muscle fibers.' *Society for Neuroscience, 5th Annual Meeting, New York* Abstract no. 945

DIENGOTT, D., ROZSA, O., LEVY, N. and MUAMMAR, S. (1964). 'Hypokalaemia in barium poisoning.' *Lancet* **ii**, 343–344

DILLON, J. B., FIELDS, J., GUMAS, T., JENDEN, D. J. and TAYLOR, D. B. (1955). 'An isolated human voluntary muscle preparation.' *Proceedings of the Society of Experimental Biology and Medicine*, **90**, 409

DOUGLAS, W. B. (1972). 'Sciatic cross-innervation of parabiotic mice. I. Surgical method and comments on animal care.' *Laboratory Animal Science*, **22**, 559–56

DOUGLAS, W. B. (1975). 'Sciatic cross-innervation of normal and dystrophic muscles in parabiotic mice: isometric contractile responses of reinnervated tibialis anticus and triceps surae.' *Experimental Neurology* **48**, 647–663

DOUGLAS, W. B. and COSMOS, Ethel (1975). 'Histochemical responses of dystrophic murine muscles cross innervated by sciatic nerves of normal mice.' In *Exploratory Concepts in Muscle (II)*. Ed. by A. T Milhorat, pp. 374–380. Amsterdam: Excerpta Medica

DOWNES, J. M., GREENWOOD, B. M. and WRAY, S. H. (1966). 'Autoimmune aspects of myasthenia gravis.' *Quarterly Journal of Medicine*, **35**, 85–105

DRACHMAN, D. B., MURPHY, S. R., NIGAM, M. P. and HILLS, J. R. (1967). 'Myopathic changes in chronically denervated muscles.' *Archives of Neurology*, **16**, 14–24

DRACHMAN, D. B., TOYKA, K. V. and MYER, E. (1974). 'Prednisone in Duchenne muscular dystrophy.' *Lancet* **ii**, 1409–1412

DRAHOTA, Z., and GUTMANN, E. (1961). 'The influence of age on the course of reinnervation of muscle.' *Gerontologia*, **5**, 88–109

DRAHOTA, Z. and GUTMANN, E. (1963). 'Long-term regulatory influence of the nervous system on some metabolic differences in muscles of different function.' *Physiologia Bohemoslovaca*, **12**, 339–348

DROZ, B. and LEBLOND, C. P. (1963). 'Axonal migration of proteins in the central nervous system and peripheral nerves as shown by radioautography. *Journal of Comparative Neurology*, **121**, 325–346

DUBOIS-DALCQ, M., BUYSE, M., BUYSE, G. and GORCE, F (1971). 'The action of Guillain-Barré syndrome serum on myelin. A tissue culture and electron microscopic analysis.' *Journal of the Neurological Sciences*, **13** 67–83

DUBOWITZ, V. (1965). 'Enzyme histochemistry of skeletal muscle. Part II. Developing human muscle.' *Journal of Neurology, Neurosurgery and Psychiatry*, **28**, 519–524

DUBOWITZ, V. (1967). 'Cross innervated mammalian skeletal muscle: histochemical, physiological and biochemical observations.' *Journal of Physiology*, **193**, 481–496

DUBOWITZ, V. (1969). 'Chemical and structural changes in muscle. The importance of the nervous system.' In *Some Inherited Disorders of Brain and Muscle*. Ed. by J. D. Allan and D. N. Raine, p. 32. Edinburgh: Livingstone

DUBOWITZ, V. (1974). 'Histochemical aspects of muscle disease.' In *Disorders of Voluntary Muscle*. Ed. by J. N. Walton, 3rd edn., pp. 310–359. Edinburgh: Churchill Livingstone

DUBOWITZ, V. and BROOKE, M. H. (1973). *Muscle Biopsy: a Modern Approach*. London: Saunders

DUBOWITZ, V. and CROME, L. (1969). 'The central nervous system in Duchenne muscular dystrophy.' *Brain*, **92**, 805–808

DUBOWITZ, V. and PEARSE, A. G. E. (1960). 'Reciprocal relationship of phosphorylase and oxidative enzymes in skeletal muscle.' *Nature (London)*, **185**, 701–702

DUCHEN, L. W. (1970a). 'Changes in motor innervation and cholinesterase localization induced by botulinum toxin in skeletal muscle of the mouse: differences between fast and slow muscles.' *Journal of Neurology, Neurosurgery and Psychiatry*, **33**, 40–54

DUCHEN, L. W. (1970b). 'The effect in the mouse of nerve crush and regeneration on the innervation of skeletal muscles paralysed by Clostridium botulinum toxin.' *Journal of Pathology*, **102**, 9–14

DUCHEN, L. W. (1971). 'An electronmicroscopic study of the changes induced by botulinum toxin in the motor end-plates of slow and fast skeletal muscle fibres of the mouse.' *Journal of Neurological Sciences*, **14**, 47–60

DUCHEN, L. W. and STEFANI, E. (1971). 'Electrophysiological studies of neuromuscular transmission in hereditary "motor end-plate disease" of the mouse.' *Journal of Physiology*, **212**, 535–548

DUCHEN, L. W., STOLKIN, C. and TONGE, D. A. (1972). 'Light and electronmicroscopic changes in slow and fast skeletal muscle fibres and their motor end-plates in the mouse after the local injection of tetanus toxin.' *Journal of Physiology*, **222**, 136–137P

DUCHENNE, G. B. (1861, 1872). *De l'électrisation localisée et son application a la pathologie et a la thérapeutique*. 2nd and 3rd edns. Paris: Baillière et fils

DULHUNTY, Angela F. and FRANZINI-ARMSTRONG, Clara (1975). 'The relative contributions of the folds and caveolae to the surface membrane of frog skeletal fibres at different sarcomere lengths.' *Journal of Physiology*, **250**, 513–539

DULHUNTY, Angela F. and GAGE, P. W. (1973). 'Differential effects of glycerol treatment on membrane capacity and excitation-contraction coupling in toad sartorius fibres.' *Journal of Physiology*, **234**, 373–408

DUNCAN, D. (1934). 'A determination of the number of nerve fibres in the eighth thoracic and the largest lumbar ventral roots of the albino rat.' *Journal of Comparative Neurology*, **59**, 47–60

DURACK, D. T., GUBBAY, S. S. and KAKULAS, B.A. (1969). 'Electrophysiological studies in the Rottnest quokka with nutritional myopathy.' *Australian Journal of Experimental Biology and Medical Science*, **47**, 581–588

DYCK, R. J. and LAMBERT, E. H. (1968a). 'Lower motor and primary sensory neuron diseases with peroneal muscular atrophy. I. Neurologic, genetic and electrophysiologic findings in hereditary polyneuropathies.' *Archives of Neurology*, **18**, 603–618

DYCK, P. J. and LAMBERT, E. H. (1968b). 'Lower motor and primary sensory neuron diseases with peroneal muscular atrophy. II. Neurologic, genetic and electrophysiologic findings in various neuronal degenerations.' *Archives of Neurology*, **18**, 619–625

DYKEN, M. L., SMITH, D. M. and PEAK, R. L. (1967). 'An electromyographic diagnostic screening test in McArdle's disease and a case report.' *Neurology (Minneapolis)*, **17**, 45–50

EARL, C. J., FULLERTON, Pamela, WAKEFIELD, G. S. and SCHUTTA, H. S. (1964). 'Hereditary neuropathy, with liability to pressure palsies.' *Quarterly Journal of Medicine*, **33**, 481–498

EATON, L. M. and LAMBERT, E. H. (1957). 'Electromyography and electric stimulation of nerves in diseases of motor unit: observations on the myasthenic syndrome associated with malignant tumours.' *Journal of the American Medical Association*, **163**, 1117–1124

EBERSTEIN, A. and SANDOW, A. (1963). 'Fatigue mechanisms in muscle fibres.' In *The Effect of Use and Disease on Neuromuscular Functions*, pp. 516–526. Ed. by E. Gutmann and P. Hnik. Amsterdam: Elsevier

ECCLES, J. C., ECCLES, R. M. and LUNDBERG, A. (1958). Action potentials of alpha motoneurones supplying fast and slow muscles. *Journal of Physiology*, **142**, 275–291

ECCLES, J. C., LIBET, B. and YOUNG, R. R. (1958). 'The behaviour of chromatolysed motoneurones studied by intracellular recording.' *Journal of Physiology*, **143**, 11–40

ECCLES, J. C. and SHERRINGTON, C. S. (1930). 'Numbers and contraction values of individual motor units examined in some muscles of the limb.' *Proceedings of the Royal Society, Series B.*, **106**, 326–357

EDSTRÖM, L. (1970a). 'Selective changes in the sizes of red and white muscle fibres in upper motoneurone lesions and Parkinsonism.' *Journal of Neurological Sciences*, **11**, 537–550

EDSTRÖM, L. (1970b). 'Selective atrophy of red muscle fibres in the quadriceps in long-standing knee-joint dysfunction. Injuries to the anterior cruciate ligament.' *Journal of the Neurological Sciences*, **11**, 551–558

EDSTRÖM, L. and EKBLOM, B. (1972). 'Differences in sizes of red and white muscle fibres in vastus lateralis of musculus quadriceps femoris of normal individuals and athletes. Relation to physical performance.' *Scandinavian Journal of Clinical and Laboratory Investigations*, **30**, 175–181

EDSTRÖM, L. and KUGELBERG, E. (1968). 'Histochemical composition, distribution of fibres and fatiguability of single motor units. Anterior tibial muscle of the rat.' *Journal of Neurology, Neurosurgery and Psychiatry*, **31**, 424–433

EDWARDS, R. H. T., HILL, D. K. and MCDONNELL, M. (1972). 'Myothermal and intramuscular pressure measurements during isometric contractions of the human quadriceps muscle.' *Journal of Physiology*, **224**, 58–59P

EISEN, A., KARPATI, G., CARPENTER, S. and DANON, J. (1974). 'The motor unit profile of the rat soleus in experimental myopathy and reinnervation.' *Neurology (Minneapolis)*, **24**, 878–884

EISENBERG, Brenda R. (1974). 'Quantitative ultrastructural analysis of adult mammalian skeletal muscle fibres.' In *Exploratory Concepts in Muscular Dystrophy II*. Ed. by A. T. Milhorat. New York: Excerpta Medica

EISENBERG, R. S. and GAGE, P. W. (1969). 'Ionic conductances of the surface and transverse tubular membranes of frog sartorius fibres.' *Journal of General Physiology*, **53**, 279–297

EKSTEDT, J. (1964). 'Human single muscle fibre action potentials.' *Acta Physiologica Scandinavica*, **61**, Suppl. 226, 1–96

EKSTEDT, J. and STÅLBERG, E. (1967). 'Myasthenia gravis. Diagnostic aspects by a new electrophysiological method.' *Opuscula Medica*, **12**, 73–76

ELLIS, K. O. and CARPENTER, J. F. (1972). 'Studies on the mechanism of action of Dantrolene sodium.' *Naunyn-Schmiedebergs Archives of Pharmacology*, **275**, 83–94

ELMQVIST, D., HOFMANN, W. W., KUGELBERG, J. and QUASTEL, D. M. J. (1964). 'An electrophysiological investigation of neuromuscular transmission in myasthenia gravis.' *Journal of Physiology*, **174**, 417–434

ELMQVIST, D. and JOSEFSSON, J-O (1962). 'The nature of the neuromuscular block produced by neomycine.' *Acta Physiologica Scandinavica*, **54**, 105–110

ELSBERG, C. A. (1917). 'Experiments on motor nerve regeneration and the direct neurotization of paralysed muscles by their own and foreign nerves.' *Science, N.Y.*, **45**, 318–320

ELUL, R., MILEDI, R. and STEFANI, E. (1968). 'Neurotrophic control of contracture in slow muscle fibres.' *Nature (London)*, **217**, 1274–1275

EMERY, A. E. H. (1963). 'Clinical manifestations in two carriers of Duchenne Muscular Dystrophy.' *Lancet*, **i**, 1126–1128

ENDO, M. (1966). 'Entry of fluorescent dyes into the sarcotubular system of the frog muscle.' *Journal of Physiology*, **185**, 224–238

ENGEL, A. G. (1966). 'Electron microscopic observations in thyrotoxic and corticosteroid myopathies.' *Mayo Clinic Proceedings*, **41**, 785–796

ENGEL, A. G. (1972). 'Neuromuscular manifestation of Graves' disease.' *Mayo Clinic Proceedings*, **47**, 919–925

ENGEL, A. G. and ANGELINI, C. (1973). 'Carnitine deficiency of human skeletal muscle with associated lipid storage myopathy: a new syndrome.' *Science, N.Y.*, **179**, 899–901

ENGEL, A. G., GOMEZ, M. R., SEYBOLD, M. E. and LAMBERT, E. H. (1973). 'The spectrum and diagnosis of acid maltase deficiency.' *Neurology (Minneapolis)*, **23**, 95–106

ENGEL, A. G. and LAMBERT, E. H. (1969). 'Calcium activation of electrically inexcitable muscle fibres in primary hypokalemic periodic paralysis.' *Neurology (Minneapolis)*, **19**, 851–858

ENGEL, A. G., POTTER, C. S. and ROSEVEAR, J. W. (1967) 'Studies on carbohydrate metabolism and mitochondria respiratory activities in primary hypokalemic periodic paralysis.' *Neurology (Minneapolis)*, **17**, 329–336

ENGEL, A. G., TSUJIHATA, M., LINDSTROM, J. and LENNON vanda A. (1976). 'The motor end plate in myasthenia gravis and in the experimental autoimmune myasthenia.' *Annals of the New York Academy o Sciences*. **274**, 60–79

ENGEL, W. K. (1962). 'The essentiality of histo- and cytochemical studies of skeletal muscle in the investigation of neuromuscular disease.' *Neurology (Minneapolis)*, **12**, 778–794

ENGEL, W. K. (1971a). 'Myotonia. A different point of view.' *California Medicine*, **114**, 32–37

ENGEL, W. K. (1971b). 'Nouvelle hypothèse sur la pathogénie de la dystrophie musculaire pseudo-hypertrophique de Duchenne.' *Revue Neurologique*, **124** 291–298

ENGEL, W. K. and BROOKE, M. H. (1966). 'Histochemistry of the myotonic disorders.' In *Progressive Muskel dystrophie, Myotonie, Myasthenie*. Ed. by E. Kuhn pp. 203–222. Heidelberg: Springer

ENGEL, W. K., HOGENHUIS, L. A. H., COLLIS, W. J. SCHALCH, D. S., BARLOW, M. H., GOLD, G. N. and DORMAN, J. D. (1969). 'Metabolic studies and thera peutic trials in amyotrophic lateral sclerosis.' In *Moto Neuron Diseases*. Ed. by F. H. Norris, Jr and L. T Kurland, pp. 199–208. New York: Grune and Stratton

ENGEL, W. K. and WARMOLTS, J. R. (1971). 'Myasthenia gravis: a new hypothesis of the pathogenesis and a new form of treatment.' In *Myasthenia Gravis*. Ed. by W. S. Fields. *Annals of the New York Academy o Sciences*, **183**, 72–87

ENGEL, W. K. and WARMOLTS, J. R. (1973). 'The motor unit. Disease affecting it *in toto* or *in portio*.' In *New Developments in Electromyography and Clinical Neurophysiology*. Ed. by J. E. Desmedt. Vol. 1, pp 141–177. Basel: Karger

ENTIN, M. A. (1968). 'Carpal tunnel syndrome and its variants.' *Surgical Clinics of North America*, **48** 1097–1112

ERB, W. (1879). 'Über einen neuen, wahrscheinlich bulbären Symptamenkomplex.' *Archiv für Psychiatrie und Nervenkrankheiten*, **9**, 336–350

ERB, W. H. (1876). 'Diseases of the peripheral cerebro spinal nerves.' In H. S. Von Ziemssen, *Cyclopaedia o the Practice of Medicine*, trans. by A. H. Buck. Vol. 11 London: Sampson Low

ERB, W. H. (1884). 'Über die "juvenile Form" der progressiven muskelatrophie ihre beziehungen zur sogenante pseudohypertrophie der muskeln.' *Deutsches Archiv für klinische Medecin*, **34**, 466–519

ERB, W. H. (1891). 'Dystrophia muscularis progressiva Klinische und pathologischanatomische Studien. *Deutsche Zeitschrift für Nervenheilkunde*, **1**, 173–261

ERNSTER, L., IKKOS, D. and LUFT, R. (1959). 'Enzymi studies of human skeletal muscle mitochondria: a too in clinical metabolic research.' *Nature (London)*, **184** 1851–1854

EXNER, S. (1885). 'Notiz zu der Fage von der Faserverthelung mehreren nerven in einem Muskeln.' *Pfluegers Archiv. European Journal of Physiology*, **36**, 572–576

AMBROUGH, D. M. (1970). 'Acetylcholine sensitivity of muscle fibre membranes: mechanism of regulation by motoneurones.' *Science N.Y.*, **168**, 372–373

AMBROUGH, D. M., DRACHMAN, D. B. and SATYAMURTI, S. (1973). 'Neuromuscular junction in myasthenia gravis: decreased acetylcholine receptors.' *Science, N.Y.*, **182**, 293–295

AMBROUGH, D., HARTZELL, H. C., RASH, J. E. and RITCHIE, AILEEN K. (1974). 'Receptor properties of developing muscle.' In *Trophic Functions of the Neuron*. Ed. by D. B. Drachman. *Annals of the New York Academy of Sciences*, **228**, 47–61

ARMER, T. W., BUCHTHAL, F. and ROSENFALCK, P. (1960). 'Refractory period of human muscle after the passage of a propagated action potential.' *Electroencephalography and Clinical Neurophysiology*, **12**, 455–466

ATT, P. and KATZ, B. (1951). 'An analysis of the end-plate potential recorded with an intracellular electrode.' *Journal of Physiology*, **115**, 320–370

ATT, P. and KATZ, B. (1952). 'Spontaneous subthreshold activity of motor nerve endings.' *Journal of Physiology*, **117**, 109–128

EASBY, T. E. and BROWN, W. F. (1974). 'Variation of motor unit size in the human extensor digitorum brevis and thenar muscles.' *Journal of Neurology, Neurosurgery and Psychiatry*, **37**, 916–926

EINSTEIN, B., LINDEGÅRD, B., NYMAN, E. and WOHLFART, G. (1955). 'Morphologic studies of motor units in normal human muscles.' *Acta Anatomica*, **23**, 127–142

ENICHEL, G. M., DAROFF, R. B. and GLASER, G. H. (1964). 'Hemiplegic atrophy: histological and etiologic considerations.' *Neurology (Minneapolis)*, **14**, 883–890

ENICHEL, G. M. and SHY, G. M. (1963). 'Muscle biopsy experience in myasthenia gravis.' *Archives of Neurology*, **9**, 237–243

EUDELL, P. and FISHER, W. (1956). 'Tropische und vasomotorische Storungen bei kapsulaen Hemiplegien.' *Deutsches Archiv für klinische Medecin*, **203**, 117–134

EX, S., SONESSON, B., THESLEFF, S. and ZELENÁ, JIRINA (1966). 'Nerve implants in botulinum poisoned mammalian muscles.' *Journal of Physiology*, **184**, 872–882

IEHN, W. and PETER, J. B. (1971). 'Properties of the fragmented sarcoplasmic reticulum from fast twitch and slow twitch muscles.' *Journal of Clinical Investigation*, **50**, 570–573

ILOGAMO, G. and GABELLA, G. (1966). 'Cholinesterase behaviour in the denervated and reinnervated muscles.' *Acta anatomica*, **63**, 199–214

ISCHBACH, G. D., NAMEROFF, M. and NELSON, P. G. (1971). 'Electrical properties of chick skeletal muscle fibres developing in cell culture.' *Journal of Cellular Physiology*, **78**, 289–300

ISCHBACH, G. D. and ROBBINS, N. (1969). 'Changes in contractile properties of disused soleus muscles.' *Journal of Physiology*, **201**, 305–320

ISCHMAN, D. A. (1972). 'Development of striated muscle.' In *The Structure and Function of Muscle*, 2nd edn. Ed. by G. H. Bourne, pp. 75–148. New York: Academic Press

LACKE, W. E., BLUME, R. P., SCOTT, W. R., FOLDES, F. F. and OSSERMAN, K. E. (1971). 'Germine mono- and diacetate in myasthenia gravis.' In *Myasthenia Gravis*. Ed. by W. S. Fields. *Annals of the New York Academy of Sciences*, **183**, 316–333

FLOYD, W. F., KENT, P. and PAGE, F. (1955). 'An electromyographic study of myotonia.' *Electroencephalography and Clinical Neurophysiology*, **7**, 621–630

FORD, L. E. and PODOLSKY, R. J. (1972). 'Intracellular calcium movements in skinned muscle fibres.' *Journal of Physiology*, **223**, 21–33

FORSTER, F. M. and ALPERS, B. J. (1944). 'Site of origin of fasciculations in voluntary muscle.' *Archives of Neurology and Psychiatry (Chicago)*, **51**, 264–267

FORSTER, F. M., BORKOWSKI, W. J. and ALPERS, B. J. (1946). 'Effects of denervation on fasciculations in human muscle.' *Archives of Neurology and Psychiatry (Chicago)*, **56**, 276–283

FRANK, E., JANSEN, J. K. S., LØMO, T. and WESTGAARD, R. (1974). 'Maintained function of foreign synapses on hyperinnervated skeletal muscle fibres of the rat.' *Nature (London)*, **247**, 375–376

FRANK, E., JANSEN, J. K. S., LØMO, T. and WESTGAARD, R. (1975). 'The interaction between foreign and original motor nerves innervating the soleus muscle of rats.' *Journal of Physiology*, **247**, 725–743

FRANK, G. B. (1958). 'Inward movement of calcium as a link between electrical and mechanical events in contraction.' *Nature (London)*, **182**, 1800–1801

FRANZINI-ARMSTRONG, C. and PORTER, K. R. (1964). 'Sarcolemmal invaginations constituting the T-system on fish muscle fibres.' *Journal of Cell Biology*, **22**, 675–696

FRASER, D. C., PALMER, A. C., SENIOR, J. E. B., PARKES, J. D. and YEALLAND, M. F. T. (1970). 'Myasthenia gravis in the dog.' *Journal of Neurology, Neurosurgery and Psychiatry*, **33**, 431–437

FRIEDMAN, A. P. and FREEDMAN, D. (1950). 'Amyotrophic lateral sclerosis.' *Journal of Nervous and Mental Diseases*, **111**, 1–18

FRYKHOLM, R. (1951). 'Cervical nerve root compression resulting from disc degeneration and root-sleeve fibrosis. A clinical investigation.' *Acta Chirugica Scandinavica*, Suppl. 160, 1–149

FUKUHARA, N., TAKAMORI, M., GUTMANN, L., and CHOU, S. M. (1972). 'Eaton-Lambert Syndrome. Ultrastructural study of the motor end-plates.' *Archives of Neurology*, **27**, 67–78

FULKS, R. M., LI, J. B. and GOLDBERG, A. L. (1975). 'Effects of insulin, glucose and amino acids on protein turnover in rat diaphragm.' *Journal of Biological Chemistry*, **250**, 290–298

FULLERTON, Pamela M. (1969). 'Electrophysiological and histological observations on peripheral nerves in acrylamide poisoning in man.' *Journal of Neurology, Neurosurgery and Psychiatry*, **32**, 186–192

FULLERTON, Pamela M. and GILLIATT, R. W. (1967). 'Median and ulnar neuropathy in the guinea pig.' *Journal of Neurology, Neurosurgery and Psychiatry*, **30**, 393–402

FULTON, J. F. (1936). 'The interrelation of cerebrum and cerebellum in the regulation of somatic and autonomic functions.' *Medicine (Baltimore)*, **15**, 247–306

FULTON, J. F. (1949). *Physiology of the Nervous System*, 3rd ed. New York: Oxford University Press

GAGE, P. W. and EISENBERG, R. S. (1969a). 'Capacitance of the surface and transverse tubular membrane of frog sartorius muscle fibres.' *Journal of General Physiology*, **53**, 265–278

GAGE, P. W. and EISENBERG, R. S. (1969b). 'Action potentials, after potentials, and excitation-contraction coupling in frog sartorius fibres without transverse tubules.' *Journal of General Physiology*, **53**, 298–310

GALAVAZI, G, and SZIRMAI, J, A. (1971). 'Cytomorphometry of skeletal muscle: the influence of age and testosterone on the rat m. levator ani.' *Zeitschrift fur Zellforschung und Mikrokopische Anatomie*, **121**, 507–530

GALLUP, belinda and DUBOWITZ, V. (1973). 'Failure of "dystrophic" neurones to support functional regeneration of normal or dystrophic muscle in culture.' *Nature (London)*, **243**, 287–289

GAMSTORP, ingrid (1956). 'Adynamia episodica hereditaria.' *Acta Paediatrica*, **45** (Suppl. 108), 1–126

GAMSTORP, ingrid (1973). 'Involvement of peripheral nerves in disorders causing progressive cerebral symptoms and signs in infancy and childhood.' In *New Developments in Electromyography and Clinical Neurophysiology* Ed. by J. E. Desmedt. Vol. 2, pp. 306–312. Basel: Karger

GAMSTORP, ingrid and WOHLFART, G. (1959). 'A syndrome characterized by myokymia, myotonia, muscle wasting and increased perspiration.' *Acta Psychiatrica et Neurologica Scandinavica*, **34**, 181–194

GARÇIN, R., FARDEAU, M. and GODET-GUILLAIN, MME (1965). 'A clinical and pathological study of a case of alternating and recurrent external ophthalmoplegia with amyotrophy of the limbs observed for forty-five years: discussion of the relationship of this condition with myasthenia gravis.' *Brain*, **88**, 739–752

GARDNER, E. (1940). 'Decrease in human neurones with age.' *Anatomical Record*, **77**, 529–536

GARLAND, T. O. and PATTERSON, M. W. H. (1967). 'Six case of acrylamide poisoning.' *British Medical Journal*, **4**, 134–138

GEREN, B. B. (1954). 'The formation from the Schwann cell surface of myelin in the peripheral nerves of chick embryos.' *Experimental Cell Research*, **7**, 558–562

GIBBS, C. J. Jr and GAJDUSEK, D. C. (1969). 'Kuru—a prototype subacute infectious disease of the nervous system as a model for the study of amyotrophic lateral sclerosis.' In *Motor Neuron Diseases*. Ed. by F. H. Norris, Jr and L. T. Kurland, pp. 269–279

GILBERT, J. J., STEINBERG, Marta C. and BANKER, Betty Q. (1973). 'Ultrastructural alterals of the motor end-plate in myotonic dystrophy of the mouse (dy²ʲ/ dy²ʲ).' *Journal of Neuropathology and Experimental Neurology*

GILLESPIE, C. A., SIMPSON, D. R. and EDGERTON, V. R. (1974). 'Motor unit recruitment as reflected by muscle fibre glycogen loss in a prosimian (bushbaby) after running and jumping.' *Journal of Neurology, Neurosurgery and Psychiatry*, **37**, 817–824

GILLIATT, R. W. (1973). 'Recent advances in the pathophysiology of nerve conduction.' In *New Developments in Electromyography and Clinical Neurophysiology* Ed. by J. E. Desmedt. Vol. 2, pp. 2–18. Basel: Karger

GILLIATT, R. W. and HJORTH, R. J. (1972). 'Nerve conduction during Wallerian degeneration in the baboon.' *Journal of Neurology, Neurosurgery and Psychiatry*, **35**, 335–341

GILLIATT, R. W. and WILLISON, R. G. (1962). 'Peripheral nerve conduction in diabetic neuropathy.' *Journal of Neurology, Neurosurgery and Psychiatry*, **25**, 11–18

GITLIN, G. and SINGER, M. (1974). 'Myelin movements in mature mammalian peripheral nerve fibres.' *Journal of Morphology*, **143**, 167–186

GLATT, H. R. and HONEGGER, C. G. (1973). 'Retrograde axonal transport for cartography of neurones.' *Experientia*, **29**, 1515–1517

GLEES, P. and CLARK, W. E. LE GROS (1941). 'The termination of optic fibres in the lateral geniculate body of the monkey.' *Journal of Anatomy*, **75**, 295–308

GOLDBERG, A. L. (1968). 'Role of insulin in work induced growth of skeletal muscle.' *Endocrinology*, **83** 1071–1073

GOLDBERG, A. L. and GOODMAN, H. M. (1969). 'Relationship between growth hormone and muscular work in determining muscle size.' *Journal of Physiology*, **200** 655–666

GOLDBY, F. (1957). 'A note on transneuronal atrophy in the human lateral geniculate body.' *Journal of Neurology, Neurosurgery and Psychiatry*, **20**, 202–207

GOLDFLAM, S. (1895). 'Weitere Mittheilung über die paroxysmale, familiäre Lähmung.' *Deutsche Zeitschrift für Nervenheilkunde*, **7**, 1–31

GOLDKAMP, O. (1967). 'Electromyography and nerve conduction studies in 116 patients with hemiplegia.' *Archives of Physical Medicine*, **48**, 59–63

GOLDMAN, D. E. (1943). 'Potential, impedance and rectification in membranes.' *Journal of General Physiology*, **27**, 37–60

GOLDSPINK, G. (1965). 'Cytological basis of decrease in muscle strength during starvation.' *American Journal of Physiology*, **209**, 100–114

GOLDSPINK, G. (1970). 'The proliferation of myofibres during muscle fibre growth.' *Journal of Cell Science* **6**, 593–603

GOLDSPINK, G. (1972). 'Postembryonic growth and development of striated muscle.' In *The Structure and Function of Muscle*, 2nd edn. Ed. by G. H. Bourne. pp. 179–236. New York: Academic Press

GOLDSPINK, G. and ROWE, R. W. D. (1968). 'The growth and development of muscle fibres in normal and dystrophic mice.' In *Research in Muscular Dystrophy. Proceedings of the Fourth Symposium of the Muscular Dystrophy Group*, pp. 116–218. London: Pitman Medical

GOLDSTEIN, G. and HOFMANN, W. W. (1968). 'Electrophysiological changes similar to those of myasthenia gravis in rats with experimental autoimmune thymitis.' *Journal of Neurology, Neurosurgery and Psychiatry*, **31**, 453–459

GOLDSTEIN, G. and MANGANARO, A. (1971). 'Thymin: a thymic polypeptide causing the neuromuscular block of myasthenia gravis.' In *Myasthenia Gravis*. Ed. by W. S.

Fields. *Annals of the New York Academy of Sciences,* **183**, 230–240

GOLDSTEIN, G. and WHITTINGHAM, S. (1966). 'Experimental autoimmune thymitis. An animal model of human myasthenia gravis.' *Lancet,* **ii**, 315–318

GOLLNICK, P. D., KARLSSON, J., PIEHL, Karin and SALTIN, B. (1974). 'Selective glycogen depletion in skeletal muscle fibres of man following sustained contraction.' *Journal of Physiology,* **241**, 59–67

GOLLNICK, P. D., PIEHL, Karin and SALTIN, B. (1974). 'Selective glycogen depletion in human muscle fibres after exercise of varying intensity and at varying pedalling rates.' *Journal of Physiology,* **241**, 45–57

GOMBAULT, A. (1880). 'Contribution a l'étude anatomique de la névrite parenchymateuse subaiguë at chronique. Névrite segmentaire péri-axile.' *Archives de Neurologie,* Paris, **1**, 11–38

GONZÁLEZ-SERRATOS, H. (1971). 'Inward spread of activation in vertebrate muscle fibres.' *Journal of Physiology,* **212**, 777–799

GORDON, A. M., HUXLEY, A. F., and JULIAN, F. J. (1966). 'The variation in isometric tension with sarcomere length in vertebrate muscle fibres.' *Journal of Physiology,* **184**, 170–192

GORDON, E. E. (1967). 'Anatomical and biochemical adaptations of muscles to different exercises.' *Journal of the American Medical Association,* **201**, 755–758

GOTOH, F., KITAMURA, A., KOTO, A., KATAOKA, K. and ATSUJI, H. (1972). 'Abnormal insulin secretion in amyotrophic lateral sclerosis.' *Journal of the Neurological Sciences,* **16**, 201–207

GOWERS, W. H. (1899). *A Manual of Diseases of the Nervous System.* London: Churchill

GOWERS, W. R. (1902). 'On myopathy and a distal form.' *British Medical Journal,* **ii**, 89–92

GRAMPP, W., HARRIS, J. B. and THESLEFF, S. (1972). 'Inhibition of denervation changes in skeletal muscle by blockers of protein synthesis.' *Journal of Physiology,* **221**, 743–754

GRANIT, R., PHILLIPS, C. G., SKOGLUND, S. and STEG, G. (1957). 'Differentiation of tonic from phasic alpha ventral horn cells by stretch, pinna and crossed extensor reflexes.' *Journal of Neurophysiology,* **20**, 470–481

GRIMBY, L. and HANNERZ, J. (1970). 'Differences in recruitment order of motor units in phasic and tonic flexion reflex in "spinal man".' *Journal of Neurology, Neurosurgery and Psychiatry,* **33**, 562–570

GROB, D., JOHNS, R. J. and LILJSETRAND, A. (1957). 'Potassium movements in patients with familial periodic paralysis.' *American Journal of Medicine,* **23**, 356–375

GRUENER, R., MCARDLE, B., RYMAN, Brenda E. and WELLER, R. O. (1968). 'Contracture of phosphorylase deficient muscle.' *Journal of Neurology, Neurosurgery and Psychiatry,* **31**, 268–283

GRUENER, R., STERN, L. Z., PAYNE, Claire and HANNAPEL, Linda (1975). 'Hyperthyroid myopathy. Intracellular electrophysiological measurements in biopsied human skeletal muscle.' *Journal of Neurological Sciences,* **24**, 339–349

GRUNDFEST, H. (1936). 'Effects of hydrostatic pressures on the excitability, the recovery and the potential sequence of frog nerve.' *Cold Spring Harbour Symposia on Quantitative Biology,* **4**, 177–187

GUEDEL, A. E. (1937). *Inhalation Anaesthesia.* New York: Macmillan

GUTH, L., ALBERS, R. W. and BROWN, W. C. (1964). 'Quantitative changes in cholinesterase activity of denervated muscle fibres and sole plates.' *Experimental Neurology,* **10**, 236–250

GUTH, L., WATSON, Phyllis K. and BROWN, W. C. (1968). 'Effects of cross-innervation on some chemical properties of red and white muscles of rat and cat.' *Experimental Neurology,* **20**, 52–69

GUTH, L. and WELLS, J. (1974). 'Physiological and histochemical properties of the soleus muscle after denervation of its antagonists.' *Experimental Neurology,* **36**, 463–471

GUTH, L. and YELLIN, H. (1971). 'The dynamic nature of the so-called "fibre types" of mammalian skeletal muscles.' *Experimental Neurology,* **31**, 277–300

GUTMANN, E. (1971). 'Histology of degeneration and regeneration.' In *Electrodiagnosis and Electromyography,* 3rd edn. Ed. S. Licht, pp. 113–133. Baltimore: Waverly Press

GUTMANN, E., GUTMAN, L., MEDAWAR, P. B. and YOUNG, J. Z. (1942). 'The rate of regeneration of nerve.' *Journal of Experimental Biology,* **19**, 14–44

GUTMANN, E. and HANZLÍKOVÁ, V. (1966). 'Motor unit in old age.' *Nature (London),* **209**, 921–922

GUTMANN, E. and HANZLÍKOVÁ, V. (1972). *Age changes in the neuromuscular system.* Bristol: Scientechnica

GUTMANN, E., HANZLÍKOVÁ, V. and VYSKOČIL, F. (1971). 'Age changes in cross-striated muscle of the rat.' *Journal of Physiology,* **219**, 331–343

GUTMANN, E. and SANDOW, A. (1965). 'Caffeine induced contracture and potentiation of contraction in normal and denervated muscle.' *Life Sciences,* **4**, 1149–1156

GUTMANN, E., SCHIAFFINO, S. and HANZLÍKOVÁ, vera (1971). 'Mechanism of compensatory hypertrophy in skeletal muscle of the rat.' *Experimental Neurology,* **31**, 451–464

GUTMANN, E., VODIČKA, Z. and ZELENÁ, Jirina (1955). 'Veranderungen im quergestreiften. Muskel bei Durchtrennung in Abhängigkeit von der Länge des peripheren Stumpfes.' *Physiologia Bohemoslovaca,* **4**, 200–204

GUTMANN, E. and ŽAK, R. (1961). 'Nervous regulation of nucleic acid level in cross-striated muscle changes in denervated muscle.' *Physiologia Bohemoslovaca,* **10**, 493–500

GUYTON, A. C. and MACDONALD, M. A. (1947). 'Physiology of botulinus toxin.' *Archives of Neurology and Psychiatry (Chicago),* **57**, 578–592

HAGGAR, R. A. and BARR, M. L. (1950). 'Quantitative data on the size of synaptic end-bulbs in the cat's spinal cord.' *Journal of Comparative Neurology,* **93**, 17–35

HÁJEK, I., GUTMANN, E. and SYROVÝ, I. (1964). 'Proteolytic activity in denervated and reinnervated muscle.' *Physiologia Bohemoslovaca,* **13**, 32–38

HALL-CRAGGS, E. C. B. (1970). 'The longitudinal division of fibres in overloaded rat skeletal muscle.' *Journal of Anatomy,* **107**, 459–470

HAMBURGH, M., BORNSTEIN, M. B., PETERSON, E. R., CRAIN, S. M., MASUROVSKY, E. B. and KIRK, C. (1973).

'In vitro studies of regeneration and innervation of muscle from dystrophic (dy²ʲ) mutant mice.' In *Progress in Brain Research.* Ed. by D. H. Ford. Vol. 40, pp. 497–508. Amsterdam: Elsevier

HANNERZ, J. (1974). 'Discharge properties of motor units in relation to recruitment order in voluntary contraction.' *Acta Physiologica Scandinavica*, **91**, 374–384

HARMAN, J. B. and RICHARDSON, A. T. (1954). 'Generalized myokymia in thyrotoxicosis. Report of a case.' *Lancet*, **ii**, 473–474

HARPER, P. S. and DYKEN, P. R. (1972). 'Early onset dystrophia myotonica. Evidence supporting a maternal environmental factor.' *Lancet*, **ii**, 53–55

HARRIMAN, D. G. F., TAVERNER, D. and WOOLF, A. L. (1970). 'Ekbom's syndrome and burning paraesthesiae. A biopsy study by vital staining and electron microscopy of the intramuscular innervation with a note on age changes in motor nerve endings in distal muscles.' *Brain*, **93**, 393–406

HARRIS, A. J. and MILEDI, R. (1971). 'The effect of type D botulinum toxin on frog neuromuscular junctions.' *Journal of Physiology*, **217**, 497–515

HARRIS, J. B. and LUFF, A. R. (1970). 'The resting membrane potentials of fast and slow skeletal muscle fibres in the developing mouse.' *Comparative Biochemistry and Physiology*, **33**, 923–931

HARRIS, J. B. and MARSHALL, M. W. (1973). 'A study of action potential generation in murine dystrophy with reference to "functional denervation".' *Experimental Neurology*, **41**, 331–344

HARRIS, J. B. and MONTGOMERY, A. (1975). 'Some mechanical and electrical properties of distal hind limb muscles of genetically dystrophic mice (C57 BL/6 Jdy²ʲ/dy²ʲ).' *Experimental Neurology*, **48**, 569–585

HARRIS, J. B. and THESLEFF, S. (1972). 'Nerve stump length and membrane changes in denervated skeletal muscle.' *Nature New Biology*, **236**, 60–61

HARRIS, J. B., WALLACE, C. and WING, J. (1972). 'Myelinated nerve fibre counts in the nerves of normal and dystrophic mouse muscle.' *Journal of the Neurological Sciences*, **15**, 245–249

HARRIS, J. B. and WARD, M. R. (1975). 'Some electrophysiological properties of isolated extensor digitorum longus muscles from normal and genetically dystrophic hamsters.' *Experimental Neurology*, **46**, 103–114

HARRIS, J. B. and WILSON, P. (1971). 'Mechanical properties of dystrophic mouse muscle.' *Journal of Neurology, Neurosurgery and Psychiatry*, **34**, 512–520

HARVEY, A. M. (1939). 'The peripheral action of tetanus toxin.' *Journal of Physiology*, **96**, 348–365

HARTWIG. (1874). 'Inaugural dissertation.' In *Centralblatt für die medecinischen Wissenschaften*, **26**, 428 (1875)

HASHIMOTO, K. and ALDRIDGE, W. N. (1970). 'Biochemical studies on acrylamide: a neurotoxic agent.' *Biochemical Pharmacology*, **19**, 2591–2604

HASHIMOTO, K. and ANDO, K. (1973). 'Alteration of amino acid incorporation into proteins of the nervous system *in vitro* after administration of acrylamide to rats.' *Biochemical Pharmacology*, **22**, 1057–1066

HATHAWAY, P. W., ENGEL, W. K. and ZELLWEGER, H. (1970). 'Experimental myopathy after microarterial embolization. Comparison with childhood X-linked pseudohypertrophic muscular dystrophy.' *Archives of Neurology*, **22**, 365–378

HAUSMANOWA-PETRUSEWICZ, Irena and JEDRZEJOWSKA, Hanna (1971). 'Correlation between electromyographic findings and muscle biopsy in cases of neuromuscular disease.' *Journal of the Neurological Sciences*, **13**, 85–106

HAVARD, C. W. H., CAMPBELL, E. D. R., ROSS, H. B. and SPENCE, A. W. (1963). 'Electromyographic and histological findings in the muscles of patients with thyrotoxicosis.' *Quarterly Journal of Medicine*, **32**, 145–163

HAY, Elizabeth D. (1970). 'Regeneration of muscle in the amputated amphibian limb.' In *Regeneration of striated muscle, and myogenesis.* Ed. by A. Mauro, S. A. Shafiq and A. T. Milhorat, pp. 3–24. Amsterdam: Excerpta Medica

HAYFLICK, L. (1965). 'The limited *in vitro* lifetime of human diploid cell strains.' *Experimental Cell Research*, **37**, 614–636

HEILBRONN, E., MATTSON, C., STÅLBERG, E. and HILTON-BROWN, P. (1975). 'Neurophysiological signs of myasthenia in rabbits after receptor antibody development.' *Journal of the Neurological Sciences*, **24**, 59–64

HEILBRUNN, L. V. and WIERCINSKI, F. J. (1947). 'The action of various cations on muscle protoplasm.' *Journal of Cellular and Comparative Physiology*, **29**, 15–32

HENNEMAN, E., SOMJEN, G. and CARPENTER, D. O. (1965). 'Functional significance of cell size in spinal motoneurones.' *Journal of Neurophysiology*, **28**, 560–580

HENRIKSEN, J. D. (1956). 'Conduction Velocity of Motor Nerves in Normal Subjects and Patients with Neuromuscular Disorders.' M.S. (Phys. Med.) Thesis University of Minnesota

HESS, A. (1957). 'The experimental embryology of the foetal nervous system.' *Biological Reviews*, **32**, 231–260

HEUSER, J. E., REESE, T. S., and LANDIS, D. M. D. (1974). 'Functional changes in frog neuromuscular junctions studied with freeze-fracture.' *Journal of Neurocytology*, **3**, 109–131

HEWER, R. L. (1968). 'Study of fatal cases of Friedreich's ataxia.' *British Medical Journal*, **3**, 649–652

HILL, D. K. (1964). 'The space accessible to albumin within the striated muscle fibre of the toad.' *Journal of Physiology*, **175**, 275–294

HIRANO, A., KURLAND, L. T. and SAYRE, G. P. (1967). 'Familial amyotrophic lateral sclerosis. A subgroup characterized by posterior and spinocerebellar tract involvement and hyaline inclusions in the anterior horn cells.' *Archives of Neurology*, **6**, 232–242

HIRANO, A., MALAMUD, N., KURLAND, L. T. and ZIMMERMAN, H. M. (1969). 'A review of the pathologic findings in amyotrophic lateral sclerosis.' In *Motor Neuron Diseases.* Ed. by F. H. Norris, Jr and L. T. Kurland, pp. 51–60. New York and London: Grune and Stratton

HIRONAKA, T. and MIYATA, Y. (1975). 'Transplantation of skeletal muscle in normal and dystrophic mice.' *Experimental Neurology*, **47**, 1–15

HNÍK, P. (1972). 'Changes in function of muscle afferents during muscle atrophy (de-efferentation or tenotomy).' In Symposium on *Structure and Function of Normal and Disease Muscle and Peripheral Nerve* (Programme

Abstract No. 20), Kazimierz. Warsaw: Polish Academy of Sciences

HODES, R. (1948). 'Electromyographic study of defects of neuromuscular transmission in human poliomyelitis.' *Archives of Neurology and Psychiatry (Chicago)*, **60**, 457–473

HODES, R., LARRABEE, M. G. and GERMAN, W. (1948). 'The human electromyogram in response to nerve stimulation and the conduction velocity of motor axons. Study on normal and on injured peripheral nerves.' *Archives of Neurology and Psychiatry*, **60**, 340–365

HODGKIN, A. L. and HUXLEY, A. F. (1952a). 'Currents carried by sodium and potassium ions through the membrane of the giant axon of *Loligo*.' *Journal of Physiology*, **116**, 449–472

HODGKIN, A. L. and HUXLEY, A. F. (1952b). 'A quantitative description of membrane current and its application to conduction and excitation in nerve.' *Journal of Physiology*, **117**, 500–544

HODGKIN, A. L. and HOROWICZ, P. (1959). 'The influence of potassium and chloride ions on the membrane potentials of single fibres.' *Journal of Physiology*, **148**, 127–160

HOFFMAN, H. (1950a). 'Fate of interrupted nerve fibres regenerating into partially denervated muscles.' *Australian Journal of Experimental Biology and Medical Science*, **29**, 211–219

HOFFMAN, H. (1950b). 'Local re-innervation in partially denervated muscle: a histophysiological study.' *Australian Journal of Experimental Biology and Medical Science*, **28**, 383–397

HOFFMANN, J. (1893). 'Uber chronische spinale Muskelatrophie im Kindsalter, auf familiärer Basis.' *Deutsche Zeitschrift für Nervenheilkunde*, **3**, 427

HOFMANN, W. W., ALSTON, W. and ROWE, G. (1966). 'A study of individual neuromuscular junctions in myotonia.' *Electroencephalography and Clinical Neurophysiology*, **21**, 521–537

HOFMANN, W. W. and DENYS, E. H. (1972). 'Effects of thyroid hormone at the neuromuscular junction.' *American Journal of Physiology*, **223**, 283–287

HOFMANN, W. W., KUNDIN, J. E. and FARRELL, D. F. (1967). 'The pseudomyasthenic syndrome of Eaton and Lambert: an electrophysiological study.' *Electroencephalography and Clinical Neurophysiology*, **23**, 214–224

HOFMANN, W. W. and RUPRECHT, E. O. (1973). 'Observations on the efficiency of dystrophic muscle *in vitro*.' *Journal of Neurology, Neurosurgery and Psychiatry*, **36**, 565–573

HOFMANN, W. W. and SMITH, R. A. (1970). 'Hypokalemic periodic paralysis studies *in vitro*.' *Brain*, **93**, 445–474

HOFMANN, W. W. and THESLEFF, S. (1972). 'Studies on the trophic influence of nerve on skeletal muscle.' *European Journal of Pharmacology*, **20**, 256–260

HOGAN, E. L., DAWSON, D. M. and ROMANUL, F. C. A. (1965). 'Enzymatic changes in denervated muscle. II. Biochemical studies.' *Archives of Neurology*, **13**, 274–282

HOH, J. F. Y. (1975). 'Selective and non-selective re-innervation of fast-twitch and slow-twitch rat skeletal muscle.' *Journal of Physiology*, **251**, 791–801

HOLLIDAY, T. A., VAN METER, J. R., JULIAN, L. M. and

AMUNDSON, V. S. (1965). 'Electromyography of chickens with inherited muscular dystrophy.' *American Journal of Physiology*, **209**, 871–876

HOLTZER, H. (1970). In *Cell Differentiation*. Ed. by O. Schjeide and J. de Vellis, pp. 476–503. Princeton, N.Y.: Van Nostrand-Reinhold

HOPF, H. C. (1962). 'Untersuchungen über die Unterschiede in der Leitgeschwindigkeit motorischer Nervenfasern beim Menschen.' *Deutsches Zeitschrift für Nervenheilkunde*, **183**, 579–588

HOPF, H. C. (1963). 'Electromyographic study in so-called mononeuritis.' *Archives of Neurology (Chicago)*, **9**, 307–312

HOPF, H. C. and LUDIN, H. P. (1968). 'Neurogene Muskelatrophien, aufgetreten in Verlauf einer vornehmlich ocularen Myasthenia gravis.' *Nervenarzt*, **39**, 416–421

HOPKINS, A. (1970). 'The effect of acrylamide on the peripheral nervous system of the baboon.' *Journal of Neurology, Neurosurgery and Psychiatry*, **33**, 805–816

HOPKINS, A. P. and GILLIATT, R. W. (1971). 'Motor and sensory nerve conduction velocity in the baboon, normal values and changes during acrylamide neuropathy.' *Journal of Neurology, Neurosurgery and Psychiatry*, **34**, 415–426

HUANG, K. N. (1943). 'Pa Ping (transient paralysis simulating family periodic paralysis).' *Chinese Medical Journal*, **61**, 305–312

HUBBARD, J. I. and WILSON, D. F. (1973). 'Neuromuscular transmission in a mammalian preparation in the absence of blocking drugs and the effect of D-tubocurarine.' *Journal of Physiology*, **228**, 307–325

HUDGSON, P. and MASTAGLIA, F. L. (1974). 'Ultrastructural studies of disease muscle.' In *Disorders of Voluntary Muscle*. Ed. by J. N. Walton, 3rd edn., pp. 360–416. Edinburgh: Churchill Livingstone

HUIZAR, P., KUNO, M. and MIYATA, Y. (1975). 'Electrophysiological properties of spinal motoneurones of normal and dystrophic mice.' *Journal of Physiology*, **248**, 231–246

HULL, K. L. Jr and ROSES, A. D. (1976). 'Stoichiometry of sodium and potassium transport in erythrocytes from patients with myotonic muscular dystrophy.' *Journal of Physiology*, **254**, 169–181

HUMPHREY, J. G. and RICHARDSON, J. C. (1962). 'Myotonia associated with hypothyroidism.' *Canadian Medical Association Journal*, **87**, 1084

HUMPHREY, J. G. and SHY, G. M. (1962). 'Diagnostic electromyography: clinical and pathological correlation in neuromuscular disorders.' *Archives of Neurology*, **6**, 339–352

HUTCHINSON, J. (1879). 'On ophthalmoplegia externa, or symmetrical paralysis of the ocular muscles.' *Lancet*, **i**, 229

HUTTER, O. F. and NOBLE, D. (1960). 'The chloride conductance of frog skeletal muscle.' *Journal of Physiology*, **151**, 89–102

HUXLEY, A. F. (1959a). 'Local activation in muscle.' *Annals of the New York Academy of Sciences*, **81**, 446–452

HUXLEY, A. F. (1959b). 'Muscle structure and theories of contraction.' *Progress in Biophysics*, **7**, 255–318

HUXLEY, A. F. (1974). 'Muscular contraction (Review lecture).' *Journal of Physiology*, **243**, 1–43

HUXLEY, A. F. and NIEDERGERKE, R. (1954). 'Structural changes in muscle during contraction. Interference microscopy of living muscle fibres.' *Nature (London)*, **173**, 971–973

HUXLEY, A. F. and SIMMONS, R. M. (1971). 'Mechanical properties of the cross-bridges of frog striated muscle.' *Journal of Physiology*, **218**, 59–60P

HUXLEY, A. F. and TAYLOR, R. E. (1958). 'Local activation of striated muscle fibres.' *Journal of Physiology*, **144**, 426–441

HUXLEY, H. E. (1964). 'Evidence for continuity between the central elements of the triads and extracellular space in frog sartorius muscle.' *Nature (London)*, **202**, 1067–1071

HUXLEY, H. E. and HANSON, Jean (1954). 'Changes in the cross-striations of muscle during contraction and stretch and their structural interpretation.' *Nature (London)*, **173**, 973–976

IKAI, M., YABE, K. and ISCHII, K. (1967). 'Muskelkraft und Muskulare Ermudung bei Willkurlicher Anspannung und Elektrischer Reizung des Muskels.' *Sportarzt und Sportmedizin*, **5**, 197

IONASESCU, V. and LUCA, N. (1964). 'Studies on carbohydrate metabolism in amyotrophic lateral sclerosis and hereditary proximal spinal muscular atrophy.' *Acta Neurologica Scandinavica*, **40**, 45–57

IONESESCU, V., ZELLWEGER, H. and CONWAY, T. W. (1971). 'A new approach for carrier detection in Duchenne muscular dystrophy.' *Neurology (Minneapolis)*, **21**, 703–709

ISAACS, E. R., BRADLEY, W. G. and HENDERSON, G. (1973). 'Longitudinal fibre splitting in muscular dystrophy: a serial cinematographic study.' *Journal of Neurology, Neurosurgery and Psychiatry*, **36**, 813–819

ISAACS, H. (1961). 'A syndrome of continuous muscle fibre activity.' *Journal of Neurology, Neurosurgery and Psychiatry*, **24**, 319–325

ISAACS, H. and BARLOW, M. B. (1973). 'Malignant hyperpyrexia. Further muscle studies in asymptomatic carriers identified by creatinine phosphokinase screening.' *Journal of Neurology, Neurosurgery and Psychiatry*, **36**, 228–243

ISAACS, H. (1964). 'Quantal quander.' *South African Journal of Laboratory and Clinical Medicine*, **10**, 93–95

ISCH, F., ISCH TREUSSARD, C. and JESEL, M. (1972). 'Electromyographic features in muscular glycogenosis.' In *Structure and Function of Normal and Diseased Muscle and Peripheral Nerve* Abstract no. 79. Kazimierz, Poland: Polish Academy of Sciences

IWAYAMA, T. and OHTA, M. (1969). 'Morphology in neuromuscular function in myasthenia gravis.' *Proceedings of Myasthenia gravis Symposium* (Kyoto), **1**, 41–46

JABLECKI, C. and BRIMIJOIN, S. (1974). 'Reduced axoplasmic transport of choline acetyltransferase activity in dystrophic mice.' *Nature (London)*, **250**, 151–154

JACOBSON, S. and GUTH, L. (1965). 'An electrophysiological study of the early stages of peripheral nerve regeneration.' *Experimental Neurology*, **11**, 48–60

JANSEN, J. K. S., LØMO, T., NICOLAYSEN, K. and WESTGAARD, R. H. (1973). 'Hyperinnervation of skeletal muscle fibres: dependence on muscle activity.' *Science, N.Y.*, **181**, 559–561

JASMIN, G. and BOKDAWALA, F. (1970). 'Muscle transplantation in normal and dystrophic hamsters.' *Revu canadienne de biologie*, **29**, 197–201

JAYAM, A. V., RAJU, T. N. K., PANDYA, S. S. and DESAI A. D. (1970). 'Motor nerve conduction in the Duchenn type of muscular dystrophy.' *Neurology (India)*, **18** 8–12

JĘDRZEJOWSKA, Hanna (1968). 'Badania histopato logiczne wewnątrzmięśniowych rùchowych wtokie nerwowych w postępującej dystrofii mięśniowej. *Neuropatologia polska*, **6**, 359–402

JĘDRZEJOWSKA, H., JOHNSON, A. G. and WOOLF, A. L (1965). 'The intramuscular nerve endings in muscula dystrophy.' *Acta neuropathologica (Berlin)*, **5** 225–242

JĘDRZEJOWSKA-KUFAKOWSKA, Hanna, HAUSMANOWA-PETRUSEWICZ, Irena, GAWLIK, Z., RAFALOWSKA Janina and SLUCKA, Cecylia (1968). 'Zweryfi kowany sekeyjnie przypadek postępującej dystrofi mięśniowej typu Duchenne A.' *Neuropatologi. Polska*, **6**, 71–85

JENNEKENS, F. G. I., TOMLINSON, B. E. and WALTON, J. N (1971). 'Data on the distribution of fibre types in fiv human limb muscles. An autopsy study.' *Journal of th Neurological Sciences*, **14**, 245–257

JENNEKENS, F. G. I., TOMLINSON, B. E. and WALTON, J. N (1972). 'The extensor digitorum brevis: histological anc histochemical aspects.' *Journal of Neurology, Neuro surgery and Psychiatry*, **35**, 124–132

JERUSALEM, F., ENGEL, A. G. and GOMEZ, M. R. (1974a) 'Duchenne dystrophy. I. Morphometric study of the muscle microvasculature.' *Brain*, **97**, 115–122

JERUSALEM, F., ENGEL, A. G. and GOMEZ, M. R. (1974b) 'Duchenne dystrophy. II. Morphometric study of motor end-plate fine structure.' *Brain*, **97**, 123–130

JOHNS, R. J., GROB, D. and HARVEY, A. M. (1956). 'Studies in neuromuscular function. II. Effects of nerve stimulation in normal subjects and in patients with myasthenia gravis.' *Bulletin of the Johns Hopkins Hospital*, **99**, 125–135

JOHNS, T. R. and THESLEFF, S. (1961). 'Effects of motor inactivation on the chemical sensitivity of skeletal muscle.' *Acta Physiologica Scandinavica*, **51**, 136–141

JOHNSON, A. G. and WOOLF, A. L. (1965). 'Replacement at the neuromuscular synapse of the terminal axonic expansion by the Schwann cell.' *Acta neuropathologica*, **4**, 436–441

JOHNSON, H. A. and ERNER, S. (1972). 'Neurone survival in the ageing mouse.' *Experimental Gerontology*, **7**, 111–117

JOHNSON, M. A. and MONTGOMERY, A. (1975). 'Parabiotic reinnervation in normal and dystrophic mice. Part 2. Morphological studies.' *Journal of the Neurological Sciences*, **26**, 425–441

JOHNSON, M. A. and MONTGOMERY, A. (1976). 'Parabiotic reinnervation in normal and myopathic (BIO 14.6) hamsters.' *Journal of the Neurological Sciences*, **27**, 201–215

JOHNSON, Margaret A., POLGAR, J., WEIGHTMAN D. and APPLETON, D. (1973). 'Data on the distribution of fibre types in thirty-six human muscles.' *Journal of the Neurological Sciences*, **18**, 111–129

JOHNSON, R. T. (1969). 'Virologic studies and summary of Soviet experiments on the transmission of amyotrophic lateral sclerosis (ALS) to monkeys.' In *Motor Neuron Diseases*. Ed. by F. H. Norris, Jr and L. T. Kurland, pp. 280–283. New York: Grune and Stratton

JOLLY, F. (1895). 'Uber Myasthenia gravis pseudo-paralytica.' *Berliner klinische Wochenschrift*, **32**, 1–7

JONES, S. F. and KWANBUNBUMPEN, S. (1970). 'The effects of nerve stimulation and hemicholinium on synaptic vesicles at the mammalian neuromuscular junction.' *Journal of Physiology*, **207**, 31–50

JOSEFSSON, J. O. and THESLEFF, S. (1961). 'Electromyographic findings in experimental botulinum intoxication.' *Acta Physiologica Scandinavica*, **51**, 163–168

JUNTUNEN, J. and TERAVAINEN, H. (1972). 'Structure development of myoneural junctions in the human embryo.' *Histochemie*, **32**, 107–112

KAESER, H. E. and SANER, A. (1970). 'The effect of tetanus toxin on neuromuscular transmission.' *European Neurology*, **3**, 193–205

KAKULAS, B. A. (1966). 'Destruction of differentiated muscle cultures by sensitized cells.' *Journal of Pathology and Bacteriology*, **91**, 495–503

KALDEN, J. R., WILLIAMSON, W. G., JOHNSTON, R. J. and IRVINE, W. J. (1969). 'Studies on experimental autoimmune thymitis in guinea pigs.' *Clinical and Experimental Immunology*, **5**, 319–340

KALOW, W. A., BRITT, B. A., TERREAU, M. E. and HAIST, C. (1970). 'Metabolic error of muscle metabolism after recovery from malignant hyperthermia.' *Lancet*, **ii**, 895–898

KALYANARAMAN, K., SMITH, B. H. and CHADHA, A. L. (1973). 'Evidence for neuropathy in myotonic muscular dystrophy.' *Bulletin of the Los Angeles Neurological Societies*, **38**, 188–196

KAO, C. Y. (1966). 'Tetrodotoxin, saxitonin and their significance in the study of excitation phenomena.' *Pharmacological Reviews*, **18**, 997–1049

KARPATI, G., CARPENTER, S. and EISEN, A. A. (1972). 'Experimental core-like lesions and nemaline rods. A correlative morphological and physiological study.' *Archives of Neurology*, **27**, 237–251

KARPATI, G. and ENGEL, W. K. (1968). 'Correlative histochemical study of skeletal muscle after suprasegmental denervation, peripheral nerve section and skeletal fixation.' *Neurology (Minneapolis)*, **18**, 681–692

KATZ, B. (1966). *Nerve, Muscle and Synapse*. New York: McGraw-Hill

KATZ, B. and MILEDI, R. (1965). 'Propagation of electric activity in motor nerve terminals.' *Proceedings of the Royal Society*, B, **161**, 453–482

KATZ, B. and MILEDI, R. (1972). 'The statistical nature of the acetylcholine potential and its molecular components.' *Journal of Physiology*, **224**, 665–699

KELLERTH, J. O. (1973). 'Intracellular staining of cat spinal motoneurones with procion yellow for ultrastructural studies.' *Brain Research*, **50**, 415–418

KELLY, A. M. and ZACKS, S. I. (1969). 'The fine structure of motor end plate morphogenesis.' *Journal of Cell Biology*, **42**, 154–169

KERNAN, R. P. (1963). 'Resting potential of isolated rat muscles measured in plasma.' *Nature (London)*, **200**, 474–475

KEYNES, R. D., RITCHIE, J. M. and ROJAS, E. (1971). 'The binding of tetrodoxin to nerve membranes.' *Journal of Physiology*, **213**, 235–254

KLAUS, W., LÜLLMANN, H. and MUSCHOLL, E. (1960). 'Der Kalium-flux des normalen und denervierten rattenzwerchfells.' *Pflügers Archiv: European Journal of Physiology*, **271**, 761–775

KLINKERFUSS, G. H. and HAUGH, M. J. (1970). 'Sisuse atrophy of muscle. Histochemistry and electron microscopy.' *Archives of Neurology*, **22**, 309–320

KNOWLES, M., CURRIE, S., SAUNDERS, M., WALTON, J. N. and FIELD, E. J. (1969). 'Lymphocyte transformation in the Guillain-Barré syndrome.' *Lancet*, **ii**, 1168–1170

KOERNER, D. R. (1952). 'Amyotrophic lateral sclerosis on Guam.' *Annals of Internal Medicine*, **37**, 1204–1220

KOMIYA, Y. and AUSTIN, L. (1974). 'Axoplasmic flow of protein in the sciatic nerve of normal and dystrophic mice.' *Experimental Neurology*, **43**, 1–12

KOPEC, J., HAUSMANOWA-PETRUSEWICZ, I., RAWSKI, M. and WOLYNSKI, M. (1973). 'Automatic analysis in electromyography.' In *New Developments in Electromyography and Clinical Neurophysiology*. Ed. by J. E. Desmedt. Vol. 2, pp. 477–481. Basel: Karger

KOPELL, H. P. and THOMPSON, W. A. L. (1963). '*Peripheral entrapment neuropathies.*' Baltimore: Williams and Wilkins

KOZICKA, Anna, PROT, Janina and WASILEWSKI, R. (1971). 'Mental retardation in patients with Duchenne progressive muscular dystrophy.' *Journal of the Neurological Sciences*, **14**, 209–213

KRABBE, K. H. (1934). 'The myotonia acquista in relation to the postneuritic muscular hypertrophies.' *Brain*, **57**, 184–194

KRISTENSSON, K. and OLSSON, Y. (1971). 'Retrograde axonal transport of protein.' *Brain Research*, **29**, 363–365

KRNJEVIĆ, K. and MILEDI, R. (1958). 'Failure of neuromuscular propagation in rats.' *Journal of Physiology*, **140**, 440–461

KRULL, G. H., LEIJNSE, B., VIËTOR, W. P. J., VLEIGER, M. D., BRAAK, J. W. G. Ter and GERBRANDY, J. (1966). 'Myotonia produced by an unknown humoral substance.' *Lancet*, **ii**, 668–672

KUFFLER, S. W. and YOSHIKAMI, D. (1975). 'The number of transmitter molecules in a quantum: an estimate from iontophoretic application of acetylcholine at the neuromuscular synapse.' *Journal of Physiology*, **251**, 465–482

KUGELBERG, E., EDSTRÖM, L. and ABBRUZZESE, M. (1970). 'Mapping of motor units in experimentally reinnervated rat muscle. Interpretation of histochemical and atrophic fibre patterns in neurogenic lesions.' *Journal of Neurology, Neurosurgery and Psychiatry*, **33**, 319–329

KUGELBERG, E. and WELANDER, L. (1956). 'Heredofamilial juvenile muscular atrophy simulating muscular dystrophy.' *Archives of Neurology and Psychiatry*, **75**, 500–509

KUHN, E. (1973). 'Myotonia. The clinical evidence.' In *New Developments in Electromyography and Clinical Neurophysiology*. Ed. by J. E. Desmedt, Vol. 1, pp. 413–419. Basel: Karger

KUNO, M., MIYATA, Y. and MUÑOZ-MARTINEZ, E. J.

(1974a). 'Differential reaction of fast and slow α-moto-neurones to axotomy.' *Journal of Physiology*, **240**, 725–739

KUNO, M., MIYATA, Y. and MUÑOZ-MARTINEZ, E. J. (1974b). 'Properties of fast and slow alpha moto-neurones following motor reinnervation.' *Journal of Physiology*, **242**, 273–288

KUNZE, D., REICHMANN, G., EGGER, E., LEUSCHNER, G. and ECKHARDT, H. (1973). Erythrozytenlipide bei Pro-gressiver Muskeldystrophie.' *Clinica Chimica Acta*, **43**, 333–341

KURLAND, L. T., CHOI, N. W. and SAYRE, G. P. (1969). 'Implications of incidence and geographic patterns on the classification of amyotrophic lateral sclerosis.' In *Motor Neuron Diseases*. Ed. by F. H. Norris, Jr and L. T. Kurland, pp. 28–50. New York: Grune and Stratton

KURLAND, L. T. and MULDER, D. W. (1954). 'Epi-demiologic investigations of amyotrophic lateral sclerosis. 2. Familial aggregations indicative of dominant inheritance. Parts 1 and 2.' *Neurology (Minneapolis)*, **5**, 182–196 and 249–268

KUSUI, K. (1962). 'Epidemiological study on amyotrophic lateral sclerosis (ALS) and other neighbouring motor neurone diseases in Kii peninsula (Japanese).' *Psychiatria et Neurologia Japonica*, **64**, 85–99

LA COUR, D., JUUL-JENSEN, P. and RESKE-NIELSEN, EDITH (1973). 'Central and peripheral mechanisms in malig-nant hyperthermia.' In *Malignant Hyperthermia (Symposium)*. Ed. by R. A. Gordon *et al.*, pp. 380–386. Springfield, Ill.: Thomas

LAIRD, J. L. and TIMMER, R. F. (1965). 'Homotrans-plantation of dystrophic and normal muscle.' *Archives of Pathology*, **80**, 442–446

LAMBERT, E. H. (1969). 'The accessory deep peroneal nerve. A common variation in innervation of extensor digitorum brevis.' *Neurology (Minneapolis)*, **19**, 1169–1176

LAMBERT, E. H. and ELMQVIST, D. (1971). 'Quantal com-ponents of end-plate potentials in the myasthenic syn-drome.' In *Myasthenia Gravis*. Ed. by W. S. Fields. *Annals of the New York Academy of Sciences*, **183**, 183–199

LAMBERT, E. H., ELMQVIST, D. and GOLDSTEIN. (1969). Unpublished observations cited by E. H. Lambert. In *Motor Neurone Diseases*. Ed. by F. H. Norris Jr and L. T. Kurland, p. 144. New York: Grune and Stratton

LAMBERT, E. H., LINDSTROM, J. M. and LENNON, VANDA A. (1975). 'End-plate potentials in experimental auto-immune myasthenia.' *Annals of the New York Academy of Sciences*, **274**, 300–318

LAMBERT, E. H., UNDERDAHL, L. O., BECKETT, SYBIL and MEDEROS, L. O. (1951). 'A study of the ankle jerk in myxoedema.' *Journal of Clinical Endocrinology*, **11**, 1186–1205

LAMPERT, P. W. (1969). 'Mechanism of demyelination in experimental allergic neuritis.' *Laboratory Investiga-tion*, **20**, 127–138

LANARI, A. (1947). 'La contracción miotónica en el hombre después de curarizacion.' *Medicina (Buenos Aires)*, **7**, 21–26

LANDMESSER, Lynn (1971). 'Contractile and electrical responses of vagus-innervated frog sartorius.' *Journal of Physiology*, **213**, 707–725

LANDMESSER, Lynn (1972). 'Pharmacological properties, cholinesterase activity and anatomy of nerve-muscle junctions in vagus-innervated frog sartorius.' *Journal of Physiology*, **220**, 243–256

LANDMESSER, Lynn and MORRIS, Deborah G. (1975). 'The development of functional innervation in the hind limb of the chick embryo.' *Journal of Physiology*, **249**, 301–326

LANDON, D. N. and LANGLEY, O. K. (1971). 'The local chemical environment of nodes of Ranvier: a study of cation binding.' *Journal of Anatomy*, **108**, 419–432

LANDOUZY, L. J. and DÉJÉRINE, J. (1886). 'Nouvelles recherches clinique et anatomopathologiques sur la myopathie atrophique progressive à propos de six observations nouvelles, dontune avec autopsie.' *Revue de médecin (Paris)*, **6**, 977–1027

LAPRESLE, J. and FARDEAU, M. (1965). 'Diagnostic histo-logique des atrophies et hypertrophies musculaires.' In *Proceedings of the 8th International Congress of Neurology, Vienna, 1965.* Neuromuscular Diseases, pp. 47–66. Vienna: Wiener

LAPRESLE, J., FARDEAU, M. and SAID, G. (1973). 'L'hyper-trophie musculaire vraie secondaire à une atteinte ner-veuse périphérique. Etude clinique et histologique d'une observation d'hypertrophie du mollet con-secutive à une sciatique.' *Revue Neurologique*, **128**, 153–160

LAW, P. K. and ATWOOD, H. L. (1972). 'Nonequivalence of surgical and natural denervation in dystrophic mouse muscle.' *Experimental Neurology*, **34**, 200–209

LAW, P. K. and ATWOOD, H. L. (1974). 'Does axonal sprouting occur in dystrophic mouse muscles?' *Experientia*, **30**, 155–156

LAW, P. K., COSMOS, Ethel, BUTLER, Jane and MCCOMAS, A. J. (1976). 'The absence of dystrophic characteristics in normal muscles successfully cross-reinnervated by nerves of dystrophic genotype: physiological and cytochemical study of crossed solei of normal and dystrophic parabiotic mice.' *Experimental Neurology*, **51**, 1–21

LeDOUARIN, Nicole (1973). 'A biological cell labelling technique and its use in experimental embryology.' *Developmental Biology*, **30**, 217–222

LEKSELL, L. (1945). 'The action potential and excitatory effects of the small ventral root fibres to skeletal muscle.' *Acta Physiological Scandinavica*, **10**, Suppl. 31, 1–84

LENMAN, J. A. R. (1959). 'Quantitative electromyographic changes associated with muscular weakness.' *Journal of Neurology, Neurosurgery and Psychiatry*, **22**, 306–310

LENNON, Vanda A., LINDSTROM, J. M. and SEYBOLD, Marjorie E. (1975). 'Experimental autoimmune myasthenia (EAMG): a model of myasthenia gravis in rats and guinea pigs.' *Journal of Experimental Medicine* **141**, 1365–1375

LENNON, Vanda A., LINDSTROM, J. M. and SEYBOLD, Marjorie E. (1976). 'Experimental autoimmune myasthenia: cellular and humoral immune responses.' *Annals of the New York Academy of Sciences*. In press

LENTZ, T. L., ROSENTHAL, Jean and MAZURKIEWICZ, J. E.

(1975). 'Cytochemical localization of acetylcholine receptors by means of peroxidase-labelled α-bungarotoxin.' *Society for Neuroscience, 5th Annual Meeting, New York.* Abstract No. 976

LESCH, M., PARMLEY, W. W., HAMOSH, Margit, KAUFMAN, S. and SONNENBLICK, E. H. (1968). 'Effects of acute hypertrophy on the contractile properties of skeletal muscle.' *American Journal of Physiology,* **214,** 685–690

LEVI-MONTALCINI, Rita and ANGELETTI, P. U. (1961). 'Growth control of sympathetic system by a specific protein factor.' *Quarterly Review of Biology,* **36,** 99–108

LEVIN, P. M. and BRADFORD, F. K. (1938). 'The exact origin of the cortico-spinal tract in the monkey.' *Journal of Comparative Neurology,* **68,** 411–422

LEWIS, D. M. (1972). 'The effect of denervation on the mechanical and electrical responses of fast and slow mammalian twitch muscle.' *Journal of Physiology,* **222,** 51–95

LEYBURN, P. and WALTON, J. N. (1959). 'The treatment of myotonia: a controlled trial.' *Brain,* **82,** 81–91

LEYDEN, E. (1876). *Klinik der Ruckenmarks-krankheiten,* **2,** p. 531. Berlin: Hirschwald

LINDSLEY, D. (1935). 'Electrical activity of human motor units during voluntary contraction.' *American Journal of Physiology,* **114,** 90–99

LINDSTROM, J. M., LENNON, vanda, SEYBOLD, Marjorie E. and WHITTINGHAM, S. (1976). 'Experimental autoimmune myasthenia and myasthenia gravis: biochemical and immunochemical aspects.' *Annals of the New York Academy of Sciences.* In press

LINKHART, T. A., YEE, G. W. and WILSON, B. W. (1975). 'Myogenic defect in acetylcholinesterase regulation in muscular dystrophy of the chicken.' *Science, N.Y.,* **187,** 549–550

LIPICKY, R. J. and BRYANT, S. H. (1973). 'A biophysical study of the human myotonias.' In *New Developments in Electromyography and Clinical Neurophysiology.* Ed. by J. E. Desmedt, pp. 451–463. Basel: Karger

LIPICKY, R. J., BRYANT, S. H. and SALMON, J. H. (1971). 'Cable parameters, sodium, potassium, chloride, and water content, and potassium efflux in isolated external intercostal muscle of normal volunteers and patients with myotonia congenita.' *Journal of Clinical Investigation,* **50,** 2091–2103

LISHMAN, W. A. and RUSSELL, W. R. (1961). 'The brachial neuropathies.' *Lancet,* **ii,** 941–946

LIVERSEDGE, L. A. (1959). 'Cervical spondylosis.' *Postgraduate Medical Journal,* **35,** 380–383

LIVERSEDGE, L. A. and CAMPBELL, M. J. (1974). 'Motor neurone diseases.' In *Disorders of Voluntary Muscle,* 3rd ed. Ed. by J. N. Walton, pp. 775–803. Edinburgh: Churchill Livingstone

LØMO, T. and ROSENTHAL, Jean (1972). 'Control of ACh sensitivity of muscle activity in the rat.' *Journal of Physiology,* **221,** 493–513

LOWENBERG-SCHARENBERG, K. (1962). 'Degeneration of peripheral nerves and muscles in myasthenia gravis.' *Transactions of the American Neurological Association,* **87,** 235–237

LUBINSKA, Liliana and NIEMIERKO, stella (1970). 'Velocity and intensity of bidirectional migration of

acetylcholinesterase in transected nerves.' *Brain Research,* **27,** 329–342

LUCO, J. V. and EYZAGUIRRE, C. (1955). 'Fibrillation and hypersensitivity to ACh in denervated muscle. Effect of length of degenerating nerve fibres.' *Journal of Neurophysiology,* **18,** 65–73

LUDIN, H. P. (1970). 'Microelectrode study of dystrophic human skeletal muscle.' *European Neurology,* **3,** 116–121

LUDIN, H. P., SPIESS, H. and KOENIG, M. P. (1969). 'Neuromuscular dysfunction associated with thyrotoxicosis.' *European Neurology,* **2,** 269–278

LUFT, R., IKKOS, D., PALMIERI, G., ERNSTER, L. and AFZELIUS, B. (1962). 'A case of severe hypermetabolism of nonthyroid origin with a defect in the maintenance of mitochondrial respiratory control: a correlated clinical, biochemical and morphological study.' *Journal of Clinical Investigation,* **41,** 1776–1804

LÜTTGAU, H. C. (1965). 'The effect of metabolic inhibitors on the fatigue of the action potential in single muscle fibres.' *Journal of Physiology,* **178,** 45–67

LYON, Mary F. (1961). 'Gene action in the X-chromosomes of the mouse. (*Mus. musculus L.*).' *Nature (London),* **190,** 372–373

MCARDLE, B. (1951). 'Myopathy due to a defect in muscle glycogen breakdown.' *Clinical Science,* **10,** 13–33

MCARDLE, B. (1962). 'Adynamia episodica hereditaria and its treatment.' *Brain,* **85,** 121–148

MCARDLE, B. (1974). 'Metabolic and endocrine myopathies.' In *Disorders of Voluntary Muscle.* Ed. by J. N. Walton, 3rd ed., pp. 726–759. Edinburgh: Churchill Livingstone

MCARDLE, J. J. and ALBUQUERQUE, E. X. (1973). 'A study of the reinnervation of fast and slow mammalian muscles.' *Journal of General Physiology,* **61,** 1–23

MACCALLUM, J. B. (1898). 'On the histogenesis of the striated muscle fibre, and the growth of the human sartorius muscle.' *Bulletin of Johns Hopkins Hospital,* **9,** 208–215

MCCOMAS, A. J. (1975). 'The neural hypothesis. In Workshop on the aetiology of Duchenne muscular dystrophy.' In *Recent Advances in Myology* (Proceedings of the 3rd International Congress on Muscle Diseases). Ed. by W. G. Bradley, D. Gardner-Medwin and J. N. Walton. pp. 152–158. Amsterdam: Excerpta Medica

MCCOMAS, A. J., CAMPBELL, M. J. and SICA, R. E. P. (1971). 'Electrophysiological study of dystrophia myotonica.' *Journal of Neurology, Neurosurgery and Psychiatry,* **34,** 132–139

MCCOMAS, A. J., FAWCETT, P. R. W., CAMPBELL, M. J. and SICA, R. E. P. (1971a). 'Electrophysiological estimation of the number of motor units within a human muscle.' *Journal of Neurology, Neurosurgery and Psychiatry,* **34,** 121–131

MCCOMAS, A. J., JORGENSEN, P. B. and UPTON, A. R. M. (1974). 'The neurapraxic lesion: a clinical contribution to the study of trophic mechanisms.' *Canadian Journal of Neurological Sciences,* **1,** 170–179

MCCOMAS, A. J. and MOSSAWY, S. J. (1965). 'Electrophysiological investigation of normal and dystrophic muscles in mice.' In *Research in Muscular Dystrophy. Proceedings of the Third Symposium of the Muscular*

Dystrophy Group, pp. 317–341. London: Pitman Medical

McCOMAS, A. J. and MROŻEK, K. (1967). 'Denervated muscle fibres in hereditary mouse dystrophy.' *Journal of Neurology, Neurosurgery and Psychiatry*, 30, 526–530

McCOMAS, A. J. and MROŻEK, K. (1968). 'The electrical properties of muscle fibre membranes in dystrophia myotonia and myotonia congenita.' *Journal of Neurology, Neurosurgery and Psychiatry*, 31, 441–447

McCOMAS, A. J., MROŻEK, K. and BRADLEY, W. G. (1968). 'The nature of the electrophysiological disorder in adynamia episodica.' *Journal of Neurology, Neurosurgery and Psychiatry*, 31, 448–452

McCOMAS, A. J., MROŻEK, K., GARDNER-MEDWIN, D. and STANTON, W. H. (1968). 'Electrical properties of muscle fibre membranes in man.' *Journal of Neurology, Neurosurgery and Psychiatry*, 31, 434–440

McCOMAS, A. J. and SICA, R. E. P. (1970). 'Muscular dystrophy: myopathy or neuropathy?' *Lancet*, i, 1119

McCOMAS, A. J., SICA, R. E. P. and BROWN, J. C. (1971). 'Myasthenia gravis: evidence for a "central" defect.' *Journal of Neurological Sciences*, 13, 107–113

McCOMAS, A. J., SICA, R. E. P. and CAMPBELL, M. J. (1971). '"Sick" motoneurones. A unifying concept of muscle disease.' *Lancet*, i, 321–325

McCOMAS, A. J., SICA, R. E. P., CAMPBELL, M. J. and UPTON, A. R. M. (1971b). 'Functional compensation in partially denervated muscles.' *Journal of Neurology, Neurosurgery and Psychiatry*, 34, 453–460

McCOMAS, A. J., SICA, R. E. P. and CURRIE, S. (1970). 'Evidence for a neural factor in muscular dystrophy.' *Nature (London)*, 226, 1263–1264

McCOMAS, A. J., SICA, R. E. P. and CURRIE, S. (1971). 'An electrophysiological study of Duchenne dystrophy.' *Journal of Neurology, Neurosurgery and Psychiatry*, 34, 461–468

McCOMAS, A. J., SICA, R. E. P., MCNABB, A. R., GOLDBERG, W. M. and UPTON, A. R. M. (1973a). 'Neuropathy in thyrotoxicosis.' *New England Journal of Medicine*, 289, 219–220

McCOMAS, A. J., SICA, R. E. P., MCNABB, A. R., GOLDBERG, W. M. and UPTON, A. R. M. (1974a). 'Evidence for reversible motoneurone dysfunction in thyrotoxicosis.' *Journal of Neurology, Neurosurgery and Psychiatry*, 37, 548–558

McCOMAS, A. J., SICA, R. E. P. and PETITO, F. (1973). 'Muscle strength in boys of different ages.' *Journal of Neurology, Neurosurgery and Psychiatry*, 36, 171–173

McCOMAS, A. J., SICA, R. E. P. and UPTON, A. R. M. (1974). 'Multiple muscle analysis of motor units in muscular dystrophy.' *Archives of Neurology*, 30, 249–251

McCOMAS, A. J., SICA, R. E. P., UPTON, A. R. M. and AGUILERA, Nidia (1973b). 'Functional changes in motoneurones of hemiparetic muscles.' *Journal of Neurology, Neurosurgery and Psychiatry*, 36, 183–193

McCOMAS, A. J., SICA, R. E. P., UPTON, A. R. M., AGUILERA, Nidia and CURRIE, S. (1971c). 'Motoneurone dysfunction in patients with hemiplegic atrophy.' *Nature New Biology*, 233, 21–23

McCOMAS, A. J., SICA, R. E. P., UPTON, A. R. M. and PETITO, F. (1974b). 'Sick motoneurones and muscle disease.' In *Trophic Functions of the Neuron*. Ed. by

D. B. Drachman. *Annals of the New York Academy of Sciences*, 228, 261–279

McCOMAS, A. J. and THOMAS, A. C. (1968a). 'Fast and slow twitch muscles in man.' *Journal of the Neurological Sciences*, 7, 301–307

McCOMAS, A. J. and THOMAS, A. C. (1968b). 'A study of the muscle twitch in the Duchenne type muscular dystrophy.' *Journal of the Neurological Sciences*, 7, 309–312

McCOMAS, A. J., UPTON, A. R. M. and JORGENSEN, P. B. (1975a). 'Patterns of motoneurone dysfunction and recovery.' *Canadian Journal of Neurological Sciences*, 2, 5–15

McCOMAS, A. J., UPTON, A. R. M. and JORGENSEN, P. B. (1975b). 'Serial studies of sick motoneurones: the silent synapses.' In *Recent Advances in Myology* (Proceedings of the 3rd International Congress on Muscle Diseases). Ed. by W. G. Bradley, D. Gardner-Medwin and J. N. Walton. pp. 84–90. Amsterdam: Excerpta Medica

McCOMAS, A. J., UPTON, A. R. M. and SICA, R. E. P. (1973). 'Motoneurone disease and ageing.' *Lancet*, ii, 1477–1480

MacCONNACHIE, H. F., ENESCO, M. and LEBLOND, C. P. (1964). 'The mode of increase in the number of skeletal muscle nuclei in the postnatal rat.' *American Journal of Anatomy*, 114, 245–253

McCOUCH, G. P., AUSTIN, G. M., LIU, C. N. and LIU, C. Y. (1958). 'Sprouting as a cause of spasticity.' *Journal of Neurophysiology*, 21, 205–216

MacDERMOT, violet (1960). 'The changes in the motor end-plates in myasthenia gravis.' *Brain*, 83, 24–36

MacDERMOT, violet (1961). 'The histology of the neuromuscular junction in dystrophia myotonica.' *Brain*, 84, 75–84

McDONALD, W. I. (1963a). 'The effects of experimental demyelination on conduction in peripheral nerve: a histological and electrophysiological study. I. Clinical and histological observations.' *Brain*, 86, 481–500

McDONALD, W. I. (1963b). 'The effects of experimental demyelination on conduction in peripheral nerve: a histological and electrophysiological study. II. Electrophysiological observations.' *Brain*, 86, 501–524

McINTYRE, A. R., BENNET, A. L. and BRODKEY, J. S. (1959). 'Muscular dystrophy in mice of the Bar Harbor strain.' *Archives of Neurology and Psychiatry*, 81, 678–683

McLELLAN, D. L. and SWASH, M. (1976). 'Longitudinal sliding of the median nerve during movements of the upper limb.' *Journal of Neurology, Neurosurgery and Psychiatry*, 39, 566–570

MacLENNAN, D. H. and HOLLAND, P. C. (1975). 'Calcium transport in sarcoplasmic reticulum.' *Annual Review of Biophysics and Bioengineering*, 4, 377–404

McPHEDRAN, A. M., WUERKER, R. B. and HENNEMAN, E. (1965). 'Properties of motor units in heterogeneous pale muscle (m. gastrocnemius) of the cat.' *Journal of Neurophysiology*, 28, 85–99

McPHERSON, A. and TOKUNAGA, J. (1967). 'The effects of cross-innervation on the myoglobin concentration of tonic and phasic muscles.' *Journal of Physiology*, **188**, 121–129

MARIE, P. and FOIX, C. (1913). 'Atrophie isolée de l'éminence thénar d'origine névritique. Rôle du ligament annulaire antérieur du carpe dans la pathogénie de la lésion.' *Revue Neurologique*, **26**, 647–649

MAROTTE, L. R. and MARK, R. F. (1970). 'The mechanism of selective reinnervation of fish eye muscle. I. Evidence from muscle function during recovery.' *Brain Research*, **19**, 41–51

MARSDEN, C. D. and MEADOWS, J. C. (1970). 'The effect of adrenaline on the contraction of human muscle.' *Journal of Physiology*, **207**, 429–448

MARSDEN, C. D., MEADOWS, J. C. and MERTON, P. A. (1971). 'Isolated single motor units in human muscle and their rate of discharge during maximal voluntary effort.' *Journal of Physiology*, **217**, 12–13P

MARSHALL, M. W., MOORE, M. J. and WILSON, P. (1974). 'Acetylcholine contractures in murine dystrophy and the neurogenic hypothesis.' *Experimental Neurology*, **44**, 329–332

MATHESON, D. W. and HOWLAND, J. L. (1974). 'Erythrocyte deformation in human muscular dystrophy.' *Science, N.Y.*, **184**, 165–166

MATTHEWS, M. R., COWAN, W. M. and POWELL, T. P. S. (1960). 'Transneuronal cell degeneration in the lateral geniculate nucleus of the macaque monkey.' *Journal of Anatomy*, **94**, 145–169

MATTHEWS, P. B. C. (1972). *Mammalian Muscle Receptors and their Central Actions*. London: Arnold

MAURO, A. (1961). 'Satellite cell of skeletal muscle fibres.' *Journal of Biophysical and Biochemical Cytology*, **9**, 493–495

MAXWELL, M. H. and KLEEMAN, C. R. (1952). *Clinical Disorders of Fluid and Electrolyte Metabolism*. New York: McGraw-Hill

MAYER, R. F. and DOYLE, A. M. (1970). 'Studies of the motor unit in the cat. Histochemistry and topology of anterior tibial and extensor digitorum longus muscles.' In *Muscle Diseases*. Ed. by J. N. Walton, N. Canal and G. Scarlato, pp. 159–163. Amsterdam: Excerpta Medica

MECHLER, F. (1974). 'Changing electromyographic findings during the chronic course of polymyositis.' *Journal of the Neurological Sciences*, **23**, 237–242

MELLANBY, Jane and THOMPSON, P. A. (1972). 'The effect of tetanus toxin at the neuromuscular junction in the goldfish.' *Journal of Physiology*, **224**, 407–419

MELNICK, S. C. (1963). '38 Cases of the Guillian-Barré syndrome: an immunological study.' *British Medical Journal*, **1**, 368–373

MENDELL, J. R., ENGEL, W. K. and DERRER, E. C. (1971). 'Duchenne muscular dystrophy: functional ischaemia reproduces its characteristic lesions.' *Science, N.Y.*, **172**, 1143–1145

MERTON, P. A. (1954). 'Voluntary strength and fatigue.' *Journal of Physiology*, **123**, 553–564

MERYON, E. (1852). 'On granular and fatty degeneration of the voluntary muscles.' *Medico-Chirurgical Transactions*, **35**, 73–84

MEYER, P. (1881). 'Anatomische Untersuchungen uber diphtheritische Lahmung.' *Virchows Archiv für patologische Anatomie und Physiologie*, **85**, 181–226

MIDDLETON, P. J., ALEXANDER, Rosalie M. and ZYMANSKI, M. T. (1970). 'Severe myositis during recovery from influenza.' *Lancet*, **ii**, 533–535

MIGLIETTA, O. E. (1971). 'Myasthenic-like response in patients with neuropathy.' *American Journal of Physical Medicine*, **50**, 1–16

MILEDI, R. (1960a). 'The acetylcholine sensitivity of frog muscle fibres after complete or partial denervation.' *Journal of Physiology*, **151**, 1–23

MILEDI, R. (1960b). 'Properties of regenerating neuromuscular synapses in the frog.' *Journal of Physiology*, **154**, 190–205

MILEDI, R. and SLATER, C. R. (1969). 'Electron-microscopic structure of denervated skeletal muscle.' *Proceedings of the Royal Society of London, Series B.*, **174**, 253–269

MILEDI, R. and SLATER, C. R. (1970). 'On the degeneration of rat neuromuscular junctions after nerve section.' *Journal of Physiology*, **207**, 507–528

MILLER, J. F. A. P. (1961). 'Immunological function of the thymus.' *Lancet*, **ii**, 748–749

MILLER, S. E., ROSES, A. D. and APPEL, S. H. (1976). 'Scanning electron microscopy studies in muscular dystrophy.' *Archives of Neurology*, **33**, 172–174

MILNER-BROWN, H. S., STEIN, R. B. and LEE, R. G. (1974a). 'Contractile and electrical properties of human motor units in neuropathies and motor neurone disease.' *Journal of Neurology, Neurosurgery and Psychiatry*, **37**, 670–676

MILNER-BROWN, H. S., STEIN, R. B. and LEE, R. G. (1974b). 'Pattern of recruiting human motor units in neuropathies and motor neurone disease.' *Journal of Neurology, Neurosurgery and Psychiatry*, **37**, 665–669

MILNER-BROWN, H. S., STEIN, R. B. and YEMM, R. (1973a). 'The orderly recruitment of human motor units during voluntary isometric contractions.' *Journal of Physiology*, **230**, 359–370

MILNER-BROWN, H. S., STEIN, R. B. and YEMM, R. (1973b). 'Changes in firing rate of human motor units during linearly changing voluntary contractions.' *Journal of Physiology*, **230**, 371–390

MINES, G. R. (1913). On functional analysis of the action of electrolytes.' *Journal of Physiology*, **46**, 188–235

MITCHELL, S. W., MOREHOUSE, G. R. and KEEN, W. W. (1864). *Gunshot Wounds and Other Injuries of Nerves*. Philadelphia, Pa.: Lippincott

MÖBIUS, P. J. (1879). 'Uber die heriditaren nervenkrankheiten.' *Sammlung Klinischer Vorträge*, **171**, 1505–1531

MONTGOMERY, A. (1972). 'A study of the effects of disuse upon the isometric characteristics of fast twitch and slow twitch mammalian skeletal muscle.' Ph. D. thesis, University of Bristol, Bristol, England

MONTGOMERY, A. (1975). 'Parabiotic reinnervation in normal and dystrophic mice. 1. Muscle weight and physiological studies.' *Journal of the Neurological Sciences*, **26**, 401–423

MOORE, J. W., NARAHASHI, T. and SHAW, T. I. (1967). 'An upper limit to the number of sodium channels in nerve membrane?' *Journal of Physiology*, **188**, 99–105

MOSHER, C. G., GERLACH, R. L. and STUART, D. G. (1972).

'Soleus and anterior tibial motor units of the cat.' *Brain Research*, **44**, 1–11

MUKOYAMA, M. and SOBUE, I. (1975). 'Changes in the spinal roots in Duchenne muscular dystrophy and other neuromuscular disorders.' In *Recent Advances in Myology* (Proceedings of the 3rd International Congress on Muscle Diseases). Ed. by W. G. Bradley, D. Gardner-Medwin and J. N. Walton, pp. 144–147. Amsterdam: Excerpta Medica

MULDER, D. W. (1957). 'The clinical syndrome of amyotrophic lateral sclerosis.' *Proceedings of the Mayo Clinic*, **32**, 427

MULDER, D. W. and ESPINOSA, R. E. (1969). 'Amyotrophic lateral sclerosis: comparison of the clinical syndrome in Guam and the United States.' In *Motor Neurone Diseases*. Ed. by F. H. Norris, Jr and L. T. Kurland, pp. 12–20. New York and London: Grune and Stratton

MULDER, D. W., LAMBERT, E. H. and EATON, L. M. (1959). 'Myasthenic syndrome in patients with amyotrophic lateral sclerosis.' *Neurology (Minneapolis)*, **9**, 627–631

MURPHY, D. L., MENDELL, J. R. and ENGEL, W. K. (1973). 'Serotonin and platelet function in Duchenne muscular dystrophy.' *Archives of Neurology*, **28**, 239–242

MURRAY, J. M. and WEBER, ANNEMARIE (1974). 'The cooperative action of muscle proteins.' *Scientific American*, **230**, ii, 58–71

MUSICK, J. and HUBBARD, J. I. (1972). 'Release of protein from mouse motor nerve terminals.' *Nature (London)*, **237**, 279–281

NAKAO, K., KITO, S., MURO, T., TOMONAGA, M. and MOZAI, T. (1968). 'Nervous system involvement in progressive muscular dystrophy.' *Proceedings of the Australian Association of Neurologists*, **5**, 557–564

NAMBA, T., ABERFELD, D. C. and GROB, D. (1970). 'Chronic proximal spinal muscular atrophy.' *Journal of the Neurological Sciences*, **11**, 401–423

NAMBA, T., SCHUMAN, M. H. and GROB, D. (1971). 'Conduction velocity in the ulnar nerve in hemiplegic patients.' *Journal of the Neurological Sciences*, **12**, 177–186

NASTUK, W. C., STRAUSS, A. J. L. and OSSERMAN, K. E. (1959). 'Search for a neuromuscular blocking agent in the blood of patients with myasthenia gravis.' *American Journal of Medicine*, **26**, 394–409

NEARY, D., OCHOA, J. and GILLIATT, R. W. (1975). 'Subclinical entrapment neuropathy in man.' *Journal of the Neurological Sciences*, **24**, 283–298

NEERUNJUN, J. S. and DUBOWITZ, V. (1974a). 'Muscle transplantation and regeneration in the dystrophic hamster. Part I. Histological studies.' *Journal of the Neurological Sciences*, **23**, 505–519

NEERUNJUN, J. S. and DUBOWITZ, V. (1974b). 'Muscle transplantation and regeneration in the dystrophic hamster. Part II. Histochemical studies.' *Journal of the Neurological Sciences*, **23**, 521–536

NEERUNJUN, J. S. and DUBOWITZ, V. (1975). 'Identification of regenerated dystrophic minced muscle transplanted in normal mice.' *Journal of the Neurological Sciences*, **24**, 33–38

NELSON, T. E. (1973). 'Porcine stress syndromes.' In *Malignant Hyperthermia (Symposium)*. Ed. by R. A. Gordon *et al.*, pp. 191–197. Springfield, Ill.: Thomas

NISSL, F. (1892). 'Über die veränderungen der Ganglien-zellen am Facialiskern des kaninchens nach Aureissung der nerven.' *Allgemeine Zeitschrift fur Psychiatrie*, **48**, 197–198

NORRIS, F. H. Jr (1962). 'Unstable membrane potential in human myotonic muscle.' *Electroencephalography and Clinical Neurophysiology*, **14**, 197–201

NORRIS, F. H. Jr and ENGEL, W. K. (1964). 'Neoplasms in patients with amyotrophic lateral sclerosis.' *Transactions of the American Neurological Association*, **89**, 238

NORRIS, F. H. and GASTEIGER, E. L. (1955). 'Action potentials of single motor units in normal muscle.' *Electroencephalography and Clinical Neurophysiology*, **7**, 115–126

NORRIS, F. H. Jr, MCMENEMY, W. H. and BARNARD, R. O. (1969). 'Anterior horn cell pathology in carcinamatons neuromyopathy compared with other forms of motor neurone disease.' In *Motor Neurone Disease*. Ed. by F. H. Norris, Jr and L. T. Kurland, pp. 100–112. New York: Grune and Stratton

NOTERMANS, S. L. H. (1968), 'EMG in patients with so-called parietal atrophy.' *Electroencephalography and Clinical Neurophysiology*, **25**, 405P

OCHOA, J., DANTA, G., FOWLER, T. J. and GILLIATT, R. W. (1971). 'Nature of the nerve lesion caused by a pneumatic tourniquet.' *Nature (London)*, **233**, 265–266

OCHOA, J., FOWLER, T. J. and GILLIATT, R. W. (1972). 'Anatomical changes in peripheral nerves compressed by a pneumatic tourniquet.' *Journal of Anatomy*, **113**, 433–455

OCHOA, J. and MAIR, W. G. P. (1969). 'The normal sural nerve in man. 2. Changes in the axons and Schwann Cells due to ageing.' *Acta Neuropathologica (Berlin)*, **13**, 217–239

OCHOA, J. and MAROTTE, L. (1973). 'The nature of the nerve lesion caused by chronic entrapment in the guinea-pig.' *Journal of the Neurological Sciences*, **19**, 491–495

OCHS, S. (1972). 'Fast transport of materials in mammalian nerve fibres.' *Science, N.Y.*, **176**, 252–260

OCHS, S. (1974). 'Systems of material transport in nerve fibres (axoplasmic transport) related to nerve function and trophic control.' In *Trophic Functions of the Neuron*. Ed. by D. B. Drachman. *Annals of the New York Academy of Sciences*, **228**, 202–223

OCHS, S. and RANISH, N. (1969). 'Characteristics of the fast transport system in mammalian nerve fibres.' *Journal of Neurobiology*, **1**, 247–261

OFFERIJNS, F. G. J., WESTERINK, D. and WILLEBRANDS, A. F. (1958). 'The relation of potassium deficiency to muscular paralysis by insulin.' *Journal of Physiology*, **141**, 377–384

OGG, Elizabeth (1971). *Milestones in Muscle Disease Research*. New York: Muscular Dystrophy Associations of America, Inc.

OKINAKA, S., SHIZUME, K., IIONO, S., WATANABE, A., IRIE, M., NOGUCHI, A., KUMA, S., KUMA, K. and ITO, T. (1957). 'The association of periodic paralysis and hyperthroidism in Japan.' *Journal of Clinical Endocrinology*, **17**, 1454–1459

OLSON, Camille B. and SWETT, C. P. Jr (1969). 'Speed of contraction of skeletal muscle. The effect of hypoactivity and hyperactivity.' *Archives of Neurology*, **20**, 263–270

OLSSON, Y. and SJÖSTRAND, J. (1969). 'Origin of macrophages in Wallerian degeneration of peripheral nerves demonstrated autoradiographically.' *Experimental Neurology*, **23**, 102–112

OOSTERHUIS, H. and BETHLEM, J. (1973). 'Neurogenic muscle involvement in myasthenia gravis. A clinical and histopathological study.' *Journal of Neurology, Neurosurgery and Psychiatry*, **36**, 244–254

OOSTERHUIS, H. J. G. H., FELTKAMP, T. E. W. and VAN DER GELD, H. R. W. (1966). 'Muscle antibodies in myasthenic mothers and their babies.' *Lancet*, **ii**, 1226–1227

O'SULLIVAN, D. J. and SWALLOW, M. (1968). 'The fibre size and content of the radial and sural nerves.' *Journal of Neurology, Neurosurgery and Psychiatry*, **31**, 464–470

OTSUKA, M. and OHTSUKI, I. (1965). 'Mechanism of muscle paralysis by insulin with particular reference to familial periodic paralysis.' *Nature (London)*, **207**, 300–301

ÖZDEMIR, C. and YOUNG, R. R. (1971). 'Electrical testing in myasthenia gravis.' In *Myasthenia Gravis*. Ed. by W. S. Fields. *Annals of the New York Academy of Sciences*, **183**, 287–302

PADYKULA, Helen A. and GAUTHIER, G. F. (1966). 'Morphological and cytochemical characteristics of fiber types in normal mammalian skeletal muscle.' In *Exploratory Concepts in Muscular Dystrophy and Related Disorders*, edited by A. T. Milhorat, pp. 117–128

PADYKULA, Helen A. and GAUTHIER, G. F. (1967). 'Ultrastructural features of three fiber types in the rat diaphragm.' *Anatomical Record*, **157**, 157–296

PANAYIOTOPOULOS, C. P. and SCARPALEZOS, S. (1975). 'Electrophysiological estimation of motor units in limb-girdle muscular dystrophy and chronic spinal muscular atrophy.' *Journal of the Neurological Sciences*, **24**, 95–107

PANAYIOTOPOULOS, C. P. and SCARPALEZOS, S. (1976). 'Dystrophia myotonica, peripheral nerve involvement and pathogenetic implications.' *Journal of the Neurological Sciences*, **27**, 1–16

PANAYIOTOPOULOS, C. P., SCARPALEZOS, S. and PAPAPETROPOULOS, T. (1974). 'Electrophysiologic estimation of motor units in Duchenne muscular dystrophy.' *Journal of the Neurological Sciences*, **23**, 89–98

PANSE, F. (1930). *Die Schadigungen des Nervern systems durch techische Elektrizitat*. Berlin. Cited by M. Critchley in *Proceedings of the Royal Society of Medicine*, **55**, 1032–1033

PAPAPETROPOULOS, T. A. and BRADLEY, W. G. (1972). 'Spinal motoneurones in murine muscular dystrophy and spinal muscular atrophy. A quantitative histological study.' *Journal of Neurology, Neurosurgery and Psychiatry*, **35**, 60–65

PARK, J. H., CHOU, T. H., PINSON, R., ROELOFS, R. I. and OLSON, W. H. (1974). 'Beneficial effects of penicillamine treatment on hereditary muscular dystrophy.' *3rd International Congress on Muscle Diseases, Newcastle-upon-Tyne* (Abstract 132). Amsterdam: Excerpta Medica

PARKER, J. M. and MENDELL, J. R. (1974). 'Proximal myopathy induced by 5-HT-imipramine stimulates Duchenne dystrophy.' *Nature (London)*, **247**, 103–104

PARKES, J. D. and MCKINNA, J. A. (1966). 'Neuromuscular blocking activity in the blood of patients with myasthenia gravis.' *Lancet*, **i**, 388–391

PARSONS, R. L., HOFMANN, W. W. and FEIGEN, G. A. (1966). 'Mode of action of tetanus toxin on the neuromuscular junction.' *American Journal of Physiology*, **210**, 84–90

PATRICK, J. and LINDSTROM, J. (1973). 'Autoimmune response to acetylcholine receptor.' *Science*, **180**, 871–872

PATTEN, B. M., BILEZIKIAN, J. P., MALLETTE, L. E., PRINCE, A., ENGEL, W. K. and AURBACH, G. D. (1974). 'Neuromuscular disease in primary hyperparathyroidism.' *Annals of Internal Medicine*, **80**, 182–193

PATTEN, B. M., HART, A. and LOVELACE, R. (1972). 'Multiple sclerosis associated with defects in neuromuscular transmission.' *Journal of Neurology, Neurosurgery and Psychiatry*, **35**, 385–394

PAUL, C. V. and POWELL, Jeanne A. (1974). 'Organ cultures of coupled fetal cord and adult muscle from normal and dystrophic mice.' *Journal of the Neurological Sciences*, **21**, 365–379

PAULSON, O. B., ENGEL, A. G. and GOMEZ, M. R. (1974). 'Muscle blood flow in Duchenne type muscular dystrophy, limb-girdle dystrophy, polymyositis and in normal controls.' *Journal of Neurology, Neurosurgery and Psychiatry*, **37**, 685–690

PAYAN, J. (1970). 'Anterior transposition of the ulnar nerve: an electrophysiological study.' *Journal of Neurology, Neurosurgery and Psychiatry*, **33**, 157–165

PEACHEY, L. D. (1965). 'The sarcoplasmic reticulum and transverse tubules of the frog's sartorius.' *Journal of Cell Biology*, **25**, 209–231

PEACOCK, J. H. and NELSON, P. G. (1973). 'Synaptogenesis in cell cultures of neurones and myotubes from chickens with muscular dystrophy.' *Journal of Neurology, Neurosurgery and Psychiatry*, **36**, 389–398

PEARCE, G. W. and WALTON, J. N. (1963). 'A histological study of muscle from the Bar Harbor strain of dystrophic mice.' *Journal of Pathology and Bacteriology*, **86**, 25–33

PEARSE, A. G. E. (1969). 'Cytochemistry and ultrastructure of polypeptide hormone-producing cells of APUD series and embryologic, physiologic and pathologic implications.' *Journal of Histochemistry and Cytochemistry*, **17**, 303–313

PEARSON, C. M. (1963). 'The periodic paralyses: Differential features and pathological observations in permanent myopathic weakness.' *Brain*, **87**, 341–354

PEARSON, C. M. and CURRIE, S. (1974). 'Polymyositis and related disorders.' In *Disorders of Voluntary Muscle*. Ed. by J. N. Walton, 3rd edn., pp. 614–652. Edinburgh: Churchill Livingstone

PELLERGRINO, C. and FRANZINI, clara (1963). 'An electron microscope study of denervation atrophy in red and white skeletal muscle fibres.' *Journal of Cell Biology*, **17**, 327–349

PENFIELD, W. and BOLDREY, E. (1937). 'Somatic motor and sensory representation in the cerebral cortex of man as studied by electrical stimulation.' *Brain*, **60**, 389–443

PENNES, H. H. (1949). 'Temperature of skeletal muscle in cerebral hemiplegia and paralysis agitans.' *Archives of Neurology and Psychiatry (Chicago)*, **62**, 269–279

PENROSE, L. S. (1948). 'The problem of anticipation in pedigrees of dystrophia myotonica.' *Annals of Eugenics*, **14**, 125–132

PERLOFF, J. K., DELEON, A. C. and O'DOHERTY, D. (1966). 'The cardiomyopathy of progressive muscular dystrophy.' *Circulation*, **33**, 625–648

PESTRONK, A., DRACHMAN, D. B. and GRIFFIN, J. W. (1976). 'Disuse of muscle: partial denervation effect on ACh receptors.' *Nature (London)*. In press

PETAJAN, J. H. and PHILIP, Betty A. (1969). 'Frequency control of motor unit action potentials.' *Electroencephalography and Clinical Neurophysiology*, **27**, 66–72

PETER, J. B., BARNARD, R. J., EDGERTON, V. R., GILLESPIE, CYNTHIA A. and STEMPEL, K. E. (1972). 'Metabolic profiles of three fibre types of skeletal muscle in guinea pigs and rabbits.' *Biochemistry*, **11**, 2627–2633

PETER, J. B. and FIEHN, W. (1973). 'Diazacholesterol myotonia: accumulation of desmosterol and increased adenosine triphosphastase activity of sarcolemma.' *Science, N.Y.*, **179**, 910–912

PETER, J. B., FIEHN, W., NAGATOMO, T., ANDIMAN, R., STEMPEL, K. and BOWMAN, R. (1974). 'Studies of sarcolemma from normal and diseased skeletal muscle.' In *Exploratory Concepts in Muscular Dystrophy, II*. Ed. by A. T. Milhorat, pp. 479–490. Amsterdam: Excerpta Medica

PETER, J. B. and WORSFOLD, M. (1969). 'Muscular dystrophy and other myopathies: sarcotubular vesicles in early disease.' *Biochemical Medicine*, **2**, 364–371

PETERSON, A. C. (1974). 'Chimaera mouse study shows absence of disease in genetically dystrophic muscle.' *Nature (London)*, **248**, 561–564

PETTE, D., SMITH, Margaret E., STAUDTE, H. W. and VRBOVÁ, Gerta (1973). 'Effects of long-term electrical stimulation on some contractile and metabolic characteristics of fast rabbit muscle.' *Pfluegers Archiv; European Journal of Physiology*, **338**, 257–272

PEYRONNARD, J. M. (1975). 'An experimental evaluation of the motor unit counting technique.' *Canadian Journal of Neurological Sciences*, **2**, 332

PHALEN, G. S. (1966). 'The carpal-tunnel syndrome. Seventeen years' experience in diagnosis and treatment of six hundred fifty-four hands.' *Journal of Bone and Joint Surgery*, **48**, 211–228

PICTET, R. L., RALL, L. B., PHELPS, PATRICIA and RUTTER, W. J. (1976). 'The neural crest and the origin of the insulin producing and other gastrointestinal hormone-producing cells.' *Science*, **191**, 191–192

PILZ, H., PRILL, A. and VOLLES, E. (1974). 'Kombination von myotonischer Dystrophie mit 'idiopathischer' Neuropathie: Mitteilung klinischer Befunde bei 10 Fällen mit gleichzeitiger Proteinvermehrung im Liquor.' *Zeitschrift für Neurologie*, **206**, 263–265

PITTINGER, C. and ADAMSON, R. (1972). 'Antibiotic blockade of neuromuscular function.' *Annual Review of Pharmacology*, **12**, 169–184

PLEASURE, D. E., MISCHLER, K. C. and ENGEL, W. K. (1969). 'Axonal transport of proteins in experimental neuropathies.' *Science, N.Y.*, **166**, 524–525

PODOLSKY, R. J. (1964). 'The maximum sarcomere length for contraction of isolated myofibrils.' *Journal of Physiology*, **170**, 110–123

POLGAR, J. G., BRADLEY, W. G., UPTON, A. R. M., ANDERSON, J., HOWAT, J. M. L., PETITO, F., ROBERTS, D. F. and SCOPA, J. (1972). 'The early detection of dystrophia myotonica.' *Brain*, **95**, 761–776

POLLARD, J. D., KING, R. H. M. and THOMAS, P. K. (1975). 'Recurrent experimental allergic neuritis. An electron microscope study.' *Journal of the Neurological Sciences*, **24**, 365–383

POLLOCK, M. and DYCK, P. J. (1976). 'Peripheral nerve morphometry in myotonic dystrophy.' *Archives of Neurology*, **33**, 33–39

PORTER, C. W. and BARNARD, E. A. (1975). 'The density of cholinergic receptors at the end-plate postsynaptic membrane: ultrastructural studies in two mammalian species.' *Journal of Membrane Biology*, **20**, 31–49

PORTER, K. R. (1956). 'The sarcoplasmic reticulum in muscle cells in Amblystoma larvae.' *Journal of Biophysical and Biochemical Cytology*, **2**, 163–170

POSKANZER, D. C., KANTOR, H. M. and KAPLAN, GAIL S. (1969). 'The frequency of preceding poliomyelitis in amyotrophic lateral sclerosis.' In *Motor Neuron Diseases*. Ed. by F. H. Norris, Jr and L. T. Kurland, pp 286–288. New York: Grune and Stratton

POSKANZER, D. C. and KERR, D. N. S. (1961). 'A third type of periodic paralysis with normokalemia and favourable response to sodium chloride.' *American Journal of Medicine*, **31**, 328–342

POTTER, L. T. (1970). 'Synthesis, storage and release of [^{14}C] acetylchole in isolated rat diaphram muscles.' *Journal of Physiology*, **206**, 145–166

PRABHU, V. G. and OESTER, Y. T. (1962). 'Electromyographic changes in skeletal muscle due to tetanus toxin.' *Journal of Pharmacology and Experimental Therapeutics*, **138**, 241–248

PRESWICK, G. (1965). 'The myasthenic syndromes and their reactions.' *Proceedings of the Australian Association of Neurologists*, **3**, 61–69

PREWITT, Margaret A. and SALAFSKY, B. (1967). 'Effect of cross-innervation on biochemical characteristics of skeletal muscles.' *American Journal of Physiology*, **213**, 295–300

PRIDGEN, J. E. (1956). 'Respiratory arrest thought to be due to intraperiotoneal neomycin.' *Surgery*, **40**, 571–574

PRINEAS, J. (1969a). 'The pathogenesis of dying-back polyneuropathies. Part I. An ultrastructural study of experimental tri-orth-cresyl phosphate intoxication in the cat.' *Journal of Neuropathology and Experimental Neurology*, **28**, 571–597

PRINEAS, J. (1969b). 'The pathogenesis of dying-back polyneuropathies. Part II. An ultrastructural study of experimental acrylamide intoxication in the cat.' *Journal of Neuropathology and Experimental Neurology*, **28**, 598–621

PROSSER, E. Jane, MURPHY, E. G. and THOMPSON, Margaret W. (1969). 'Intelligence and the gene for Duchenne muscular dystrophy.' *Archives of Disease in Childhood*, **44**, 221–230

PURVES, D. and SAKMANN, B. (1974). 'Membrane properties underlying spontaneous activity of denervated muscle fibres.' *Journal of Physiology*, **239**, 125–153

QUICK, D. T. and GREER, M. (1967). 'Pancreatic dysfunction in amyotrophic lateral sclerosis.' *Neurology (Minneapolis)*, **17**, 112–116

RAFTERY, M. A. (1973). 'Isolation of acetylcholine receptor alpha-bungarotoxin complexes from *Torpedo Californica* electroplax.' *Archives of Biochemistry and Biophysics*, **154**, 270–276

RAGAB, A. H. M. F. (1971). 'Motor end-plate changes in mouse muscular dystrophy.' *Lancet*, **ii**, 815–816

RAISMAN, G. and FIELD, P. M. (1973). 'A quantitative investigation of the development of collateral reinnervation after partial deafferentation of the septal nuclei.' *Brain Research*, **50**, 241–264

RAMSAY, I. D. (1966). 'Muscle dysfunction in hyperthyroidism.' *Lancet*, **ii**, 931–935

RAMSAY, I. D. (1969). 'Thyrotoxic muscle disease.' *Postgraduate Medical Journal*, **44**, 385

RAMSEY, R. W. and STREET, S. F. (1942). 'Absence of fatigue of the contractile mechanism in single muscle fibres.' *Federation Proceedings*, **1**, 70

RANVIER, L. (1873). 'Propriétés et structures différents des muscles rouges et des muscles blancs, chez les lapins et chez les raies.' *Comptes Rendus hebdomadaires des Seances de l'Academie des Sciences: D. Sciences Naturelles (Paris)*, **77**, 1030–1034

RASMINSKY, M. (1973). 'The effects of temperature on conduction in demyelinated single nerve fibres.' *Archives of Neurology*, **28**, 287–292

RASMINSKY, M., BRAY, G. M. and AGUAYO, A. J. (1975). 'Abnormal conduction in morphologically normal peripheral nerves: an electrophysiologic light and electron microscope experimental study.' *Tenth Canadian Congress of Neurological Sciences (London, Ontario).* Abstract No. 40

RASMINSKY, M. and SEARS, T. A. (1972). 'Internodal conduction in undissected demyelinated nerve fibres.' *Journal of Physiology*, **227**, 323–350

RATHBONE, M. P., DIMOND, PATRICIA A. and VETRANO, F. (1975). 'Dystrophic spinal cord transplants induce abnormal thymidine kinase activity in normal muscles.' *Science, N.Y.*, **189**, 1106–1107

REDFERN, P. A. (1970). 'Neuromuscular transmission in new-born rats.' *Journal of Physiology*, **209**, 701–709

REIER, P. J. and HUGHES, A. (1972). 'Evidence for spontaneous axon degeneration during peripheral nerve maturation.' *American Journal of Anatomy*, **135**, 147–152

RELTON, J. E. S. (1973). 'Malignant hyperthermia—anaesthetic techniques and agents.' In *Malignant Hyperthermia*. Ed. by R. A. Gordon *et al.*, pp. 425–429. Springfield, Ill.: Thomas

RESKE-NIELSEN, Edith, DALBY, Agnes and DALBY, M. (1965). 'Studies on the innervation of muscles in muscular and neuromuscular diseases. An attempt of diagnosis by comparing biopsy and endplate studies with clinical and electromyographic findings.' *Acta Neurologica Scandinavica*, **41**, Suppl. 13, 289–296

RESKE-NIELSEN, Edith, HARMSEN, A. and OVESEN, N. (1971). 'Pathological study of muscle biopsies from the legs in patients with fractures of the cervical spine.'

In *Actualités de Pathologie Neuro-musculaire*, pp. 509–521. Paris: Expansion Scientifique

REZNIK, M. (1970). 'Satellite cells, myoblasts and skeletal muscle regeneration.' In *Regeneration of Striated Muscle, and Myogenesis*. Ed. by A. Mauro, S. A. Shafiq and A. T. Milhorat, pp. 133–153. Amsterdam: Excerpta Medica

RICKER, K., MEINCK, H-M. and STUMPF, H. (1973). 'Neurophysiologische Untersuchungen uber das Stadium passagerer Lahmung bei Myotonia congenita und Dystrophia myotonica.' *Zeitschrift fur Neurologie*, **204**, 135–148

RIECKER, G. and BOLTE, H. D. (1966). 'Membranpotentiale einzelner Skeletmuskelzellen bei hypokaliämischer Muskelparalyse.' *Klinische Wochenschrift*, **44**, 804–807

RIECKER, G., DOBBELSTEIN, H., RÖHL, D. and BOLTE, H. D. (1964). 'Messungen des Membranpotentials einzelner quergestreifter Muskelzellen bei Myotonia congenita (Thomsen).' *Klinische Wochenschrift*, **42**, 519–522

RINGER, S. (1883). 'A further contribution regarding the influence of different constituents of the blood on the contraction of the heart.' *Journal of Physiology*, **4**, 29–42

ROBBINS, N. and YONEZAWA, T. (1971). 'Physiological studies during formation and development of rat neuromuscular junctions in tissue culture.' *Journal of General Physiology*, **58**, 467–481

ROBERT, E. D. and OESTER, Y. T. (1970). 'Absence of supersensitivity to acetylcholine in innervated muscle subjected to a prolonged pharmacologic block.' *Journal of Pharmacology and Experimental Therapeutics*, **174**, 133–140

ROMANUL, F. C. A. (1964). 'Enzymes in muscle. I. Histochemical studies of enzymes in individual muscle fibres.' *Archives of Neurology*, **11**, 355–368

ROMANUL, F. C. A. and HOGAN, E. L. (1965). 'Enzymatic changes in denervated muscle. I. Histochemical studies.' *Archives of Neurology*, **13**, 263–273

ROMANUL, F. C. A. and POLLOCK, M. (1969). 'The parallelism of changes in oxidative metabolism and capillary supply of skeletal muscle fibres.' In *Modern Neurology: Papers in Tribute to Derek Denny-Brown*. Ed. by S. Locke

ROMANUL, F. C. A. and VAN DER MEULEN, J. P. (1966). 'Reversal of the enzyme profiles of muscle fibres in fast and slow muscles by cross-innervation.' *Nature (London)*, **212**, 1369–1370

ROSE, A. L. and WILLISON, R. G. (1967). 'Quantitative electromyography using automatic analysis: studies in healthy subjects and patients with primary muscle disease.' *Journal of Neurology, Neurosurgery and Psychiatry*, **30**, 403–410

ROSES, A. D. and APPEL, S. H. (1973). 'Protein kinase activity in erythrocyte ghosts of patients with myotonic dystrophy.' *Proceedings of the National Academy of Sciences of the United States of America*, **70**, 1855–1859

ROSES, A. D. and APPEL, S. H. (1974). 'Muscle membrane protein kinase in myotonic muscular dystrophy.' *Nature (London)*, **250**, 245–247

ROSES, A. D., HERBSTREITH, M. H. and APPEL, S. H. (1975). 'Membrane protein kinase alteration in

Duchenne muscular dystrophy.' *Nature (London)*, **254**, 350–351

ROSES, A. D., ROSES, M. J., MILLER, S. E., HULL, K. L. Jr and APPEL, S. H. (1975). Carrier detection in Duchenne muscular dystrophy. *New England Journal of Medicine*, **294**, 193–198

ROSMAN, N. P. and KAKULAS, B. A. (1966). 'Mental deficiency associated with muscular dystrophy. A neuropathological study.' *Brain*, **89**, 769–788

ROSSELLE, N. and STEVENS, A. (1973). 'Unexpected incidence of neurogenic atrophy of the extensor digitorum brevis muscle in young normal adults.' In *New Developments in Electromyography and Clinical Neurophysiology*. Ed. by J. E. Desmedt. Vol. 1, pp. 69–70. Basel: Karger

ROWLAND, L. P., ARAKI, S. and CARMEL, P. (1965). 'Contracture in McArdle's disease.' *Archives of Neurology*, **13**, 541–544

RUBINSTEIN, L. J. (1960). 'Ageing changes in muscles.' In *The Structure and Function of Muscle*. Ed. by G. H. Bourne. Vol. 3, pp. 209–226. New York: Academic Press

RÜDEL, R. and SENGES, J. (1972): 'Experimental myotonia in mammalian skeletal muscle: Changes in membrane properties.' *Pfuegers Archiv: European Journal of Physiology*, **331**, 324–334

RUDEL, R. and TAYLOR, S. R. (1973). 'Aqueorin luminescence during contraction of amphibian skeletal muscle.' *Journal of Physiology*, **233**, 5–6 P

RUSSELL, DOROTHY S. (1953). 'Histological changes in the striped muscles in myasthenia gravis.' *Journal of Pathology and Bacteriology*, **65**, 279–289

RUSTIGIAN, R. and PAPPENHEIMER, A. W. (1949). 'Myositis in mice following intramuscular injection of viruses of the mouse encephalomyelitis group and of certain other neurotropic viruses.' *Journal of Experimental Medicine*, **89**, 69–92

SALAFSKY, B. (1971). 'Functional studies of regenerated muscles from normal and dystrophic mice.' *Nature (London)*, **229**, 270–272

SALMONS, S. and VRBOVÁ, Gerta (1969). 'The influence of activity on some contractile characteristics of mammalian fast and slow muscles.' *Journal of Physiology*, **201**, 535–549

SAMAHA, F. J. and GERGELY, J. (1969). 'Biochemical abnormalities of the sarcoplasmic reticulum in muscular dystrophy.' *New England Journal of Medicine*, **280**, 184–188

SAMAHA, F. J., GUTH, L. and ALBERS, R. W. (1970). 'The neural regulation of gene expression in the muscle cell.' *Experimental Neurology*, **27**, 276–282

SAMAHA, F. J., SCHROEDER, J. M., REBEIZ, J. and ADAMS, R. D. (1967). 'Studies on myotonia.' *Archives of Neurology*, **17**, 22–33

SANDERS, F. K. and YOUNG, J. Z. (1946). 'The influence of peripheral connexion on the diameter of regenerating nerve fibres.' *Experimental Biology*, **22**, 203–212

SANDERSON, K. V. and ADEY, W. R. (1952). 'Electromyographic and endocrine studies in chronic thyrotoxic myopathy.' *Journal of Neurology, Neurosurgery and Psychiatry*, **15**, 200–205

SANDOW, A. (1965). 'Excitation-contraction coupling in skeletal muscle.' *Pharmacological Reviews*, **17**, 265–320

SANDOW, A. and BRUST, M. (1958). 'Contractility of dystrophic mouse muscle.' *American Journal of Physiology*, **194**, 557–563

SANTA, T., ENGEL, A. G. and LAMBERT, E. H. (1972a). 'Histometric study of neuromuscular junction ultrastructure. I. Myasthenia gravis.' *Neurology (Minneapolis)*, **22**, 71–82

SANTA, T., ENGEL, A. G. and LAMBERT, E. H. (1972b). 'Histometric study of neuromuscular junction ultrastructure. II. Myasthenic syndrome.' *Neurology (Minneapolis)*, **22**, 370–376

SCARPALEZOS, S. and PANAYIOTOPOULOS, C. P. (1973). 'Duchenne muscular dystrophy: reservations to the neurogenic hypothesis.' *Lancet*, **ii**, 458

SCHAUMBURG, H. H., SPENCER, P. S., WIŚNIEWSKI, H., GHETTI, B. and COOK, R. D. (1973). 'Experimental acrylamide neuropathy—a light microscope, ultrastructural and clinical study.' *Journal of Neuropathology and Experimental Neurology*, **32**, 17

SCHAUMBURG, H. H., WIŚNIEWSKI, H. and SPENCER, P. S. (1974). 'Ultrastructural studies of the dying-back process. I. Peripheral nerve terminal and axon degeneration in systemic acrylamide intoxication.' *Journal of Neuropathology and Experimental Neurology*, **33**, 260–284

SCHOTT, G. D. and MCARDLE, B. (1974). 'Barium-induced skeletal muscle paralysis in the rat, and its relationship to human familial periodic paralysis.' *Journal of Neurology, Neurosurgery and Psychiatry*, **37**, 32–39

SCHRÖDER, J. M. (1972). 'Altered ratio between axon diameter and myelin sheath thickness in regenerated nerve fibres.' *Brain Research*, **45**, 49–65

SCHULTZE, F. (1895). 'Beitrage zur Muskel pathologie.' *Deutsche Zeitschrift fur Nervenheilkunde*, **6**, 65–70

SCHWARTZ, O. and JAMPEL, R. S. (1962). 'Congenital blepharophimosis associated with a unique generalized myopathy.' *Archives of Ophthalmology*, **68**, 52–57

SCHWARZ, R. A., ARCHIBALD, K. C. and HAGSTRON, J. W. C. (1966). 'Correlative findings by electromyography and muscle biopsy in neuromuscular disorders.' *Archives of Physical Medicine*, **47**, 653–658

SCOTT, sheryl A. (1975). 'Maintained functional hyperinnervation of goldfish extraocular muscles.' In *Society for Neuroscience, 5th Annual Meeting, New York*. Programme Abstract no. 1161

SCOVILLE, W. B. (1946). In discussion of paper by J. J. Michelsen and W. J. Mixter, entitled 'Diagnostic aspects of unilateral ruptured cervical disk'. *Archives of Neurology and Psychiatry (Chicago)*, **56**, 722–723

SEDAL, L., MCLEOD, J. G. and WALSH, J. C. (1973). 'Ulnar nerve lesions associated with the carpal tunnel syndrome.' *Journal of Neurology, Neurosurgery and Psychiatry*, **36**, 118–123

SEDDON, H. J. (1943). 'Three types of nerve injury.' *Brain*, **66**, 237–288

SEDDON, H. (1972). *Surgical Disorders of the Peripheral Nerves*. Edinburgh: Churchill Livingstone

SEGAWA, M., FUKUYAMA, Y., ITOH, K. and UONO, M. (1970). 'Congenital muscular dystrophy (with progressive development of joint contracture, mental retardation and facial involvement). 1. Clinical Studies.' *Brain and Development (Tokyo)*, **2**, 439

SELANDER, P. (1950). 'Dermatomyositis in early childhood.' *Acta Medical Scandinavica*, Supplement **246**, 187–203

SEMMES, R. E. and MURPHY, F. (1943). 'The syndrome of unilateral rupture of the sixth cervical intervertebral disk with compression of the seventh cervical nerve root.' *Journal of the American Medical Association*, **121**, 1209–1214

SERRATRICE, G., GASTAUT, G. L., PELLISSIER, J. F., BARET, J., ROUX, H. and CARTOUZOU, G. (1975). 'Amyotrophies et dépopulations neuronales d'origine encéphalique.' *Revue Neurologique*, **131**, 185–192

SERRATRICE, G., ROUX, H. and AQUARON, R. (1968). 'Proximal muscle weakness in elderly subjects. Report of 12 cases.' *Journal of the Neurological Sciences*, **7**, 275–299

SHA'AFI, R. I., RODAN, S. B., HINTZ, R. L., FERNANDEZ, S. M. and RODAN, G. A. (1975). 'Abnormalities in membrane microviscosity and ion transport in genetic muscular dystrophy.' *Nature (London)*, **254**, 525–526

SHAHANI, B., DAVIES-JONES, G. A. B. and RUSSELL, W. R. (1971). 'Motor neurone disease. Further evidence for an abnormality of nerve metabolism.' *Journal of Neurology, Neurosurgery and Psychiatry*, **34**, 185–191

SHAHANI, B. and RUSSELL, W. R. (1969). 'Motor neurone disease. An abnormality of nerve and metabolism.' *Journal of Neurology, Neurosurgery and Psychiatry*, **32**, 1–5

SHAINBERG, A., YAGIL, G. and YAFFE, D. (1969). 'Control of myogenesis *in vitro* by Ca²⁺ concentration in nutritional medium.' *Experimental Cell Research*, **58**, 163–167

SHARMA, A. K. and THOMAS, P. K. (1975). 'Peripheral nerve regeneration in experimental diabetes.' *Journal of the Neurological Sciences*, **24**, 417–424

SHEARD, C. (1951). 'Dermatomyositis.' *Archives of Internal Medicine*, **88**, 640–658

SHERRINGTON, C. S. (1929). 'Some functional problems attaching to convergence.' *Proceedings of the Royal Society, Series B*, **105**, 332–362

SHIBUYA, N., HAZAMA, R., KURASHIGE, Y. and NAKAZAWA, Y. (1975). 'Effect of incomplete ligation of peripheral nerves on neuromuscular transmission. Appearance of myasthenic phenomenon.' *Journal of the Neurological Sciences*, **25**, 463–471

SHIRAKI, H. (1969). 'The neuropathology of amyotrophic lateral sclerosis (ALS) in the Kii peninsula and other areas of Japan.' In *Motor Neurone Diseases*. Ed. by F. H. Norris, Jr and L. T. Kurland, pp. 80–84. New York and London: Grune and Stratton

SHY, G. M., ENGEL, W. K., SOMERS, J. E. and WANKO, T. (1963). 'Nemaline myopathy. A new congenital myopathy.' *Brain*, **86**, 793–810

SHY, G. M., GONATAS, N. K. and PEREZ, M. (1966). 'Two childhood myopathies with abnormal mitochondria. I. Megaconial myopathy. II. Pleoconial myopathy.' *Brain*, **89**, 133–158

SHY, G. M. and MAGEE, K. R. (1956). 'A new congenital non-progressive myopathy.' *Brain*, **79**, 610–620

SHY, G. M., WANKO, T., ROWLEY, P. T. and ENGEL, A. G. (1961). 'Studies in familial periodic paralysis.' *Experimental Neurology*, **3**, 53–121

SICA, R. E. P. and AGUILERA, Nidia (1972). 'Electro-physiological studies in hypokalemic periodic paralysis.' *Medicina (Buenos Aires)*, **32**, 93–99

SICA, R. E. P. and MCCOMAS A. J. (1971a). 'Fast and slow twitch units in a human muscle.' *Journal of Neurology, Neurosurgery and Psychiatry*, **34**, 113–120

SICA, R. E. P. and MCCOMAS, A. J. (1971b). 'An electrophysiological investigation of limb-girdle and facio-scapulohumeral dystrophy.' *Journal of Neurology, Neurosurgery and Psychiatry*, **34**, 469–474

SICA, R. E. P., MCCOMAS, A. J., UPTON, A. R. M. and LONGMIRE, D. (1974). 'Estimations of motor units in small muscles of the hand.' *Journal of Neurology, Neurosurgery and Psychiatry*, **37**, 55–67

SIEGEL, I. M., MILLER, R. E. and RAY, R. D. (1974). 'Failure of corticosteroids in the treatment of Duchenne (pseudo-hypertrophic) muscular dystrophy. Report of a clinical matched three year double-blind study.' *Illinois Medical Journal*, **145**, 32–33

SILVERSTEIN, A. (1931). 'Atrophy of the limbs as a sign of involvement of the parietal lobe.' *Archives of Neurology and Psychiatry (Chicago)*, **26**, 237–240

SILVERSTEIN, A. (1955). 'Diagnostic localizing value of muscle atrophy in parietal lobe lesions.' *Neurology (Minneapolis)*, **5**, 30–55

SIMONS, D. J. (1937). 'A note on the effect of heat and of cold upon certain symptoms of multiple sclerosis.' *Bulletin of the Neurological Institute of New York*, **6**, 385–386

SIMPSON, J. A. (1958). 'An evaluation of thymectomy in myasthenia gravis.' *Brain*, **81**, 112–144

SIMPSON, J. A. (1960). 'Myasthenia gravis: a new hypothesis.' *Scottish Medical Journal*, **5**, 419–436

SIMPSON, J. A. (1966). 'Myasthenia gravis as an auto-immune disease: clinical aspects.' In *Myasthenia Gravis* (Symposium). Ed. by K. E. Osserman. *Annals of the New York Academy of Sciences*, **135**, 506–516

SIMPSOM, J. A. (1974). 'Myasthenia gravis and myasthenic syndromes.' In *Disorders of Voluntary Muscle*. Ed. by J. N. Walton, 3rd edn., pp. 653–692. London: Churchill Livingstone

SINGER, H. D. and GOODBODY, F. W. (1901). 'A case of family periodic paralysis with a critical digest of the literature.' *Brain*, **24**, 257–285

SKOU, J. C. (1957). 'The influence of some cations on an adenosine triphosphatase from peripheral nerves.' *Biochimica et Biophysica Acta*, **23**, 394–401

SLOMÍC, A., ROSENFALCK, Annelise and BUCHTHAL, F. (1968). 'Electrical and mechanical responses of normal and myasthenic muscle with particular reference to the staircase phenomenon.' *Brain Research*, **10**, 1–78 (Special issue)

SPENCER, P. S. (1971). 'Light and electromicroscopic observations on localized peripheral nerve injuries.' 2 vols. Ph.D. Thesis, University of London, London. Cited by P. S. Spencer and H. H. Schaumburg. *Canadian Journal of Neurological Sciences*, **1**, 152–169

SPENCER, P. S. (1972). 'Reappraisal of the model for "bulk axoplasmic flow".' *Nature New Biology*, **240**, 283–285

SPENCER, P. S. and SCHAUMBURG, H. H. (1974). 'A review of acrylamide neurotoxicity. Part I. Properties, uses and human exposure.' *Canadian Journal of Neurological Sciences*, **1**, 143–150

SPIRO, A. J., SHY, G. M. and GONATAS, N. K. (1966). 'Myotubular myopathy.' *Archives of Neurology*, **14**, 1–14

SRETER, F. A., GERGELY, J., SALMONS, S. and ROMANUL, F. (1973). 'Synthesis by fast muscle of myosin light chains characteristic of slow muscle in response to long-term stimulation.' *Nature (New Biology)*, **241**, 17–18

STAAL, A. (1970). 'The entrapment neuropathies.' In *Diseases of Nerves*, vol. 7 of *Handbook of Clinical Neurology*. Ed. by P. J. Vinken and G. W. Bruyn, pp. 285–325. Amsterdam: North Holland

STÅLBERG, E. (1966). 'Propagation velocity in human muscle fibres *in situ*.' *Acta Physiologica Scandinavica*, **70**, Supp. **287**, 1–112

STÅLBERG, E. (1974). *Single fibre electromyography*. Copenhagen: Disa Information Department

STÅLBERG, E., EKSTEDT, J. and BROMAN, A. (1974). 'Neuromuscular transmission in myasthenia gravis studied with single fibre electromyography.' *Journal of Neurology, Neurosurgery and Psychiatry*, **37**, 540–547.

STÅLBERG, E. and THIELE, Barbara (1972). 'Transmission block in terminal nerve twigs: a single fibre electromyographic finding in man.' *Journal of Neurology, Neurosurgery and Psychiatry*, **35**, 52–59

STÅLBERG, E., TRONTELJ, J. V. and JANKO, M. (1972). 'Single fibre EMG findings in muscular dystrophy.' In *Symposium on Structure and Function of Normal and Diseases of Muscle and Peripheral Nerve* (Abstract, no. 76). Kazimierz, Poland

STEIDL, R. M., OSWALD, A. J. and KOTTKE, F. J. (1962). 'Myasthenic syndrome with associated neuropathy.' *Archives of Neurology*, **6**, 451–461

STEIN, J. M. and PADYKULA, Helen A. (1962). 'Histochemical classification of individual skeletal muscle fibres of rat.' *American Journal of Anatomy*, **110**, 103–123

STEINBACH, J. H. and HEINEMANN, S. (1974). 'Nerve-muscle interaction in clonal cell culture.' In *Exploratory Concepts in Muscular Dystrophy II*. Ed. by A. T. Milhorat, pp. 161–169. Amsterdam: Excerpta Medica

STEINBERG, S. and BOTELHO, Stella (1962). 'Myotonia in a horse.' *Science, N.Y.*, **137**, 979–980

STEINERT, H. (1909). 'Myopathologische beitrage: 1.Über das klinische und anatomische bild des muskelschwunds der myotoniker.' *Deutsche Zeitschrift fur Nervenheilkunde*, **37**, 38–104

STEINKE, J. and TYLER, R. H. (1964). 'The association of amyotrophic lateral sclerosis (motor neuron disease) with carbohydrate intolerance, a clinical study.' *Metabolism*, **13**, 1376–1381

STEPHENS, J. A. and STUART, D. G. (1975). 'The motor units of cat medial gastrocnemius: speed-size relations and their significance for the recruitment order of motor units.' *Brain Research*, **91**, 177–195

STEPHENS, J. A. and TAYLOR, A. (1972). 'Fatigue of maintained voluntary muscle contraction in man.' *Journal of Physiology*, **220**, 1–18

STERN, G. M., HALL, Judith M. and ROBINSON, D. C. (1964). 'Neonatal myasthenia gravis.' *British Medical Journal*, **ii**, 284–286

STIEL, J. N. (1967). 'The incidence of gastrectomy and gastric secretion in motor neuron disease.' *Australasian Annals of Medicine*, **16**, 176–177

STIRLING, C.A. (1975). 'Experimentally induced myelination of amyelinated axons in dystrophic mice.' *Brain Research*, **87**, 130–135

STONNINGTON, H. H. and ENGEL, A. G. (1973). 'Normal and denervated muscle. A morphometric study of fine structure.' *Neurology (Minneapolis)*, **23**, 714–724

STRAUSS, A. J. L., SEEGAL, BEATRICE C., HSU, K. C., BURKHOLDER, P. M., NASTUK, W. L. and OSSERMAN, K. E. (1960). 'Immunofluorescence demonstration of a muscle binding, complement-fixing serum globulin fraction in myasthenia gravis.' *Proceedings of the Society for Experimental Biology and Medicine*, **105**, 184–191

STRICKHOLM, A. (1974). 'Intracellular generated potentials during excitation coupling in muscle.' *Journal of Neurobiology*, **5**, 161–187

STURUP, G., BOLTAN, B., WILLIAMS, D. J. and CARMICHAEL, E. A. (1935). 'Vasomotor responses in hemiplegic patients.' *Brain*, **58**, 456–459

STUDITSKY, A. N. (1952). 'Restoration of muscle by means of transplantation of minced muscle tissue (Russian).' *Dok. Akad. Nauk. SSSR*, 84/2 389

STUDITSKY, A. N., ZHENEVSKAYA, R. B. and RUMYANTSEVA, O. N. (1963). 'The role of neurotrophic influences upon the restitution of structure and function of regenerating muscles.' In *The Effect of Use and Disuse on Neuromuscular Functions*. Ed. by E. Gutman and P. Hnik, pp. 71–81. Prague: Publishing House of the Czechoslovak Academy of Sciences

SUGITA, H., OKIMOTO, K., EBASHI, S. and OIMAKA, S. (1967). 'Biochemical alterations in progressive muscular dystrophy with special reference to the sarcoplasmic reticulum.' In *Exploratory Concepts in Muscular Dystrophy and Related Disorders*. Ed. by A. T. Milhorat, pp. 321–332. Amsterdam: Excerpta Medica

SUMNER, A. J. (1975). 'Preservation of early discharge of muscle afferents in acrylamide neuropathy,' *Journal of Physiology*, **246**, 277–288

SUNDERLAND, S. (1947). 'Rate of regeneration in human, peripheral nerves. Analysis of the interval between injury and onset of recovery.' *Archives of Neurology and Psychiatry (Chicago)*, **58**, 251–295

SUNDERLAND, S. (1951). 'A classification of peripheral nerve injuries producing loss of function.' *Brain*, **74**, 491–516

SUNDERLAND, S. (1968). *Nerves and Nerve Injuries*. Edinburgh: Livingstone

SUNDERLAND, S. and RAY, L. J. (1950). 'Denervation changes in mammalian striated muscle.' *Journal of Neurology, Neurosurgery and Psychiatry*, **13**, 159–177

SWALLOW, M. (1966). 'Fibre size and content of the anterior tibial nerve of foot.' *Journal of Neurology, Neurosurgery and Psychiatry*, **29**, 205–213

SWIFT, T. R. and LAMBERT, E. H. (1974). Unpublished observations cited by M. Tsujihata, A. G. Engel, and E. H. Lambert, *Neurology (Minneapolis)*, **24**, 849–856

TABARY, J. C., TABARY, C., TARDIEU, C., TARDIEU, G. and GOLDSPINK, G. (1972). 'Physiological and structural changes in the cat's soleus muscle due to immobilization at different lengths by plaster casts.' *Journal of Physiology*, **224**, 231–244

TAKAMORI, M., GUTMANN, L. and SHANE, S. R. (1971). 'Contractile properties of human skeletal muscle.' *Archives of Neurology*, **25**, 535–546

TAKEUCHI, A. and TAKEUCHI, N. (1960). 'On the permeability of end-plate membrane during the action of transmitter. *Journal of Physiology*, **154**, 52–67

TANG, B. Y., KOMIYA, Y. and AUSTIN, L. (1974). 'Axoplasmic flow of phospholipids and cholesterol in the sciatic nerve of normal and dystrophic mice.' *Experimental Neurology*, **43**, 13–20

TANJI, J. and KATO, M. (1972). 'Discharge of single motor units at voluntary contraction of abductor digiti minimi muscle in man.' *Brain Research*, **45**, 590–593

TASAKI, I. (1953). *Nervous Transmission*. Springfield, Ill.: Thomas

THESLEFF, S. (1960). 'Supersensitivity of skeletal muscle produced by botulinum toxin.' *Journal of Physiology*, **151**, 598–607

THESLEFF, S. (1962). 'Spontaneous electrical activity in denervated rat skeletal muscle.' In *The Effect of Use and Disuse on Neuromuscular Functions*. Ed. by E. Gutmann and P. Hnik, pp. 41–51. Amsterdam: Elsevier

THESLEFF, S. (1963). 'Spontaneous electrical activity in denervated rat skeletal muscle.' In *The Effect of Use and Disuse on Neuromuscular Functions*. Ed. by E. Gutmann and P. Hnik, pp. 41–51. Prague: Czechoslovak Academy of Sciences

THESLEFF, S. and WARD, M. R. (1975). 'Studies on the mechanism of fibrillation potentials in denervated muscle.' *Journal of Physiology*, **244**, 313–323

THESLEFF, S., ZELENA, Jirina and HOFMANN, W. W. (1964). 'Restoration of function in botulinum paralysis by experimental nerve regeneration.' *Proceedings of the Society for Experimental Biology and Medicine*, **116**, 19–20

THOMAS, P. K. (1970). 'The cellular response to nerve injury. 3. The effect of repeated crush injuries.' *Journal of Anatomy*, **106**, 463–470

THOMAS, P. K., SEARS, T. A. and GILLIATT, R. W. (1959). 'The range of conduction velocity in normal motor nerve fibres to the small muscles of the hand and foot.' *Journal of Neurology, Neurosurgery and Psychiatry*, **22**, 175–181

THOMAS, R. C. (1972). 'Electrogenic sodium pump in nerve and muscle cells.' *Physiological Reviews*, **52**, 563–594

TOMLINSON, B. E., WALTON, J. N. and IRVING, Dorothy (1974). 'Spinal cord limb motor neurones in muscular dystrophy.' *Journal of the Neurological Sciences*, **22**, 305–327

TOMLINSON, B. E., WALTON, J. N. and REBEIZ, J. J. (1969). 'The effects of ageing and of cachexia upon skeletal muscle. A histopathological study. *Journal of the Neurological Sciences*, **9**, 321–346

TONGE, D. A. (1974a). 'Synaptic function in experimental dually innervated muscle in the mouse.' *Journal of Physiology*, **239**, 96–97P

TONGE, D. A. (1974b). 'Physiological characteristics of reinnervation of skeletal muscle in the mouse.' *Journal of Physiology*, **241**, 141–153

TOOP, J. (1975). 'The histochemical development of human skeletal muscle and its motor innervation.' In *Recent Advances in Myology* (Proceedings of the 3rd International congress on Muscle Diseases). Ed. by W. G. Bradley, D. Gardner-Medwin and J. N. Walton pp. 322–329. Amsterdam: Excerpta Medica

TORRES, J., IRIARTE, L. L. G. and KURLAND, L. T. (1957). 'Amyotrophic lateral sclerosis among Guamanians in California.' *California Medicine*, **86**, 385–388

TOWER, S. S. (1937). 'Trophic control of non-nervous tissues by the nervous system: a study of muscle and bone innervated from an isolated and quiescent region of spinal cord.' *Journal of Comparative Neurology*, **67**, 241–267

TOWER, Sarah (1939). 'The reaction of muscle to denervation.' *Physiological Reviews*, **19**, 1–48

TOYKA, K. V., DRACHMAN, D. B., PESTRONK, A. and KAO, I. (1975). 'Myasthenia gravis: passive transfer from man to mouse.' *Science (New York)*, **190**, 397–399

TROJABORG, W. and BUCTHAL, F. (1965). 'Malignant and benign fasciculations.' *Acta Neurologica Scandinavica*, **41**, Suppl. **13**, 251–254

TSUJIHATA, M., ENGEL, A. G. and LAMBERT, E. H. (1974). 'Motor end-plate fine structure in acrylamide dying-back neuropathy: A sequential morphometric study.' *Neurology (Minneapolis)*, **24**, 849–856

TSUKIYAMA, K., NAKAI, A., MINE, R. and KITANI, T. (1959). 'Studies on a myasthenic substance present in the serum of a patient with myasthenia gravis.' *Medical Journal of Osaka University*, **10**, 159

TYLER, F. H., STEVENS, F. E., GUNN, F. D. and PERKOFF, G. T. (1951). 'Studies in disorders of muscle. VII. Clinical manifestations and inheritance of a type of periodic paralysis without hypopotassemia.' *Journal of Clinical Investigation*, **30**, 492–502

TUFFERY, A. R. (1971). 'Growth and degeneration of motor end-plates in normal cat hind limb muscles.' *Journal of Anatomy*, **110**, 221–247

UNIVERSITY OF CALIFORNIA (1947). *Fundamental Studies of Human Locomotion and Other Information relating to the Design of Artificial Limbs*. Vol. 2

UNVERRICHT, H. (1887). 'Polymyositis acuta progressiva.' *Zeitschrift für klinische Medecin*, **12**, 533–549

UPRUS, V., GAYLOR, J. B., WILLIAMS, D. J. and CARMICHAEL, E. A. (1935). 'Vasodilation and vasoconstriction in response to warming and cooling the body. A study in patients with hemiplegia.' *Brain*, **58**, 448–455

UPTON, A. R. M. and MCCOMAS, A. J. (1973). 'The double crush in nerve entrapment syndromes.' *Lancet*, **ii**, 359–362

UPTON, A. R. M., MCCOMAS, A. J. and BIANCHI, F. A. (1973). 'Neuropathy in McArdle's syndrome.' *New England Journal of Medicine*, **289**, 750–751

UTTERBACK, R. A., CUMMINS, A. J., CAPE, C. A. and GOLDENBERG, J. (1970). 'Pancreatic function in amyotrophic lateral sclerosis.' *Journal of Neurology, Neurosurgery and Psychiatry*, **33**, 544–547

VAN ESSEN, D. and JANSEN, J. K. S. (1974). 'Re-innervation of the rat diaphragm during perfusion with α-bungarotoxin. *Acta Physiologica Scandinavica*, **91**, 571–573

VERATTI, E. (1902). 'Richerche sulla fine struttura della

fibra muscolare striata.' *Memorie Reale Istituto Lombardi*, **19**, 87–133

VIZOSO, A. D. (1950). 'The relationship between internodal length and growth in human nerves.' *Journal of Anatomy*, **84**, 342–353

VRBOVÁ, Gerta (1963). 'The effect of motoneurone activity on the speed of contraction of striated muscle.' *Journal of Physiology*, **169**, 513–526

WACHSTEIN, M. and MEISEL, E. (1955). 'The distribution of demonstrable succinic dehydrogenase and mitochondria in tongue and skeletal muscles.' *Journal of Biophysical and Biochemical Cytology*, **1**, 483–488

WAGNER, E. (1863). 'Fall einer seltnen Muskelkrankheit.' *Archiv der Heilkunde (Leipzig)*, **4**, 282–283

WAINMAN, P. and SHIPOUNOFF, G. C. (1941). 'The effects of castration and testosterone propionate on the striated peroneal musculature in the rat.' *Endocrinology*, **29**, 975–978

WAKSMAN, B. H. and ADAMS, R. D. (1955). 'Allergic neuritis: an experimental disease of rabbits induced by the injection of peripheral nervous tissue and adjuvants.' *Journal of Experimental Medicine*, **102**, 213–236

WALD, I., LOESCH, D. and WOCHNIK, D. (1962). 'Concerning the relationship between dystrophia myotonica and peroneal muscular atrophy.' *Psychiatria et Neurologia*, **143**, 392–397

WALKER, M. B. (1934). 'Treatment of myasthenia gravis with progstigmine.' *Lancet*, **226**, 1200–1201

WALLER, A. (1850). 'Experiments on the section of the glossopharyngeal and hypoglossal nerves of the frog, and observation on the alteration produced thereby in the structure of their primitive fibres.' *Philosophical Transactions of the Royal Society, London*, **140**, 423

WALLIS, W. E., POZNAK, A. V. and PLUM, F. (1970). 'Generalized muscular stiffness, fasciculations and myokymia of peripheral nerve origin.' *Archives of Neurology*, **22**, 430–439

WALSHE, F. M. R. (1945). 'On ''acroparaesthesia'' and so-called ''neuritis'' of the hands and arms in women. Their probable relation to brachial plexus pressure by normal first ribs.' *British Medical Journal*, **ii**, 596–599

WALTON, J. N. and GARDNER-MEDWIN, D. (1974). 'Progressive muscular dystrophy and the myotonic disorders.' In *Disorders of Voluntary Muscle*. Ed. by J. N. Walton, 3rd ed., pp. 561–613. Edinburgh: Churchill Livingstone

WARMOLTS, J. R. and ENGEL, W. K. (1972). 'Open-biopsy electromyography. 1. Correlation of motor unit behaviour with histochemical muscle fibre type in human limb muscle.' *Archives of Neurology*, **27**, 512–517

WARTENBERG, R. (1944). 'Brachialgia statica paresthetica' *Journal of Nervous and Mental disease*, **99**, 877–887

WATSON, W. E. (1968a). 'Observations on the nucleolar and total cell body nucleic acid of injured nerve cells.' *Journal of Physiology*, **196**, 655–676

WATSON, W. E. (1968b). 'Centripetal passage of labelled molecules along mammalian motor axons.' *Journal of Physiology*, **196**, 122P–123P

WATSON, W. E. (1969). 'The response of motor neurones to intramuscular injection of botulinum toxin.' *Journal of Physiology*, **202**, 611–630

WATSON, W. E. (1970). 'Some metabolic responses of axotomized neurones to contact between their axons and denervated muscle.' *Journal of Physiology*, **210**, 321–343

WATSON, W. E. (1972). 'Some quantitative observations upon the responses of neuroglial cells which follow axotomy of adjacent neurones.' *Journal of Physiology*, **225**, 415–435

WEBSTER, H. de F., SPIRO, D., WAKSMAN, B. and ADAMS, R. D. (1961). 'Phase and electron microscopic studies of experimental deyelination. II. Schwann cell changes in guinea pig sciatic nerves during experimental diptheritic neuritis.' *Journal of Neuropathology and Experimental Neurology*, **20**, 5–34

WECHSLER, I. S., BROCK, S. and WEIL, A. (1929). 'Amyotrophic lateral sclerosis with objective and subjective (neuritic) sensory disturbance.' *Archives of Neurology and Psychiatry (Chicago)*, **21**, 299–310

WEICHERT, R. F. (1970). 'The neural ectodermal origin of the peptide-secreting endocrine glands.' *American Journal of Medicine*, **49**, 232–241

WEINSTOCK, I. M. and DJU, M. Y. (1971). 'Thymidine phosphorylation and thymidylate kinase in developing breast muscle of normal and dystrophic chickens.' *Biochima et Biophysica Acta*, **232**, 5–13

WEISS, P. (1944). 'Damming of axoplasm in constricted nerve: a sign of perpetual growth in nerve fibres.' *Anatomical Records*, **88**, 464

WEISS, P. (1969). 'Neuronal dynamics.' In *Neurosciences Research Symposium Summaries*. Ed. F. O. Schmitt et al. Vol. 3, pp. 255–299. Cambridge, Mass.: M.I.T. Press

WEISS, P. and CAVANAUGH, MARGARET W. (1959). 'Further evidence of perpetual growth of nerve fibres: recovery of fibre diameter after the release of prolonged constrictions.' *Journal of Experimental Zoology*, **142**, 461–473

WEISS, P. and DAVIS, H. (1943). 'Pressure block in nerves provided with arterial sleeves.' *Journal of Neurophysiology*, **6**, 269–286

WEISS, P. and EDDS, M. V. Jr (1945). 'Spontaneous recovery of muscle following partial denervation.' *American Journal of Physiology*, **145**, 587–607

WEISS, P. and HISCOE, H. (1948). 'Experiments on the mechanism of nerve growth.' *Journal of Experimental Zoology*, **107**, 315–395

WERDNIG, G. (1891). 'Zwei frühinfantile hereditäre Fälle von progressiver Muskelatrophie unter dem Bilde der Dystrophie, aber auf neurotischer Grundlage.' *Archiv. Psychiat. Nervenkr.* **22**, 437–480

WESTALL, F., ROBINSON, A. B., CACCAM, Juanita, JACKSON, J. and EYLAR, E. H. (1971). 'Essential chemical requirements for induction of allergic encephalomyelitis.' *Nature (London)*, **229**, 22–24

WHITFIELD, A. G. W. and HUDSON, W. A. (1961). 'Chronic thyrotoxic myopathy.' *Quarterly Journal of Medicine*, **30**, 257–267

WHITTAKER, V. P., MICHAELSON, I. A. and KIRKLAND, R. J. A. (1964). 'The separation of synaptic vesicles from nerve-ending particles (''synaptosomes'').' *Biochemical Journal*, **90**, 293–303

WILLIAMS, E. R. and BRUFORD, Anne (1970). 'Creatine phosphokinase in motor neurone disease.' *Clinica Chimica Acta*, **27**, 53–56

WILLIAMS, P. E. and GOLDSPINK, G. (1971). 'Longitudinal growth of striated muscle fibres.' *Journal of Cell Science*, **9**, 751–767

WILLIAMS, P. L. and HALL, susan, M. (1971a). 'Prolonged *in vivo* observations of normal peripheral nerve fibres and their acute reactions to crush and deliberate trauma.' *Journal of Anatomy*, **108**, 397–408

WILLIAMS, P. L. and HALL, susan M. (1971b). 'Chronic Wallerian degeneration—an *in vivo* and ultrastructural study.' *Journal of Anatomy*, **109**, 487–503

WILLIAMS, P. L. and LANDON, D. N. (1967). In *Gray's Anatomy*, 34th edn., p. 62. London: Longmans Green

WILLIAMSON, E. and BROOKE, M. H. (1972). 'Myokymia and the motor unit.' *Archives of Neurology*, **26**, 11–16

WILLIS, T. (1672). *De Anima Brutorum*. 400 pp. Amsterdam: Blaeus

WILSON, A. and STONER, H. B. (1944). 'Myasthenia Gravis: a consideration of its causation in a study of fourteen cases.' *Quarterly Journal of Medicine*, **13**, 1–18

WIŚNIEWSKI, H. M., BROSTOFF, S. W., CARTER, H. and EYLAR, E. H. (1974). 'R-current experimental allergic polyganglioradiculoneuritis.' *Archives of Neurology*, **30**, 347–358

WOCHNER, R. D., DREWS, Genevieve, STROBER, W. and WALDMAN, T. A. (1966). 'Accelerated breakdown of immunoglobulin G (IgG) in myotonic dystrophy: a hereditary error of immunoglobulin catabolism.' *Journal of Clinical Investigation*, **45**, 321–329

WOHLFART, G. (1942). 'Zwei Falle von Dystrophia musculorum progressiva mit fibrillaren Zuckungen und atypischen Muskelbefund.' *Deutsche Zeitschrift für Nervenheilkunde*, **153**, 189–204

WOOLF, A. L. and COËRS, C. (1974). 'Pathological anatomy of the intramuscular nerve endings.' In *Disorders of Voluntary Muscle*. Ed. by J. N. Walton, 3rd edn., pp. 274–309. Edinburgh: Churchill Livingstone

WRAY, shirley H. (1969). 'Innervation ratios for large and small limb muscles in the baboon.' *Journal of Comparative Neurology*, **137**, 227–250

WRIGHT, T. L., O'NEILL, J. A. and OLSON, W. H. (1973). 'Abnormal intramyofibrillar monoamines in sex-linked muscular dystrophy.' *Neurology (Minneapolis)*, **23**, 510–517

WRIGHT, E. A. and SPINK, Jean M. (1959). 'A study of the loss of nerve cells in the central nervous system in relation to age.' *Gerontologia*, **3**, 277–287

YELLIN, H. (1967). Neural regeneration of enzymes in muscle fibres of red and white muscle.' *Experimental Neurology*, **19**, 92–103

YELLIN, H. and GUTH, L. (1970). The histochemical classification of muscle fibers. *Experimental Neurology*, **26**, 424–432

YOUNG, I. J. (1966). 'Morphological and histochemical studies of partially and totally deafferented spinal cord segments.' *Experimental Neurology*, **14**, 238–248

YUNIS, E. J., STUTMAN, O. and GOOD, R. A. (1971). 'Thymus, immunity and autoimmunity.' In *Myasthenia Gravis*. Ed. by W. S. Fields. *Annals of the New York Academy of Sciences*, **183**, 205–220

ZACKS, S. I., BAUER, W. C. and BLUMBERG, J. J. (1961). 'Abnormalities in the fine structure of the neuromuscular junction in patients with myasthenia gravis.' *Nature (London)*, **190**, 280–281

ZACKS, S. I., BAUER, W. C. and BLUMBERG, J. J. (1962). 'The fine structure of the myasthenic neuromuscular junction.' *Journal of Neuropathology and Experimental Neurology*, **21**, 335–347

ZACKS, S. I. and SAITO, A. (1969). 'Uptake of exogenous horseradish peroxidase by coated vesicles in mouse neuromuscular junctions.' *Journal of Histochemical and Cytochemistry*, **17**, 161–170

ZACKS, S. I., SHIELDS, D. R. and STEINBERG, S. A. (1966). 'A myasthenic syndrome in the dog: a case report with electron microscope observations on motor end plates and comparisons with the fine structure of end plates in myasthenia gravis.' In *Myasthenia Gravis*. Ed. by K. E. Osserman. *Annals of the New York Academy of Sciences*, **135**, 79–97

ZAJAC, F. E. and YOUNG, J. (1975). 'Motor unit discharge patterns during treadmill walking and trotting in the cat.' *Society for Neuroscience, 5th Annual Meeting, New York*. Abstract No. 255

ZELLWEGER, H. and NIEDERMEYER, E. (1965). 'Central nervous system manifestations in childhood muscular dystrophy (CMD). 1. Psychometric and electroencephalographic findings.' *Annales Paediatrici (Basel)*, **205**, 25–42

ZIEGLER, T. F. (1969). 'Acrylamide toxicity: residue in rat urine.' In American Cyanamid Company Interoffice Correspondence. Cited, with permission by P. S. Spencer and H. H. Schaumburg (1974)

ZIERLER, K. L. (1959). 'Effect of insulin on membrane potential and potassium content of rat muscle.' *American Journal of Physiology*, **197**, 515–522

ZIERLER. K. L. (1961). 'Potassium flux and further observations on aldolase flux in dystrophic mouse muscle.' *Bulletin of Johns Hopkins Hospital*, **108**, 208–215

ZIERLER, K. L. and ANDRES, R. (1957). 'Movement of potassium into skeletal muscle during spontaneous attack in family periodic paralysis.' *Journal of Clinical Investigation*, **36**, 730–737

ZIL'BER, L. A., BAJDAKOVA, Z. L., GARDAS'JAN, A. N., KONOVALOV, N. V., BUNINA, T. L. and BARABADZE, E. M. (1963). 'Study of the etiology of amyotrophic lateral sclerosis.' *Bulletin of the World Health Organization*, **29**, 449–456

ZILKHA, K. J. (1962). In 'Discussion on motor neurone disease.' *Proceedings of the Royal Society of Medicine*, **55**, 1028

SUPPLEMENTARY RECENT ARTICLES (CITED IN TEXT)

BRAY, J. J., HAWKEN, M. J. HUBBARD, J. I., POCKETT, susan and WILSON, Leona (1976). 'The membrane potential of rat diaphragm muscle fibres and the effect of denervation.' *Journal of Physiology*, **255**, 651–667

DI MAURO, S., BONILLA, E., LEE, C. P., SCHOTLAND, D. L., CARPA, A., CONN, H. Jr., and CHANCE (1976). 'Luft's disease: further biochemical and ultrastructural studies of skeletal muscle in the second case.' *Journal of the Neurological Sciences*, **27**, 217–232

DRACHMAN, D. B. and FAMBROUGH, D. M. (1976). 'Are muscle fibres denervated in myotonic dystrophy?' *Archives of Neurology.* **33**, 485–488

DROZ, B., RAMBOURG, A., and KOENIG, H. L. (1975). 'The smooth endoplasmic reticulum: structure and role in the renewal of axonal membrane and synaptic vesicles by fast axonal transport. *Brain Research.* **93**, 1–13

ENGEL, A. G. (1970). 'Evolution and content of vacuoles in primary hypokalaemic periodic paralysis.' *Mayo Clinic Proceedings.* **45**, 774–814

FEIBEL, J. H. and CAMPA, J. F. (1976). 'Thyrotoxic neuropathy (Basedow's paraplegia).' *Journal of Neurology, Neurosurgery and Psychiatry.* **39**, 491–497

GRAFSTEIN, Bernice (1971). 'Transneuronal transfer of radioactivity in the central nervous system.' *Science,* **172**, 177–179

GRUENER, R. (1977). '*In vitro* membrane excitability of diseased human muscle.' In *Exploratory Concepts in Muscular Dystrophy III.* Ed. by L. P. Rowland. Amsterdam: Excerpta Medica. In press

HEUSER, J. E. and REESE, T. S. (1973). 'Evidence for recycling of synaptic vesicle membrane during transmitter release at the frog neuromuscular junction.' *Journal of Cell Biology.* **57**, 315–344

ITO, Y., MILEDI, R., MOLENAAR, P. C., VINCENT, Angela, POLAK, R. L., VAN GELDER, Monique and DAVIS, J. N. (1976). 'Acetylcholine in human muscle.' *Proceedings of the Royal Society. B.* **192**, 475–480

KAMOSHITA, S., KONISHI, Y., SEGAWA, M. and FUKUYAMA, Y. (1976). 'Congenital muscular dystrophy as a disease of the central nervous system.' *Archives of Neurology.* **33**, 513–516

LOCKE, S. and SOLOMON, H. C. (1967). 'Relation of resisting potential of rat gastrocnemius and soleus muscles to innervation, activity and the Na–K pump.' *Journal of Experimental Zoology.* **166**, 377–386

MOKRI, B. and ENGEL, A. G. (1975). 'Duchenne dystrophy: electron microscopic findings pointing to a basic or early abnormality in the plasma membrane of the sarcolemma,' *Neurology (Minneapolis),* **25**, 111–1120

NATORI, R. (1975). 'The electrical potential change of internal membrane during propagation of contraction in skinned fibre of toad skeletal muscle.' *Japanese Journal of Physiology.* **25**, 51–63

RASMINSKY, M. and KEARNEY, R. E. (1976). 'Continuous conduction in large diameter bare axons in spinal roots of dystrophic mice.' *28th Annual Meeting of the American Academy of Neurology. Toronto. Abstracts.* p. 80

SCHWARTZ, M. S. and STÅLBERG, E. (1975). 'Single fiber electromygraphic studies in myasthenia gravis with repetitive nerve stimulation.' *Journal of Neurology, Neurosurgery and Psychiatry.* **38**, 678–682

STÅLBERG, E. (1977). 'Electrogenesis in human dystrophic muscle.' In *Exploratory Concepts in Muscular Dystrophy III.* Ed. by L. P. Rowland. Amsterdam: Excerpta Medica

SUNDERLAND, S. (1976). 'The nerve lesion in the carpal tunnel syndrome.' *Journal of Neurology, Neurosurgery and Psychiatry.* **39**, 615–626

THESLEFF, S. (1975). 'Discussion on neurotrophic mechanisms.' In *Exploratory Concepts in Muscular Dystrophy II.* Ed. by A. T. Milhorat, pp. 465–466. Amsterdam: Excerpta Medica

INDEX

A-band, 5, 35, 39, 93
  antibody, 207, 208
Absolutely refractory period, 24
Accommodation of excitable membranes, 24, 124, 130, 137, 138
Acetate, 31
Acetazolamide, 134, 135
Acetylcholine (ACh), 8, 27, 29, 30–32, 68, 71, 75, 77, 84, 93, 95, 124, 127
  diffusion, 30, 205, 206
  hydrolysis, 30, 32
  membrane sensitivity, 75–77, 83–88, 93, 95, 106
  quanta, 31
  receptor (AChR), 5, 30, 33, 75, 87, 88, 92, 93, 202–208, 224
  receptor antibodies in myasthenia, 202–208
  release, 29–33, 84
    after antibiotic application, 212, 213
    after nerve section, 222
    in botulism, 215
    in Eaton-Lambert Syndrome, 211, 212
    in myasthenia gravis, 198–202, 205–207
    in quantal squander myokymia, 214
    in tetanus, 216, 217
  synthesis, 31
Acetylcholinesterase, 5, 15, 33, 34, 95, 196, 198, 205, 206
Aconitine, 129
Acrylamide, 71
  electrophysiological studies in neuropathy, 276
  metabolism, 275
  neuropathy, 274–276, 283
  toxicity, 275
Actin, 35–38, 43–46, 58, 78, 92, 93
Action potential (impulse),
  block by nerve compression, 251, 258, 259
  conduction velocity measurement, 25, 305–307
  effect of demyelination, 239–242
  effect of local anaesthetics, 83
  failure, 68, 69
  in axotomized motoneurone, 89, 90
  in denervated muscle fibre, 74, 75, 78
  in developing muscle cells, 93
  in divided axons, 221
  in dystrophic mice, 239
  in idiopathic polyradiculoneuritis, 235
  in myasthenia gravis, 195, 199–202, 205–207
  in myotonia, 123, 125–132
  in periodic paralysis, 135–138
  in peroneal muscular atrophy, 239
  in regenerated axons, 224

Action potential (impulse), continued
  in terminal motor axon, 28, 30, 68, 69, 71, 77, 84, 114, 118
  in transverse tubular (T) system, 38–40
  intracellular recording, 20–22
  ionic mechanism, 11, 18, 20, 21
  propagation, 24–26
  velocity in muscle fibre, 25
  velocity in nerve fibre, 26 (see also under various disorders)
Actinomycin D, 88
Active complex, 38
Active state, 41, 42, 74, 78
  in thyrotoxicosis, 286, 287
Activity of muscle, as trophic influence, 86
Actomyosin, 15
Adenosine disphosphate (ADP), 37, 38
Adenosine triphosphatase (ATPase),
  calcium-magnesium, 5, 41, 187
  myosin, 58, 59, 61, 62, 67, 78, 81, 83, 98, 106, 151, 152, 165, 229
  sodium-potassium, 5, 11, 23, 26, 74, 123, 131, 138
Adenosine triphosphate (ATP), 7, 11, 15, 23, 27, 37, 38, 41–43, 58, 59, 70, 78
  in McArdle's disease, 189
  in malignant hyperthermia, 187
  in mitochondrial myopathy, 189
Adrenaline, 42
Adynamia episodica hereditaria (see Familial periodic paralysis, hyperkalaemic)
After-potential, 20
After-spasm, 125, 126
Ageing, 101–108, 215, 233, 234
  effects on muscle, 297, 298, 300, 302
  neuromuscular studies in animals, 106–108
  neurophysiological studies, 103
Albumin, 15, 39, 91
Aldolase, 146, 185, 313
Aldosterone, 140
Alternation phenomenon, 51, 311
Alzheimer's disease, 271
Amino acids, 16
Amyotrophic lateral sclerosis (see Motoneurone disease)
Anabolic steroids, 96
Anaesthetic,
  general, 82
  general, in malignant hyperthermia, 184
  local, 23, 63, 83, 85, 114
  muscle action, 42
Andersen's disease, 188

Anions, 16, 18, 123, 139 (*see also* Chloride)
  lyotropic, 42
Anoxia, 69, 123
Antibiotics, causing pseudomyasthenic syndrome, 212, 213
Antibody,
  in experimental allergic myasthenia gravis, 203–205
  in experimental allergic neuritis, 236, 237
  in myasthenia gravis, 196, 206–208
  to acetylcholine receptor, 196, 203–208
Anticholinesterase, 34, 71, 195–198, 210, 212, 214, 264, 317
Anticipation, in myotonic dystrophy, 314
Antiviral drugs, 264
Aquerin, 40
Arylsulphatase A deficiency, 285
Athletics, 96
  and motoneurone disease, 269, 271
Atrophy, 71–73, 82–84, 96–101 (*see also* Grouped muscle fibre atrophy)
  denervation, 72–73, 282, 296
  disuse, 82–84
  in Duchenne dystrophy, 145, 148, 153
  in hemiplegia, 294
  in limbgirdle dystrophy, 160
  in motoneurone disease, 263, 264
  in myasthenia gravis, 197, 198, 205
  in myotonic dystrophy, 165
  in periodic paralysis, 134
  in polymyositis, 179
  in thyrotoxicosis, 285, 286
  progressive muscular, 263
  spinal muscular, 160–165, 272, 273
Atropine, 196
Autograft, 98
Axolemma, 9, 10, 171
Axon (nerve fibre),
  autonomic (cholinergic), 77
  compression,
    clinical syndromes, 244, 245
    effects of, 83–86, 106, 212, 233, 234, 243–252
    EMG findings, 255, 256
    experimental studies, 244, 245
  cutaneous, 26
  cylinder, 10
  density, 103
  demyelination, 233–242
  diameter, 10, 11, 26, 53, 67
  effects of ligation, 212
  effects of section, 89, 114, 126, 127, 221–222
    on motoneurone, 89, 90
  hillock, 10, 67, 89, 91
  in muscle development, 94, 95
  in Wallerian degeneration, 107, 221, 222, 233, 234, 236
  injury, effects of, 243–252
    types, 243
  motor nerve terminal, 28, 30, 68, 69, 71, 77, 84, 102, 106, 114, 118
  muscle, 26
  neurapraxic lesion, 83, 84, 86, 243–249
  numbers in ageing, 103, 106
  regeneration, 30, 222–224

Axon (nerve fibre), continued
  sprouting, 87, 89, 90, 102, 106, 107, 113–115, 223–232, 243, 297
    in hemiplegia, 293
    stimulus for, 225–227
    types, 224, 225
  squid, 21, 23
  unmyelinated, 26
Axoplasmic transport (flow), 12, 33, 80, 83, 85–88, 107, 212, 222, 271, 295, 296
  block, 83, 85
  centripetal, 15, 91
  contents, 14, 15, 86
  fast, 13, 14
  in dying-back neuropathy, 283
  in murine dystrophy, 172, 173
  in nerve compression, 251, 258, 259
  in thyrotoxicosis, 288
  measurement, 13
  mechanism, 14, 15
  modulation, 14
Axonotmesis, 243

Bacterial neurotoxins, 214–217
Band of Bungner, 222, 223, 276
Barium toxicity, 140
Basement membrane, 5, 27, 92, 93, 100, 182
Basophilia, 73
Batrachatoxin, 24, 217
Becker dystrophy, 145
Beta (β)-adrenergic receptors, 42, 287
Bicarbonate, 16, 185
Black widow spider venom, 32, 217
Blastema, 99
Blastula, 92
Blocking factor,
  in myasthenia, 196, 202–205
  in serum from patients with multiple sclerosis, 241
Blood flow in hemiplegic limbs, 294
Blood vessels in regenerating muscle, 98
Body-building, 80, 96
Bone-pinning, 84
Bornholm disease (epidemic myalgia), 183
Botulinum toxin, 84, 85, 90, 114, 214, 215, 228
Botulism, 214, 215
Boutons termineaux, 10, 89, 90
Brachial neuralgia (*see* Paraesthesiae in upper limb)
Brachial plexus lesion, 253, 256, 257
Brancher enzyme, 188
Bromide, 42
Bronchial carcinoma, 209, 210
Bungarotoxin (BTX), 33, 84, 93, 202, 206, 217, 227
Bushbaby (*Galago senegalensis*), 67

Caffeine, 42, 70, 76, 185, 189
Calcium, 16
  in cell fusion, 93
  in Eaton-Lambert syndrome, 211
  in excitation-contraction coupling, 40–42, 138
  in McArdle's disease, 189
  in malignant hyperthermia, 187

Calcium, continued
  in muscle contraction, 38, 40–42, 70
  in muscular dystrophy, 148, 313
  in myotonia, 130, 131
  in neuromuscular transmission, 29–31, 33
  in periodic paralysis, 138
  pump, 41, 42, 70
Calcium gluconate, 135
Calsequestrin, 41
Capacitance,
  membrane, 19, 24
  myelin sheath, 239
Capillary, muscle, 59, 62, 81, 82
Carbamezapine, 214
Carbohydrate metabolism, 134, 135, 139, 187–189, 268
Carbon tetrachloride poisoning, 270
Carcinoma, 101, 103, 234
  and motoneurone disease, 268
  remote effects on nervous system, 209, 210
Carcinomatous neuropathy (see Eaton-Lambert syndrome)
Cardiac failure, 45, 188
  in dystrophy, 148, 158, 160, 165
Carpal tunnel syndrome, 249–259
  EMG studies, 255–257
  pathogenesis, 251, 252
Carrier detection in Duchenne dystrophy, 146
Carrier molecules, 5, 23
Cartilage, 92, 99
Castration, effects on muscle, 96
Cataracts, 124, 125
Cations, 16, 18 (see also Calcium, Magnesium, Potassium and Sodium)
Caveolae, 3
Central core disease, 190
'Central' myotonia (see After-spasm)
Centronuclear myopathy, 190
Ceramide trihexosidase deficiency, 285
Cervical rib, 253
Cervical root lesion, 253–257, 259
Cervical spondylosis, 131
Charcot-Marie-Tooth disease (Peroneal muscular atrophy), 238, 239
Chicken dystrophy (see Muscular dystrophy in Animals)
Chimaera experiment, 177, 178, 301
Chloride, 18, 19, 20
  permeability of membrane, 16, 18–20, 74, 138
  in myotonia, 128, 129, 132
Chlorthiazide, 134
Cholesterol, 131
Choline, 21, 31
Choline acetyltransferase, 14, 31
Cholinesterase, 30, 32–34, 75, 77, 86, 93, 95
Cholistin, 213
Chondrogenic cells in development, 92
Chromosomes, 9
Cirrhosis of the liver, 103
Classification of muscle fibre types, 61, 62
Cleft, synaptic, 27, 33, 34, 95, 99
  in Eaton-Lambert syndrome, 212
  in myasthenia gravis, 197, 206
Clofibrate, 125

Coaxial (concentric) needle electrode, 49, 75, 115, 125
  (see also Electromyography)
Cobrotoxin, 217
Coenzyme A, 31
Colchicine, 85, 100
Collateral reinnervation, 30, 113–115, 224–232, 265, 297
  effectiveness, 230–232
  in botulism, 215
  in Duchenne dystrophy, 300, 302
  in hemiplegia, 293
  in limbgirdle and facioscapulohumeral dystrophies, 162, 163, 300
  in motoneurone disease, 265, 272
  in myasthenia gravis, 197
  in myotonic dystrophy, 165
  in tetanus, 217
  in thyrotoxicosis, 286
  in toxic and metabolic neuropathies, 282, 283
  stimulus for, 227
  types of sprouting, 224, 225
Compression of nerve (see Axon, compression)
Conduction velocity of impulse (see also Action potential),
  in axon, 26
  in muscle fibre, 25, 26
  techniques for measurement, 25, 305–307
Congenital hypotonia, 128
Congenital muscular dystrophy, 300, 301
Connective tissue, muscle, 83, 98, 113
  after denervation, 73, 157, 158
  in ageing, 101
  in Duchenne dystrophy, 145, 148, 157, 158
  in polymyositis, 180, 181
Continuous muscle fibre activity (see Quantal squander myokymia)
Contraction of muscle,
  failure, 68–70
  isometric, 43–46 (see also below)
  isotonic, 43, 44, 80, 97
  single fibre, 44, 45
  tetanic, 42–46, 59–62, 69, 70, 74, 85, 95
  twitch, 41, 45, 46, 54, 57, 60–62, 77, 78, 81–83, 85
    in ageing, 101, 104, 105, 106
    in denervation, 73, 74
    in development, 93, 96, 98
    in Duchenne dystrophy, 151, 152
    in hemiplegia, 291
    in hypothyroidism, 286
    in limbgirdle dystrophy, 163, 164
    in myotonic dystrophy, 167, 168
    in thyrotoxicosis, 286
  voluntary, 43, 63–70, 80, 81, 96, 97, 124 (see also under diseases)
Contracture,
  knot, 148
  pathological, 43, 145
  physiological, 40, 42, 43, 70, 77, 84, 313
    in McArdle's disease, 188, 189
    in malignant hyperthermia, 185–187
Conversion of muscle fibre types, 61, 62, 81
Cooling, 20, 42, 125, 129, 137
Correlation of muscle fibre characteristics, 59–62
Corticosteroids, 132, 135, 145, 196, 208
Cramps, muscle, 264, 318

Creatine phosphokinase (CPK), 15
  in Duchenne dystrophy, 146
  in Duchenne dystrophy carriers, 146
  in limbgirdle dystrophy, 160, 310
  in malignant hyperthermia, 185
  in myotonic dystrophy, 165
  in polymyositis, 181
Cristae, 6
Critical membrane depolarization, 21, 24, 128, 130, 137
Critical membrane potential, 30
Cross-bridge, 37, 38, 43–46
Crotoxin, 217
Crush injury of nerve, 106, 228 (see also Axon, compression)
Curare (and D-tubocurarine), 33, 34, 75, 84, 126, 187, 193, 198, 212
Cyanide, sodium, 69
Cyclic AMP, 5
Cycloheximide, 14, 93

Damming of axoplasm, 13, 259
Dantrolene sodium, 42, 185
Debrancher enzyme, 188
Decamethonium, 34, 198
Decremental response of muscle, 118
  in botulism, 215
  in Eaton-Lambert Syndrome, 210
  in limbgirdle dystrophy, 163, 164
  in myasthenia gravis, 195, 200
  in myopathies, 212, 213
  in myotonic dystrophy, 167
  in nerve compression, 212, 249
  in neuropathies, 71, 212, 213
Degeneration of axon (see Axon, in Wallerian degeneration)
Degeneration of muscle fibre,
  in ageing, 101
  in animal models of dystrophy, 170–172
  in central core disease, 190
  in centronuclear myopathy, 190
  in denervation, 73
  in Duchenne dystrophy, 145
  in glycogen storage diseases, 188, 189
  in limbgirdle dystrophy, 160
  in mitochondrial myopathies, 189
  in myasthenia gravis, 197, 198
  in myotonic dystrophy, 165
  in periodic paralysis, 1, 34
  in polymyositis, 181, 182
  in tetanus, 217
Déjérine-Sottas neuropathy, 234, 239
Delay, synaptic, 29
Dementia, 169, 271
Demyelination, 233–242, 244, 252
  after diphtheria toxin, 237, 238
  effect on impulse conduction, 239–242
  in experimental allergic neuritis (EAN), 235–237
  in idiopathic polyradiculoneuritis, 234, 235
  in neuropathies, 233, 234
  in peroneal muscular atrophy, 238, 239

Denervation of muscle, 53, 61, 64, 72–79, 83–86, 114, 131
  biochemical and histochemical changes, 73, 79
  connective tissue changes, 73, 157, 158
  contractile changes, 73, 74
  degeneration of fibres, 73
  during progressive motoneurone dysfunction, 113–119, 281–283, 296, 297
  functional, 151, 171, 182, 282
  impulse conduction velocity, 25, 74
  in ageing, 102–108
  in botulism, 215
  in Duchenne dystrophy, 153
  in extensor digitorum brevis, 53, 307
  in hemiplegia, 291–293
  in idiopathic polyradiculoneuritis, 234
  in limbgirdle and facioscapulohumeral dystrophy, 160–164
  in motoneurone disease, 263–267
  in myasthenia gravis, 198, 201
  in myotonic dystrophy, 165–169
  in nerve injuries, 245–251
  in peroneal muscular atrophy, 238
  in polymyositis, 182
  in spinal muscular atrophy, 160–165, 272, 273
  in tetanus, 216, 217
  in thyrotoxicosis, 285–288
  in toxic and metabolic neuropathies, 276–284
Deoxyribonucleic acid (DNA), 9, 10, 87, 88, 97, 100, 107, 314
Depolarization, 18, 129, 135, 139
  axonal, 28, 68, 69, 71, 77
  block, 137
  motoneurone, 67–68
  of end-plate, 31
  T-tubules, 38
Dermatomyositis (see Polymyositis)
Desheathed muscle fibre, 40, 138
Desmesterol, 131
Diiosopropyl fluorophosphate (DFP), 227
Diabetes mellitus, 101, 233, 234, 242
  neuropathy in, 251–258
Diameters, of nerve fibres, 10, 11, 26, 53, 67
Diazacholesterol, 125, 128, 131
Dichlorphenamide, 134
Dichlorphenoxyacetate, 125
Dinitrophenol (DNP), 14
Diphenylhydantoin, 132, 214
Diphtheria, 233, 234, 237
  effects of toxin on nerve, 237–242
Disuse, effects on muscle, 80, 82–86, 101, 294
Dive-bomber discharge, 127
Docasadienoic acid, 131
Donnan equilibrium, 16, 18
Dopamine-β-hydroxylase, 14, 283
Dorsal roots, 83, 126, 171, 293
Double crush syndrome, 253–259
Doublet, in motoneurone discharge, 65
Duchenne dystrophy, 43, 71, 113, 116, 117, 118, 119, 143–158
  cardiomyopathy, 148, 158
  carrier detection, 146
  cerebral malformation, 155

Duchenne dystrophy, continued
  clinical features, 145–146
  EEG abnormalities, 155
  EMG findings, 151, 156
  erythrocyte studies, 146, 148, 313
  incidence, 145
  membrane hypothesis, 148–150, 313
  mental retardation, 143, 153, 154
  microelectrode recordings, 151
  motoneurones, 150, 151, 156
  motor unit counting studies, 152, 153, 299–301, 310
  multielectrode recordings, 151, 156
  muscle fibre impulse conduction velocity, 25
  muscle morphology, 147–150
  muscle twitch, 151–152
  mutation rate, 146
  nerve conduction studies, 152, 154
  neural hypothesis, 153–158
  neuromuscular junction, 150, 157, 158
  serum enzyme levels, 146–158
  special investigations, 146–153
  treatment, 145, 146
  vascular hypothesis, 312, 313
'Dying-back' neuropathy, 71, 228, 274–284, 290
Dystrophia myotonica (see Myotonic dystrophy)
Dystrophic mice (see Muscular dystrophy in animals)
  amyelination of roots, 239

Eaton-Lambert Syndrome, 209–212
  clinical features, 209–210
  electrophysiological investigations, 210–212
  microelectrode recordings, 211–212
  morphological studies, 212
  repetitive nerve stimulation, 210–211
  treatment, 210
Echinocytes, 148, 313
Ectoderm, 92
Edrophonium chloride, 34, 195
Elasticity of muscle, 41, 46
Electric organ, eel, 31, 33
Electroencephalogram (EEG)
  in Duchenne dystrophy, 155, 301
  in myotonic dystrophy, 169
Electrogenic pump, 21 (see also Sodium pump)
Electromyography (EMG), 48, 63, 75, 86, 104, 115
  in botulism, 215
  in carpal tunnel syndrome, 255, 256
  in cramp, 318
  in Duchenne dystrophy, 150, 151,
  in Eaton-Lambert syndrome, 210, 211
  in fasciculations, 317
  in idiopathic polyradiculoneuritis, 235
  in limbgirdle and facioscapulohumeral dystrophies, 160–165
  in malignant hyperthermia, 187
  in myopathy, 309
  in myotonic dystrophy, 167
  in neurapraxia, 246–249
  in 'normal' extensor digitorum brevis muscle, 307
  in peroneal muscular atrophy, 239
  in polymyositis, 182
  in quantal squander myokymia, 214

Electromyography (EMG), continued
  in spinal muscular atrophy, 160–165, 273
  in thyrotoxicosis, 286
  in Werdnig-Hoffman disease, 273
Embryonic development of muscle, 92–98
En grappe innervation, 227
Endoneurium, 12, 77, 224, 243
Endoplasmic reticulum, 5, 92
  axonal, 15
End-plate (see also Neuromuscular Junction), 27, 28, 51, 75–77, 83, 90, 127, 222
  after nerve section, 222
  in acrylamide neuropathy, 71, 276
  in ageing, 106
  in animal dystrophies, 171
  in antibiotic neurotoxicity, 213
  in botulism, 215
  in Eaton-Lambert syndrome, 211
  in myasthenia gravis, 198–200, 202
  in tetanus, 215, 216
End-plate potential (EPP), 30, 31, 69, 95, 106
  miniature (MEPP), 31, 32, 77
Entoderm, 92
Entrapment neuropathies, 249–252
Epineurium, 12
Equilibrium potential, 129
  chloride, 18
  potassium, 17, 18, 20
  sodium, 18, 21
Erythrocyte, in dystrophy, 131, 146, 313
Evans blue, 15, 91
Excitability, persistence after nerve section, 221–223
Excitation-contraction coupling, 38–42, 68–70, 124
  in Duchenne dystrophy, 151
  in malignant hyperthermia, 187
  in periodic paralysis, 138
Exercise, 62–71, 80–82, 134
  effect in Eaton-Lambert syndrome, 209
Exophthalmos, 208
Experimental allergic neuritis (EAN), 235–237
Extrinsic membrane proteins, 4

Facioscapulohumeral dystrophy, 116, 117, 118, 143, 145, 160–165 (see also Limbgirdle dystrophy)
Familial periodic paralysis, 123, 128, 133–140, 189
  biochemistry, 135–137
  clinical features, 133, 134
  depolarization in, 137–140
  hyperkalaemic, hypokalaemic, normokalaemic, 123, 124, 130, 132–140
  microelectrode recording, 135–137
  treatment, 134, 135
Fasciculation,
  benign syndrome, 317, 318
  potential, 263, 264, 317, 318
Fasciculi, nerve, 12
Fast-twitch,
  motor unit, 57, 59, 61, 62, 67, 106
  muscle, 77, 78, 79, 82, 83, 98, 286, 287
Fatigue,
  muscle, 59–61, 62, 68–71

Fatigue, continued
  in neuromuscular diseases, 71, 195
Fatty acids, 7, 71, 131, 132
Ferritin, 39
Fibre-type grouping, 229–231
  in ageing, 102
Fibrillation, 153, 182, 245, 277–280, 282, 293, 307, 317
Fibroblast, 92, 107, 108
Flexor retinaculum (see Transverse carpal ligament)
Fluidity, membrane, 131, 313
Force-velocity curve, 43, 58
Fragility, membrane, 131
Freund's adjuvant, 183, 203, 235, 236
Friedreich's ataxia, 158, 234, 268
Frontal baldness, 124
Fructose, 188, 189
  1 : 6 diphosphate, 139
Functional denervation, 151, 171, 182, 282
Fusion of myoblasts, 93
F-wave, 308, 309

Galactose, 188
Gamstorp's syndrome, 134 (see also Familial periodic paralysis, hyperkalaemic)
Gap substance, 11, 25
Gastric resection and motoneurone disease, 265, 267
Gate permeability, 23
Genes, 9, 78, 132
Genetic influence on motoneurone, 268
Germine acetate, 24, 198, 214
Glial cells, 10, 89, 90
Globulin, 123
Glove-and-stocking sensory loss, 234, 239
Glucosamine, 93
Glucose, 58, 134, 135, 137, 139, 188, 189
Glycolytic muscle fibre, 59, 62
Glycerol, 19, 39, 129, 139
Glycine, 145
Glycogen, 7, 59, 67, 70, 71, 188, 189
  breakdown, 58
  depletion in muscle fibres (method), 54, 56, 59
  enzyme, 86
  in thyrotoxic myopathy, 286
  storage diseases, 125, 187–189
Glycosides, cardiac, 23
Goat myotonia, 125, 128, 130, 311, 312
Goldman equation, 18, 21, 129
Golgi apparatus, 10, 14, 92
Gonyalaux catanella, 23
Gower's sign, 144, 145
Grana, 40
Grip strength, 101
Grouped muscle fibre atrophy, 30, 102, 115
  in Duchenne dystrophy, 153
  in myasthenia gravis, 198, 206, 207
Growth cone of axon, 222, 223
Growth hormone, 95, 97
Guam, form of motoneurone disease, 269, 272
Guanidine, 210, 211, 214, 264
Guillain-Barré syndrome (idiopathic polyradiculo-neuritis), 61, 234, 235

Halothane, 185
Hamster dystrophy (see Muscular dystrophy in animals)
Hemicholinium, 31, 32
Hemiplegia,
  effects on motoneurones, 289–294
  muscle atrophy in, 71, 289–294
Herpes zoster, 317
Hers's disease, 189
Hexose-6-phosphate, 139
High affinity calcium binding protein (HABP), 41
Histochemistry of muscle, 55, 57–62, 78
  after denervation, 73, 79, 229–231
  during development, 98
  in Duchenne dystrophy, 150–152
  in McArdle's disease, 189
  in myotonic dystrophy, 165
Histrionicotoxin, 33
Homograft, 98
Horse myotonia (Stringhalt), 125
Horseradish peroxidase (HRP), 15, 33, 39, 91, 148
Hot bath test, 241
'Hot spot' in membrane, 93
Hyaline degeneration, 148
Hydrochlorthiazide, 134
Hypermetabolic myopathy, 189
Hyperpolarization, 18
Hyperthermia (hyperpyrexia), malignant (see Malignant hyperthermia)
Hyperthyroidism, 125, 269 (see also Thyrotoxicosis)
Hypertonic saline, 69
Hypertrophy of muscle, 61, 72, 80, 81, 96, 101, 112, 124, 125, 181
  in chicken dystrophy, 175
  in Duchenne dystrophy, 148, 150, 157, 158
H-zone, 5, 35

I-band, 5, 35, 39, 93
Imipramine, 313
Immunoglobulin, 165, 195, 202–205, 207, 208, 234, 235, 237
Impulse (see Action potential)
Induction during embryological development, 178, 301
Influenza virus, 183
Injury of muscle, 99, 100
'In portio' disorder, 119
Input resistance, 67
Insulin secretion in motoneurone disease, 268
Interference pattern, 48, 151, 161, 182, 246–248
Internode (of axon), 11, 12, 221, 222, 224, 238–242
Interstitial fluid, 16, 18, 123, 129
'In toto' disorder, 119
Intracellular stimulation,
  axon, 21, 22
  motoneurone, 54, 59, 69
  muscle, 19, 20, 128, 129, 135, 136, 151, 303
Intracellular recording (see Microelectrode recording)
Intrafusal muscle fibres, 3
Intravital staining of motor nerve endings,
  in ageing, 102
  in Duchenne dystrophy, 150, 158
  in Eaton-Lambert syndrome, 212
  in myotonic dystrophy, 165

ravital staining of motor nerve endings, continued
  n myasthenia gravis, 196, 197, 205
  n upper motoneurone lesions, 293
  method, 102
  rinsic proteins, 4
  vagination of node of Ranvier, 244
  doacetate, 69
  n conductance modulator, 33
  n exchange resin, 132
  nophores, 5, 23, 295
  ntophoresis,
    acetylcholine, 30, 32, 93, 171, 198–200, 206, 213
    calcium, 138, 189
  ac's syndrome (see Quantal squander myokymia)
  haemia, 70, 71, 99, 101, 105
  plated spinal cord (Tower) preparation, 82, 83, 289, 290
  ometric contraction (see Contraction of muscle, iso-
      metric)
  otonic contraction (see Contraction of muscle, isotonic)

  tter', in neuromuscular transmission, 200
  int fixation, 62, 84, 85
  nctional folds, 3 (see also Synaptic cleft)

  anamycin, 213
  i Peninsula, 269
  nase,
    protein, 4, 131, 148, 313
    thymidine, 175, 176
  nee injury, 84
  ugelberg-Welander syndrome, 114, 116–118, 272, 273
      (see also Spinal muscular atrophy)

  actic acid, 58, 139, 185, 188
  actic dehydrogenase, 58
  atent period in muscle shortening, 43
  ateral sac, 6, 40, 42
  ead poisoning, 233, 234, 267
  engthening of muscle, 43–45
  ength-tension curve, 95, 101
  eprosy, 234
  eucine, labelled, 13, 14
  eukaemia, 277
  eukodystrophy, 234
  imb amputation experiments, 99
  imbgirdle and facioscapulohumeral dystrophies, 116,
      117, 118, 143, 145, 212
    clinical features 159, 160
    electromyography, 160–164
    microelectrode studies, 160
    motoneurones, 302
    motor unit studies, 162–164, 299–301, 310
    muscle morphology, 160
    muscle twitch, 163, 164
    neural hypothesis, 160–165
    repetitive nerve stimulation, 163–164
  ipid,
    axonal, 14
    membrane, 3

Lipid, continued
  muscle, 7
  storage myopathy, 190
Lipofucsin, 10, 101
Lipoprotein deficiency, 285
Lipoproteinaemia, 234
Local anaesthesia, 125, 214
Lyon hypothesis, 146
Lymphocyte,
  infiltration,
    in experimental allergic neuritis, 236, 237
    in idiopathic polyradiculoneuritis, 234
    in muscle transplant, 98
    in myasthenia gravis, 197, 198, 203–205, 207
    in polymyositis, 182, 183
    in thyrotoxicosis, 286
  sensitization,
    in Duchenne dystrophy, 154
    in experimental allergic neuritis, 237
    in myasthenia gravis, 203, 205
    in polymyositis, 183

McArdle's syndrome, 42, 188, 189, 212, 300
Macrophage, 98, 148, 197, 222, 234, 237
Magnesium, 5, 16, 29, 41
Malic dehydrogenase, 56, 59, 62
Malignant hyperthermia (hyperpyrexia), 184–187, 300,
    302
  associated musculoskeletal abnormalities, 184
  biochemical studies, 185
  calcium in, 87
  clinical features, 184, 185
  detection of trait, 185
  electromyography, 187
  in animals, 187
  induction by anaesthetics, 184
  motor unit counting studies, 187
  muscle morphology, 185, 187
  non-rigid form, 185
  pathogenesis of hyperthermic reaction, 187
Maltose, 188
Manganese poisoning, 267
Maximum evoked muscle response (M wave) in ageing,
    101, 102
Median nerve, compression (see Carpal tunnel syndrome)
Megaconial myopathy, 189
Membrane (see also Axolemma and Sacrolemma),
  basement, 4, 5, 27, 28, 100
  capacitance, 19, 24, 239
  electrical analogue, 18
  erythrocyte, 148, 313
  excitability, 20–24
  hypothesis for dystrophy, 313
  in periodic paralysis, 137–140
  myotonic, 128–132
  permeability, 16, 18, 19, 21, 138
  potential (see Action potential and Resting potential)
  pump (see Adenosine triphosphatase)
  resistance, 18, 24, 128, 129, 138, 239
Mental retardation,
  in Duchenne dystrophy, 143, 154, 155, 301
  in myotonic dystrophy, 124, 169

Mesenchyme, 92
Mesoderm, 92
Metabolism,
    aerobic (oxidative), 6, 59, 61, 62, 82, 86
    anaerobic (glycolytic), 7, 58, 61, 62, 70
    disorders of glycogen, 187–189
    in malignant hyperthermia, 185
    in mitochondrial myopathies, 189
    in periodic paralysis, 139
    rate, 187, 189, 214, 295, 296
Metachromatic leukodystrophy, 234
Methylene blue, 102
Methylsulphate, 19, 42, 128
Microelectrode recordings,
    axon, 21–22
    motoneurone, 59, 239
    muscle, 16–20, 31–33, 38–41
        after botulinum toxin administration, 215
        after nerve section, 74–76, 85, 222
        after tetanus toxin administration, 216, 217
        in acrylamide neuropathy, 276
        in ageing, 106
        in animal models of dystrophy, 171
        in antibiotic neurotoxicity, 213
        in developing muscle, 93–95
        in disuse, 84
        in Duchenne dystrophy, 151
        in Eaton-Lambert syndrome, 211, 212
        in limbgirdle dystrophy, 160
        in myasthenia gravis, 198–200, 202
        in myotonia, 127–130
        in myotonic dystrophy, 168
        in periodic paralysis, 135–137
        in thyrotoxicosis, 287
        techniques in man, 303, 304
Miniature end-plate potentials (MEPP) (see End plate
    potential, miniature)
Mitochondria,
    axonal, 12, 14, 15, 29, 31, 32, 222
    muscle, 6, 10, 27, 56, 57, 59, 61, 62, 67, 73, 79, 81,
        92, 93, 97, 98, 100 (see also under muscle morpho-
        logy sections of diseases)
    myopathy, 189, 190
Mitosis,
    muscle fibre nuclei, 72, 93, 97–100
    Schwann cell, 222, 223, 238
M-line, 5, 6, 35
Mobilization of transmitter, 29, 201
Monocarboxylic aromatic acid, 125, 128, 129
Morula, 92
Mosaic (chequer board) pattern of muscle fibres, 229, 230
Motoneurone, 8, 54, 59, 65, 67, 69, 72, 77, 80, 82, 86, 88,
        89, 98, 105, 106, 107, 125, 127
    after tetanus toxin administration, 216
    alpha-, 9
    chromatolysis, 89–91
    'dead', 113–119, 282, 296, 297
    degenerative disorders, 263–273
    dysfunction, 111, 113, 115, 116, 282, 285–288, 296,
        297
    gamma-, 9
    'healthy', 113–119
    in Duchenne dystrophy, 150–151

Motoneurone, continued
    in embryo, 94
    in hemiplegia, 290–294
    in limbgirdle dystrophy, 164, 165
    in murine dystrophy, 172
    in toxic and metabolic disorders, 274–284
    'reversible dysfunction in thyrotoxicosis, 285–288
    'sick', 113–119, 282, 296, 297
    trans-synaptic degeneration, 289–294
Motoneurone disease (Amyotrophic lateral sclerosis), 71,
        212, 230, 231, 233, 263–272
    aetiology, 267–273
    ageing hypothesis, 269–273
    case histories, 265–267
    clinical features, 263, 264
    fasciculations, 318
    motor unit estimates, 265–267
    sick motoneurone hypothesis, 113–118
    treatment, 264
Motor axon terminal (see under Axon and Neuro-
    muscular junction)
Motor cortex and trophic influence, 293, 294
Motor end-plate (see End-plate)
Motor end-plate disease (Med) in mice, 30, 69, 84
Motor unit, 8, 47–62
    amplitude of potential, 50, 51
    architecture, 54, 55
    conversion of types, 61, 62
    counting techniques, 49–53, 307–311
    discharges, 125
    effect of immobilization, 84, 85
    estimates of number, 47–53
    fast-twitch, 57, 59, 61, 62, 67
    features predicted in disease, 112, 113, 117
    firing frequency, 63–67, 70
    number in ageing, 107
    phasic, 65
    recruitment, 63–67, 81, 232
    size, 53–54, 116, 117, 118
    slow-twitch, 57, 59, 61, 62, 67
    tonic, 65
    twitch, 57, 59–62, 64–66, 231, 232 (see also Contrac-
        tion of muscle)
    types, 56–62, 63–67
Motor unit counting,
    criticisms of technique, 307–311
    disulfiram neuropathy, 280, 281
    electrophysiological technique, 49–53, 307–311
    in ageing, 103
    in animals, 308, 310
    in Duchenne dystrophy, 152–153, 299–300
    in familial periodic paralysis, 140
    in hemiplegia, 290–293
    in limbgirdle and facioscapulohumeral dystrophies,
        162–164, 299, 300
    in malignant hyperthermia, 299, 302, 310
    in motoneurone disease, 230, 231, 265–267
    in myasthenia gravis, 201, 202
    in myotonia congenita, 132
    in myotonic dystrophy, 168–170, 299, 300
    in nerve compression, 247, 248
    in polymyositis, 183

Motor unit counting, continued
  in renal failure, 278, 279
  in thyrotoxicosis, 286–288
  in vincristine neuropathy, 277
M-response (wave), 50–52, 101, 102, 277–281, 286
Mucopolysaccharide, 11
Multielectrode studies, 151, 200
Multiple sclerosis, 71, 241
Murine dystrophy (*see* Muscular dystrophy in animals)
Muscle biopsy, 66, 67, 102, 143 (*see also under muscle
    morphology sections of diseases and also* Intravital
    staining of motor nerve endings)
Muscle contraction (*see* Contraction of muscle)
Muscle fibre,
  action potential, 20–24, 68, 74, 75, 78
  atrophy (*see* Atrophy)
  classification of types, 61
  conversion of types, 61
  correlation of properties, 59–62
  degeneration in disease (*see under muscle morphology
    sections of diseases*)
  denervated, 72–79, 83–86, 88
  desheathed, 40, 138, 189
  development, 92–100, 174
  disused, 82–85
  histochemistry (*see* Histochemistry of muscle)
  hypertrophy, 61, 72, 80, 81, 96, 101, 112, 124, 125,
    148, 150, 157, 158, 175
  in ageing, 101–108
  injury, 99–100
  ionic composition, 16, 18, 138–140
  lengthening, 43–45
  morphology, 3–7, 35
  necrosis, 83, 99–100, 101
  pale, 56, 62
  red, 56, 62
  regeneration, 98–100, 148, 153, 181
  reinnervation, 76–79, 153, 224–232
  splitting, 62, 68, 80, 81, 101, 148, 171, 172, 190
  transplantation, 98, 99
  types, 58–62
Muscle growth, 92–100, 174
Muscle injury experiments, 99–100
Muscle ischaemia, 70
Muscle spindle, 84
  in acrylamide neuropathy, 276, 283
  reinnervation, 229, 281
Muscle stretch, 65, 80
Muscle transplantation, 98, 99, 175
Muscular dystrophy, 30, 71, 111, 112, 114, 143–178
    (*see also under each type*)
  classifications, 145
  historical observations, 143–144
  pathogenesis, 299–301
Muscular dystrophy in animals, 170–178, 301
  abnormal myelination, 171–172
  axoplasmic transport, 172–173
  clinical features, 170
  electrophysiological studies, 170–171
  experimental hyperinnervation, 173
  functional denervation, 171
  limb-bud transplantation, 175
  motoneurones, 172

Muscular dystrophy in animals, continued
  mouse chimaera study, 177, 178
  muscle morphology, 171–172
  muscle transplantation, 175
  neural hypothesis, 173–178
  neural tube transplantation, 175–177
  neuromuscular junction, 171
  parabiosis, 173–174
  pathogenesis, 173–178
  tissue culture, 174
Muscular rigidity in malignant hyperthermia, 184–187
Mutation rate in Duchenne dystrophy, 146
Myasthenia gravis, 30, 71, 111, 113, 114, 116, 119, 193–
    208, 209, 211, 225, 300, 302, 310, 317
  acetylcholine receptor antibody model, 203–205
  clinical features, 193–195
  electrophysiological tests, 195
  Goldstein model, 203
  historical survey, 193
  immunological studies, 196, 202–206
  in the dog, 205
  incidence, 193
  microelectrode recordings, 198, 199, 206
  motor unit counting studies, 201, 202, 206
  multielectrode recordings, 200
  muscle morphology, 197, 198
  nature of lesion, 207–208
  neuromuscular blocking agent, 202–206
  neuromuscular junction, 196
  pharmacological studies, 195, 198
  prognosis, 196
  site of lesion, 193, 205–207
  thymoma in, 195
  thyroid disorders in, 195
  thyrotoxicosis, 285
  treatment, 196
Myasthenic syndrome (*see* Eaton-Lambert syndrome)
Myelin basic proteins, 236, 237
Myelin sheath, 10–12, 25–27, 95, 111
  after nerve section, 221, 222
  effect of demyelination on impulse conduction, 239–242
  in acrylamide neuropathy, 276
  in demyelinating disorders, 233–242, 274
  in diphtheria, 237–238
  in experimental allergic neuritis, 236, 237
  in idiopathic polyradiculoneuritis, 234, 235
  in muscular dystrophy, 154, 171, 172, 239, 241
  in nerve compression, 244, 245, 251
  in nerve regeneration, 224
  in peroneal muscular atrophy, 238, 239
Myoblast, 92–94, 98–100, 174
Myofibril, 5, 35, 40, 41, 57, 61, 72, 73, 80, 92, 93, 97, 100,
    101, 148, 197
  formation, 97
  over-contraction, in dystrophy, 148
  splitting, 80, 96
Myofilament, 35–38, 43, 165
Myoglobin, 56, 59, 73, 79
Myoglobinuria, 185, 188
Myokymia, 54, 315–317 (*see also* Quantal squander myo-
    kymia)
Myonucleus, 4–6, 28, 72, 73, 77, 81, 82, 88, 92–94, 98–
    100, 148, 165, 166, 175, 177, 178, 181, 190, 197

'Myopathic EMG', 151, 156, 160, 161, 167, 182, 187, 211, 248
Myopathic-myasthenic syndrome (see Eaton-Lambert syndrome)
Myopathy, 102, 111–119, 141, 299–302
  animal models of dystrophy, 170–178
  central core disease, 190
  centronuclear, 190
  Duchenne dystrophy, 143–159
  familial periodic paralysis, 133–140
  glycogen storage diseases, 187–189
  limbgirdle and facioscapulohumeral dystrophies, 159–165
  lipid storage, 190
  malignant hyperthermia, 184–187
  mitochrondrial, 189, 190
  myotonic, 165–170
  nemaline, 190
  polymyositis (and dermatomyositis), 179–181
  thyrotoxic, 285, 286
Myophosphorylase deficiency, 42, 188
Myosin, 35–38, 43–46, 58, 78, 82, 86, 93
Myosin ATPase (see Adenosine triphosphatase, myosin)
Myotonia, 20, 123–132, 137
  biochemistry of membrane, 131
  clinical features, 124, 125
  congenita, 71, 124, 125, 127, 128, 130, 131, 212, 225, 300
  in goats, 311, 312
  induction, 125, 128, 132
  microelectrode recordings, 127–130
  peripheral, 20
  possible membrane defects, 128–131
  treatment, 132
Myotonic dystrophy (Dystrophia myotonica, Steinert's disease), 116–119, 124, 127, 128, 130, 131, 145, 165–170, 212, 225, 299–302
  anticipation, 314
  blood group linkage, 165
  cataracts, 165
  clinical features, 165, 166
  coaxial electrode recordings, 167
  creatine phosphokinase, 165
  endocrine abnormalities, 165
  immunoglobulins, 165
  insulin, 165
  intracellular recordings, 168
  motor innervation, 165–167
  motor unit studies, 168–170, 299–301
  muscle morphology, 165, 166
  muscle twitch, 167, 168
  myotonia in, 165
  nerve conduction studies, 167
  neural hypothesis, 168–170
  repetitive nerve stimulation, 167
Myotube, 92–94, 98, 100, 174, 190

Necrosis,
  muscle, 99, 100, 101, 181, 185
Negative after-potential, 129
Nemaline myopathy, 190
Nembutal, 82

Neomycin, 213
Nernst equation, 17, 23, 139
Nerve fibre (see Axon)
Neural tube,
  inductive influence, 178
  transplantation, 175–177
Neurapraxia, 83–84, 86, 243–249
  clinical case reports, 246–248
Neurofilaments, 10, 15, 27, 258
Neuroma, 227
Neuromuscular junction, 8, 27–34
  after botulinum toxin administration, 215, 226
  after tetanus toxin administration, 216, 217, 225
  effects of nerve compression, 249
  effects of nerve section, 222
  in acrylamide neuropathy, 276
  in developing muscle, 94, 95
  in Duchenne dystrophy, 150, 151
  in Eaton-Lambert syndrome, 211, 212
  in hemiplegia, 293
  in myasthenia gravis, 193, 196–200
  in myotonic dystrophy, 165, 167
  in regenerating muscle, 98, 99
  in reinnervation, 223–232
  in thyrotoxicosis, 286
  in toxic and metabolic neuropathies, 281–284
  morphology, 27
  non-transmitting ('silent'), 77, 84, 229, 249, 281, 282, 293
  transmission, 27–34
    block, 84, 86
Neuromyotonia (see Quantal squander myokymia)
Neuropathy, 111–119
  acrylamide, 274–276
  ageing, 102, 105
  Bassen–Kornweig's disease, 285
  causing pseudomyasthenic syndrome, 212
  demyelinating types, 233, 234
  diabetic, 285
  disulfiram, 279–281
  'dying-back', 71, 274, 282, 283, 290
  experimental allergic neuritis (EAN), 235–237
  Fabry's disease, 285
  Guillain–Barré, 61, 234, 235
  hepatic, 285
  hypoglycaemic, 285
  hyperparathyroidism, 285
  hypertrophic and non-hypertrophic types, 238, 239
  metachromatic leukodystrophy, 285
  peripheral, 71, 111
  porphyria, 285
  renal, 278, 279, 285
  Tangier disease, 285
  thyrotoxic, 285–288, 302
  toxic, 274–284
  vincristine, 276–277, 318
Neurotmesis, 243
Neurotoxin, 91, 214,–217
Neurotrophic influence (see Trophic influence)
Neurotubules, 10, 15, 27, 89, 258
Nissl substance, 10, 89, 90, 107, 293
Nitrate, 42
Nodal sprouting, 224

Node of Ranvier, 9, 11, 12, 25, 26
  in acrylamide neuropathy, 276
  in demyelinating disorders, 233, 237, 239–242
  in nerve compression, 244, 252
  in nerve degeneration, 221, 224
  in nerve regeneration, 224, 225, 227
Non-transmitting ('silent') synapse, 77, 84, 229, 249, 279, 281, 283, 293
Noradrenaline, 313
Nuclear chain, 72, 93
Nucleolus, 10, 72, 90, 92
Nucleus,
  muscle fibre, (see Myonucleus)
  motoneurone, 9, 10, 15, 87–91, 227
Numbers of muscle fibres, 3, 4, 73, 93–95, 101, 106, 148, 151, 171

Ocular muscular dystrophy, 143, 145
Oculopharyngeal muscular dystrophy, 145
Ohm's law, 19
Oligodendroglial cells, 10
'Onion bulb', 237, 238
Opisthotonos, 215
Optic nerve, 107
Ouabain, 23
Overloading of muscle, 61, 62
Oxidative (aerobic) metabolism (see Metabolism, aerobic)

Pa Ping (disease), 140
Pacinian corpuscle, 276
'Pale' muscle, 56
Pancreas, in motoneurone disease, 264, 268
Panhypopituitarism, 95
Papain, 37
Parabiotic cross-innervation experiment, 127, 173, 174, 301, 304
Paraesthesiae in upper limb, 253–258
  causes, 253, 254
  electrophysiological investigation, 255–257
  treatment, 254
Paralysis (see under appropriate disorder)
Paramyotonia congenita, 124, 125, 131
Parietal lobe, and trophic influence, 293, 294
Pargyline, 14
Parkinsonism, 81
Penicillamine, 145
Permeability, membrane (see also under appropriate ion), 16, 18, 19, 21
Perikaryon, 8
Perineurium, 12, 243, 251
Peripheral myotonia, 127, 128
Peripheral neuropathy (see Neuropathy)
Peroneal muscular atrophy (Charcot-Marie-Tooth disease), 238, 239, 272
Peroneal nerve compression, 251
Phagocytosis, 73, 98, 99, 101, 148, 197, 222, 234, 237
Phalen's sign, 250
Phasic motor unit, 65
Phosphate, 16, 18, 37, 38
Phospholipid, 41

Phosphorylase, 41, 56, 58, 62, 148, 150, 188, 189
Phytanic acid, 239
Picornavirus, 183
Pinocytosis, 91
Plasticity of muscle, 83, 100
Pleiotropic gene expression, 158, 170, 301
Pleoconial myopathy, 189
Poliomyelitis, 47, 71, 108, 150, 212, 267, 272
  and Duchenne dystrophy, 312
Polymyositis (and Dermatomyositis), 71, 179–184, 212, 300
  aetiology and pathogenesis, 183, 184
  association with malignancy, 181, 183, 184
  blood tests, 181
  clinical features, 179–181
  cutaneous manifestations, 179–181
  electrophysiological studies, 182
  experimental model, 183
  motor unit estimates, 183
  muscle morphology, 181, 182
  role of viruses, 183
  treatment and prognosis, 181
Polymyxin, 213
Polyneuritis, 125, 132, 234, 235
Polyneuronal innervation of muscle, 95, 227–230, 283
Polyneuropathy (see Neuropathy)
Polyradiculoneuritis, idiopathic (Guillain-Barré syndrome), 61, 234, 235
Polyribosomes, 7, 93, 97, 146
Polysaccharide, axonal, 14
Pompe's disease, 188
Positive sharp wave, 75, 182, 217
Potassium, 11, 16–23, 77, 92, 123, 124, 129, 134–137
  channels (carriers), 23, 24
  depletion, 140
  equilibrium potential, 42
  permeability of membrane, 16–23, 30
  sequestration, 139, 140
Potentiation, post-tetanic, 42, 200, 201, 210–212, 215
Prednisone, 181, 196, 208, 317
Pressure, intramuscular during exercise, 70
Presynaptic failure, 30, 68, 69, 84, 198, 199, 205–207
  (see also Pseudomyasthenic syndromes and Non-transmitting ('silent') synapse)
Procaine, 136, 185
Procaineamide, 132, 185
Procion yellow, 8
Progressive bulbal palsy, 263
Progressive muscular atrophy, 263
Prolapsed intravertebral disc, 253
Proline, 289
Protein, 16, 123
  kinase, 131, 146
  synthesis, 10, 14, 78, 86–88, 90, 93, 95, 97, 146, 283
Pseudobulbar palsy, 263
Pseudohypertrophy of muscle, 144–146, 157, 158, 160
Pseudomyasthenic syndromes, 209, 217, 268
Pseudomyotonia (see Quantal squander myokymia)
Pseudomyotonic discharge, 182
Puberty, 96
Pump, membrane (see under Adenosine triphosphatase (ATPase))
Puromycin, 14, 88

Purkinje cell, 107
Pyruvic acid, 139, 185

Quanta, acetylcholine (*see also* Acetylcholine), 71, 95
Quantal squander myokymia (Isaac's syndrome; con-
    tinuous muscle fibre activity; neuromyotonia;
    myokymia with impaired muscle relaxation;
    pseudomyotonia and myokymia), 208, 213, 214,
    315–317
  case report, 315–317
Quinine, 132

Radial nerve, 103, 250
Raynaud's phenomenon, 181, 207
Rectifier, membrane, 20
Red cell (*see* Erythrocyte)
Red muscle, 56, 62, 72, 73
Red tide, 23
Reflex,
    activity, 126
    cutaneous, 65
    in axotomized motoneurone, 89
    phasic, 65
    tonic, 65
Refractoriness of membrane, 24, 124, 130, 137, 138
Refractory period, 24
Refsum neuropathy, 239
Regeneration of muscle, 98–100, 148, 153, 181
Reinnervation of muscle, 76–79, 84, 89, 90, 113, 115,
    223–232
    collateral (*see* Collateral reinnervation)
    cross-reinnervation, 77–79, 127, 173, 174, 301, 304
    self-reinnervation, 76, 77
Relaxation, muscle, 41
Renal failure, 101, 233, 234
    neuropathy, 251, 258, 278, 279
Renaut body, 251
Renshaw cell, 216
Repetitive firing of muscle, 24, 198 (*see also* Myotonia)
Repetitive nerve stimulation, 32, 42–46, 54, 59–62, 69,
    70, 81–83, 114, 118
    after nerve ligation, 212
    in botulism, 215
    in Eaton-Lambert syndrome, 210–211
    in hemiplegia, 291
    in limbgirdle dystrophy, 163, 164
    in myasthenia gravis, 195, 196, 200, 201
    in myopathies and neuropathies, 212
    in myotonic dystrophy, 167
Resistance, membrane, 18, 24, 128, 129, 138
    input, 19
    myelin sheath, 239
Resting potential, 16–18, 23, 86
    fall after denervation, 74, 77, 84–86
    in ageing, 106
    in axotomized motoneurone, 89
    in developing muscle, 92, 93, 98
    in Duchenne dystrophy, 151
    in familial periodic paralysis, 135–137
    in limbgirdle dystrophy, 160

Resting potential, continued
    in murine dystrophy, 177
    in myotonia, 127–130
    in myotonic dystrophy, 168
    in thyrotoxicosis, 287
    ionic basis, 16
    techniques for measurements in man, 303, 304
Reticulosis, 234
Retrograde degeneration of motoneurone, 77, 89–91
Rheumatoid arthritis, 181, 207
Ribonucleic acid (RNA), 7, 10, 13, 88–90, 92, 148, 181,
    227 (*see also* Ribosomes)
Ribosomes, 7, 73, 92, 97, 148
Rigor, 43
Ringbinden, 101
'Ringed' muscle fibres, 83
Risus sardonicus, 215
Rottnest quokka, 125

Safety factor,
    for impulse at node of Ranvier, 242
    in neuromuscular transmission, 206, 207
Saltatory conduction, 26, 239–241
Sarcolemma, 3–5, 19, 27–30, 33, 34, 121 (*see also* Neuro-
    muscular junction)
    after denervation, 74–76, 84, 85
    after reinnervation, 76, 77, 83
    in development, 93–95
    in Duchenne dystrophy, 148, 150, 313
    in myotonic dystrophy, 165, 313
    in periodic paralysis, 135–140
    in thyrotoxicosis, 286
    myotonic, 123–132
    potential across (*see* Resting potential *and* Action
      potential)
Sarcomere, 5, 35, 45, 78, 79, 86, 95, 97
Sarcoplasmic reticulum (SR), 5, 38–42, 57, 70, 73, 97,
    131
    in dystrophy, 313
    in familial periodic paralysis, 139, 140
Satellite cell, 5, 100
Saxitonin, 23, 217
Scalenus anterior syndrome, 253
Schmidt–Lanterman incisures (clefts), 11, 12, 221, 222
Schwann cell, 10, 11, 25, 26, 27, 77, 95, 233, 234, 241–
    243, 295 (*see also* Myelin sheath)
    in acrylamide neuropathy, 276
    in diphtheritic neuropathy, 237, 238
    in experimental allergic neuritis, 237
    in idiopathic polyradiculoneuritis, 235
    in nerve degeneration, 221, 222
    in nerve regeneration, 223, 224, 227
    in peroneal muscular atrophy, 239
Scleroderma, 181, 207, 300
Secondary myopathy, 102
Segmental demyelination (*see* Demyelination)
Sensory nerves, 103, 234, 235, 249, 255, 256, 277, 283,
    307
Series elastic component, 41, 46
Sharp wave, 293, 307
Shell-fish poisoning, 23
Shunting of action potential currents, 51

ick motoneurone (hypothesis), 113–119, 299–301
   in animal dystrophies, 173–178
   in Duchenne dystrophy, 153–158
   in hemiplegia, 291
   in limbgirdle and facioscapulohumeral dystrophies, 160–165
   in myotonic dystrophy, 168–170
   in thyrotoxicosis, 285–288
   in toxic and metabolic neuropathies, 250, 251, 274–284
ignal averaging, 64, 65
Silent' synapse (see Non-transmitting ('silent') synapse)
Sink' (current), 24
ize principle of motoneurone activation, 67
izes of muscle fibres, 3
keletal abnormalities, in malignant hyperthermia, 184
kin effects of denervation, 289
kin rash, in dermatomyositis, 179
liding filament hypothesis, 35–38
liding of peripheral nerves, 251, 258
lowing of muscle contraction, 82, 84
low-twitch motor unit/muscle, 57, 59, 61, 62, 67, 77–79, 82, 83, 98, 105
Slow' virus in motoneurone disease, 267
Snake-coil' muscle fibres, 83
odium, 11, 16, 21, 23, 33, 75, 123, 135, 138
   'carrier', 23, 24, 83, 87, 124, 137
   in familial periodic paralysis, 138–140
   permeability, 16, 18, 21, 23, 24, 30, 75, 92, 93, 123, 129, 130, 136
   pump, 5, 11, 23, 26, 74, 123, 131, 138
ole-plate, 27, 76, 95
oma, 8–10, 13–15, 87–91 (see also Motoneurone)
ource (current), 24
peech, 133
Speeding-up' of muscle contraction, 84, 85
pinal cord, 89, 91, 94, 107, 113, 114, 126, 133
   isolated preparation, 82, 83
pinal muscular atrophy, 114, 160–165, 272, 273, 310
plitting,
   of muscle fibre, 62, 68, 80, 81, 101, 148, 171, 172, 190
   of myofibril, 80, 96
prouting of axon (see Axon, sprouting)
taircase phenomenon, 42
tarvation, 96, 98
tiffness of muscle, 124
timulation, intracellular (see also Intracellular stimulation),
   of denervated muscle, 82, 83, 85, 86
   nerve (see under Action potential)
   repetitive (see Repetitive nerve stimulation)
tomatocyte, 146
Stop-flow' technique, 14, 283
treptomycin, 213
treptozotocin, 239
tretching of muscle, 84–87, 97, 129
tump, nerve, 85, 86
uccinic dehydrogenase, 56, 58, 59, 62
uccinylcholine, 34, 84, 184, 187, 209, 214
Suppressed' synapse (see also Non-transmitting ('silent') synapse), 227–230
ural nerve, 103, 234, 235, 249, 255, 256, 277, 283, 307
wallowing, 133

Synapse,
   neuromuscular (see Neuromuscular junction)
   on motoneurone, 8–10, 89, 291–294
Synaptic (see also Neuromuscular junction),
   cleft, 27–30, 32–34, 95, 99, 196, 205, 206, 212, 222
   transmission, 27–34, 106, 193, 195–217, 222
   vesicle, 27–33, 106, 150, 196, 197, 205, 206, 212, 222

Temperature, effect on impulse conduction in demyelinated nerve, 241, 242
Tenotomy, 61, 62, 84, 85, 145, 146, 190
Tensilon test (see Edrophonium chloride)
Terminal cistern (lateral sac), 6, 40, 42
Terminal motor latency,
   in Duchenne dystrophy, 152
   in investigation of brachialgia, 256
   in limbgirdle and facioscapulohumeral dystrophies, 164
   in myasthenia gravis, 201, 206
   in myotonic dystrophy, 167
   in sick motoneurones, 114
Terminal sprouting, 224, 225
Tetanus,
   contraction, 42–46, 59–62, 69, 70, 74, 85, 95
   disease, 215–217
   stimulation (see Repetitive nerve stimulation)
   toxin, 215–217
   -twitch ratio, 46, 74
Testosterone, 96, 97, 98
Tetany, 123, 130
Tetracycline, 213
Tetrodotoxin (TTX), 23, 39, 74, 75, 83–88, 217, 304, 305
Thionin, 107
Thorium oxide, 39
Threshold of motor axon, 45–51
Thymectomy, 196
Thymidine kinase, 175, 176
Thymin, 203
Thymitis, 203
Thymoma, 195, 317
Thymotoxin, 203
Thymus, 195, 196, 203, 207, 317
Thyroid,
   dysfunction in familial periodic paralysis, 140
   dysfunction in myasthenia gravis, 195
Thyrotoxicosis, 140, 195, 215, 300, 302, 317
   electrophysiological studies, 286–288
   morphological studies, 286
   myopathy, 285, 286
   neuropathy, 285–288
Time constant, membrane, 138
Tinel's sign, 250, 254
Tip potential in microelectrode recording, 304
Tonic motor unit, 65
Tower preparation, 82, 83, 289, 290
Toxic neuropathies, 274–284
Toxins, affecting neuromuscular junction, 214–217
Transcription of DNA, 88
Translation of RNA, 88
Transmission, neuromuscular (see Neuromuscular junction)
Transmitter (see Acetylcholine)

Transplantation of muscle, 90, 98, 174, 175, 178
Transport filament, 15
Transverse carpal ligament (flexor retinaculum), 250–252, 254
Transverse tubular (T) system, 6, 19, 20, 38, 39, 42, 70, 73
    disruption by glycerol, 19, 39, 129
    in developing muscle, 93
    in excitation–contracting coupling, 38, 39, 70
    in familial periodic paralysis, 129
    in myotonia, 129
    permeability of, 19
Trauma, nerve, 83, 84, 86, 243–249
Triad, 6, 42
Tricarboxylic acid, 6
Triorthocresyl phosphate (TOCP) neuropathy, 274
Triparanol, 125
Trophic influence(s),
    in botulism, 215
    in central nervous system, 119, 289–294
    in muscular dystrophy, 113–119, 178, 301
    in neurapraxia, 249, 258
    in toxic and metabolic neuropathies, 281–284
    muscle on nerve, 89–91
    nerve on muscle, 12–15, 34, 62, 72–91, 98, 102, 108, 111, 113–119, 295, 296
Tropomyosin, 38, 40
Troponin, 38, 40
Tuberculosis, 103
Tubocurarine, 34, 84, 126, 184, 195, 198, 209, 214, 227
    regional perfusion, 212
Twitch contraction (*see* Contraction of muscle)
Types of muscle fibre, 58–62

Ulnar nerve compression, 250, 251, 257, 258
Uncoupling of respiration, 187, 189
Universal gas constant, 17
Unmyelinated nerve fibres, 26
Upper motoneurone lesion, 81, 263, 264, 271, 272, 289–294
Use (exercise) of muscle, 56, 59, 62, 63–71, 80–82, 86, 87, 105, 124, 134

Vacuole,
    in degenerating axon, 222

Vacuole, continued
    in muscle fibre, 33, 73, 101, 134, 138, 139, 148, 188
Vascular hypothesis of Duchenne dystrophy, 312, 313
Ventral roots, 102, 103, 106, 154, 239, 240
Veratrine, 24, 129
Vesicle,
    coated, 27, 91
    release sites, 33
    synaptic, 27–33, 106, 150, 196, 197, 205, 206, 212, 222
Vincristine neuropathy, 276, 277
Virus,
    infection, 99, 234
    neurotrophic, 91, 208
    poliomyelitis (*see* Poliomyelitis)
    possible role in polymyositis, 183
Vitamin B_{12}, 264
    deficiency, 234
Vitamin E, 125, 145, 264
Voltage clamp, 39
    experiments, 21
Von Gierke's disease, 188

Walking in decerebrate cat, 65
Wallerian degeneration, 107, 291
    after nerve section, 221, 222
    in acrylamide neuropathy, 276
    in compressive lesions, 247, 249, 250
    in demyelinating disorders, 233, 234, 236
    in motoneurone dysfunction, 282
    in vincristine neuropathy, 278
Weightlifting, 80, 96
Werdnig–Hoffman disease, 272, 273
Wheatstone bridge, 20, 136, 304
White muscle fibre, 72, 73
'Wobbler' disease of mice, 272

X-irradiation, 99

Z-disc (line), 5, 35, 39, 57, 62, 73, 93, 96
    in Duchenne dystrophy, 148
    in malignant hyperthermia, 185
    in nemaline myopathy, 190
Zellreizung, 90
Zinc, 42
Zygote, 92